Gender-Based Violence: A Comprehensive Guide

Parveen Ali • Michaela M. Rogers
Editors

Gender-Based Violence: A Comprehensive Guide

Springer

Editors
Parveen Ali
The Health Sciences School
University of Sheffield
SHEFFIELD, UK

Michaela M. Rogers
Department of Sociological Studies
University of Sheffield
SHEFFIELD, UK

ISBN 978-3-031-05639-0 ISBN 978-3-031-05640-6 (eBook)
https://doi.org/10.1007/978-3-031-05640-6

This Springer imprint is published by the registered company Springer Nature Switzerland AG
The registered company address is: Gewerbestrasse 11, 6330 Cham, Switzerland

Foreword

I am honoured to have been asked to write the foreword to this important and groundbreaking book. There is now greater recognition of gender-based violence, and a much better appreciation of the forms and impact of a range of harmful behaviours. It is increasingly recognised that gender-based violence is endemic, universal and multidimensional, and intersects across the intimate, interpersonal and structural dimensions of society. And yet, we still have an incomplete knowledge base to inform how we should understand and respond.

Over the four decades I have been involved in addressing gender-based violence as a practitioner, a policy maker and as a researcher, I wish I had a book like this to support my work. In recent years I have seen an increasing recognition by professionals, and a greater acceptance among wider society of the many forms that gender-based violence can take in private, public and virtual spheres, and the immediate and longer term impacts. However, there remain many misconceptions about what causes and sustains such harms, and the types of responses and interventions that are likely to make a difference. As such, having a comprehensive book such as this is extremely helpful, especially at a time when some of the protections, for women and girls in particular, are being rolled back or challenged in many countries.

The editors are to be commended for bringing together such a learned collective of contributors on a wide range of forms of gender-based violence. It is refreshing to see contributions on such a diverse, yet inter-connected range of issues, and to have work from across the globe. Scholars from low- and middle-income countries have added greatly to our understanding about the many ways in which women and girls especially can experience violence and abuse from intimate partners, family members, members of their communities and even the State. The growing body of work about gender-based violence has been enriched by such contributions, much of which has highlighted the intersection between various forms of harm and a range of social and health inequalities. A key message from many of the chapters in this book is that gender-based violence can never be truly addressed without creating greater gender equality, alongside addressing the misogyny that is so prevalent across societies. This new scholarship is helping to make important advances in the field of gender-based violence.

Health professionals have a specific opportunity to identify and intervene in situations where individuals may be experiencing, or causing, harm. This book is therefore well placed to support practitioners in responding in ways which are likely to be experienced as helpful, and to support professionals to think about how services and practice responses reduce the potential barriers to disclosure and increase the opportunities for providing effective help.

Thank you to all the contributors for sharing their insights and wisdom, and to the editors for all the hidden work that goes into producing such a landmark text that is likely to become a key reference point for many years to come.

University of Edinburgh
Edinburgh, UK

John Devaney,

Contents

Contributors

Anum S. Hussaini Clinical Trials Unit at the Aga Khan University, Karachi, Pakistan

Parveen Ali Health Sciences School, University of Sheffield, Sheffield, UK

Tazeen Saeed Ali School of Nursing and Midwifery, The Aga Khan University, Karachi, Pakistan

Department of Community Health Sciences, The Aga Khan University, Karachi, Pakistan

Rachel Alsop Centre for Women's Studies at the University of York, York, UK

Lisa Fontes Department of Interdisciplinary, University of Massachusetts, Amherst, MA, USA

Kim Barker Law School, The Open University, Milton Keynes, UK

Sadiq Bhanbhro Health Research Institute, Sheffield Hallam University, Sheffield, UK

Khatidja Chantler Department of Nursing, Manchester Metropolitan University, Manchester, UK

Nida Usman Chaudhary Independent Researcher, Lahore, Pakistan

Punita Chowbey College of Health, Wellbeing and Life Sciences at Sheffield Hallam University, Sheffield, UK

Laura Connelly Department of Sociological Studies, The University of Sheffield, Sheffield, UK

Silvia Fraga Dominguez Department of Psychology, Faculty of Business, Law, and Social Sciences, Birmingham City University, Birmingham, UK

Colleen Fisher School of Population and Global Health, University of Western Australia, Perth, WA, Australia

Debbie Hager School of Population Health, University of Auckland, Auckland, New Zealand

Abby Hare Forensic Psychology, University of Kent, Kent, UK

Susan Heward-Belle Sydney School of Education and Social Work at the University of Sydney, Sydney, NSW, Australia

Kathryn Hinsliff-Smith Faculty of Health and Life Sciences, Leicester School of Nursing and Midwifery, De Montfort University, Leicester, UK

Matt Hopkins School of Criminology, University of Leicester, Leicester, England, UK

Moninuola Ifayomi Health Science School, University of Sheffield, Sheffield, UK

Romina Istratii School of History, Religions and Philosophies, SOAS University of London, London, UK

Susie Jacobs Sociology at Manchester Metropolitan University, Manchester, England, UK

Zohra Jetha School of Nursing and Midwifery, Aga Khan University, Nairobi, Kenya

Joyce Jiang University of York, York, UK

Carolyn Harris Johnson University of Western Australia, Perth, WA, Australia

Olga Jurasz Faculty of Business and Law, Law School, The Open University, Milton Keynes, UK

Monica Majumdar Queen Mary University of London, London, UK

Julieta Marotta UNU-MERIT, United Nations University, Maastricht, The Netherlands

Kaveri Mayra Birth Place Lab, University of British Columbia and a Subject Matter Expert at the WHO HQ, Vancouver, BC, Canada

Global Health, Obstetric Violence in India, University of Southampton, Southampton, UK

Sue McAndrew Mental Health and Young People, University of Salford, Salford, UK

Mental Health and Young People at the University of Salford, Salford, England, UK

Julie McGarry Health Sciences School, University of Sheffield and Sheffield Teaching Hospitals NHS Foundation Trust, Sheffield, UK

Kirsty McGregor School of Humanities and Social Science, University of Brighton, Brighton, UK

Peggy Mulongo Mental Health Nursing & Practice, University of Central Lancashire (UCLan), Preston, Lancashire, UK

Equality, Diversity and Inclusion, School of Nursing, University of Central Lancashire (UCLan), Preston, Lancashire, UK

School of Nursing, Faculty of Health & Wellbeing, University of Central Lancashire (UCLan), Preston, Lancashire, UK

Neil Murphy School of Health and Society, University of Salford, Salford, UK

Lucy Neville School of Criminology, University of Leicester, Leicester, England, UK

Ikenna Fernandez Nnoli Department of Nursing Science, University of Benin, Benin, Edo State, Nigeria

Madhumita Pandey Helena Kennedy Centre for International Justice, Department of Law and Criminology, Sheffield Hallam University, Sheffield, UK

Shagufta Parveen Health Sciences School, University of Sheffield, Sheffield, UK

Afroditi Pina Centre for Research and Education in Forensic Psychology (CORE-FP), University of Kent, Kent, UK

Nasrin Rahman Federation University Australia, Varendra University, Rajshahi, Bangladesh and Rajshahi Judges Court, Rajshahi, Bangladesh

Michaela M. Rogers Department of Sociological Studies, University of Sheffield, Sheffield, UK

Andrew Rowland Manchester, England, UK

Children's Rights, Law, and Advocacy, University of Salford, Salford, UK

M'Lop Tapang, Sihanoukville, Cambodia

SicKids Charity, London, UK

Sam Rowlands Department of Medical Science & Public Health, Bournemouth University, Bournemouth, UK

Teela Sanders School of Criminology, University of Leicester, Leicester, England, UK

Judit Montenegro Sebastian Survivors' Network, Sussex, UK

Nicola Sharp-Jeffs Surviving Economic Abuse, London, UK

Jennifer E. Storey Forensic Psychology in the School of Psychology, University of Kent, Kent, UK

School of Psychology at the University of Kent, Kent, UK

Sally Sutherland Radical Methodologies Research Group, University of Brighton, Brighton, UK

Emma Tomalin School of Philosophy, Religion and History of Science, University of Leeds, Leeds, UK

Signe Uldbjerg Department of Cultural Sciences, The Faculty of Humanities, Southern Danish University, Odense, Denmark

Aarhus University, Aarhus, Denmark

Rodante van der Waal Care Ethics Department, University for Humanistic Studies, Utrecht, The Netherlands

Laura Viliardos Counselling and Psychotherapy, University of Salford, Salford, UK

Abu Naser Md. Wahid Department of Law, Rajshahi University, Rajshahi, Bangladesh

Susan Walker School of Nursing & Midwifery, Anglia Ruskin University, Chelmsford, UK

Chris Waugh Department of Sociology, The University of Manchester, Manchester, UK

Department of Strategy, Enterprise and Sustainability, Manchester Metropolitan University, Manchester, UK

University of Law, Manchester, UK

Richard Whitecross Law, The Business School, Edinburgh Napier University, Edinburgh, UK

Lisa Wiebesiek Centre for Visual Methodologies for Social Change, University of KwaZulu-Natal, UKZN, Durban, KwaZulu-Natal, South Africa

Abbreviations

ACAS	Advisory, Conciliation and Arbitration Service
AFP	Australian Federal Police
AGTR	Asociación Grupo De Trabajo Redes
ANC	African National Congress (Republic of South Africa)
APPG	All Party Parliamentary Group
ARCHES	Addressing Reproductive Coercion in Health Settings
ASF	Acid Survivors' Foundation
ASTI	Acid Survivors' Trust International
BAME	Black, Asian and minority ethnic
BC	Before Christ
BDSM	Bondage, Domination, Sadism, Masochism
BME	Black and minority ethnic
BPD	Borderline personality disorder
CAID	Child Abuse Image Database
CAMHS	Child & Adolescent Mental Health Services
CDC	Centres for Disease Control and Prevention
CDW	Child domestic worker
CEDAW	Convention for the Elimination of All Forms of Discrimination Against Women
Convention of Belém do Pará	Inter-American Convention on the Prevention, Punishment and Eradication of Violence against Women
CPO	Child protection operation
CSA	Child sexual abuse
CSE	Child sexual exploitation
CSEC	Commercial sexual exploitation of children
CSEW	Crime Survey for England and Wales
CTS	Conflict Tactic Scale
CWDM	Community Watch Dog Model (for monitoring women's land rights)
DfE	Department for Education

DSA	Digital sexual assault
DSM	Diagnostic & Statistical Manual
DVA	Domestic violence and abuse
EU	European Union
EZLN	*Ejército Zapatista de Liberación Nacional*, of Chiapas, Mexico ('Zapatista' Army of National Liberation)
FAO	Food and Agriculture Organization of the United Nations
FBI	Federal Bureau of Investigation
FMPO	Forced Marriage Protection Order
FV	Family violence
GAATW	Global Alliance Against Traffic in Women
GBV	Gender-based violence
GCC	Global commodity chain
GPS	Global positioning system
GVC	Global value chain
HCPs	Healthcare professionals
Het-cis	Heterosexual and cisgender
HIV	Human immunodeficiency virus
HRW	Human Rights Watch
IBSA	Image-based sexual abuse
IDWN	International Domestic Workers Network
IFAD	International Fund for Agricultural Development of the United Nations
IICSA	Independent Inquiry into Child Sexual Abuse
IIED	International Institute for Environment and Development
ILO	International Labour Organization
IOM	International Organization for Migration
IPC	Indian Penal Code
IPV	Intimate partner violence
ITUC	International Trade Union Confederation
Law 26485	Law on the Right of Women to Live Free of Violence
LGB	Lesbian, Gay, Bisexual
LGBTIQ+	Lesbian, Gay, Bisexual, Trans, Intersex, Queer …
LGBTQI+	Lesbian, gay, bisexual, transgender, queer and intersex
LMIC	Low- and middle-income countries
MDW	Migrant domestic worker
MILF	Mum I'd like to fuck
MSM	Men who have sex with men
NCCR	Non-consensual condom removal

NGO	Non-governmental organisation
NPCC	National Police Chief's Council [UK]
NRM	National Referral Mechanism
NSPCC	National Society for the Prevention of Cruelty to Children
NYU	New York University
OAM	Older adult mistreatment
ODW	Overseas domestic worker
ONS	Office of National Statistics
OSCE	Organization for Security and Co-operation in Europe
OVAW	Online violence against women
Pact of San José	American Convention on Human Rights
pH	Power of hydrogen
PPV	Pay per view
PSC	Project Safe Childhood
PTSD	Post-traumatic stress disorder
RAINM	Rape, Abuse and Incest National Network
RCA	Reproductive coercion and abuse
SARC	South Asian Association for Regional Cooperation
SGBV	Sexual and gender-based violence
SRHR	Sexual and reproductive health and rights
SSA	Sub-Saharan Africa
STI	Sexually transmitted infection
TBA	Text-based abuse
TBSA	Text-based sexual abuse
TFA	Technology-facilitated abuse
UK	United Kingdom
UKCCIS	UK Council for Child Internet Safety
UN	United Nations
UNCRC	United Nations Convention on the Rights of the Child
UNCRPD	United Nations Convention on the Rights of Persons with Disability
UNDP	United Nations Development Programme
UN ESCAP	United Nations Economic and Social Commission for Asia and the Pacific
UNFPA	United Nations Population Fund
UNHRC	United Nations Human Rights Convention on the Rights of the Child
UNICEF	United Nations International Children's Emergency Fund
UNODC	United Nations Office on Drugs and Crime
UNRHCO	United Nations Resident and Humanitarian Coordinator's Office

VAWG	Violence against women and girls
VoDW	Voice of domestic workers
WHO	World Health Organization
WOLTS	Women and Land Tenure Security project
WSW	Women who have sex with women

Part I

Introduction

Understanding Gender-Based Violence

Michaela M. Rogers and Parveen Ali

Learning Objectives
After reading this chapter, the reader will be able to

- Define gender and understand how it is theorised.
- Define gender-based violence.
- Identify various types of gender-based violence.
- Understand the terminologies and typologies used in this book.

Introduction

Gender-based violence (GBV) is a public health and human right concern that affects millions of individuals, families and communities across the globe. It is endemic, universal and multi-dimensional and operates as intimate, interpersonal and structural violence (Aghtaie and Gangoli 2018). A substantial body of evidence demonstrates the serious health, social and economic consequences of GBV for victims and their families as well as considerable social and economic costs to communities and economies (European Institute for Gender Equality (EIGE) 2021;

M. M. Rogers (✉)
Department of Sociological Studies, University of Sheffield, Sheffield, UK
e-mail: m.rogers@sheffield.ac.uk

P. Ali
Health Sciences School, University of Sheffield, Sheffield, UK
e-mail: parveen.ali@sheffield.ac.uk

P. Ali, M. M. Rogers (eds.), *Gender-Based Violence: A Comprehensive Guide*,
https://doi.org/10.1007/978-3-031-05640-6_1

Oliver et al. 2019). The global nature and concern about GBV are reflected by the principles that everyone has the right to live free from violence, and these principles are upheld by international agreements such as the *Convention of the Elimination of All Forms of Discrimination Against Women* and the *UN Declaration on the Elimination of Violence Against Women* (UN Women n.d.).

It is critical to note that this book was written during the COVID-19 pandemic, which, globally, has resulted in long-term negative consequences and has caused widespread loss. By the first week of March 2020, many countries had reported cases of COVID-19, and on the 11 March 2020, the World Health Organization (WHO) declared a global pandemic and a public health emergency of international concern (Al Jazeera 2021). Subsequently, the world experienced a global lockdown to limit the spread of COVID-19 within and across countries. Numerous negative impacts were reported on health, education, economic and social life as the United Nations described the COVID-19 pandemic as the 'worst crisis' since World War II (Al Jazeera 2021).

Importantly, the impact of the pandemic on GBV has been widely reported. A report by UN Women (2021) summarised survey data in 13 countries representing all regions of the world (including Kenya, Thailand, Ukraine, Cameroon, Albania, Bangladesh, Colombia, Paraguay, Nigeria, Cote D'Ivoire, Morocco, Jordan, and Kyrgyzstan) highlighting that:

1. Whilst rates vary across countries and demographics, overall, the pandemic increased women's experiences of violence and eroded their feelings of safety.
2. Violence against women had a significant impact on mental health of those experiencing it during the pandemic.
3. Socioeconomic factors play a significant role in women's experiences of violence.
4. Age is no barrier in violence against women, with similar rates found across various age ranges.
5. While most women will seek informal support (around half surveyed), rather than professional support, when they do access services, this can be a crucial turning point.

This introduction provides a backdrop to the remaining chapters in this book which, in combination, illustrate the diversity and complexity of GBV. In particular, we are pleased to include under-researched or emerging practices in contemporary contexts. We do, however, wish to emphasise that the spectrum of GBV covered in this book is not exhaustive, but we do offer a comprehensive overview in terms of its wide-ranging presentation, plethora of victim and perpetrator characteristics, relationship dynamics, diverse causes and consequences. The chapters also highlights various policy and practice frameworks that address GBV in different parts of the world.

In this chapter, we start by summarising current theoretical debates about gender before exploring the term 'gender-based violence'. This offers a foundational understanding about how we employ this umbrella term in this book. We then set out some definitions about forms of violence, propose a typology of GBV to illuminate its complexity and reach in terms of private, public and virtual environments. Building on this introduction, the ways in which GBV can be theoretically and conceptually examined are set out in the next chapter titled 'Theorising Gender-Based Violence'.

What Is Gender?

It is important to recognise current debates about gender to understand the phenomenon of GBV. The word 'gender' refers to the social and cultural differences that are associated with identifying as a man, woman or a minority gender identity and includes things such as norms, roles, presentation and behaviour. It is essential that there is clarity about the distinction between gender and sex as these terms, often used interchangeably, are not interchangeable. The term 'sex' refers to the physical or physiological characteristics of a body (e.g. genitalia, chromosomes, and the endocrine system) that are usually attributed to a male or female sex.

Since the influential feminist scholarship of the 1970s, it has generally been agreed that gender is a social construct. It is an idea created and shaped through social interactions and, therefore, it is clearly discernible from sex. Contemporary literature conceptualises gender as multi-dimensional in that it can be an identity category; a means of identification; and as having a performative quality in that it is something that we simply 'do' (Butler 1990; West and Zimmerman 2009). Gender can be understood on an individual level as an aspect of one's identity or, on a structural level, it can be thought of as a form of social organisation and classification (Rogers and Ahmed 2017).

Mostly gender is considered to be binary; that is, it has two categories—man and woman. However, as gender is largely considered a social construct, it is possible to conceptualise gender as a spectrum that offers a plethora of gender identities (Rogers and Ahmed 2017). In recent years, there has been an expansion of scholarship that explores this idea and a notable growth in work on trans and non-binary identities and experiences (Rogers and Ahmed 2017).

Trans is an umbrella term that refers to people whose gender identity differs from what was assigned at birth and includes a range of identities that align with the gender binary, including trans woman, trans man, transgender woman, transgender man, male to female (MtF), female to male (FtM), and a woman or man with a transgender history (Bachmann and Gooch 2018). Non-binary is also a catchall term, falling under the trans umbrella. It includes identities that do not conform to the man/woman binary including queer, genderqueer, genderfluid, gender neutral, gender diverse, gender questioning, and gender non-conforming (Bachmann and Gooch 2018). Scholarship pertaining to gender identity recognises that identity is not predetermined nor fixed, nor is it binary; identity is multiple, shifting, contingent and intersectional. A person whose gender identity remains the same as that ascribed at birth is commonly referred to as cisgender (or its shorthand 'cis') (Schilt and Westbrook 2009).

The identities listed here are merely indicative, not exhaustive, and terminology in this field changes frequently. It is also important to acknowledge the multiplicity and diversity of trans identities (Dargie et al. 2014) and that a person's experience of gender identity is subjective and should not be reduced to the biological or physical presentation of their sexed body. Nor should one assume someone's gender identity merely by reading their behaviour or presentation. Finally, just as sex and gender are not interchangeable, gender and sexuality are different elements of identity, but one should not confuse or conflate the two. Just as cis people can be heterosexual, homosexual, bisexual, or queer, so can trans and non-binary people.

Most chapters in this book refer to identities tied to the gender binary; that is, they refer to men and women. However, it is important to contextualise the harmful practices, abuses and harms explored in this work in relation to these evolving, dynamic and, often, politicised debates about gender identity. It is also important to note that gender-based violence occurs for people identifying across the gender spectrum (including boys, men, trans and non-binary people) despite the focus on women in many of the chapters contained herein for reasons set out in this chapter. Finally, whilst gender is central to the analysis in this book, we concurrently seek to acknowledge the intersectional nature of identity, which is constituted by multiple components (Crenshaw 1989). While the overlapping effects of gender, sex and ethnicity have been widely explored in the feminist literature (Crenshaw 1989; Ahmed 2017), it is also important to be mindful of other intersecting aspects of social location such as migration status, sexual orientation, age, marriage status, disability and socio-economic status to name a few. We acknowledge intersectional identities in the consideration of GBV, and these are represented in the diversity of practices and forms of GBV examined in this book.

Gender-Based Violence

Gender-based violence refers to acts of maltreatment that are directed toward an individual or community because of their gender. It is rooted in gender inequality and reflects harmful norms and practices (UNHCR 2021). The European Commission's definition also identifies GBV as violence that affects persons of a particular gender disproportionately. GBV is an abuse of power and constitutes one of the most serious human rights violations within all societies (EIGE 2022). While people of any gender can experience GBV, the majority of victims are women and girls, and most violence is inflicted by men who are current or former intimate partners. In addition, the abuse that women experience is often repeated, systematic, more severe and more likely to result in injury or death. For this reason, the terms GBV and violence against women (VAW) are often used interchangeably. It is important to note, however, that GBV intersects the boundaries of gender, age, ability, socioeconomic class and sexual identity as well as those denoted by culture, religion and ethnicity. As such, an intersectional lens should be used to understand GBV in any context (Crenshaw 1989; Thiara et al. 2011).

GBV can be enacted in personal or family relationships, or through institutional practices. It can be perpetrated by one or more individuals (for example, see chapter 'Forced Marriage' or chapter 'Obstetric Violence'). It can occur in marital, cohabiting, separated, heterosexual as well as same-sex relationships (for example, see chapter 'Post-Separation Abuse', or chapter 'Domestic Violence and Abuse in LGBTQ+ Communities', which explores abuse in LGBTQ relationships). GBV can be perpetrated against victims/survivors of childhood, adolescence, early and middle adulthood as well as in later life (see, for example, chapter 'Childhood Sexual Abuse' and chapter 'Older Adult Maltreatment'). However, as shown throughout this book, GBV is also perpetrated by acquaintances and strangers, particularly when examining public and virtual environments (for example, see chapter 'Sexual harassment' or chapter 'Technology-Facilitated Abuse' exploring online text-based sexual abuse). The landscape of GBV is extensive and multifaceted as this book demonstrates.

Existing research illustrates this point. For example, the World Health Organization (WHO) undertook a study using available databases to measure two forms of GBV: intimate partner violence (IPV) and sexual violence by non-intimate partners (García-Moreno and Pallioto 2013). Findings indicate that the global prevalence of IPV was 30–33% and found to be highest in African, Eastern Mediterranean and South-East Asian regions where 37% of women reported experiencing IPV. For non-partner sexual violence, the study found that globally 7% of all women report experiencing this form of GBV, with the highest rates found in Africa (11.9%) and the Americas (10.7%). Authors of the study did acknowledge the paucity of reliable data on non-partner sexual violence in conflict areas and in several regions of the world.

The WHO study explored two forms of GBV, but as an umbrella term, it presents in myriad forms such as IPV, female genital mutilation, forced marriage, hate crime, grooming and child sexual exploitation. The study of the European Union countries found that since the age of 15, 1 in 3 women had experienced physical and/or sexual violence; 1 in 2 women had experienced sexual harassment; 1 in 20 women had been raped; 1 in 5 women had experienced stalking; and 95% of victims trafficked for sexual exploitation in the EU are women (European Union Agency for Fundamental Rights 2015). These statistics perpetuate the notion that GBV is a problem that exists in the *epidemic* of male violence toward women (Heise 1994).

We do not dispute that the majority of victims/survivors are female and that the most serious impacts are experienced by women (including fatalities). However, there is a barrier to the wider conversations about male victimisation, which is upheld by notions of masculinity that position men as perpetrators rather than victims/survivors. There is, increasingly, scholarship that illustrates men as both victims and perpetrators, which poses a challenge to feminist theoretical explanations of GBV (Williamson 2018; Huntley et al. 2019). There has been a distinct growth in studies focusing on general population experiences of domestic violence and abuse (DVA) (Archer 2002) and not just women's experiences. Often these studies rely on the controversial Conflict Tactics Scale (Straus et al. 1996), but the findings do suggest that more men experience DVA than previously thought.

Whilst many of these studies are often criticised on methodological grounds, e.g. studies tend to measure incidents not patterns of abuse and that studies do not adequately measure impacts (Myhill 2017; Williamson 2018), this body of work has undoubtedly been disruptive to feminist scholarship and activism. Every reader of this book will make up their own mind having considered a range of practices, causes and impacts that are examined in this book using a gendered lens. Furthermore, establishing the scale and extent of GBV across any population is fraught with difficulties as terminology in this field can be confusing as there are several terms in operation; some are distinct, and some are used interchangeably to refer to the same or similar phenomenon. Across the literature, this creates challenges when researchers use different terms, definitions, measures and methodologies. It can mean that making generalisations or comparisons is problematic. In addition, different contexts have varied understandings of GBV, and in some, it may be so normalised that it is impossible to measure.

A Note on Terminology

In a similar way to GBV, 'domestic violence and abuse' is a common umbrella term that integrates various forms of maltreatment, including child abuse, IPV and older adult mistreatment. In setting out these umbrella terms and diverse forms of abuse, it is evident that GBV is complex and can be understood in diverse ways, and across scholarship, the terms GBV, VAW, DVA and IPV are often used interchangeably too, which can be confusing for the reader. Whilst there are some similarities and overlaps across these concepts, there are important distinctions. For example, DVA is a broad concept that incorporates a range of abuse and violence that occurs within a domestic context. The perpetrator of DVA might be a partner or other family member; however, in cases of some forms of GBV, as noted above, it is also likely that the perpetrator is a stranger or a community member or may belong to an institution. Another problem is that the term 'violence' is often conflated with the act of physical violence, whereas the term 'abuse' includes all forms of maltreatment whether it is physical, sexual, psychological or coercive and controlling behaviour. However, these terms are also used interchangeably within the literature, often referring to the same behaviour.

Victims or Survivors

The debate about the different terms 'victim' and 'survivor' ensues, albeit the combined term 'victim/survivor' has gained traction in recent years. This debate is important because at its core is the consequences about having the power to name and frame someone as one thing or another. The terms 'victim' and 'survivor' are evocative and can be understood in binary opposition as being labelled as a 'victim' can be associated with weakness and passivity whereas labelling someone as a 'survivor' is suggestive of valour and having strength to overcome adversity (Gavey 1999; Gupta 2014). Intrinsically, this debate is rooted in political and social concerns. Gupta (2014) argues that the term 'survivor' is important as it recognises the agency of women, and in this way, it centres individual capacity. However, Gupta (2014) also argues, the term 'victim' should be reclaimed by feminist politics in order to shift the focus from the individual and to foreground the structural and systemic influences associated with and that sustain GBV. Notwithstanding this argument, the term 'survivor' is positive and evocative of the empowerment model adopted in the DVA and VAW field (Women Against Abuse 2021). Throughout this book, contributors use all three terms ('victim', 'survivor', and 'victim/survivor'), which reflect the different geographical, social and political contexts and practices in which women work and live. This also reflects the diverse disciplinary backgrounds of the contributors as, for example, criminologists and victimologists may prefer to adopt the term 'victim' whereas feminists in other disciplines might prefer 'survivor' (Hoyle 2007).

Forms of GBV

The notion that GBV is a continuum is reflected by the UN Secretary General's report on violence against women. GBV can include physical, sexual, mental, psychological, material and economic harm inflicted in private, public or online environments (see Fig. 1). It can include neglectful or coercive and controlling behaviours such as threats of violence and manipulation. Individuals can be subjected to one or more forms at any one time, a phenomenon known as polyvictimisation (WHO 2013; Wolfe 2018). Highlighting the complexity and diversity of GBV, the chapters in this book illustrate the ways in which these forms of violence are experienced and perpetrated by different groups in disparate contexts. For clarity, here we include some basic definitions of types of maltreatment.

Physical violence/abuse refers to the use of physical force to inflict pain, physical suffering or injury to the victim. Examples of physical violence include pinching, scratching, pushing, slapping, spanking, beating, biting, kicking, dragging, stabbing, hitting with a fist or object to inflict pain or injury, burning, strangling, use or threat of use of a gun, knife or other weapon (García-Moreno et al. 2005).

Sexual violence/abuse includes unwanted sex, coerced sex, rape or attempted rate as a result of force, threat of force or inability to give consent due to

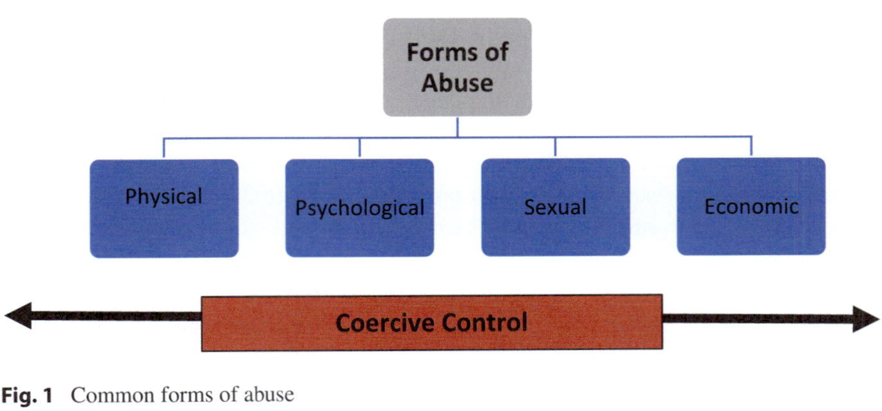

Fig. 1 Common forms of abuse

intoxication, forced sex without protection, forced or coerced use of pornography, and degrading or humiliating sex (WHO 2014; Kennedy et al. 2021). More recently, digital forms of GBV have emerged that fall under the umbrella of technology-facilitated sexual violence, e.g. non-consensual sharing of sexually explicit images via social media (including so-called 'revenge porn'), online grooming, cyberstalking and cyberflashing to name a few (McGlynn and Johnson 2021; Stonard 2021).

Psychological violence/abuse can take the form of, inter alia, blackmail, constant criticism, defamation, verbal insults and/or threats, harassment, yelling or screaming at a partner, acts of humiliation, monitoring and surveillance, restricting the victim's access to their social environment, network, financial resources, vehicle, or telephone (WHO 2002; EIGE 2017).

Economic abuse refers to controlling a person's ability to acquire, use and maintain their own money and resources. An abuser may prevent a woman from working to earn her own money (not letting her go to work or sabotaging job interviews), taking and controlling income from work or welfare benefits, using another's money without consent, building up debts in a woman's name, damaging property, and possessions, withholding maintenance payments (Johnson 2021; EIGE 2022).

Neglect is a form of abuse by individuals resulting from inadequate attention, especially through carelessness or disregard for the needs of others. When in the context of caregiving, where the perpetrator is a carer for someone who is unable to care for themselves, neglect is the failure to provide care and meet the other person's needs.

Coercive control is any act or a pattern of acts of assault, threats, humiliation and intimidation or other abuse that is used to harm, punish or frighten their victim (Stark 2007).

Gender-Based Violence and Power, Privilege and Positionality

GBV happens in public or private as well as digital spheres. The concepts of power and control have always been central to GBV. However, we extend the conceptual underpinning by also drawing attention to privilege and positionality as these are different to power and control, but integral to an understanding of GBV (see Fig. 2, and Box 1 for a case study that applies these concepts). Here is a short description of each one of these aspects:

Power: Refers to the ability, of someone, to control access to resources, opportunities, privileges and decision-making processes of another individual or group. Power is the ability of an individual or group to achieve their own goals or aims; however, it can be used negatively to prevent another (the victim/survivor in the context of GBV) from making their own decisions and exercising their personal right and powers on themselves.

Privilege: By privilege we refer to a special right, advantage or immunity, granted or available, accessible only to a particular person or group, and this privilege is usually because of their position.

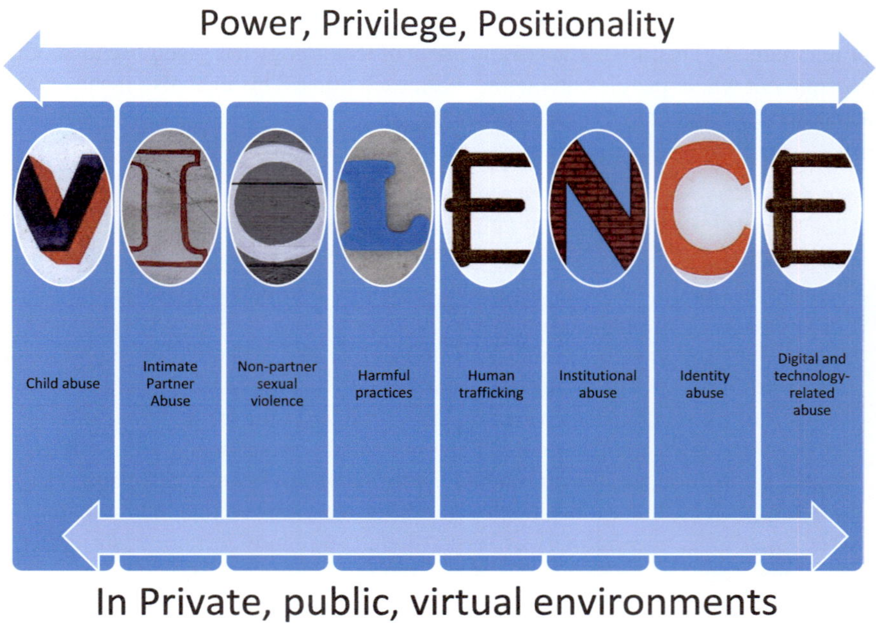

Fig. 2 A typology of gender-based violence

Positionality: By positionality, or positionalities, we refer to 'placement within a set of relations' as well as 'practices that implicate identification and "performativity" or action' (Anthias 2002: 501). This includes an understanding of social positioning (as a process, practice or action) as well as social position (as an outcome). 'Positioning' is a useful conceptual tool in examining the synergy between social structures and individual agency (Rogers and Ahmed 2017). In this way, it is central to an analysis of GBV in which social structures and individual/community identities, practices and norms collide. For example, the power, privilege and positionality of a legal advocate play a significant role in the experience of a rape survivor in court proceedings. Another example is of the difference of power, privilege and positionality between a woman and a girl in a community that accepts female genital mutilation as part of its culture. These examples highlight the multiple positionalities that people have in terms of professional identity, personal identity, age and gender as well as the structures that affect people's experiences (the legal system, community culture and norms).

It is also important to understand the concepts of **public, private and virtual environments** in which GBV occurs. Often rationales have been given to justify abuse and GBV-related practices. For example, historically, DVA has been considered a private phenomenon, something that happens with private spheres of home and therefore not a focus of government policy. It happens in public spaces, such as streets, places of worship, places of work and not enough is done to prevent abuse and protect victims. Victims, mostly women, are often criticised for being in public spaces and presenting in particular ways or at certain times of the day, and GBV is (problematically) justified. The advancement of technology has given rise to another environment where people can interact with each other. This then also means that it is another space where GBV can take place.

Box 1 Case Study Using the PPP-PPV Framework to Understand Older Adult Mistreatment

Three years ago, at 82 years old, Sarah went to live with her daughter, Martha, when she became unable to manage on her own due to decreased physical functioning and mobility resulting from arthritis and an immunity suppressing condition. An only daughter, Martha and her husband, Malcolm, felt obliged to make space in their home for Sarah and transformed their dining room into a downstairs bedroom. They lived in a cottage in an idyllic village in the countryside, and this room had lovely views out towards farmland. The move went well, but within months Sarah felt very unwelcome and unhappy (she sensed she was 'in the way' even though she rarely left her room). She also missed the hustle and bustle of city living.

Malcolm and Martha both felt frustrated and resentful of having to change their lifestyle (both had recently retired) to incorporate Sarah's needs such as medical appointments (and these were a fair distance to drive to). On days when Sarah's health conditions flared up, she needed help with daily activities (washing and dressing). Sarah found it increasingly difficult to ask for help on the days that she needed it. Malcolm had set up Sarah's online banking prior to her move and began accessing her money to compensate him for hospitality and care (without Sarah's knowledge and Sarah was not very good with technology and had forgotten how to log in anyway). Relationships broke down and Malcolm became verbally and emotionally abusive to Sarah. He called her 'the old pest', not to her face but openly and certainly while in her company. Sarah felt that Martha colluded with Malcolm and did nothing to stand up to him.

One day, Sarah's former neighbour, Mrs. Hampson, called round to see her; she did so periodically but had not called for a couple of months. Mrs. Hampson was in the area and thought she'd call on the off chance. She was shocked at the sight of Sarah; she was unkempt and smelly. Her fingernails and hair were unclean, as were her clothes. Her room smelled too as though the bedclothes had not been washed for some time. She looked like she had lost weight. Sarah was subdued and Mrs. Hampson was deeply upset when she left. She made a telephone call to adult social services to discuss her concerns, who reassured her that she was not unduly worrying and that they would make a home visit to establish what was happening and to see how Sarah was.

Understanding Sarah's experiences

Dynamics

Power: As an older woman moving into the home of her daughter and son-in-law, Sarah has little power over everyday living conditions or decision-making. She does not know anyone else in the village. She has no access to transport and so relies on Martha and Malcolm to meet her everyday needs as well as her long-term health needs.

Privilege: Malcolm is the head of the household. He is the rule maker and decision-maker. It has always been the case as he was a businessman who brought all the income into the family home and it was accepted that, therefore, he is in charge. In this way, Malcolm has always invoked his male privilege in family practices that reflect patriarchal ideology (that is, reflect notions of male dominance).

Positionality: On a micro (personal/individual) level, the relations between Sarah, Martha and Malcolm, Sarah is positioned in such a way that she has been stripped of her ability to make everyday decisions (decisions about when she eats, what she eats, where she goes, what she watches on television are made for her). Malcolm's opinion counts above Martha and Sarah. He sees them as subordinate as they have never financially contributed to the household. Martha views Malcolm as 'boss' as he is the head of the household and therefore any decision he makes, she stands by. Any request he makes, she fulfils. Martha thinks Sarah should view Malcolm in the same way. Such beliefs exist on a macro (structural) level, which view men and women as different with patriarchy positioning men as superior and dominant. In addition, ageist stereotypes underpin Malcolm's views about Sarah and he sees her as a drain on his finances. His views underpin his behaviour towards Sarah and constitute a **harmful practice** on the grounds of age and calling her 'the old pest' is a form of **identity abuse**.

Contexts

Public: Martha and Malcolm do go out for an occasional pub meal but do not take Sarah with them. Sarah only leaves the house to go to medical appointments.

Private: The case study gives brief information about the situation but clearly demonstrates the neglect and abuse of Sarah in the private setting of a family home.

Virtual: Malcolm has access to Sarah's online banking and he has been transferring Sarah's money to his own online account without her knowledge or permission; this constitutes financial abuse.

Summary

After considerable involvement from adult social care services, during which they attempted to work with Martha and Malcolm to care for Sarah, Sarah was relocated to more appropriate accommodation due to concerns about neglect, financial and emotional abuse.

This book covers various aspects of GBV, including child abuse, intimate partner abuse, non-partner sexual violence, harmful practices, human trafficking, institutional abuse, identity abuse, and digital and technology-related abuse. Figure 2 illustrates the categories which we have used to type each form of GBV. Some of the types of GBV overlap and could be located in more than one category; we have made a pragmatic decision under which category they best fit and organised them accordingly into different sections of the book. Chapters are intended as an introduction, rather than as an in-depth analysis, with a focus on defining the topic or practice and then by offering a brief outline of historical contexts, international comparison, prevalence, risk and protective factors, impact, and implications for policy and practice. Reflecting the diversity of topics, not all chapters will follow the same structure, but each contains a relevant and up-to-date overview of the topic or practice. Each chapter pays attention, where possible, to structural and individual influences, explanations and/or key theories and concepts and may include case studies to really bring life to the discussion.

Summary

- Gender is a social construct and impacts how women and men (and other identities) are positioned in society.
- Gender as a spectrum offers a plethora of gender identities ranging from man and women to trans and non-binary identities.
- GBV affects people all across the world.
- GBV can affect any gender, but the most common victim remains women.

References

Aghtaie N, Gangoli G (2018) Key issues in researching gender based violence. In: Aghtaie N, Gangoli G (eds) Understanding gender based violence: national and international contexts. Taylor and Francis, London

Ahmed S (2017) Living a feminist life. Duke University Press, London

Al Jazeera (2021) Timeline: how the new coronavirus spread. https://www.aljazeera.com/news/2020/12/31/timeline-how-the-new-coronavirus-spread. Accessed 22 Apr 2022

Anthias F (2002) Where do I belong: narrating collective identity and translocational positionality. Ethnicities 2(4):491–514

Archer J (2002) Sex differences in physically aggressive acts between heterosexual partners: a meta-analytic review. Aggress Violent Behav 7:313–351

Bachmann CL, Gooch B (2018) LGBT in Britain: trans report. Stonewall, London

Butler J (1990) Gender trouble: feminism and the subversion of identity. Routledge, New York

Crenshaw K (1989) Demarginalizing the intersection of race and sex: a black feminist critique of antidiscrimination doctrine: feminist theory and antiracist politics. University of Chicago, Legal Forum, Chicago, pp 138–167

Dargie E, Blair KL, Pukall CF, Coyle SM (2014) Somewhere under the rainbow: exploring the identities and experiences of trans persons. Can J Hum Sex 23(2):60–74

European Institute for Gender Equality (2017) Glossary of definitions of rape, femicide and intimate partner violence. European Institute for Gender Equality, Vilnius

European Institute for Gender Equality (2021) The costs of gender-based violence in the European Union. European Institute for Gender Equality, Vilnius

European Institute for Gender Equality (2022) What is gender-based violence. https://eige.europa.eu/gender-based-violence/what-is-gender-based-violence

European Union Agency for Fundamental Rights (2015) Violence against women: an EU-side—results at a glance. https://fra.europa.eu/en/publication/2014/violence-against-women-eu-wide-survey-main-results-report. Accessed 1 Apr 2022

García-Moreno C, Pallioto C (2013) Global and regional estimates of violence against women: prevalence and health effects of intimate partner violence and non-partner sexual violence. https://www.who.int/publications/i/item/9789241564625. Accessed 1 Apr 2022

García-Moreno C, Jansen HADM, Ellsberg M, Heise L, Watts C (2005) WHO multi-country study on women's health and domestic violence against women: initial results on prevalence, health outcomes and women's responses. World Health Organization, Geneva

Gavey N (1999) "I wasn't raped, but …" revisiting definitional problems in sexual victimisation. In: Lamb S (ed) New versions of victims: feminists struggle with the concept. New York University Press, New York

Gupta R (2014) 'Victim' vs 'survivor': feminism and language. Open Democracy. https://www.opendemocracy.net/en/5050/victim-vs-survivor-feminism-and-language/. Accessed 31 Mar 2022

Heise L (1994) Gender-based abuse: the global epidemic. Caderno Saúde Pública 10(1):135–145

Hoyle C (2007) Feminism, victimology and domestic violence. In: Walklate S (ed) Handbook of victims and victimology. Routledge, London, pp 146–174

Huntley A, Potter L, Williamson E, Malpass A, Szilassy E, Feder G (2019) Help-seeking by male victims of domestic violence and abuse (DVA): a systematic review and qualitative evidence synthesis. BMJ Open 9(6):e021960. https://doi.org/10.1136/bmjopen-2018-021960

Johnson L (2021) Economic abuse in intimate relationships. In: Devaney J, Bradbury-Jones C, Macy RJ, Øverlien C, Holt S (eds) The Routledge International handbook of domestic violence and abuse. Routledge, Abingdon

Kennedy AC, Meier E, Saba J (2021) Sexual violence within intimate relationships. In: Devaney J, Bradbury-Jones C, Macy RJ, Øverlien C, Holt S (eds) The Routledge international handbook of domestic violence and abuse. Routledge, Abingdon

McGlynn C, Johnson K (2021) Cyberflashing: recognising harms, reforming laws. Bristol University Press, Bristol

Myhill A (2017) Measuring domestic violence: context is everything. J Gender-Based Viol 1(1):33–44

Oliver R, Alexander B, Roe S, Wlasny M (2019) The economic and social costs of domestic abuse, research report 107. Home Office, London

Rogers M, Ahmed A (2017) Interrogating trans and sexual identities through the conceptual lens of translocational positionality. Sociol Res Online 22(1):81. http://www.socresonline.org.uk/22/1/contents.html

Schilt K, Westbrook L (2009) Doing gender, doing heteronormativity: 'gender normals', transgender people, and the social maintenance of heterosexuality. Gend Soc 23(4):440–464

Stark E (2007) Coercive control: the entrapment of women in personal life. Oxford University Press, New York.

Stonard KE (2021) Technology-assisted abuse within intimate relationships. In: Devaney J, Bradbury-Jones C, Macy RJ, Øverlien C, Holt S (eds) The Routledge International handbook of domestic violence and abuse. Routledge, Abingdon

Straus MA, Hamby SL, Boney-McCoy S, Sugarman D (1996) The revised conflicts tactics scale (CTS2)—development and preliminary pscyhometric data. J Fam Issues 17:283–316

Thiara R, Schroettle M, Condon S (2011) Violence against women and ethnicity: commonalities and differences across Europe: a reader. Barbara Budrich Publishers, Berlin

UN Women (2021) Measuring the shadow pandemic: violence against women during COVID-19. https://data.unwomen.org/sites/default/files/documents/Publications/Measuring-shadow-pandemic.pdf. Accessed 22 Apr 2022

UN Women (n.d.) Ending violence against women. https://www.unwomen.org/en/what-we-do/ending-violence-against-women. Accessed 31 Mar 2022

UNHRC (2021) Gender-based violence. https://www.unhcr.org/uk/gender-based-violence.html Accessed 31 Mar 2022

West C, Zimmerman DH (2009) Accounting for doing gender. Gend Soc 23(1):112–122

WHO (2002) World report on violence and health: summary. WHO, Geneva. https://www.who.int/violence_injury_prevention/violence/world_report/en/summary_en.pdf. Accessed 31 Mar 2022

WHO (2013) Global and regional estimates of violence against women: prevalence and health effects of intimate partner violence and non-partner sexual violence. WHO, Geneva. https://www.who.int/publications/i/item/9789241564625. Accessed 31 Mar 2022

WHO (2014) Health care for women subjected to intimate partner violence or sexual violence: a clinical handbook. WHO, Geneva. https://www.who.int/reproductivehealth/publications/violence/vaw-clinical-handbook/en/. Accessed 31 Mar 2022

Williamson E (2018) Heterosexual men as victims of domestic violence and abuse: prevlance, help seeking, and challenges to feminist theoretical frameworks. In: Aghtaie N, Gangoli G (eds) Understanding gender based violence: national and international contexts. Taylor and Francis, London, pp 147–162

Wolfe DA (2018) Why polyvictimization matters. J Interpers Violence 33(5):832–837

Women Against Abuse (2021) The language we use. https://www.womenagainstabuse.org/education-resources/the-language-we-use. Accessed 31 Mar 2022

Michaela Rogers, PhD is a Senior Lecturer in Social Work in the Department of Sociological Studies at the University of Sheffield. Her research examines interpersonal violence with a focus on marginalized groups, impacts, help-seeking, service access and service responses.

Parveen Ali, PhD is a Professor of Gender Based Violence and Professor of Nursing in the Health Sciences School, the University of Sheffield and Doncaster and Bassetlaw Teaching Hospitals. Her research examines gender-based violence, inequalities in health related to gender and ethnicity, and professionals preparedness to support victims of gender based violence.

Theorising Gender-Based Violence

Michaela M. Rogers and Parveen Ali

Learning Objectives
After reading this chapter, the reader will be able to

- Understand how gender-based violence is theorised and explained over time.
- Explore biological and psychological explanations of gender-based violence.
- Understand feminist and sociological explanations of gender-based violence.
- Explore ecological perspectives on gender-based violence.

Introduction

This chapter provides an overview of the common theoretical perspectives used to explain gender-based violence (GBV). Over a few decades, theories and frameworks have been proposed to explain and understand GBV and subsequently some have been developed further, and some have fallen out of favour.

M. M. Rogers (✉)
Department of Sociological Studies, University of Sheffield, Sheffield, UK
e-mail: m.rogers@sheffield.ac.uk

P. Ali
Health Sciences School, University of Sheffield, Sheffield, UK
e-mail: parveen.ali@sheffield.ac.uk

P. Ali, M. M. Rogers (eds.), *Gender-Based Violence: A Comprehensive Guide*,
https://doi.org/10.1007/978-3-031-05640-6_2

The aim of this chapter is to provide an overview of both those that have been influential and those that are currently deemed useful in explaining GBV within contemporary global contexts. The chapter explores common approaches to understanding GBV including feminist, sociological and psychological and biological theoretical frameworks.

Theorising Gender-Based Violence

Over the past few decades, many theories have been proposed to explain GBV, and these include the biological perspective (aggression resulting from structural and chemical changes in the brain due to, for example, trauma or head injury) and psychopathological theories (psychopathology, mental illness, attachment problems, inability to manage anger and hostility, deficiency in various skills and abilities such as management of anger and hostility, lack of assertiveness, self-esteem and communication skills). Also commonly found are the feminist perspective (patriarchal structure of the societies, power and control issues and learned helplessness) and sociological perspective (violence in the family of origin, differences in the resources, and resourcefulness, of men and women in a marital or intimate relationship, conflict and stress in the family, and an ecological perspective). In the following discussion, a brief description of these perspectives, as indicated in Table 1, is presented.

Table 1 Perspectives on gender-based violence

Biological perspectives	Psychological perspectives	Feminist perspectives	Sociological perspectives
• Head injury • Neurotransmitters • Genetics • Infection	• Psychopathology • Personality theories • Attachment • Anger/hostility • Self-esteem • Communication skills and assertiveness • Substance and alcohol use	• Cycle of violence • Learned helplessness • Battered women syndrome • Power and control wheel • Coercive control • Patriarchy • Heteropatriarchy	• Social learning theory • Resource theory • Culture and religion • Nested ecological framework • Social norms

Biological Perspectives

Earlier explanations of GBV centred around the biological causes or explanations, and these included genetic, congenital, and organic causes of aggressive or violent behaviour. Researchers explored the role of genetic defects, brain injury, neuropathology, brain infections, and medical illnesses affecting brain and structural or functional changes in the brain secondary to trauma in the development of violent and aggressive behaviours (Ali and Naylor 2013a, 2013b).

Head Injury

Head injury is known to result in negative consequences for the survivor of the injury and their family. While survivors face difficulties with behaviour, anger management, and self-monitoring, partners and family members report changes in the survivor's personality, irritability, rage outbursts and reduced impulse control as long-term consequences of head injury (Wood et al. 2005). The association between violent and abusive behaviour and head injury was first explored by Rosenbaum and Hoge (1989) who found a history of head injury in 61.3% of their participants ($N = 31$) who were perpetrators of IPV. Rosenbum and colleagues conducted further research to explore this association (Gosling and Oddy 1999; Rosenbaum et al. 1994; Warnken et al. 1994) and concluded that head injury might affect impulse control (thereby increasing aggressive behaviour) and cause personality changes (thereby affecting the quality of relationship), which in turn may increase the risk of aggressive behaviour. However, this explanation is criticised as not all violent men have a history of head injury, and not all men with a history of head injury are violent (Godwin et al. 2011).

Neurotransmitters

Researchers also tried to explore the link between various neurotransmitters, such as testosterone and serotonin, with aggressive behaviours. Men with high testosterone levels tend to be more aggressive, have difficulty in maintaining good marital relationships, are more prone to having extramarital affairs and have lower-quality marital interactions than men with low testosterone levels. Testosterone has also been found to be positively associated with verbal and physical aggression (Soler et al. 2000), dominance, sensation seeking, and criminal, violent and/or antisocial behaviour (Cohan et al. 2003; Romero-Martínez et al. 2016). At the same time, a lower level of serotonin is identified as predictive of impulsive and violent behaviour (Badawy 2003). Decreased serotonin levels have also been found to have a negative effect on mood and behaviour, whereas increased serotonin levels have been found to result in improved social interaction and decreased aggression.

Overall research examining the relationship between neurotransmitters and GBV/intimate partner violence (IPV) is scarce and inconsistent. Some studies report a strong positive association (Soler et al. 2000), some a moderate or weak association (Archer 2006), while some could not identify any association at all (Carré and McCormick 2008). In addition, many studies on neurotransmitters have been conducted on animals and are dated. More research is needed to understand the role of neurotransmitters in causing violent and aggressive behaviour.

Other Biological Causes

Very limited research has been conducted to explore the association between genetics and violence (Saudino and Hines 2007). Evidence from some studies on twins suggests that aggression and the ability to control aggression are genetically influenced characteristics. Certain people, due to their genotype, may act more aggressively than others (Carey and Goldman 1997). Evidence also suggests that genetic factors combined with environmental influences increase the risk of aggressive, antisocial, and criminal behaviour (Miles and Carey 1997).

Evidence, although there is modest and it is dated, suggests that there is an association between some infections/illnesses, such as encephalitis, meningitis, syphilis, herpes simplex, tuberculosis, and violent behaviour (Tardiff 1992). In summary, very little attention has been paid to looking at the biological determinants of GBV. One reason for this could be the fear of providing men with an excuse for their violent behaviour. Further research is needed to determine the links between biological factors and GBV.

Psychological Perspectives

There is a vast body of psychological research that examines factors in relation to GBV. This literature explores the role of various psychological and psychiatric conditions (e.g. psychopathology, trauma, and attachment needs) as well as individual attributes (e.g. assertiveness, communication, and problem-solving skills). Many studies explore the broader psychosocial outcomes of being exposed to GBV whilst others look more specifically at the associations between GBV and the diagnosis of one or more mental disorders. Psychological explanations can examine factors affecting both the individual perpetrator or the victim/survivor. However, Kessi and Boonzaier (2018) argue that the discipline of psychology has done little to attend to questions of historically contextualised and situated, gendered, raced, and localised understandings of trauma and GBV.

Psychopathology

Early theories on the intersection of psychopathology and violence emerged from research conducted on imprisoned violent men or women who had left violent relationships and were accommodated in refuges/shelters. This scholarship led to conclusions that mental health problems (e.g. depression, borderline antisocial personality disorders) are experienced by both violent men and women who experience violence (Chester and DeWall 2018). Due to the limited sample of people included in this body of work, the findings of such studies have limited generalisability. In addition, not everyone with psychopathology reacts violently towards their partners, families, or communities; and not every violent person has a psychopathological disorder. Scholars have problematised this approach in that positioning psychopathology as the primary or sole cause of violence is unhelpful and serves to disregard other factors including social and cultural norms as well as structural inequalities that influence violent behaviour.

Attachment Theory

Another influential theory, but again one that is focused on the individual (rather than on family or communities), attachment theory proposes that violence and abuse could be a result of a dysfunctional attachment to another (Bowlby 1988). Attachment theory emerged in studies of child development. It is described as a process by which an infant attaches to an adult (the attachment figure) who is a constant source of care in their initial period of life and who responds sensitively to the infant's needs. Through social interaction and meeting the infant's needs, trust is built in the attachment figure as they are experienced by the infant as available, accessible, and reliable. The infant seeks closeness, or proximity, to the mother (or substitute caregiver), particularly in situations that are experienced as distressing or threatening. The process of attachment continues during infancy and childhood and then adolescence and the expectations developed during infancy remain relatively static throughout life (Bowlby 1973). The attachment experiences of the infant result in the development of an internal working model, which serves as a template for an individual's beliefs and expectations about future relationships.

For infants who do not have positive early attachment experiences, that is, for whom their needs are unmet or disturbed, or for whom there has been a real or perceived threat of separation or loss of the attachment figure, feelings of grief, rage or fear abound (Bowlby 1973). Repetition of these experiences during childhood, Bowlby argued, may lead to poor or insecure attachment patterns in adult relationships. Research underpinned by attachment theory can help understand dysfunctional and abusive relationships and the reasons that people behave in particular ways (Gormley 2005). Applied in this way, however, attachment theory has its limitations as it does not explain why children from one family do not all behave in the same way (Ali and Naylor 2013a). Attachment theory is relevant in an analysis where violence exists in a household as there can be severe disruptions and challenges to forming a positive, secure attachment by an infant to a mother. However, research has shown that while the space and time for mothers and infants to form strong attachments can be disrupted due to violence, sustained violence can also result in mothers prioritising the protection and well-being of the child/ren (Buchanan 2018).

Adult Attachment, Relationship Behaviours and Communication Skills

Communication skills can be examined from an attachment perspective, as the formation of internal working models in childhood influence cognition and affect, as well as behaviour in later relationships (Simpson et al. 2010). These working models reflect behaviours as securely attached individuals (i.e. people with low attachment anxiety and avoidance) tend to show independence and ease with intimacy, whereas insecurely attached people tend to display an array of dysfunctional thoughts and feelings about the self and others (Sierau and Herzberg 2012). Specifically, people with insecure attachment can show a strong need for intimacy and fear of rejection by their partners, whereas highly avoidant people tend to show emotional detachment and self-sufficiency (Bonache et al. 2019). Thus, people with these flawed thoughts and behaviours often favour the use of destructive conflict resolution strategies (Sierau and Herzberg 2012). Clearly adult attachment style influences the way in which conflict is addressed, which may lead to its resolution or a deteriorating situation. This is significant as dysfunctional conflict resolution skills can be destructive and/or abusive. In contrast, it might mean that an individual avoids conflict and withdraws from an abusive relationship.

There is a body of work to suggest that when comparing non-violent men with those who use violence in their intimate relationships, violent men tend to have poor communication skills, and display aversive, offensive or defensive behaviour (Berns et al. 1999; Waltz et al. 2000). Moreover, the use of violence by men with poor communication skills has been said to account for a lack of conflict resolution skills (Ramos Salazar 2015). Assertiveness is a skill linked to conflict resolution, and various studies have investigated two types of assertiveness including general assertiveness (the ability to behave in an assertive manner in any given situation) and spouse-specific assertiveness (the ability to behave assertively with one's spouse). However, the results of these studies are inconsistent, meaning there is a lack of robust, reliable evidence questioning its utility in an analysis of GBV (Satyanarayana et al. 2015).

Feminist Perspectives

The achievements of the feminist movement have been transformative in terms of putting the issue of GBV on global and national agendas. Feminist work has led to the development of infrastructure of the women's sector in many countries, including the establishment of safe accommodation and advocacy for women and children fleeing domestic abuse and perpetrator programmes, as well as resulting in the politicisation of GBV and changes to legal and criminal justice systems (Bjørnholt 2021; Hague 2021). This work has also brought about enhanced theoretical and conceptual understandings of GBV. According to a feminist perspective, GBV is caused by and constitutive of gendered patterns of power and privilege in society (Bjørnholt 2021). The common central underpinning of the perspective is that GBV cannot be adequately understood through any lens that does not include gender as the central component of analysis. Feminist scholarship led to the development of various explanations of GBV, mostly in relation to intimate partner violence (IPV), including the cycle of violence, battered women syndrome, and learned helplessness (Walker 1979).

The Cycle of Violence

In the 1970s, Walker proposed the cycle of violence to explain how and why abused women remain in abusive relationships. Walker described the cycle of violence as having three phases: tension building, abuse or explosion, and honeymoon or remorse/forgiveness. In the first phase, tension builds within the couple and the abuser takes frustrations out on the wife (or partner). In this scenario, violence can take on a plethora of forms, including physical, psychological, emotional, or sexual abuse, lasting from mere moments to days. Then, the abuser is rid of the pent-up frustration. They may feel a sense of relief, start to feel remorse and apologise to the abused partner. Thereafter, the couple enjoys a so-called honeymoon period during which the victim/survivor thinks the abuser will change and that violence will stop. In some instances, the intensity of violence is decreased or ceases for some time (Walker 2006); nonetheless, the cycle continues and another period of tension soon builds up. When a victim/survivor is exposed to a cycle of violence that is relentless, this results in feelings of helplessness, reduced autonomy and constant fear (Walker 1979). The victim/survivor may blame themselves for the abuse and seek to avoid situations that have previously led to violence or abuse. The popularity of this theory was short-lived as women's experiences were not consistent with the cycle of violence. Critics highlighted flaws in an argument built upon the notion of violence resulting from tension and frustration, asking why the abuser does not vent these feelings at others.

Learned Helplessness

The term *learned helplessness* was coined in the 1960s by psychologists Seligman and Maier (1967) and refers to the state of an individual who continuously faces an adverse, uncontrollable situation and stops trying to change their circumstances, even when they have the ability to do so. Seligman and Maier were involved in animal behavioural research, which involved delivering electric shocks to dogs in a series of experiments. This research would be considered unethical now but was deemed justifiable in the 1960s. Dogs in one cage learned to accept the shock and gave up trying to escape, whereas dogs in the second cage learned to seek out a safe, shockproof place. Observing different behaviour in the dogs enabled Seligman and Maier to conclude that for one group of dogs the experience led to the development of a feeling of helplessness, inability to control and acceptance of their situation (Seligman and Maier 1967).

Subsequently, the theory of learned helplessness has been linked to IPV since Walker first proposed the concept of battered women syndrome in the late 1970s (Walker 1979). Walker (1979) concluded that a pattern of repeated abuse over time could serve to minimise a woman's motivation to respond, leading to a state of passivity (or learned helplessness). Walker suggested that IPV negatively impacts a woman's cognitive ability to perceive a scenario whereby their actions could end the abuse. Accordingly, she does not try to leave an abusive relationship. Proponents of learned helplessness also used it to explain why women may justify IPV. This is shown in research as the majority of the respondents in the World Health Organization's multi-country study justified their experiences of IPV because of reasons such as being disobedient to their husbands, refusing sex, being unfaithful, or not completing housework effectively (García-Moreno et al. 2005).

The concept of learned helplessness failed to gain traction with critics who maintain that it neglects the additional and plentiful factors that contribute to a woman's decision to stay in an abusive relationship, including social, economic, or cultural reasons (such as an inability to financially support herself and children, and a fear of rejection by the family, community, and society). It also takes a victim-blaming approach by disregarding a woman's autonomy and efforts to minimise violence towards themselves and their children. Similarly, this approach misidentifies indications of abuse such as low self-esteem, reduced decision-making, and perceived loss of control as learned helplessness. Rather than taking this victim-centred and victim-blaming approach, the problem of IPV should be attributed to the perpetrator with more focus on their behaviour as opposed to that of the victim.

Coercive Control

The concept of coercive control is both a form of abuse and a theoretical framework for understanding IPV. Moreover, it has provided the main conceptual lens for understanding violence against women in recent years (Stark 2007). As a form of abuse, the highly influential work of Stark (2012) positions coercive control as 'a liberty crime' and 'a strategic course of oppressive conduct'. In developing his thesis on coercive control, Stark drew on the abuse experiences of women to provide an explanation that countered the shortcomings of research, policy and practice at the time, which reflected a more incident-based understanding of IPV. Okun (1986) described the tactics deployed by perpetrators resulting in the isolation and exhaustion of victim-survivors, in their debilitation and in the distortion of their subjective reality.

The conceptual framework describes the basic tactics adopted in coercive control, and feminist scholarship has argued persuasively to interweave ideas about power imbalances within intimate relationships caused by structural inequalities between men and women. A clear example is the patriarchal control of the family, codified historically in legislation and capitalist regimes, that afforded women part-time and/or low-paid employment that was compatible with their disproportionate responsibility for caring, childrearing and household management (Robinson and

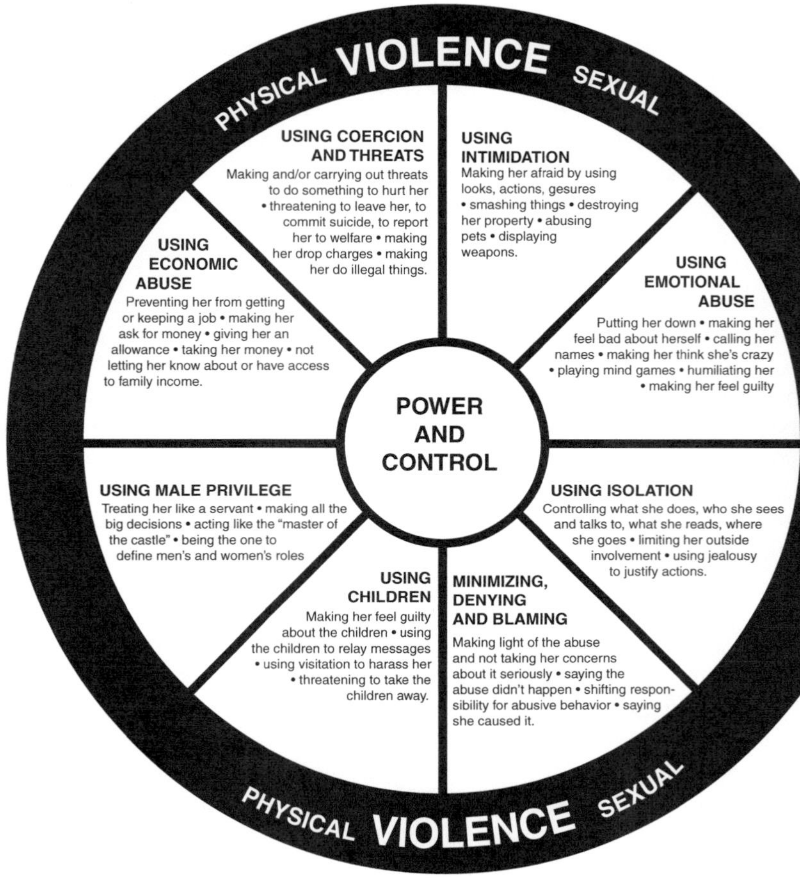

Fig. 1 The power and control wheel. (Source: Domestic Abuse Intervention Programs) Retrieved from https://www.theduluthmodel.org/wheels/). Domestic Abuse Intervention Programs (2022), East Superior Street, Duluth, Minnesota 55802; 218-722-2781

Myhill 2021). Whilst there is evidence of social change in terms of women's social position around caring, there remain many examples of social ordering and regimes that continue to privilege men and enable them to take up dominant positions in society. Indeed, the Power and Control wheel (see Fig. 1) highlights 'using male privilege' as one of the eight elements, or 'spokes', of violence against women.

Power and Control

The Duluth model is a programme of support designed to reduce violence against women and emerged from feminist activism and direct work with victim-survivors. Developed in the 1980s, the model emerged from the work of the Domestic Abuse Intervention Project (DAIP) in Duluth, MN, USA. The model explains the tactics used by abusive men to keep women in submissive positions and to maintain male power and control. Such tactics are organised into eight categories of using: intimidation; emotional use; isolation; children; male privilege; economic abuse; coercion and threats; and minimising, denying, and blaming. These are integrated into the power and control wheel (see Fig. 1). Underpinning the model is the proposition that every act of abuse is intended to control women through the exertion of the reminder of male power. Principles of the model centre on prioritising victim/survivor's safety while simultaneously holding perpetrators to account for their actions.

Patriarchy and Heteropatriarchy

A concept that is central to feminist perspectives is that of patriarchy as this describes a social system in which men hold power and privilege and dominate women (Hunnicutt 2009). Patriarchy is characterised by a value and belief system that validates male dominance while rejecting egalitarian structures in both public and private spheres of life. In the public sphere, power is shared by men, and in private spheres, the senior men exercise power over everyone else in the family, including younger men and boys (Haj-Yahia and Schiff 2007). Therefore, in patriarchal societies, a man is considered and expected to be the head of the family. The use of violence in such families is considered an acceptable mechanism for maintaining and exhibiting male dominance. Believers in patriarchal ideology tend to view wife beating [sic] not only as acceptable but also as beneficial and consider that women are responsible for the violence against them (Carter 2015).

The ground-breaking work of Dobash and Dobash (1979), which focused on IPV, highlighted that wife abuse (their terminology) is a brutal and explicit expression of male domination over women. They claimed that the patriarchal domination of women through the mechanism of wife abuse results from the long cultural history of legally sanctioned male subordination, abuse, and outright ownership of women (Lawson 2012). This history of inequality sustains wife abuse as it continues to work to embed notions of socially sanctioned male privilege through gender roles and norms. Feminist scholarship, such as that emanating from the highly influential work of Dobash and Dobash, continues supports the argument for studying violence against wives, or non-married partners, as a separate unit of analysis to be examined in its own right.

Adopting patriarchy as central to an analysis of IPV has been criticised for its stance that abuse can only be perpetrated by men against women. There is also some evidence suggesting that women can be equally or more violent (Ali and Naylor 2013b; Fiebert 2008). This argument is complex and, as several commentators, including Dobash and Dobash (2004), have highlighted in their own research, abuse is primarily an asymmetrical problem of men's violence to women, and women's violence does not equate to men's in terms of frequency, severity, consequences and the victim's sense of safety and well-being.

Contemporary feminist perspectives have also adopted the concept of heteropatriarchy, which is a socio-political system where (primarily) cisgender (or 'cis') and heterosexual males have authority over cis females as well as people with other sexual orientations and gender identities (Phipps 2020). The term is helpful in signifying that discrimination against women and lesbian, gay, bisexual and trans (LGBT) people is derived from sexism coupled with homophobia and cisgenderism, extending conceptions of patriarchy further. The notion of heteropatriarchy describes a landscape of heteropatriarchal societies in which the majority of cis, heterosexual men occupy the highest and privileged positions of power in society, causing women (including trans women), non-binary people, trans men, and other LGBT people to experience the bulk of social oppression in relation to gender and sexuality.

Other minoritized communities and black feminists maintain that oppression experienced by black women is more severe and different from that of white women and that the voices of white feminists do not speak for the oppression based on racism and classicism that mainly affects black women; issues have sharply drawn into focus in contemporary scholarship Phipps 2020; Ahmed 2017). Postcolonial feminism goes further, arguing that the positioning and perception of women from the developing world (that is, non-Western women) as oppressed, submissive, and voiceless as opposed to the Western women's positioning as educated, assertive and empowered is oppressive (Hamad 2020). This ethnocentrism is problematic and subjugating. It serves to marginalise and 'other' non-Western women. In this book, we aim to include different perspectives and international contexts to illustrate intersectionality and its relation to GBV.

Sociological Perspectives

Sociological perspectives on GBV utilise theory about the social world as the point of departure to understand the gendered nature of violence and abuse and the social contexts in which it occurs. There exists a plethora of relevant sociological perspectives, and so we have chosen a dominant few to illustrate the value of a sociological analysis and an overview is provided of social learning theory, resource theory, social–ecological theory and social norming theory.

Social Learning Theory

Social learning theory, also known as learned behaviour theory, acknowledges that the social environment plays a significant role in learning, and, in the case of violence, both the perpetration and acceptance of violence is a conditioned and learned behaviour shaped by the social setting in which it takes place (Bandura 1977). Bandura (1977) argued that observation is also central to learning, and in the case of violence, men who perpetrate abuse do so because they have seen their fathers being abusive towards their mothers. Similarly, Bandura argues that women accept abuse because they have seen their mother being abused by their father. This argument locates the family at the heart of conditioning and learning. In the case of violence, the family is the setting that not only exposes individuals to the use of violence but also serves to validate the use of violence within relationships. Social learning theory underpins the 'intergenerational cycle of violence', which proposes that children who witness violence or who have been victims of violence themselves as children are at risk of becoming perpetrators or victims of violence as adults (Black et al. 2010).

The suggestion that children who witness or have been victims of violence as children are more likely to become a perpetrator or victim has been criticised for its overly deterministic approach, which denies the agency of individuals. Indeed, it is dangerous to assume that all men who experience or witness abuse as children will become perpetrators. Equally, not all victims have a history of experiencing or witnessing abuse in childhood. Other questions have been raised about adopting this approach. For instance, studies that have employed this theory are subject to questions about the difference in adopted definitions, such as what constitutes witnessing violence as a child and how victimization and exposure to abuse in childhood are defined? Moreover, research findings are inconsistent, with some studies identifying victimisation as a stronger predictor of violence than witnessing abuse as a child while others suggest that witnessing abuse is the strongest predictor (Iverson et al. 2011). Additionally, research that investigates the role of these variables in relation to gender, when violence is perpetrated by females, remains modest.

Resource Theory

A sociological perspective that is clearly tied to the principles of patriarchy is that of resource theory. This perspective suggests that the partner with more resources in terms of income, occupational status and education may have more power and dominate in the relationship (Blood and Wolfe 1960). So, in the case of men's violence towards women, it is the lack of power, privilege, and resources that men have within a patriarchal context which results in frustration, violence and acts of domination towards women. To support this claim, research by Atkinson et al. (2005) found that violent men who were lacking in resources such as income and education, as well as having low or no occupational status, had used violence in their relationships. Furthermore, the study found that men's lack of resources was relative in that 'it is not so much men's lack of resources that predicts wife abuse, but lack of resources relative to their wives' (Atkinson et al. 2005: 1138). Providing further evidence for this theory, other studies have found that women with higher incomes or unemployed partners are more likely to be abused (Fox et al. 2002; Melzer 2002).

Disproving these findings, research by Stith et al. (2004) identified unemployment, lower incomes, and lower education as weak predictors of male physical violence. Critics have also highlighted that resource theory does not account for diverse gender ideologies and cultures that are less patriarchal and for assuming that traditional gender norms prevail; such that all men want to be the primary or sole provider for their family (Eirich and Robinson 2017). In addition, there is a certain irony that resource theory contradicts other perspectives, which propose that one way to tackle DVA is to empower women through education and enhanced employment opportunities.

Social–Ecological Theory

One of the most widely used theoretical frameworks to account for GBV is that of the social–ecological model (Bronfenbrenner 1979) (see Fig. 2). The ecological model was developed to explain a child's development and behaviours and suggests that these are influenced by interaction at various levels of social organisation. Social–ecological theory underpins variants of the original model, including the nested ecological model. The nested ecological model has value as whilst the central focus is upon the individual and their behaviour, it also prompts an analysis of those behavioural influences relating to the family, community, and wider society (Ali and Naylor 2013b). At the individual level, the biological and personal factors of a person are examined. These include a wide range of influences, including age, gender, sexual identity, ethnicity, education, income level, health, psychological problems, aggressive tendencies, and substance abuse. Next, the relationship level prompts a consideration of the interaction of the individual with others, including partners, family, friends, and workplace colleagues. The next level is related to the role of community or the neighbourhood in which the person lives and works, and in which they interact with social factors and with other people (including those

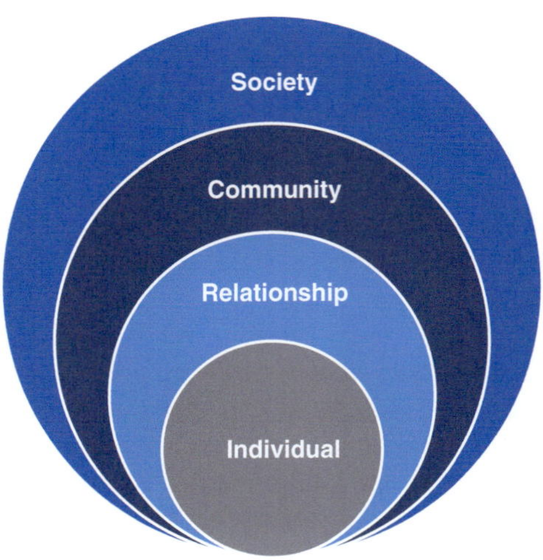

Society: norms that aggression and violence is an acceptable means of resolving conflict, and that men are meant to be head of the households and dominant to women.

Community: characterised by high unemployment, low-income families and there are few community resources that the family can access. The estate is known for ease of access to drugs and the man's whole family live on the estate.

Relationship: neither parent is employed, and both are recovering addicts. They have been together since they were 15 years old. The man often forces the woman to sex work for get money for drugs. The four children are under 10 years old. There is ongoing daily conflict, with frequent episodes of violence.

Individual: the perpetrator is male, white, 30 years old. He is on methadone and trying to overcome drug addiction. He believes that men and women and should be dominant in the home. He grew up in a household where there was domestic abuse.

Fig. 2 A social–ecological model: reflections on a perpetrator of domestic violence and abuse

identity at the 'relationship' level). The final level of the framework is the societal level that relates to the structures and systems of the society and culture where the person lives. This might include societal norms, attitudes and beliefs, family configuration and roles, healthcare systems, education and legal frameworks. The model prompts an analysis of GBV that takes factors at these different levels, and their interactions, into account and is, therefore, useful in the analysis of varied forms of GBV, and it is a common model used by researchers in studies on domestic violence and abuse.

This model is used widely, but recent studies, especially those coming from non-western cultures, have criticised the model for not having explicit mention of the family arguing that family plays an important role in the perpetration, perpetuation, and prevention of abuse. This is particularly relevant in countries where the implementation of laws to prevent GBV and availability of resources for victims may be limited and thus most responsibility of supporting victims and preventing GBV/IPV stays with the families of victims as well as perpetrators (Ali et al. 2019, 2020, 2021).

Social Norms

A sociological lens draws attention to the ways that social norms strongly influence behaviour and social interaction (Cares et al. 2021). More importantly, over the last decade social norms theory has gained momentum as a potentially useful means of understanding GBV (Cislaghi and Heise 2017), particularly as there is ample evidence of the influence of social norms related to gender and family. Social norms are shared beliefs about others and the social world that exist within social groups and are maintained through group approval and disapproval (Mackie et al. 2012). Social norms can be broadly categorised into three types:

- Actual norms: perceptions that are shown in behaviour.
- Perceived norms: perceptions about what members of a social group think others ought and ought not to do.
- Misperceived norms: situations when the perceived norm is different from the actual norm; that is, when what people think is the norm is not actually the case (Berkowitz 2012; Rogers et al. 2018).

An example to illustrate this is when victim-survivors of GBV are portrayed in the media as young, female and heterosexual; this is the misperceived norm as in reality anyone can experience some form of GBV (the actual norm). Social norms are distinct from personal attitudes and behaviour, and it might be that social norms influence an individual's behaviour more so than their personal beliefs. For example, an older victim-survivor might remain in an abusive marriage as they hold the perception that the social norm is that marriage is for life, despite feeling no love for their partner and wishing to separate. As such, age-based and gender norms have salience in relation to the roles and expectations of men and women in families and their wider communities and while there have been considerable shifts to the social institution of the family over the last few decades (including a decline in marriage rates, and increase in divorce rates), traditional gender norms and gender inequality remain and continue to be relevant in debates about GBV (Cares et al. 2021).

Summary

- Researching GBV must embed an understanding of the diversity of gender, including mainstream ideas of the gender binary as well as more contemporary debates about gender as a spectrum of identities.
- There is a plethora of theories that account for GBV, and this chapter provides a snapshot of feminist, sociological, biological, and psychological perspectives.
- Many of these theories are limited in their application as these focus on individual rather than group, community, or societal behaviours.
- Theories of GBV should include attention to individual behaviour as well as structural influences such as gender inequality.
- As the theories included in this chapter have value and limitations, it may be useful to draw on multiple explanations of GBV.

References

Ahmed S (2017) Living a Feminist Life. Duke University Press, London

Ali PA, Naylor PB (2013a) Intimate partner violence: a narrative review of the biological and psychological explanations for its causation. Aggress Violent Behav 18(3):373–382

Ali PA, Naylor PB (2013b) Intimate partner violence: a narrative review of the feminist, social and ecological explanations for its causation. Aggress Violent Behav 18(6):611–619

Ali PA, O'Cathain A, Croot E (2019) Not managing expectations: a grounded theory of intimate partner violence from the perspective of Pakistani people. J Interpers Violence 34(19):4085–4113

Ali PA, McGarry J, Maqsood A (2020) Spousal role expectations and marital conflict: perspectives of men and women. J Interpers Violence 37(9–10):NP7082–NP7108

Ali PA, O'Cathain A, Croot E (2021) Influences of extended family on intimate partner violence: perceptions of Pakistanis in Pakistan and the United Kingdom. J Interpers Violence 36(9–10):3965–3993

Archer J (2006) Testosterone and human aggression: an evaluation of the challenge hypothesis. Neurosci Biobehav Rev 30(3):319–345

Atkinson MP, Greenstein TN, Lang MM (2005) For women, breadwinning can be dangerous: gendered resource theory and wife abuse. J Marriage Fam 67:1137–1148

Badawy AAB (2003) Alcohol and violence and the possible role of serotonin. Crim Behav Ment Health 13(1):31–44

Bandura A (1977) Social learning theory. General Learning Press, New York

Berkowitz AD (2012) A grassroots' guide to fostering healthy norms to reduce violence in our communities: social norms toolkit. http://www.alanberkowitz.com/Social_Norms_Violence_Prevention_Toolkit.pdf

Berns SB, Jacobson NS, Gottman JM (1999) Demand/withdraw interaction patterns between different types of batterers and their spouses. J Marital Fam Ther 25(3):337–348

Bjørnholt M (2021) Domestic violence and abuse through a feminist lens. In: Devaney J, Bradbury-Jones C, Macy R, Øvelien C, Holt S (eds) The Routledge International handbook of domestic violence and abuse. Routledge, Abingdon, pp 11–26

Black DS, Sussman S, Unger JB (2010) A further look at the intergenerational transmission of violence: witnessing interparental violence in emerging adulthood. J Interpers Violence 25(6):1022–1042

Blood RO, Wolfe DM (1960) Husbands and wives. Free Press, Glencoe, IL

Bonache H, Gonzalez-Mendez R, Krahé B (2019) Adult attachment styles, destructive conflict resolution, and the experience of intimate partner violence. J Interpers Violence 34(2):287–309

Bowlby J (1973) Attachment and loss. In: Separation, vol 2. Basic Books, New York

Bowlby J (1988) A secure base: parent child attachment and healthy human development. Basic Books, New York

Bronfenbrenner U (1979) The ecology of human development: experiments by nature and design. Harvard University Press, Cambridge

Buchanan F (2018) Mothering babies in domestic violence: beyond attachment theory. Routledge, New York

Cares AC, Reckdenwald A, Fernandez K (2021) Domestic violence and abuse through a sociological lens. In: Devaney J, Bradbury-Jones C, Macy R, Øvelien C, Holt S (eds) The Routledge International handbook of domestic violence and abuse. Routledge, Abingdon, pp 40–54

Carey G, Goldman D (1997) The genetics of antisocial behavior. In: Stoff DM, Breiling J, Maser JD (eds) Handbook of antisocial behavior. Wiley, New York, pp 243–254

Carré JM, McCormick CM (2008) Aggressive behavior and change in salivary testosterone concentrations predict willingness to engage in a competitive task. Horm Behav 54(3):403–409

Carter J (2015) Patriarchy and violence against women and girls. Lancet 385(9978):e40–e41

Chester DS, DeWall CN (2018) The roots of intimate partner violence. Curr Opin Psychol 19:55–59. https://doi.org/10.1016/j.copsyc.2017.04.009

Cislaghi B, Heise L (2017) Measuring gender-related social norms: report of a meeting. Baltimore, Maryland, June 14-15 2016. Learning Group on Social Norms and Gender-based Violence of the London School of Hygiene and Tropical Medicine, London

Cohan CL, Booth A, Granger DA (2003) Gender moderates the relationship between testosterone and marital interaction. J Fam Psychol 17:29

Dobash RE, Dobash R (1979) Violence against wives : a case against the patriarchy. Free Press, New York

Dobash RP, Dobash RE (2004) Women's violence to men in intimate relationships: working on a puzzle. Br J Criminol 44(3):324–349

Domestic Abuse Intervention Programs (2022) The power and control wheel. https://www.theduluthmodel.org/wheels/

Eirich GM, Robinson JH (2017) Does earning more than your spouse increase your financial satisfaction? A comparison of men and women in the United States, 1982 to 2012. J Fam Issues 38(17):2371–2399

Fiebert MS (2008) References examining assaults by women on their spouses or male partners: an annotated bibliography. http://www.csulb.edu/~mfiebert/assault.htm

Fox GL, Benson ML, DeMaris AA, Wyk JV (2002) Economic distress and intimate violence: testing family stress and resources theories. J Marriage Fam 64(3):793–807

García-Moreno C, Jansen HAFM, Ellsberg M, Heise L, Watts C (2005) WHO multi-country study on women's health and domestic violence against women: initial results on prevalence, health outcomes and women's responses. World Health Organization, Geneva

Godwin EE, Kreutzer JS, Arango-Lasprilla JC, Lehan TJ (2011) Marriage after brain injury: review, analysis, and research recommendations. J Head Trauma Rehabil 26(1):43–55

Gormley B (2005) An adult attachment theoretical perspective of gender symmetry in intimate partner violence. Sex Roles 52:785–795

Gosling J, Oddy M (1999) Rearranged marriages: marital relationships after head injury. Brain Inj 13(10):785–796

Hague G (2021) History and memories of the domestic violence movement: We've come further than youthink. Policy Press, Bristol

Haj-Yahia MM, Schiff M (2007) Definitions of and beliefs about wife abuse among undergraduate students of social work. Int J Offender Ther Comp Criminol 51(2):170–190. https://doi.org/10.1177/0306624x06291457

Hamad R (2020) White tears brown scars: how white feminism betrays women of colour. Hachette UK, Dublin

Hunnicutt G (2009) Varieties of patriarchy and violence against women. Violence against women 15(5):553–573

Iverson KM, Jimenez S, Harrington KM, Resick PA (2011) The contribution of childhood family violence on later intimate partner violence among robbery victims. Violence Vict 26(1):73–87

Kessi S, Boonzaier F (2018) Centre/ing decolonial feminist pscyhology in Africa. S Afr J Psychol 48(3):299–309

Lawson J (2012) Sociological theories of intimate partner violence. Journal of human behavior in the social environment 22(5):572–590

Mackie G, Moneti F, Denny E, Shakya H (2012) What are social norms: how are they measured? University of California at San Diego. UNICEF Working Paper, San Diego

Melzer SA (2002) Gender, work, and intimate violence: men's occupational violence. J Marriage Fam 64(4):820–832

Miles DR, Carey G (1997) Genetic and environmental architecture on human aggression. J Pers Soc Psychol 72(1):207–217

Okun L (1986) Women abuse: facts replacing myths. State University of New York Press, Albany

Phipps A (2020) Me not you: the trouble with mainstream feminism. Manchester University Press, Manchester

Ramos Salazar L (2015) The negative reciprocity process in marital relationships: a literature review. Aggress Violent Behav 24:113–119. https://doi.org/10.1016/j.avb.2015.05.008

Robinson A, Myhill A (2021) Coercive control. In: Devaney J, Bradbury-Jones C, Macy R, Øvelien C, Holt S (eds) The Routledge International handbook of domestic violence and abuse. Routledge, Abingdon, pp 387–402

Rogers M, Lovatt G, Rumley T (2018) The Change Up Project: Using social norming theory with young people to address domestic abuse and promote healthy relationships. The Journal of Family Violence 34(6):507–519

Romero-Martínez Á, Lila M, Moya-Albiol L (2016) Testosterone and attention deficits as possible mechanisms underlying impaired emotion recognition in intimate partner violence perpetrators. Eur J Psychol Appl Leg Context 8:57–62

Rosenbaum A, Hoge SK (1989) Head injury and marital aggression. Am J Psychiatry 146(8):1048–1051

Rosenbaum A, Hoge SK, Adelman SA, Warnken WJ, Fletcher KE, Kane RL (1994) Head injury in partner-abusive men. J Consult Clin Psychol 62(6):1187–1193

Satyanarayana VA, Hebbani S, Hegde S, Krishnan S, Srinivasan K (2015) Two sides of a coin: perpetrators and survivors perspectives on the triad of alcohol, intimate partner violence and mental health in South India. Asian J Psychiatr 15:38–43. https://doi.org/10.1016/j.ajp.2015.04.014

Saudino K, Hines D (2007) Etiological similarities between psychological and physical aggression in intimate relationships: a behavioral genetic exploration. J Fam Violence 22(3):121–129

Seligman ME, Maier SF (1967) Failure to escape traumatic shock. J Exp Psychol 74:1–9

Sierau S, Herzberg PH (2012) Conflict resolution as a dyadic mediator: considering the partner perspective on conflict resolution. Eur J Pers 26:221–232

Simpson JA, Rholes WS, Winterheld HA (2010) Attachment working models twist memories of relationship events. Psychol Sci 21:252–259

Soler H, Vinayak P, Quadagno D (2000) Biosocial aspects of domestic violence. Psychoneuroendocrinology 25(7):721–739

Stark E (2007) Coercive control: how men entrap women in personal life. Oxford University Press, Oxford

Stark E (2012) Looking beyond domestic violence: policing coercive control. J Police Crisis Negot 12(2):199–217

Stith SM, Smith DB, Penn CE, Ward DB, Tritt D (2004) Intimate partner physical abuse perpetration and victimization risk factors: a meta-analytic review. Aggress Violent Behav 10(1):65–98
Tardiff K (1992) The current state of psychiatry in the treatment of violent patients. Arch Gen Psychiatry 49:493–499
Walker LA (1979) The battered woman. Harper & Row, New York
Walker LA (2006) Battered woman syndrome: empirical findings. Ann N Y Acad Sci 1087:142–157
Waltz J, Babcock JC, Jacobson NS, Gottman JM (2000) Testing a typology of batterers. J Consult Clin Psychol 68(4):658
Warnken WJ, Rosenbaum A, Fletcher KE, Hoge SK, Adelman SA (1994) Head-injured males: a population at risk for relationship aggression? Violence Vict 9(2):153–166
Wood RL, Liossi C, Wood L (2005) The impact of head injury neurobehavioural sequelae on personal relationships: preliminary findings. Brain Inj 19(10):845–851

Michaela Rogers, PhD is a Senior Lecturer in Social Work in the Department of Sociological Studies at the University of Sheffield. Her research examines interpersonal violence with a focus on marginalized groups, impacts, help-seeking, service access and service responses.

Parveen Ali, PhD is a Professor of Gender Based Violence and Professor of Nursing in the Health Sciences School, the University of Sheffield and Doncaster and Bassetlaw Teaching Hospitals. Her research examines gender-based violence, inequalities in health related to gender and ethnicity, and professionals preparedness to support victims of gender based violence.

Part II

Child Abuse

Child Sexual Exploitation

Moninuola Ifayomi, Parveen Ali,
and Michaela M. Rogers

Learning Objectives
After reading this chapter, the reader will be able to

- Understand the scope and nature of child sexual exploitation (CSE).
- Explore the impact of child sexual exploitation.
- Discuss the principles that should inform professional safeguarding in relation to child sexual exploitation.

Introduction

Child sexual exploitation (CSE) is a serious public health issue and an abhorrent crime across the world; it results in enduring and devastating consequences for its victims, families and societies associated with them (United Nations 2017). It is a complex form of sexual abuse, a subtype of human trafficking and criminal

M. Ifayomi (✉)
Health Science School, University of Sheffield, Sheffield, UK
e-mail: maolorunfemi1@sheffield.ac.uk

P. Ali
Health Sciences School, University of Sheffield, Sheffield, UK
e-mail: parveen.ali@sheffield.ac.uk

M. M. Rogers
Department of Sociological Studies, University of Sheffield, Sheffield, UK
e-mail: m.rogers@sheffield.ac.uk

P. Ali, M. M. Rogers (eds.), *Gender-Based Violence: A Comprehensive Guide*,
https://doi.org/10.1007/978-3-031-05640-6_3

exploitation of child/children, characterised by attempted or actual sexual exploitation of a child (NSPCC 2015; United Nations 2017). Findings from the increasing evidence base highlight failures in multi-agency partnerships and information-sharing policies, especially in education, health, and social service sectors, professionals inability to identify the child vulnerability factors and early signs of CSE (Bedford 2015; Dubowitz 2017; Sethi 2013). Research suggests that due to the transactional nature of CSE and manipulative strategies employed by perpetrators, many victims believe they are in a healthy consensual relationship, and this makes them unable to identify their experience as exploitative and one that requires support (Coy et al. 2017).

This chapter provides an overview of definitions and theories of CSE and highlights the difficulties in establishing prevalence. An international comparison is made to provide the global context. In exploring the impacts of CSE, this chapter highlights its complexity and the challenge for health and social care professionals in identifying the early signs of sexual exploitation, identifying vulnerability factors, and responding appropriately, irrespective of the heterogeneous characteristics of victims, facilitators, and perpetrators.

Defining and Understanding CSE

Although CSE has become a widespread global crime, there are various definitions in operation (Cameron et al. 2015; Kelly and Karsna 2017). The European Union focuses on understanding the scope of the activities that constitute the 'sexual exploitation of children' and on international dimensions regarding tackling sexual trafficking, child pornography, and online sexual exploitation (Cameron et al. 2015). In Sweden, emphasis has been placed on the issue of commercialization of child sexual activities; however, CSE is not always commercialized in nature. In the US-based literature, CSE is framed from two key perspectives: commercial sexual exploitation of children or trafficking; and internet sexual exploitation (Cameron et al. 2015). In the UK, although CSE is seen as a form of child sexual abuse (CSA), there is no consensus on the definition of CSE within the available practice and policy framework. The most recent guidelines in England and Wales argue that CSE cannot be separated from other forms of CSA (Brayley and Cockbain 2014; Department for Education 2017), while this can be considered appropriate, delineating its scope, nature, impacts on identification, assessment, and response. This chapter considers the most recent definition of CSE developed in England, in 2007, as the most encompassing (see Box 1).

Like other forms of CSA, CSE can affect any child (male or female), including those who have reached the age of sexual consent and can legally consent to sexual activity. The act might be contact based or non-contact based, penetrative or non-penetrative, person and/or technology mediated, and with or without the child's knowledge. The term 'CSE' broadly covers exploitative relationships, contexts, and situations, where a child or young person receives tangible or intangible benefits from a person who uses differentials in age, economic resources, intellect, or physical strength to coerce, control, manipulate, or intimidate the child into sexual activity (Department for Education 2017). The power dynamics (perpetrator's or facilitator's abuse of power and child's powerlessness) are core elements of its definition (Department for Education 2017; Pearce 2011). Owing to the complex and dynamic nature of CSE, public health approaches and policies intended to address CSE remain in a relatively nascent stage (Pearce 2011). Box 1 provides a definition of CSE as well as alternative terms and associated concepts.

Box 1 Definitions and Alternative Terminology

Definition of CSE:

> Child sexual exploitation is a form of child sexual abuse. It occurs where an individual or group takes advantage of an imbalance of power to coerce, manipulate or deceive a child or young person under the age of 18 into sexual activity (a) in exchange for something the victim needs or wants and/or (b) for the financial advantage or increased status of the perpetrator or facilitator. The victim may have been sexually exploited even if the sexual activity appears consensual. Child sexual exploitation does not always involve physical contact; it can also occur through the use of technology. (Department for Education 2017: 5)

Alternative terminology and associated concepts:

Child sexual abuse, child prostitution, child sex worker, child sex tourism, child sex trafficking victims, commercial sex trafficking, internet child pornography, internet grooming, child pornography, online child sexual exploitation, commercial sexual exploitation of children (CSEC), commercial sex trafficking, peer-to-peer and group exploitation, gang-related violence, online abuse, and sexual image exploitation (Melrose 2013; Sen 2017).

CSE usually occurs in private dwellings, hidden and difficult to detect or investigate, and victims may also experience other forms of abuse; it can be mistaken for adolescent delinquency or inappropriate behaviour. Grooming methods can mask a victim's awareness of abuse and derive benefits (Department for Education 2017). Risk factors may include children having negative past experiences of professional intervention; children, fearing reprisal by their abusers; and children being dependent on their perpetrator or facilitator for safe space, affection, protection, or even drugs (Coy et al. 2017; Gilligan 2016).

People of all backgrounds and ethnicities, gender, and of many different ages are involved in perpetrating the sexual exploitation of children and young people. According to available research evidence, the majority of CSE perpetrators are male (Cockbain 2018; Berelowitz et al. 2012). Although perpetrators of most cases are male, females can also be involved in sexually exploiting children. In several incidents, females are involved as facilitators by befriending victims and developing a network of CSE victims. Female offenders occasionally appear in organised CSE cases but only in small numbers. No child irrespective of the gender is immune against sexual exploitation, but girls have been found to be more vulnerable and victims in most reported cases of CSE.

Key Theories and Concepts

Scholars have identified a lack of theoretical development in the existing CSE literature. Since CSE has been described as a form of CSA, theories and research from other forms of CSA are deemed applicable to enhance our understanding of CSE (Selvius et al. 2018). Many theories have been used to explain its typology, criminology, victimology, and impact and to identify potential vulnerabilities, risk-taking behaviours, protective factors, or resilience among children who are sexually exploited.

Barnardo (2011) identified three relationship models as a potential typology of CSE. First, the 'inappropriate relationship' model was used to explain victims believing they are in a romantic relationship with their perpetrator. The second model was tagged the 'boyfriend' model, which begins with the perpetrator initially grooming the child into a relationship and later employing coercion, manipulation, or threats to force or persuade that child to engage in sexual activity with their gang or associates. The last model was described as the 'organised' or 'networked' form of CSE, which includes trafficking or online CSE. These models were criticized for not capturing all different characteristics of perpetrators and victims involved in CSE, as it heavily focused on female victims and adult male perpetrators. Table 1 shows other social theories and their application to CSE.

Table 1 Theories of CSE

Social theories	Application to CSE
General strain theory	– Explains social or pathological conditions that cause caregiver strain and indicates how these could result in limited or lack of nurturing or guidance, consequently increasing children and young person's susceptibility to sexual abuse – Provides the primary theoretical basis of generative factors and the mechanisms operating within the life trajectory, explaining the criminology of victimization (Agnew and Brezina 2019)
Routine activity theory	– Explains victimology of CSE – Identifies lifestyles associated with the risk of sexual assault and exploitation – Serves as a chronological approach to understanding the prevalence and prevention of CSA (Culatta et al. 2020)
Life course theory	– Identifies indicators of harmful social control processes during childhood and adolescence – The desire for acceptance and love, a better life, and fast income, as well as curiosity, have a causal relationship with CSE (Reid 2012)
Ecological systems theory	– Provides an ecological paradigm for understanding and preventing sexual exploration of children and young people – Shows the complex interplay of individual, interpersonal, social, and cultural factors that underpin sexual exploitation and abuse of children (Martinello 2020)
Feminist theory	– Conceptualises CSE as a form of gender-based violence, as it disproportionately affects females compared to males, and analyses female vulnerabilities – Feminist theory critiques current practices and policy on child protection, outlining critical feminist practice to support children and families affected with CSE in male-privileged and neoliberal society (Cooney and Rogowski 2017)

Prevalence of Child Sexual Exploitation

CSE is the second most remunerative crime in the world globally affecting approximately 5% of child and youth population with growing prevalence (Panlilio et al. 2019; Ulloa et al. 2016; United Nations 2017). The World Health Organization (WHO 2013) reported that sexual abuse is prevalent among 5.7% of boys and 13.4% of girls in Europe. In Sweden, a study on 17-year-old students reveals that 11.2% of girls and 3.1% of boys reported experiencing sexual exploitation (WHO 2013). In Canada, 14–60% of girls across each region have been sexually abused (Sethi 2013).

There are considerable challenges in identifying CSE and determining its actual prevalence. First, there are many overlapping characteristics between CSE and other forms of sexual abuse, making it difficult to distinguish one from another (Kelly and Karsna 2017). Another concern is the diverse and varied terminology employed and lack of consistency in research methodologies and design. Definitional ambiguities, the heterogeneous nature of victims and perpetrators, and the rapidly changing nature of sexual activities have masked the true scale of this crime. For example, in a systematic review of CSE, Mitchell et al. (2017) observed the lack of consistency in operational definitions of CSE in the reviewed literature and a wide range of terms employed to describe it (see Box 1). Finally, like other types of child sexual abuse, CSE is under-reported and under-identified; furthermore, a varying ability of professionals to identify CSE makes it exceedingly difficult to determine its true prevalence and scale (Beckett and Warrington 2015).

International Comparisons

Globally, the wider social and cultural context of different countries and geographical regions has framed the narrative of CSE, the definition, current practices, policy, legislation, and even the media, as well as professional narratives that construct CSE victimhood. These divergences are crucial to understanding the scope and dimension of CSE in each country (see Box 2 for an international comparison of Ireland, Australia, UK, USA, Nigeria, and Pakistan). These countries were strategically selected to present the readers with an overview of relevant policy and practices across the world.

Box 2 International Comparisons

International Comparison

Ireland

The media narrative has been dominated by high-profile cases of CSE perpetrated by clergy in the Catholic Church against children accommodated in the church-provided institutions particularly seen in Ireland, UK. Incidence has risen from 11,579 in 2006 to 21,043 in 2012 and is estimated that 1 in 4 children will experience CSE before age 18 (Cameron et al. 2015). Children

First, a national guidance document, sets out the statutory obligations of the key two agencies responsible for the protection and welfare of children: The *Tusla* (Child and family agency) and *An Garda Síochána* (police). National and professional responses have focused on child welfare and protection reform to strengthen the law and protect vulnerable institutionalised children. The Marshal report, an independent inquiry into CSE in Northern Ireland, resulted in developing a national action plan by the Department of Justice. The plan focused on strengthening the existing partnerships to actively engage young victims and communities, prosecute perpetrators, and review laws on CSE. A major reform programme also set out 99 actions to address the impacts of previous abuse, reform available services, and give young people a stronger voice.

Australia

In Australia, there is a national policy and various local ones, hence the variation in the age of consent, 16 and 17. Children with experience of CSE are portrayed as victims, and their unfortunate vulnerabilities are predominantly used to explain the occurrence of CSE. Child Wise play, one of the leading non-profit child abuse prevention organisations in Australia, plays an important role in training and providing an information package for professionals. National policies and professional responses include Tomorrow's Children: Australia's National Plan Against the CSEC, National Framework for Protecting Australia's Children 2009–2020, the Royal Commission, Australian Federal Police (AFP), Child Protection Operations (CPO) team for online, and mandatory report. Key legislations are Australian Commonwealth Criminal Code and Criminal Code Amendment (Trafficking in Persons Offences) Act 2005. There are many criticisms of the approach to CSE in Australia including an underfunded child protection system; professionals focused on responding to harm and risk rather than prevention; and a lack of a multi-agency approach (Cameron et al. 2015).

USA

CSE has been primarily framed against two narratives: the CSEC or trafficking; and internet sexual exploitation. Evidence shows 3.3 million suspected cases from 1998 to 2015 (Cameron et al. 2015). In conservative states, parents of victims are blamed for faulty upbringing. Victims are seen as exhibiting juvenile delinquency and arrested for sexual offences, rather than being seen as vulnerable and in need of support and care (Harbert and Tucker-Tatlow 2012). Like Australia, in the US the age of consent varies between 16 and 18. The criminal justice system sees young people as criminals rather than as victims, and there are ongoing programmes to avert this narrative. It has robust national policies and responses in place to respond to CSE. Furthermore, the FBI's Innocence Lost Database and the US Attorney's Office Project Safe Childhood (PSC) are national initiatives for appropriate investigation and prosecution of cases. Reflecting a criminal justice approach, rather than a welfare-centred one, the key agent is the federal judicial system, rather than the welfare system.

United Kingdom

The political, media, and professional contexts and the response have been shaped by numerous high-profile allegations against celebrities alongside reports of the persistent sexual exploitation of mainly young women across the country. A national report by the Home office in 2021 showed that 5% of boys and 15% of girls experienced atleast one form of CSA before the age of 16. A survey in Rotherham showed 1400 incidences of CSE between 1997 to 2013 (Jay 2014). The legal framework offers some consistency across the UK at the age of consent is 16. The victims are portrayed as the source of their problem, and even institutionalized children are perceived as culpable due to their troublesome behaviour and rebelliousness towards authority (Ellis 2019). Key responsible agencies are the Department for Education (DfE), which is responsible for coordinating child protection and welfare services, the UK Human Trafficking Centre, the UK Council for Child Internet Safety (UKCCIS), and the Department for Health, to mention a few. National and professional responses include numerous serious case reviews, expert reports and individual enquiries, and a focus on training professionals to identify and respond to victims. Local Safeguarding Children Board (LSCBs) also plays a critical role in ensuring multi-agency approaches. Furthermore, the Child Abuse Image Database (CAID) is a secure database used to identify the victim and perpetrator, investigate cases, and prosecute offenders. Most research published has been primarily a desk-based, drawing on a range of academic sources. In addition, HCPs are struggling with identifying the signs and securing victims' trust, and there are failures to protect children and young people and respond appropriately. Also, there are concerns regarding poor multi-agency working and information sharing.

Nigeria

In Nigeria's 1999 constitution, there is no single distinction between the rights of adults and children; it merely states that children must be protected from all forms of exploitation, abuse, and neglect. Therefore, in 2003, Nigeria adopted the Child Right Act as a predominant legislature outlining children's rights and urging all states to implement the Act. However, until date, only 23 states out of 36 states in Nigeria have adopted CRA. Apart from this, Sharia law and customary law override Child Right Act 2003 in Nigeria. Customary law does not specify the age of marriage, resulting in a predominance of childhood marriage. However, constitutionally, the age of consent is 18. It is a patriarchal society, and children and females are socially invisible. There are no national frameworks on CSA/E or specific definitions of CSE, and scholars are still relying on international definitions of CSA, although it is defined as a form of GBV. CSE victims are often blamed, stigmatized, and even punished by parents for their experience. Of concern, a survey by Positive Action for Treatment Access (year) shows that over 31.4% of girls in Nigeria disclosed that their first sexual experience had been a rape or forced sex. There is confusion regarding which key agency holds statutory responsibilities for child welfare, social services, and safeguarding children. These do not specifically address the sexual abuse of children; however, they contain important elements employed by social and healthcare professionals to support their practice. Like other African countries, Nigeria is faced with many endemic problems, such as governance challenges and national economic instability, that take government priority. There is no specific legislation that predominantly focuses on protecting children against CSE or supporting victims.

Pakistan

Pakistan has various institutions, and frequent changes in the constitution have created instability in the relationship between the country's various institutions. Defining CSA is perplexing in Pakistan since there is no existing clarity regarding the term 'child' and 'age of consent'; various legislations and authors define the upper age limit differently. Regarding prevalence, 11 cases of sexual abuse and exploitation are reported daily (Cruel Numbers 2020). Unlike Nigeria, Pakistan has a national model of plan addressing CSA/CSE, a model said to be built on several years of research and practice by academics and practitioners and on the existing international framework. National and professional responses include participating in an international congress on CSA, which include the United Nations Convention on the Rights of the Child (UNCRC) and WePROTECT Summit, relying on international framework and organizations. Effort has been made to increase awareness and sensitization programmes. Like other Asian countries, Pakistan also has governance challenges and poor implementation mechanisms.

Vulnerability Factors

Any child, regardless of gender, ethnicity, cultural background, and socio-economic class, can be a victim of CSE, which is often linked to other social problems or life experience in the life of a young person. Various research has identified several potential vulnerabilities and indicators of becoming a victim of CSE once or multiple times. Evidence has shown that children experience other forms of abuse including neglect, emotional abuse, physical abuse, and current or past lack of safe space; coming from or developing in dysfunctional home; living in an abusive home and substance abuse; and/or having a family member involved in prostitution or criminality (Brown et al. 2016; Culatta et al. 2020). In addition, a child with learning disability, physical disability, and institutionalized children either in secure or residential homes or children with interrupted care histories (Brown et al. 2016) are more at risk of experiencing CSE.

Crimes linked to CSE include child trafficking, IPV, grooming (including online grooming), obtaining and sharing abusive images of children, gang-related activities, and drugs-related or immigration-related offences (Department for Education 2017). Adverse life experiences might make some children more susceptible to child sexual exploitation. It is also important to emphasize that CSE can occur without any of the mentioned vulnerabilities and that risk factors and indicators are not conclusive. There are signs of ongoing exploitation (see Box 3).

Box 3 Indicators for CSE

Indicators for the onset or ongoing CSE

Listed below are some signs that may indicate a child is experiencing CSE.

- Running away or repeatedly missing from home, care, or education.
- Trafficked children.
- Evidence of sexual bullying.
- Association or membership of gangs.
- Early onset of sexual relationships.
- Young person self-harming.
- Unexplained physical injury.
- Possessing or receiving gifts without credible explanation or source.
- Age-inappropriate behaviour.
- Social isolation and excessive use of social media.
- Economic difficulties or homelessness.
- Sudden changes in appearance and mood.
- Withdrawn symptoms of suicidal ideation.
- Severe traumatic and dissociative symptoms.
- Contacting sexually transmitted diseases, becoming pregnant, or having an abortion (Brayley and Cockbain 2014; Brown et al. 2016; Miller and Brown 2014).

Impacts

According to the Department for Education (2017), CSE leads to short- and long-term consequences for the victim's life, family, and society at large; therefore, early identification and immediate support are critical. Health and social care practitioners, as well as other people involved in family welfare, should be aware of such effects, as this will enable them to intensify their efforts in identifying and responding to affected children and young people. Evidence highlights a wide range of consequences or even difficulties observed among victims of CSE, which can also extend to adulthood and affect different domains of victims' functioning, including physical, psychological, social, and economic aspects and interpersonal relationships. Perpetrators can be everyday family, friends, acquaintances, and even celebrities (see Box 4).

Physical Impacts

CSE occurs in contexts in which violence, psychological manipulation, fear, coercion, threats, unsafe relationships, and safety concerns are common (Bounds et al. 2015). Survivors have reported physical injury associated with penetrative sexual abuse to genital areas; anal or genital scarring; trauma; and internal injuries. Some victims have also contracted sexually transmitted diseases, including HIV and hepatitis; pelvic inflammatory disease; problems with the reproductive system and musculoskeletal system; and other unexplained medical problems (Kamiya et al. 2016). It has been linked to long-term illnesses and disabilities and a reduction in quality of life, general well-being, and daily life functioning of the affected individual (Bounds et al. 2015; Kamiya et al. 2016).

Psychological Impacts

The psychological/emotional and mental health impacts of CSE are wide ranging and diverse. Initially, it begins as an adaptive mechanism, which gradually becomes devastating to the mental and emotional well-being of the affected individual (McCrory et al. 2017). Children experiencing sexual exploitation can undergo a range of emotions, including anger, sadness, fear, guilt, confusion, dissociation, and self-blame (Perez-Gonzalez and Pereda 2015; Warrington et al. 2016). In addition, mental disorders and internalizing behaviours include anxiety, withdrawal, depression, tendency to self-harm, suicide ideation and attempt, and post-traumatic stress disorder (PTSD) (Easton and Kong 2017; Kamiya et al. 2016). Evidence shows that female victims or survivors are more likely to demonstrate internalizing behaviours compared to externalizing behaviours, which are often seen in male victims. Externalizing behaviours include misuse of substance, inappropriate sexual preferences/behaviours, anger, aggression, hostility, and antisocial behaviour (Kamiya et al. 2016; Perez-Gonzalez and Pereda 2015). Other mental illnesses associated with CSE are eating disorders, personality disorders, perinatal mental problems such as postnatal depression, and psychosis such as schizophrenia and bipolar disorder (Perez-Gonzalez and Pereda 2015).

Impacts on Interpersonal Relationships

Survivors of CSE may experience difficulties in interpersonal relationships. This can be attributed to the grooming process perpetrators and/or facilitators frequently employ to isolate, manipulate, and even coerce their victims and to the sense of betrayal, which eventually creates difficulties relating to relationships with family, friends, and other people (Casey 2015). Victims experience fear regarding their relationships and interactions with family members and friends, including the responsibility for changes to family dynamics, emotional disconnection, and interference or disruption in the well-being of family members and cycles of friendship (Casey 2015; Warrington et al. 2016).

In addition, sexual exploitation and betrayal of trust by a significant person could lead to a damaged sense of trust. Such experiences can have a profound negative effect on a victim's interpersonal relationships as they struggle to develop and/or maintain positive relationships or strong emotional bonds (Pazdera et al. 2013; Warrington et al. 2016). Survivors can experience relationship instability, issues around sexual identity and orientation, sexual function, and sex avoidance, and perpetrate interpersonal violence. The impacts on psychological, physical, and behavioural functioning can negatively affect intimate relationships (Sneddon et al. 2016). Studies show impacts when CSE survivors have children of their own as this sometimes brings about positive influence and may facilitate the recovery of victims. However, the enormous role of parenthood can also trigger a wide range of emotions and internal turmoil, including low self-esteem and lack of belief and confidence in one's own capability, ultimately resulting in negative parenting style and outcomes (Pazdera et al. 2013).

Box 4 A High-Profile Case Study of CSE

A High-Profile Case Study of Child Sexual Exploitation in the United States

On 6 July 2019, Mr. A, 66 years, an American financier with a high-profile social circle, was accused and arrested with substantial evidence for sexually exploiting and trafficking dozens of underage girls. Evidence showed that his sexual exploitation of young girls had been reported to police officers.

Mr. A hired a female to lure underage girls to one of his many residences on the basis that they had an appointment to massage him. He instructed them to strip naked and massage him. He either masturbated while being massaged or touched the girls' genitals or has forced intercourse with them. Many victims were abused on multiple subsequent occasions. He further maintained a steady supply of new victims to exploit and gained access and built a network of underage girls to abuse by paying other victims to recruit other underage girls.

In 2005, he was arrested on several charges of CSE and pleaded guilty to a crime-soliciting a minor for prostitution in 2008, which was then the least of the state charges against him. Then, the Federal investigations into his other sex crime involving minors were unexpectedly dropped and got a surprising lenient plea agreement, which was signed by the then US attorney. He served 13 month jail sentence in a private wing of county prison and was allowed to spend 12 h, 6 days a week, in his office, and he was asked to register as a sex offender. This plea deal granted him and any potential co-conspirators immunity against criminal charges. Granting his such freedom was against the Florida Law, as the law prohibits work-release programmes for convicted sex offenders. Several journalists and high-profile personnel were not exempted from his case as they witnessed the presence of young girls with him under questionable circumstances and none of them raised concerns.

He was able to evade mandatory check-ins with authorities in New York by moving his official residence to the Virgin Islands. Authorities decided that he would not be required to register as a sex offender because his victim was 17, which was considered the age of consent in that geographical area. But the truth remains that he has been sexually exploiting the victims back from 2008, when she was just 14 years. Some of his cases of child sexual exploitation known by authorities were allowed to settle out-of-court.

Socio-Economic Impacts

A wide range of evidence of socio-economic impacts exists among the victims; these impacts can start from the formative years of life and extend to adulthood. Childhood experience of sexual abuse can have negative effects on victims' and survivors' educational achievement and can lead to reduced engagement with education, less employment chances, low income, and financial instability (Barrett et al. 2014; Pereira et al. 2017). At a national level, the average annual health care and social expenses for sexually exploited individuals are more than the double of their unexploited counterparts (Barrett et al. 2014; Pereira et al. 2017). The lack of educational development of victims and loss of potential national workers stymies national development (Barrett et al. 2014). These outcomes emerge and subsequently play out and constitute a complex and dynamic situation. Outcomes can occur, or recur, at any stage of a survivor's life course: Simply because victims and survivors are not experiencing a particular outcome at one point in their lives does not mean they will not experience it at a later stage.

Policy and Practice Implication: UK Contexts

CSE is a child welfare issue requiring holistic intervention. However, several investigations and case reviews highlight a limited understanding of practitioners regarding CSE, and failures recognise early signs of exploitation, the need to work collaboratively, and lack of appropriate safeguarding procedures and information-sharing policy (Bedford 2015; Jay 2014). Evidence also suggests a lack of professional curiosity as sexually exploited children are seen as 'out of control' and treated by agencies as offenders rather than as victims. Their conceptions of vulnerability to sexual exploitation have failed to put young people's perspectives into account (Bedford 2015; Ellis 2019). These concerns call for building an understanding about the vulnerability of young people based on their real-life experiences as well as for radical re-framing of the way victims are seen and managed by working professionals and by policies written regarding CSE.

Identifying and Responding to CSE Victims

CSE is a complex, sensitive issue and a largely hidden phenomenon. Safeguarding practices require the following:

- A proactive preventative model for generating awareness, early identification, and responding to victims as well as prosecuting perpetrators.
- Agencies and practitioners to have a sound knowledge of vulnerability factors and indicators of CSE.
- Skills, professional judgement and curiosity, and a child-centred approach with an accompanying assessment of individual children's circumstances and wider context rather than routinized practice (Department for Education 2017; Sen 2017).

- Safeguarding professionals to be aware that no child is immunized against sexual exploitation and, more importantly, that even though a child has reached the age of sexual consent and can have intimate relationships with peers, it does not mean it is always consensual and the young person is not being exploited.
- A recognition that CSE is a joint responsibility that requires an integrated multi-agency approach.

Summary

- Some work has been conducted to tackle CSE, and much more is needed to tackle the issue of CSE. This chapter only highlighted some of the pertinent issues associated with the issue. The main points to remember are the following:
- Despite the dearth of empirical evidence about CSE, the limited information available illuminates our understanding of the compulsory and prompt identification and response to at-risk and victims of child sexual exploitation.
- Young people who are victims of CSE are often psychologically controlled and manipulated by facilitators and perpetrators; consequently, many victims believe they are in a healthy consensual relationship and unable to identify their experience as exploitative that requires support.
- It is important for practitioners to know that the presence of both vulnerability factors or indicators is not a confirmation that a child is being abused or exploited; it is only a call for professional curiosity, a core element for identification.
- Sexual exploitation can occur in various forms, peer to peer or adult to young person. For practitioners, it is important to know that children can be victims, perpetrators, and even facilitators at the same time and in peer-to-peer sexual exploitation, the welfare of both individuals should be the priority of care.
- In identifying cases, the priority is to support victims to escape exploitative situation, prevent harm, treat complications, and support the victim in obtaining justice in the case of prosecuting the perpetrator.
- Above all, in prevention, creating awareness, identification, and responding, practitioners should consider the wider context of the child and active engagement of the parent/guardian, stakeholder, the child's social cycle, school, and community.

References

Agnew R, Brezina T (2019) General strain theory. In: Krohn M, Hendrix N, Penly Hall G, Lizotte A, (eds) Handbook on Crime and Deviance. Handbooks of Sociology and Social Research. Springer Nature, Switzerland

Barnardo I (2011) Puppet on a string: the urgent need to cut children free from sexual exploitation. Barnardo's, Ilford

Barrett A, Kamiya Y, O'Sullivan (2014) Childhood sexual abuse and later-life economic consequences. J Behav Exp Econ 53:10–16

Beckett H, Warrington C (2015) Making justice work: experiences of criminal justice for children and young people affected by sexual exploitation as victims and witnesses. University of Bedfordshire, Luton

Bedford A (2015) Serious case review into child sexual exploitation in Oxfordshire: from the experiences of children A, B, C, D, E, and F. Oxfordshire Safeguarding Children Board, Oxford

Berelowitz S, Firmin C, Edwards G, Gulyurtlu S (2012) I thought I was the only one. The only one in the world. The Office of the Children's Commissioner's Inquiry into Child Sexual Exploitation In Gangs and Groups: Interim Report. The Office of the Children's Commissioner in England, London

Bounds D, Julion WA, Delaney KR (2015) Commercial sexual exploitation of children and state child welfare systems. Policy, Politics, & Nursing Practice 16(1–2):17–26

Brayley H, Cockbain E (2014) British children can be trafficked too: towards an inclusive definition of internal child sex trafficking. Child Abuse Rev 23(3):171–184

Brown S, Brady G, Franklin A et al (2016) Child sexual abuse and exploitation: understanding risk and vulnerability. Home Office, London

Cameron G, Sayer EM, Thomson L et al (2015) Child sexual exploitation: a study of international comparisons. The Virtual Staff College, Nottingham

Casey L (2015) Reflections on child sexual exploitation. School for Communities and Local Government. Department for Communities and Local Government, London

Cockbain (2018) Offender and victim networks in human trafficking. Routledge, London

Cooney L, Rogowski S (2017) Towards a critical feminist practice with children and families: child sexual exploitation as an exemplar. Practice 29(2):137–149

Coy M, Sharp-Jeffs N, Kelly L (2017) Key messages from research on child sexual exploitation. London Metropolitan University, London

Culatta E, Clay-Warner J, Boyle KM et al (2020) Sexual revictimization: a routine activity theory explanation. Journal of Interpersonal Violence 35(15–16):2800–2824

Department for Education (2017) Child sexual exploitation: definition and a guide for practitioners, local leaders and decision makers working to protect children from child sexual exploitation. https://assets.publishing.service.gov.uk/government/uploads/system/uploads/attachment_data/file/591903/CSE_Guidance_Core_Document_13.02.2017.pdf. Accessed 13 Apr 2021

Dubowitz H (2017) Child sexual abuse and exploitation—a global glimpse. Child Abuse Negl 66:2–8

Easton SD, Kong J (2017) Mental health indicators fifty years later: A population-based study of men with histories of child sexual abuse. Child Abuse & Neglect 63:273–283

Ellis K (2019) Blame and culpability in children's narratives of child sexual abuse. Child Abuse Rev 28(6):405–417

Gilligan (2016) Turning it around: what do young women say helps them to move on from child sexual exploitation? Child Abuse Review 25(2):115–127

Harbert A, Tucker-Tatlow J (2012) Review of child welfare risk assessments. Southern Area Consortium of Human Services, San Diego State University, San Diego

Jay A (2014) The independent inquiry into child sexual exploitation in Rotherham, 1997–2013. Rotherham Metropolitan Borough Council, Rotherham

Kamiya Y, Timonen V, Kenny RA (2016) The impact of childhood sexual abuse on the mental and physical health, and healthcare utilization of older adults. Int Psychogeriatr 28(3):415–422

Kelly L, Karsna K (2017) Measuring the scale and changing nature of child sexual abuse and child sexual exploitation. Scoping report. London Metropolitan University, London

Martinello E (2020) Applying the ecological systems theory to better understand and prevent child sexual abuse. Sex Cult 24(1):326–344

McCrory EJ, Gerin MI, Viding E (2017) Annual research review: childhood maltreatment, latent vulnerability and the shift to preventative psychiatry–the contribution of functional brain imaging. J Child Psychol Psychiatry 58(4):338–357

Melrose M (2013) Twenty-first century party people: Young people and sexual exploitation in the new millennium. Child Abuse Rev 22(3):155–168

Miller D, Brown J (2014) 'We have the right to be safe': protecting disabled children from abuse. NSPCC Munro, London

Mitchell K, Moynihan M, Pitcher C et al (2017) Rethinking research on sexual exploitation of boys: methodological challenges and recommendations to optimize future knowledge generation. Child Abuse & Neglect 66:142–151

NSPCC (2015) Protecting children from neglect. Protecting children from neglect I NSPCC learning. Accessed 13 Apr 2021

Panlilio CC, Miyamoto S, Font SA et al (2019) Assessing risk of commercial sexual exploitation among children involved in the child welfare system. Child Abuse & Neglect 87:88–99

Pazdera AL, McWey LM, Mullis A et al (2013) Child sexual abuse and the superfluous association with negative parenting outcomes: the role of symptoms as predictors. J Marital Fam Ther 39(1):98–111

Pearce JJ (2011) Working with trafficked children and young people: complexities in practice. Br J Soc Work 41(8):1424–1441

Pereira SM, Li L, Power C (2017) Child maltreatment and adult living standards at 50 years. Pediatrics 139(1):1–10

Perez-Gonzalez A, Pereda N (2015) Systematic review of the prevalence of suicidal ideation and behavior in minors who have been sexually abused. Actas Esp Psiquiatr 43(4):149–158

Reid JA (2012) Exploratory review of route-specific, gendered, and age-graded dynamics of exploitation: applying life course theory to victimization in sex trafficking in North America. Aggress Violent Behav 17(3):257–271

Selvius K, Wijkman MD, Slotboom AM et al (2018) Comparing intrafamilial child sexual abuse and commercial sexual exploitation of children: a systematic literature review on research methods and consequences. Aggress Violent Behav 41:62–73

Sen R (2017) Child Sexual Exploitation (CSE): awareness, identification, support and prevention. Sheffield, South Yorkshire Teaching Partnership

Sethi A (2013) Domestic sex trafficking of aboriginal girls in Canada: issues and implications. First Peoples Child Fam Rev 3(3):57–71

Sneddon H, Wager N, Allnock D (2016) Responding sensitively to survivors of child sexual abuse: an evidence review. Victim Support, London

Ulloa E, Salazar M, Monjaras L (2016) Prevalence and correlates of sex exchange among a nationally representative sample of adolescents and young adults. Journal of Child Sexual Abuse 25(5):524–537

United Nations (2017) United Nations glossary on sexual exploitation and abuse, 2nd edn. United Nations, New York. Published July 24, 2017. Microsoft Word—Draft 1—UN Glossary on SEA [English]. Accessed 13 Apr 2021

Warrington C, Ackerley E, Beckett H et al (2016) Making noise: children's voices for positive change after sexual abuse. University of Bedfordshire, Bedfordshire

World Health Organization (2013) Global and regional estimates of violence against women: prevalence and health effects of intimate partner violence and non-partner sexual violence. World Health Organization, Geneva

Moninuola Ifayomi is a PhD student in the Health School Science, the University of Sheffield. Her research focused on issues and challenges facing healthcare professionals in their roles of identifying and responding to sexually abused children.

Parveen Ali, PhD is a Professor of Gender Based Violence and Professor of Nursing in the Health Sciences School, the University of Sheffield and Doncaster and Bassetlaw Teaching Hospitals. Her research examines gender-based violence, inequalities in health related to gender and ethnicity, and professionals preparedness to support victims of gender based violence.

Michaela M. Rogers, PhD is a Senior Lecturer in Social Work in the Department of Sociological Studies at the University of Sheffield. Her research examines interpersonal violence with a focus on marginalised groups, impacts, help-seeking, service access and service responses.

Childhood Sexual Abuse

Laura Viliardos, Neil Murphy, and Sue McAndrew

Learning Objectives
After reading this chapter, the reader will be able to understand:

- Common features of child sexual abuse, including the physical and mental manifestations of abuse.
- Legislation in place to protect children and young people from child sexual abuse.
- How to facilitate disclosure and promote therapeutic engagement.

Introduction

Childhood sexual abuse (CSA) has been deemed an international public health problem (Pereda et al. 2009). However, determining the prevalence of CSA can be challenging due to varying definitions and how prevalence rates are measured (Gekoski and Broome 2020). CSA is associated with a range of short- and

L. Viliardos (✉)
Counselling and Psychotherapy, University of Salford, Salford, UK
e-mail: L.A.Viliardos@salford.ac.uk

N. Murphy
School of Health and Society, University of Salford, Salford, UK
e-mail: N.A.Murphy@salford.ac.uk

S. McAndrew
Mental Health and Young People, University of Salford, Salford, UK
e-mail: s.mcandrew@salford.ac.uk

P. Ali, M. M. Rogers (eds.), *Gender-Based Violence: A Comprehensive Guide*,
https://doi.org/10.1007/978-3-031-05640-6_4

long-term adverse effects, which can have a lasting impact on the psychosocial development of children and extend into adulthood (Finkelhor et al. 2007; Ingrassia 2018).

Numerous definitions of CSA exist, but most share common beliefs of what it entails.

> *Child Sexual Abuse: Any sexual contact with a child or the exploitation of a child for the sexual gratification of an adult. This may include exhibitionism, fondling of genitals or request of a child to do so, oral sex, or attempts to penetrate the vagina or anus* (National Association for Prevention of Sexual Abuse Against Children 2017).

Similarly, the World Health Organization (WHO) (1999: 15–16) defines CSA as follows:

> *The involvement of a child in sexual activity that the child does not fully comprehend; cannot give informed consent to or is not developmentally prepared for and cannot give consent. It involves activity between a child and an adult, or another child who by age or development is in a relationship of responsibility, trust or power. Child sexual abuse can include the inducement or coercion of a child to engage in any unlawful sexual activity; the exploitative use of a child in prostitution or any unlawful sexual activity; the exploitative use of a child in a pornographic performance and material.*

A systematic review found that overall, the most frequently reported prevalence rate of CSA for boys is below 10% (in 57.5% of the studies reviewed), while for girls the most frequent rate is between 10% and 20% (in 35.7% of the studies) (Chen et al. 2010). In the United Kingdom (UK), for example, the prevalence of CSA is 11% for boys and 21% for girls (May-Chahal and Cawson 2005). However, despite several high-profile cases in the UK, there is a general consensus that the tendency to under-report CSA remains problematic. Whilst high-profile cases bring the issue of CSA to the fore in the public domain, it is important to remember that for the most part CSA is familial and, as such, continues to be a secretive and taboo topic (Geanellos 2003).

Implications of CSA

CSA has been recognized as having serious adverse effects on the psychosocial development of children and young people, with the long-term effects often manifesting as mental health problems in adulthood (Mullin et al. 2000; Finkelhor et al. 2007). Numerous studies (Martin et al. 2004; Finkelhor et al. 2007) have reported that among users of mental health services there is a much higher prevalence of CSA than found in the general population. In particular, CSA, experienced by girls and boys, has been consistently linked to such mental health problems as depression, anxiety, dissociative disorder, psychosis, and suicidality (Molnar et al. 2001; Warwick 2003; Martin et al. 2004; Holm et al. 2009; Chen et al. 2010). CSA is also associated with substance misuse, which may exacerbate other emotional, behavioural, and interpersonal problems (Dube et al. 2005; Schneider et al. 2008). Likewise, post-traumatic stress disorder (PTSD) has been acknowledged as a consequence of CSA, with literature reviews (Kendall-Tackett et al. 1993), meta-analyses (Paolucci et al. 2001; Chen et al. 2010), and epidemiological and cross-cultural studies (Bruffaerts et al. 2010) all showing a direct link between CSA and PTSD.

Tyler (2002) suggests that the more extreme forms of sexual abuse, involving force and/or penetration, are linked to more harmful long-lasting effects. There is a strong correlation between CSA and suicide behaviour, which often becomes mediated by psychopathology (Martin et al. 2004; Dube et al. 2005). For some, the presence of childhood sexual abuse is considered a predictor of suicide behaviour (Molnar et al. 2001; Dube et al. 2005; Brezo et al. 2008). Molnar et al. (2001) reported that the odds of suicide attempts for sexually abused women are 2–4 times those of non-abused women, and for men they are 4–11 times more. Martin et al. (2004) found that adolescent girls who reported high levels of distress as a consequence of sexual abuse have a threefold increased risk of suicidal thoughts and plans compared with non-abused girls. Adolescent boys who have been sexually abused and who report current high levels of distress have been found to have a tenfold increased risk of suicidal plans and threats and a 15-fold increased risk of suicide attempts compared with non-abused boys.

Dube et al. (2005) found that a history of suicide attempts was more than twice as likely among both men and women who experienced CSA. Molnar et al. (2001) estimated that 8–12% of suicide attempts are linked to CSA. Similarly, Brezo et al. (2008) found that young adults with a history of CSA were 5–14 times more likely to attempt suicide. It has also been found that the earlier onset of sexual abuse and the length of duration correlate with increased suicide attempts (Lopez-Castroman et al. 2013). It has been suggested that the consequences for boys who have been sexually abused are more prolific in terms of alcohol and drug misuse, aggressive behaviour, truancy, and suicidality (Garnefski and Arends 1998). As well as being susceptible to such social and emotional problems, a growing body of research has attributed CSA to subsequent suicide attempts in adolescent and adult males (Easton 2013).

In relation to adults, previous estimates suggest that 50% of women engaged with mental health services have an abuse history and are survivors of CSA (Jacobson and Herald 1990). In adulthood, memories of CSA have also been linked to depression, anxiety, dissociative symptoms, PTSD, substance misuse, low self-esteem, and psychosis (Finkelhor et al. 2007; Chen et al. 2010). Research has also consistently demonstrated a high correlation between adult survivors of CSA and self-harming behaviour, the latter often being used as a coping mechanism for dealing with the intense emotional repercussions of the abuse (Hawton 2000; Geanellos 2003; Warne and McAndrew 2007; Rhodes et al. 2014). Unfortunately, self-harm is considered a major symptom of borderline personality disorder (BPD) in the Diagnostic and Statistical Manual (DSM) 5 (American Psychiatric Association 2013), with women who use the behaviour often being diagnosed with this condition (Geanellos 2003). Such women are subsequently labelled as being difficult and demanding, viewed pejoratively, and seen as beyond help (Cleary et al. 2002; Warne and McAndrew 2005).

CSA and the Media

As well as coming into prominence in the academic literature, CSA has recently had increasing coverage in the media at the national and international level (see Box 1). Whilst media attention has led to a growth in the number of people coming forward to seek help related to CSA, stereotypical media reports have the potential to influence social judgements of CSA in a damaging way (Collings 2002), particularly when considering the sexual abuse of males. Media coverage of CSA has been accused of focusing on individual stories from a criminal justice perspective. This can be considered a reductionist approach that offers limited understanding and ignores the socio-ethical aspects of CSA (Berkeley Media Studies Group 2011). However, exposure to media coverage may also be beneficial for some survivors. Notably, since the allegations against Jimmy Saville and other prominent media figures in the UK, many voluntary specialist organisations have reported a significant increase in the number of survivors of CSA seeking therapeutic support (Sanderson 2013).

Box 1 High Profile Case Study: The Independent Inquiry into Child Sexual Abuse

In the UK, during the last decade, several police operations focusing on CSA have been reported in the media. For example, in 2012 'Operation Yewtree' was a police investigation into sexual abuse (predominantly children) allegations against Jimmy Saville. In 2014, 'Operation Hydrant' was set up by the National Police Chief's Council (NPCC) to investigate CSA within institutions or by people in public prominence. In 2015, NPCC announced 'Operation Hydrant' and received reports of 2228 suspects being investigated by police forces in England, Wales, Scotland & Northern Ireland. Of these, 1217 suspects were 'related to institutions', and 302 were classified as people of public prominence. Following on from the above, the Independent Inquiry into Child Sexual Abuse (IICSA) was established in 2014 in order to investigate concerns around institutions in England and Wales that failed, and have continued to fail, to protect children (Ingrassia 2018). Since 2015, over 6000 people, who experienced CSA in England and Wales, have shared their experience with the Truth Project, part of the Independent Inquiry into Child Sexual Abuse. The Truth Project drew to a close in 2021 and the final report of their findings was published in October 2022 (Jay et al. 2022).

CSA and Legislation

In the UK, the Sexual Offences Act (2003) contains certain sections that specifically relate to the abuse of minors. The following parts of the Act are relevant to young people:

Part 2: Non-Consensual Offences: include rape, assault by penetration, sexual assault and causing a victim to take part in sexual activity without consent. The rule of law states that there is no defence of consent where sexual activity is alleged in relation to a child under 13 years of age or a person who has a mental disorder impeding choice.

Part 3: Offences involving Ostensible Consent: Any sexual activity involving a person below the age of consent is unlawful, notwithstanding any ostensible consent.

Part 3A: Sexual activity with children under 16—or under 18 where there is an imbalance of power (for example, within the family unit) or an absence of trust (for example between a pupil and teacher) and.

Part 3B: Sexual activity with adults who have the capacity to consent, but who by reason of, or for reasons related to, a mental disorder are susceptible to coercion and exploitation.

Part 4: Preparatory offences: sexual grooming; administering a substance with intent; committing another offence with intent; trespass with intent.

Part 5: Other Offences: prohibited adult sexual relationships, sexual activity in a public lavatory, exposure, voyeurism, intercourse with an animal, sexual penetration of a corpse.

Part 6: Exploitation Offences: broken down into 4 groups; (1) indecent photographs of children; (2) abuse of children through prostitution and pornography; (3) exploitation of prostitution and (4) trafficking.

Financial Burden of CSA

Whilst a small number of studies have been undertaken to consider the financial costs of child maltreatment, including CSA, these have mainly been carried out in the USA (Conrad 2006; Wang and Holton 2007; Fang et al. 2012). The total lifetime economic burden resulting from new cases of fatal and non-fatal child maltreatment in the United States in 2008 was approximately $124 billion. In sensitivity analysis, the total burden was estimated to be as large as $585 billion. It would appear from the evidence that compared to other health problems, the burden of child maltreatment is substantial (Fang et al. 2012). Similar approaches have been used to generate data in the UK. In 2014, the National Society for the Prevention of Cruelty to Children (NSPCC) published a review of the costs and consequences related to CSA. They estimate that the annual cost of CSA in the UK ranges from £1.6 billion (low) to £3.2 billion (central). According to the report, the cost of CSA incorporates health, services for children, criminal justice, and the labour market (Saied-Tassier 2014) but does not take into account of the cost to families of victims or third sector organisations who provide a range of support to victims and their families. In 2012/3, the total annual cost of CSA in the UK was £3.2 billion (Saied-Tassier 2014).

Common Features of CSA: Recognition, Blame, and Shame

Over the years, a range of symptoms indicative of CSA have been recognised. These include school problems, sexualised play, aggressive destructive behaviour, withdrawn/compliant behaviour, lack of trust, social isolation, running away, excessive masturbation, bedwetting, sleep disturbance, and eating problems, to name but a few. Children and young people displaying such behaviours should be listened to, supported, and given the opportunity to disclose in their own time.

As stated earlier, the experience of abuse can impact a child's development. As a consequence, children can lack personal boundaries and can be confused about the difference between a desire to be close to someone and sexual feelings (Lawrence-Mahrra 2017). Harmful sexual behaviour is characterised as developmentally inappropriate sexual behaviours displayed by children and young people, under the age of 18, which may be harmful towards the self or others. These behaviours can be abusive towards another child, young person, or adult (Hackett et al. 2015; NSPCC 2021). It is important to emphasise that most survivors of abuse do not go on to display harmful sexual behaviour. However, being exposed to neglect, trauma (Hackett 2016), or developmentally inappropriate pornography (Belton and Hollis 2016) can be a factor in the development of harmful sexual behaviour in children.

It has been found that children and young people account for around a quarter of convictions of sexual offences (Vizard et al. 2007) and around a third of sexual abuse cases reported by professional services in the United Kingdom (Erooga and Masson 2006). As a result, children and young people can adopt a dual status of victim and 'perpetrator' of acts of sexual abuse (Hackett 2016). Stigma towards children and young people who have displayed harmful sexual behaviour can increase the likelihood of reoffending (Belton and Hollis 2016). Therefore, it is imperative that young people displaying harmful sexual behaviour are acknowledged as 'persons in development' and not yet adults (Lenkiewicz and Gallagher 2016). It is advocated that interventions for children who display harmful sexual behaviours should move away from offence-focused approaches. These should be replaced with supportive, strengths-based, collaborative interventions that address issues related to the whole context of the child's life (Hackett et al. 2019). Recommended interventions include multi-systemic therapy (MST) (Letourneau et al. 2017) and trauma-focused and attachment-based models (Hackett 2016).

Often children and young people who are being abused experience entrapment on the part of the perpetrator, the latter emphasising the part the child is led to believe they play in the relationship. Common rationales for abuse, on the part of the perpetrator, include the following:

- It's just my way of showing love.
- It's not intercourse; therefore, it's not abuse.
- It doesn't hurt.
- I was abused and it did me no harm.
- The law doesn't understand the special relationship I have with my child.
- It's my stepchild; therefore, it doesn't count.
- I wanted her/him to have a proper sex education.
- He/she enjoyed it.
- It keeps the family together.
- She/he seduced me.

Keeping the 'family together' and the child 'seducing' the adult are common reasons given to the child as to why the abuse is taking place. The former gives rise to internalised guilt within the child. No matter how bad life is within a family situation, children strive for security and would rather keep the abuse secret if they believe it will keep their family together. The latter promotes a sense of shame, the blame being on the child, it being his/her 'fault' that the abuse is happening. Blame, put onto the child by the perpetrator, may then be internalised by the child. Common beliefs on the part of an abused child can involve the following:

- I must have been flirtatious.
- It was something bad in me he/she recognised.
- I was well developed for my age. I led him/her on.
- I sat on his/her knee and cuddled him/her and I liked it.
- I was the oldest/the youngest.

It has also been reported that survivors can feel that they had involvement in the sexual abuse if they experienced physical arousal. This can result in conflicting feelings of complicity, shame, and disgust (Alaggia and Millington 2008). Furthermore, as many children affected by CSA have experienced neglect, the prizing and affection expressed by the perpetrator can result in a child's feeling of 'specialness' and can reinforce the child's need for approval (Alaggia and Millington 2008).

Disclosure of CSA

When disclosure occurs, it is important to remember that the person disclosing may have been subjected to blame and shame (Bonanno et al. 2002) and is perhaps taking a risk in terms of their future and that of their family. Disclosure needs to be done in the person's own time, at their own pace, and in their own words. The person to whom they are disclosing needs to ensure that they are in a safe environment, where they are not overheard and where the person disclosing can attain a sense of security (Marchant et al. 2021). Disclosure of sexual abuse per se can promote well-being and recovery for survivors by moderating the feelings of isolation, shame, and blame and, if met with a helpful response, relieving the weight of upholding a secret

(Easton 2014). Therefore, receiving supportive and helpful responses, both emotionally and practically, can be beneficial for a survivor's well-being (Easton 2014).

Research on survivors' engagement with support services has found that, on average, there was a 12-year gap between their first disclosure of CSA and accessing a service for support for the first time (Smith et al. 2015; Gekoski et al. 2020). It has also been noted that it is common for survivors of CSA to oscillate between numerous services. On average, survivors reported that, over a 10-year period between the first service accessed and the most recent, they used between four and five services (Smith et al. 2015). A recent survey by Gekoski et al. (2020), exploring the support experiences of survivors, found that almost three-quarters of the 181 respondents (82% of the sample being female) had not accessed any support services for their experience of CSA. However, of those participants who had accessed support, the most highly rated form of support was counselling delivered by charity/voluntary organisations specialising in CSA/sexual violence.

Psychiatric Services

Within the UK, a number of services offer support for those who have experienced CSA. Such services include psychiatric services, Child and Adolescent Mental Health Services (CAMHS), and adult services. As these services generally provide care for those with diagnosed mental illness, it is questionable as to whether, or not, they are best placed to address the needs of those who have been abused. As previously alluded to, the disclosure of abuse takes time, and this is often a scarce resource in National Health Services (NHS) services, including psychiatric care. Also, within such services myths relating to CSA continue to exist. These include the following: sexual abuse is the specialist remit of psychological therapies or specialist services; survivors do not want to be asked about the abuse and those who are not survivors resent the question; abuse is a too sensitive or intrusive question to ask routinely; asking 'the question' will open up a can of worms and there are not the resources to respond; 50% of victims go on to abuse, and therefore, a significant proportion of victims/survivors are also abusers (Warne and McAndrew 2005).

Such negative attitudes on the part of those delivering mental health care have been a cause of concern over a number of years (Warwick 2003; Warne and McAndrew 2005; Havig 2008). While psychiatric services, particularly counselling, have been highlighted as being the most helpful intervention for those who have experienced CSA, lack of awareness of their needs, fear of male survivors on the part of practitioners, and a paucity of appropriate services have been identified as problematic (Warwick 2003). It has also been reported that people with a history of CSA may demonstrate a paradoxical behaviour pattern of hiding feelings and reality, while actually seeking acknowledgment of their suffering (Morse et al. 1997). This juxtaposition of survivors of abuse wanting their suffering recognised and health and social care professionals having limited knowledge and/or a fear of addressing abuse issues only perpetuates the delivery of a service not fit for purpose. The impact of CSA on mental health cannot be underestimated, and it has been suggested there is a pressing need to identify and treat all adults affected by CSA (Dube et al. 2005); however, the way in which those treatments/interventions are delivered remains critical to the process of healing.

Statutory Vs. Voluntary Services

Out of psychiatric care, other services in the UK are available to those who have experienced abuse. For example, Childline and the National Association for People Abused in Childhood (NAPAC) are both voluntary organisations offering therapeutic support for those who are, or have, experienced abuse. In a study conducted by Smith et al. (2015) with people who had experienced abuse, it was reported that over 70% of participants were more satisfied with voluntary rather than statutory services. Less than 50% of those who used social services or A&E hospital services said that they had been listened to, believed, and respected. Most participants wanted more counselling and psychotherapy services. Current problems identified included lack of availability, inadequacy of provision, insufficient free provision, long waiting lists, and too brief counselling. The impact of poor service experiences resulted in delays in accessing services in the future and longer-duration service-use. Smith et al. (2015) recommended building on the strengths of the voluntary and independent sectors as these are best placed to lead any national strategy in developing support for CSA survivors in the UK.

Further research undertaken by the NSPCC (Allnock et al. 2009) was also critical of services available. The study found the following: all too often therapeutic services are only offered to children after abuse if they are suicidal, self-harming, or developing chronic mental health problems. It was estimated that for every child identified as needing protection from abuse, another eight are suffering abuse. In a survey carried out with over 1000 professionals working with children after abuse, they found over 50% cited tight criteria to gain access to local NHS mental health services meant children are increasingly struggling to get the vital help they need. They also reported that in many cases children had to wait over 5 months to get specialised support. In the survey, 96% of professionals said there were not enough CAMHS services for children who have experienced abuse, and 75% stated it is harder to access therapeutic services than it was 5 years ago (Allnock et al. 2009).

To address some of the problems identified above and subsequently improve services for those who have or are experiencing CSA, the following principles have been suggested. Survivors of CSA will not all disclose a history of abuse when asked the question. However, they might be relieved at being asked but may want to take some time in deciding whether they wish to disclose or to what extent and to whom. Survivors have a range of needs in addition to formal therapy. To be asked, listened too, and believed can be a hugely affirming first step. Health and social care professionals should be open to learn from survivors, empower them to dictate the pace of the healing process, and enable them to stay safe when they are most distressed by their experiences of CSA (Social Care Institute for Excellence, 2008). This could be achieved by health and social care professionals hearing the story, holding the anguish, and understanding the past to contextualise the true meaning of the present. Surrogate relationships, as described by Peplau (1991), can enable a re-enactment, whereby nurturing and containing the 'child' has the potential to facilitate personal growth (Warne and McAndrew 2005).

Services and Gender

Another service is that of Rape Crisis England and Wales (RCEW). Currently, RCEW has 39 affiliated member organisations across England and Wales, and it is the national umbrella body for services offering counselling and support to survivors of sexual abuse. However, RCEW is also a feminist organisation and some services do not extend support to boys and men (RCEW, 2023). It is important to consider that it is well established that men are less likely to seek support due to the fear of stigma, vulnerability, and loss of masculinity (Pérez-Fuentes et al. 2013). Moreover, this lack of seeking help could potentially be perpetuated by the message that CSA is mainly a female issue and the subliminal message conveyed by organisations, such as RCEW, is that men and boys are rarely victims of rape and sexual violence.

The above issues raised around female-focused support services were echoed by Nelson (2009) in a study commissioned by *health in mind*, based in Scotland. The research was carried out and findings were disseminated in a report with recommendations for policy and practice. Many of the 24 male survivors of CSA interviewed conveyed frustration at the majority of rape support centres being female only, having not realised that certain services were available to men as well as women. As many of the men had been unable to locate support services for a considerable time, they felt that mental health, medical, and social work professionals needed to be more aware about where sexual abuse support services available to men are located. The participants in the study also stressed that more male-only support groups were needed. It was also found that young men in particular, who were depressed and unwell, were in urgent need of basic living skills and practical support (Nelson 2009).

While counselling and mental health services have been shown to be helpful interventions for those who have experienced CSA, lack of awareness of the needs of CSA survivors, fear of male survivors on the part of practitioners, and a paucity of appropriate services have been identified as problematic. Paradoxically, those with a history of CSA often hide feelings and reality, while actually seeking acknowledgment of their suffering. This juxtaposition of survivors of abuse wanting their suffering recognised and health and social care professionals having limited knowledge and fear of addressing abuse issues only perpetuates the delivery of an inappropriate service. The impact of CSA on mental health cannot be underestimated. There is an urgent need to identify and treat all adults affected by CSA, but the way in which those interventions are delivered remains critical to the process of healing.

Summary

- Within this chapter, we have explored various aspects of CSA:
- How various definitions and prevalence rates of CSA hinder the research process.
- There needs to be a differentiation between how CSA affects the physical and mental health of boys and girls and male and female adults.
- The financial implication of CSA needs careful consideration in terms of short- and long-term implications of CSA.
- Common features of CSA: the shame and guilt experienced by the abused and how perpetrators attribute blame to the child.
- Disclosure as being pivotal to the therapeutic endeavour.
- Available services per se and the intricacies of such services in terms of gender and appropriate support.
- It is hoped the above will provide thought and discussion as to how health and social care professionals can provide a better service for those who have experienced or are at risk of CSA.

References

Alaggia R, Millington G (2008) Male child sexual abuse: a phenomenology of betrayal. Clin Soc Work J 36(3):265–275

Allnock D, Bunting L, Price L et al (2009) Sexual abuse and therapeutic services for children and young people: the gap between provision and need. NSPCC, London

American Psychiatric Association (2013) Diagnostic and statistical manual of mental disorders (DSM-5), 5th edn. American Psychiatric Publishing, Washington, DC

Belton E, Hollis V (2016) A review of the research on children and young people who display harmful sexual behaviour online: what is developmentally appropriate online sexual behaviour, do children and young people with online versus offline harmful sexual behaviours (HSB) differ, and is there an association between online and offline HSB? NSPCC, London

Berkeley Media Studies Group 2011. Case by case: new coverage of child sexual abuse. http://www.bmsg.org/resources/publications/issue-19-case-by-case-news-coverage-of-childsexual-abuse. Accessed 21 Sept 2021

Bonanno GA, Keltner D, Noll JG et al (2002) When the face reveals what words do not: facial expressions of emotion, smiling, and the willingness to disclose childhood sexual abuse. J Pers Soc Psychol 83(1):94–110. https://doi.org/10.1037/0022-3514.83.1.94

Brezo, J., Paris, J., Vitaro, F., Hebert, M., Tremblay, R. E., & Turecki, G. (2008). Predicting suicide attempts in young adults with histories of child abuse. The British Journal of Psychiatry, 193, 134–139

Bruffaerts R, Demyttenaere K, Borges G et al (2010) Childhood adversities as risk factors for onset and persistence of suicidal behaviour. Br J Psychiatry 197(1):20–27

Chen LP, Murad MH, Paras ML et al (2010) Sexual abuse and lifetime diagnosis of psychiatric disorders: systematic review and meta-analysis. Mayo Clin Proc 85(7):618–629

Cleary M, Siegfried N, Walter G (2002) Experience, knowledge and attitudes of mental health staff regarding clients with borderline personality disorder. Int J Ment Health Nurs 11:186–191

Collings SJ (2002) Unsolicited interpretation of child sexual abuse media reports. Child Abuse Negl 26(11):1135–1147

Conrad C (2006) Measuring costs of child abuse and neglect: a mathematic model of specific cost estimations. J Health Hum Serv Adm 29(1):103–123

Dube SR, Anda RF, Whitfield CL et al (2005) Long-term consequences of childhood sexual abuse by gender of victim. Am J Prev Med 28(5):430–438

Easton SD (2013) Disclosure of child sexual abuse among adult male survivors. Clin Soc Work J 41(4):344–355

Easton SD (2014). Masculine norms, disclosure, and childhood adversities predict long-term mental distress among men with histories of child sexual abuse. Child Abuse and Neglect 38:243–251

Erooga M, Masson H (2006) Children and young people who sexually abuse others: current development and practice responses, 2nd edn. Routledge, London

Fang X, Brown DS, Curtis S et al (2012) The economic burden of child maltreatment in the United States and implications for prevention. Child Abuse Negl 36:156–165

Finkelhor D, Ormrod R, Turner H (2007) Re-victimization patterns in a national longitudinal sample of children and youth. Child Abuse Negl 31(5):479–502

Garnefski N, Arends E (1998) Sexual abuse and adolescent maladjustment: differences between male and female victims. J Adolesc 21:99–107

Geanellos R (2003) Understanding the need for personal space boundary restoration in women-client survivors of intrafamilial childhood sexual abuse. Int J Ment Health Nurs 12:186–193

Gekoski A, Broome S (2020) Victims and survivors' own stories of child sexual abuse. Cambridge Scholars Publishing, Newcastle

Gekoski A, McSweenet T, Broome S, Adler J R, Jenkins S, Georgiou D (2020) Support service for victims and survivors of child sexual abuse. Independent Inquiry into Child Sexual Abuse

Hackett S (2016) Exploring the relationship between neglect and harmful sexual behaviours in children and young people: evidence scope 3. Research in Practice NSPCC, Dartington

Hackett S, Holmes D, Branigan P (2015) Harmful sexual behaviour framework: an evidence-informed operational framework for children and young people displaying harmful sexual behaviours. NSPCC, London

Hackett S, Branigan P, Holmes D (2019) Operational framework for children and young people displaying harmful sexual behaviours, 2nd edn. NSPCC, London

Havig K (2008) The health care experiences of adult survivors of child sexual abuse: a systematic review of evidence on sensitive practice. Trauma Violence Abuse 9:19–33

Hawton K (2000) Deliberate self-harm. Medicine 28:83–86

Holm AL, Bégat I, Severinsson E (2009) Emotional pain: surviving mental health problems related to childhood experiences. J Psychiatr Ment Health Nurs 16(7):636–645

Ingrassia A (2018) The independent inquiry into child sexual abuse in the UK: reflecting on the mental health needs of victims and survivors. Br J Psychiatry 213(4):571–573

Jacobson A, Herald C (1990) The relevance of childhood sexual abuse to adult psychiatric inpatient care. Hosp Community Psychiatry 41:154–158

Jay A, Evans M, Frank I, Sharpling D (2022) The report of the independent inquiry into child sexual abuse. The independent inquiry into child sexual abuse

Kendall-Tackett KA, Williams LM, Finkelhor D (1993) Impact of sexual abuse on children: a review and synthesis of recent empirical studies. Psychol Bull 113(1):164

Lawrence-Mahrra T (2017) Working with sexually inappropriate behaviour and incest: a case study. In: Guishard-Pine J, Coleman-Oluwabusola G, McCall S (eds) Supporting the mental health of children in care: evidence-based practice. Jessica Kingsley, London, pp 73–87

Lenkiewicz J, Gallagher K (2016) Working as a therapist in a residential facility for young males with inappropriate or harmful sexual behaviours: the challenges and opportunities. NOTA News 79:10–11

Letourneau EJ, Schaeffer CM, Bradshaw CP et al (2017) Preventing the onset of child sexual abuse by targeting young adolescents with universal prevention programming. Child Maltreat 22(2):100–111

Lopez-Castroman J, Melhem N, Birmaher B et al (2013) Early childhood sexual abuse increases suicidal intent. World Psychiatry 12(2):149–154

Marchant R, Carter J, Fairhurst C (2021) Opening doors: suggested practice for medical professionals for when a child might be close to telling about abuse. Arch Dis Child 106(2):108–110. https://doi.org/10.1136/archdischild-2020-320093

Martin G, Bergen HA, Richardson AS et al (2004) Sexual abuse and suicidality: gender differences in a large community sample of adolescents. Child Abuse Negl 28:491–503

May-Chahal C, Cawson P (2005) Measuring child maltreatment in the United Kingdom: a study of the prevalence of child abuse and neglect. Child Abuse Negl 29:969–984

Molnar BE, Berkman LF, Buka SL (2001) Psychopathology, childhood sexual abuse and other childhood adversities: relative links to subsequent suicidal behaviour in the US. Psychol Med 31:965–977

Morse DS, Suchman AL, Frankel RM (1997) The meaning of symptoms in 10 women with somatization disorder and a history of childhood abuse. Arch Fam Med 6:468–476

Mullin PE, King NJ, Tonge BJ (2000) Child sex abuse: an overview. Behav Chang 17:2–14

National Association for Prevention of Sexual Abuse Against Children (2017)

National Society for the Prevention of Cruelty to Children NSPCC (2021) Protecting children from harmful sexual behaviour. Research briefing

Nelson S (2009) Care and support needs of men who survived childhood sexual abuse: report of a qualitative research project. Centre for Research on Families and Relationships, Health in Mind, Edinburgh

Paolucci EO, Genuis ML, Violato C (2001) A meta-analysis of the published research on the effects of child sexual abuse. J Psychol 135(1):17–36

Peplau HE (1991) Interpersonal relations in nursing: a conceptual frame of reference for psychodynamic nursing. Springer, Cham

Pereda N, Guilera G, Forns M et al (2009) The international epidemiology of child sexual abuse: a continuation of Finkelhor (1994). Child Abuse Negl 33:331–342

Pérez-Fuentes G, Olfson M, Villegas L et al (2013) Prevalence and correlates of child sexual abuse: a national study. Compr Psychiatry 54(1):16–27

Rape Crisis England and Wales (RCEW) (2023). https://rapecrisis.org.uk/about-us/. Accessed 26 February 2023

Rhodes AE, Bethell J, Tonmyr L (2014) Child sexual abuse and youth suicide: a review of the evidence with implications for future research. Int J Child Youth Fam Stud 5(1):113–130

Saied-Tassier A (2014) Estimating the cost of CSA in the UK. NSPCC, London. https://letterfrom-santa.nspcc.org.uk/globalassets/documents/research-reports/estimating-costs-child-sexual-abuse-uk.pdf. Accessed 29 Oct 2021

Sanderson C (2013) Counselling skills for working with trauma: healing from child sexual abuse, sexual violence and domestic abuse. Jessica Kingsley Publishers, London

Schneider R, Cronkite R, Timko C (2008) Lifetime physical and sexual abuse and substance use treatment outcomes in men. J Subst Abuse Treat 35:351–361

Smith N, Dogaru C, Ellis F (2015) Hear Me. Believe Me. Respect Me. Focus on survivors: a survey of adult survivors of child sexual abuse and their experiences of support services—executive summary. University Campus Suffolk, Ipswich

Social Care Institute for Excellence (SCIE) (2008) *Research briefing 26: Mental health and social work*. Available at https://www.scie.org.uk/publications/briefings/briefing26. Accessed 26 February 2023

The Sexual Offences Act (2003) The Stationary Office, London. https://www.legislation.gov.uk/ukpga/2003/42/contents. Accessed 21 Oct 2021

Tyler KA (2002) Social and emotional outcomes of childhood sexual abuse: a review of recent research. Aggress Violent Behav 7:567–589

Vizard E, Hickey N, French L et al (2007) Children and adolescents who present with sexually abusive behaviour: a UK descriptive study. J Forensic Psychiatry Psychol 18(1):59–73

Wang CT, Holton J (2007) Total estimated cost of child abuse and neglect in the United States. Prevent Child Abuse America, Chicago, IL

Warne T, McAndrew S (2005) The shackles of abuse: unprepared to work at the edges of reason. J Psychiatr Ment Health Nurs 12(6):679–686

Warne T, McAndrew S (2007) Bordering on insanity: Mis Nomer, reviewing the case of the condemned women. J Psychiatr Ment Health Nurs 14:155–162

Warwick I (2003) Physical examinations: the needs of adult male survivors of childhood sexual abuse. In: National organisation against male sexual victimisation conference, University of Minnesota, Minneapolis April 2003

World Health Organization (WHO) (1999) Report of the consultation on child abuse prevention (WHO/HSC/PVI/99.1). World Health Organization, Geneva

Laura Viliardos, PhD is a Lecturer in Counselling and Psychotherapy at the University of Salford. Laura is a qualified counsellor and counselling supervisor predominantly working with children and adults affected by child sexual abuse. Laura's PhD research was on the counselling and support experiences of adult male survivors of child sexual abuse.

Neil Murphy, PhD is based at University of Salford. His research interests include media representations of mental health and working with families with longer term mental health difficulties.

Sue McAndrew, PhD is an honorary Professor of Mental Health and Young People at the University of Salford. Sue's research explored gay men and suicidality, young carers and service users, childhood sexual abuse and its implications for adulthood, self-harm and suicide and therapeutic engagement.

Part III

Intimate Partner Violence

Forced Marriage

Khatidja Chantler

Learning Objectives
Having read this chapter, you should be able to understand

- Difficulties of defining forced marriage.
- International legal frameworks relating to forced marriage.
- The contextual nature of consent.
- Limitations of legal interventions in the UK to address forced marriage.
- Differences between men's and women's experiences of forced marriage.

Introduction

This chapter addresses four key issues regarding forced marriage. Forced marriage occurs when one or both parties do not consent or have been placed under duress to procure consent. First, it discusses the complexities surrounding the definition of forced marriage including child marriage. Second, it describes the legal frameworks regarding forced marriage as these are instrumental in defining forced marriage. Third, it examines the concept of consent, as this is central to marriage. Fourth, it explores the use of legal remedies for forced marriage in the UK. Lastly, it discusses the impact of forced marriage and makes recommendations for future policy, practice and research.

K. Chantler (✉)
Department of Nursing, Manchester Metropolitan University, Manchester, UK
e-mail: k.chantler@mmu.ac.uk

P. Ali, M. M. Rogers (eds.), *Gender-Based Violence: A Comprehensive Guide*,
https://doi.org/10.1007/978-3-031-05640-6_5

Child and forced marriage are often conflated on the basis that a child (defined as under 18 years) cannot fully consent to a marriage as they are not yet an adult. Full and free consent is central to a non-forced marriage. However, all these concepts, child, marriage and consent, are far from straightforward and are discussed below. See Box 1 for an overview of associated concepts.

Box 1 Associated Concepts

Forced Marriage: Duress is used to gain consent for marriage. Duress can include physical violence but also emotional and psychological pressure and can involve sexual and economic abuse. Forced marriage contravenes Article 2 of the Universal Declaration of Human Rights 1948.

Child Marriage/Early Marriage: These terms are used interchangeably to refer to a forced marriage where one or more parties are under 18 years of age. These marriages are considered to be a human rights violation under the United Nations Human Rights Convention of the Rights of the Child unless the country they live in has a marriage age of younger than 18.

Child Marriage

Child marriage (of children under 18 years) is considered to be a human rights violation by United Nations Children's Fund (UNICEF 2021). Globally, 650 million women who are alive today were married before their 18th birthday and 12 million girls under 18 are married annually (UNICEF 2020). Sub-Saharan Africa accounts for the highest prevalence of child marriages (37%). However, it is possible to prevent such marriages as seen in South Asia, which has seen a 19% drop in child marriages in the last decade (UNICEF 2020). Child marriage occurs in many cultural contexts, and there are many definitions of a child. For example, in countries where the average mortality rate is low, expectations of the age at which a child is assumed to have the maturity for adult responsibilities are lower. Furthermore, where there is no free state-funded education, children are expected to take on employment at a young age to help contribute to family finances (Chantler 2012). Hence, the notion of 'child' is heavily framed by the socio-economic, cultural and health contexts of the country and levels of gender inequality.

The United Nations Human Rights Convention on the Rights of the Child specifies that the convention applies to all under 18 s, *unless under the law applicable to the child, majority is attained earlier* (UNHRC Rights of the Child, Article 1). However, the age at which a child can marry is very diverse. In 117 countries, children can legally marry (Pew Research Center 2016) including in the United States and with parental consent for 16-year-olds in the United Kingdom. In about a third of countries, there are different marriage ages for boys and girls. For example, in Sudan, girls can marry at 10 and boys when they reach puberty. Additionally, customary laws and practices often mean that the legal age of marriage is ignored, and children are often married much earlier. The UN Sustainable Development Goals adopted in September 2015 include eliminating child marriage as a key target by 2030 for advancing gender equality. It is feared that COVID-19 has worsened the situation and placed more young girls at risk of early marriage (UNICEF 2021). Central to the age and forced marriage debate is the concept of consent as enshrined in international law.

Box 2 Countries Where Forced Marriage/Child Marriage Is Prevalent

Niger	Bangladesh	Eritrea
Chad	Mali	India
Guinea	Burkina Faso	Somalia
Mozambique	South Sudan	Sierra Leone

Source: Statista 2021

Legal Frameworks: International

This section provides a brief overview of the key pieces of international legal frameworks concerning marriage. This is important as it sets the backdrop for the recognition of forced marriage as a problem that requires solutions. Article 2 of the Universal Declaration of Human Rights 1948 states that 'Marriage shall be entered into only with the free and full consent of the intending spouses'. Article 16 states, '*Men and women of full age without any limitations due to race, nationality and religion, have the right to marry and to found a family. They are entitled to equal rights as to marriage, during marriage and at its dissolution*'. This was reiterated in 1966 in the International Covenant for Civil and Political Rights and in 1976 in the International Convention of Economic, Social and Cultural Rights. Article 10(1) of the 1976 Convention stipulates that states '*ensure that men and women have an equal right to choose if, whom and when to marry – in particular, the legal age of marriage for men and women should be the same, and boys and girls should be protected equally from practices that promote child marriage, marriage by proxy, or coercion*'.

In 1979, the Convention for the Elimination of All Forms of Discrimination Against Women (CEDAW 1994) emphasised the point that women should be treated equally to men regarding marriage and called upon nation states to introduce legislation and policy to introduce a specific age for marriage. In article 16.2 CEDAW specifies that this minimum age should be 18 and links up with the Convention on the Rights of the Child in 1989. In 2015, the UN Human Rights Council introduced a resolution to strengthen efforts to prevent and eliminate child early and forced marriage and highlighted the disproportionate impact of such marriages on girls.

The Council of Europe's Convention (Istanbul Convention) on preventing and combatting violence against women and girls was adopted in 2011 and defines and criminalises various forms of violence against women including forced marriage.

Countries that have ratified the treaty are expected to criminalise forced marriage. The UK signed the treaty in 2012 but have not yet ratified it. A key stumbling block to ratification is that the UK is unwilling to provide support to refugee and migrant women – this is an important issue for many victims of forced marriage.

Consent

As is evident from the above, the notion of full and free consent is central to differentiating forced marriage from arranged marriage. An arranged marriage is where both parties to a prospective marriage are introduced to one another by family or a matchmaker and have complete autonomy as to whether to proceed to marriage. In contrast, a forced marriage is where one or both parties do not consent or have been placed under duress to procure consent. However, authors have pointed to a 'slippage' that can occur between arranged and forced marriage and argue that the distinction between the two is not as clear cut as is sometimes posited (Gangoli et al. 2006). Furthermore, the concept of consent is also problematic as it implies an autonomy that many victim-survivors do not have. The case study below helps illustrate the contextual nature of consent. The case study is based on research interviews conducted as part of the study of Hester et al. (2007).

Case Study: Problematising Consent

Rosemary

Rosemary is from an African country, currently living in the UK. Her family were very poor and although she had dreams of going to college and making something of her life, her family could not afford to pay for her education. Often, they did not have enough to eat.

The custom of bride-wealth is where the groom's family transfer money or other forms of wealth to the bride's family on marriage. When a suitor came along and was able to offer bride-wealth for Rosemary's hand in marriage, the parents accepted as they needed the money for food and other necessities. Rosemary did not want to get married, but reported she had little choice as the bride wealth would help to feed her parents and siblings. In her country, there was no help available either at a state level or locally to help support women at risk of being forced to marry.

Rosemary married and subsequently, Rosemary and her husband moved to the UK. Rosemary experienced serious domestic abuse within her marriage. She stayed in the marriage, as according to her she would have to repay the bride-wealth to her husband should she wish to leave the marriage. She did not have access to any money of her own so she only left the relationship when she was convinced that she would be killed if she remained in the relationship.

Her situation was further complicated by her immigration status which was linked to her husband's visa. If she were to leave, she would be subject to 'no recourse to public funds', with the threat of deportation or destitution.

The case study clearly illustrates that poverty, unequal gender relations and its intersection with the cultural practice of bride-wealth were driving factors in Rosemary's forced marriage and her ability to exercise full and free consent was heavily compromised. Either she could refuse the marriage and let her parents, herself and siblings go hungry and potentially resent her, or come to their rescue by consenting to a marriage she did not want. Rosemary's context makes visible the contextual nature of consent.

Anitha and Gill (2009) also argue that consent in relation to forced marriage should be seen as contextual; that is, the choices that can be made about marriage are heavily influenced and often curtailed by factors outside the victim's immediate control. They write 'that consent and coercion in relation to marriage can be better understood as two ends of a continuum, between which lie degrees of socio-cultural expectation, control, persuasion, pressure, threat and force' (2009: 165). This is also demonstrated in Chantler and McCarry's (2020) article, based on an analysis of interviews with survivors of forced marriage in Scotland in 2016–2017. These illustrate the dynamics of socialisation into marriage from an early age, an assumption of heteronormativity and the use of culture (for example, concepts of honour and shame) to inculcate the inevitability of marriage.

Much forced marriage literature focuses on consent at the point of entry to a marriage but being free to exit the marriage is also important. In Rosemary's case, the repayment of bride-wealth was a major barrier at both entry to and exit from the forced marriage. Her immigration status and lack of available support to women with no recourse to public funds was a further barrier to leaving the marriage.

Legal Responses to Forced Marriage in the UK

The overview of the international legislative framework given above has been key to shaping forced marriage legislation in the UK. In England and Wales, the Forced Marriage (Civil Protection) Act 2007 introduced civil protection for victims of forced marriage in the form of Forced Marriage Protection Orders (FMPOs). FMPOs stipulate certain conditions intended to protect victims from being forced into marriage such as prohibiting a forced marriage or depositing passports including the victim's at a specified agency to prevent a victim being taken to another country to marry. If an FMPO was breached, it was considered a contempt of court and the perpetrator(s) was liable to serve a custodial sentence of up to 2 years, be given a fine or both. In June 2014, the government introduced the Anti-Social Behaviour, Crime and Policing Act 2014. This amended the Forced Marriage (Civil Protection) Act 2007 and created a new separate offence of Forced Marriage as well as criminalising breaches of FMPOs. The extent to which these measures have empowered victims or punished perpetrators is discussed below. Similar legislation is also in place in Scotland: The Forced Marriage (Protection and Jurisdiction; Scotland) Act 2011 provides civil protection (via FMPOs) for those at risk of forced marriage as well as those already in forced marriages. A specific criminal offence of forcing someone to marry in Scotland was created under section 122 of the Anti-Social Behaviour, Crime and Policing Act 2014.

The number of FMPOs granted in England and Wales shows a slow upward trend year by year since the introduction of the Forced Marriage (Civil Protection) Act of 2007. Overall, numbers are small: in 2018, there were 283 FMPOs granted, and in 2019, this increased to 340 (Family Court Data 2021). The national prevalence of forced marriage is estimated to be between 5 and 8000 annually (Kazimirski et al. 2009), so the numbers of FMPOs in comparison are quite small.

Problems Associated with Uptake of Legislative Responses

Although the criminalisation of forced marriage came into force in 2014, the first criminal case of forced marriage did not take place until 2018. To date, there have been very few forced marriage cases presented to criminal courts, which raises questions about the effectiveness of the legal response. To elucidate this further, the aforementioned study of Chantler and McCarry (2020) is pertinent. Whilst most survivors in this study welcomed the legal responses in Scotland (which are similar to those in England and Wales), most would not have used them as explained by the following: *Because you love them [parents/family members]. There's no way you're gonna put a criminal record against them* (Survivor 1) (see also Gangoli et al. 2006). Another survivor who had called the police regarding her impending forced marriage reported it was a lot of 'hassle' as her brothers then threatened her with violence. This illustrates the difficulties of reporting forced marriage (or any other form of gender-based violence) where the victim is still within the family context and wishes to maintain a relationship with them. The difficulties associated with moving away, particularly for younger victims who have been brought up in a close-knit family and community structure, should not be underestimated. By their nature, legal responses do not consider the needs of such victims, and other appropriate services need to be in place to offer both emotional and practical support (Chantler et al. 2017).

A further survivor who had utilised the legal remedies available via an FMPO described the difficulties of getting an FMPO. The key issue was the requirement to prove that she was being forced into a marriage. In her case, psychological and emotional methods were used to attempt to gain her consent. Psychological and emotional methods are difficult to prove. The use of physical violence is easier to evidence, and as many forced marriage cases utilise psychological and/or emotional pressure, it is perhaps not surprising that very few cases come to court or have been granted FMPOs. This survivor's experience was also that as this is a relatively new area of law (at the time of her forced marriage), legal professionals were not always prepared to respond effectively. Professionals interviewed in Chantler et al. (2017) also discussed the difficulties of using the available legal remedies. First, they reiterated the difficulties of the evidential threshold; second, they stressed the importance of conceptualising forced marriage as a process of socialisation rather than an event (the marriage) (see Chantler et al. 2021 for more details). A further concern expressed by professionals is that often victims must shoulder the financial cost of the legal process themselves. Young adults who are dependent on their families (for example, those at college or university) may not have access to resources of their own, thus hampering access to legal remedies. If an FMPO is breached, then the onus is again on the victim to bring this to the court's attention and the criminalisation of the breach of an FMPO may be a further barrier given that many victim-survivors do not want to criminalise their families.

The dearth of forced marriage cases brought forward to criminal courts in the UK indicates the ineffectiveness of this measure. The relatively low number of FMPOs strongly suggests that (1) the evidential threshold required for FMPOs needs to be reconsidered and (2) alongside legal remedies, forced marriage services offering both emotional and practical support are needed to adequately support victims of forced marriage. Policy and commissioning decisions about domestic abuse services should ensure that the vital role of Black and minoritized women's services is reinstated. Prevention of forced marriage (awareness raising within communities and amongst professionals) was seen as more valuable than legal responses (Chantler et al. 2017; Gangoli et al. 2006).

Non-Legal Interventions

As can be seen from the previous section, supporting victims of forced marriage cannot rely solely on legal remedies. The role of Black and minoritized women's organisations has been central to providing support to victims of forced marriage. However, at least 10 years of austerity means that much of the women's sector, specifically the Black and minoritized women's sector, has been decimated (Barter et al. 2018; Chantler and Thiara 2017). Many of these organisations have been at the forefront of bringing the issue of forced marriage into the public domain as well as providing services such as advocacy, emotional and practical support. They have also supported professionals by offering training and consultation about forced marriage and being involved in community-based prevention work. The lack of recognition of the specificities of forced marriage and the erosion of specialist Black and minoritized women's organisations has pushed back efforts to provide relevant and accessible support to those experiencing forced marriage. Furthermore, professionals in mainstream organisations are often reluctant to intervene in forced marriage as they see forced marriage as a cultural issue and report that cultural sensitivities hamper interventions as professionals can be fearful of being called racist or culturally insensitive. This has been termed 'race anxiety' and runs the danger of leaving victims of forced marriage unprotected (for further details, see Chantler 2012; Chantler et al. 2021).

Impact of Forced Marriage

Research has consistently shown the damaging impact of forced marriage on victims' educational opportunities and hence future earning potential as well as physical and mental health impacts (UNICEF 2020). Around 90% of adolescent pregnancies in the Global South occur within marriage (UNFPA 2015). Early or child marriage leads to adolescent pregnancies and young teenage girls are more likely to die from complications in pregnancy compared to those in their twenties. Complications arising from pregnancy and childbirth are among the leading causes of death in girls aged 15–19 (WHO 2016). Under 15s are also more likely to experience domestic violence and abuse (WHO 2016).

As early marriage is most prevalent in contexts of poverty and substantially reduces economic opportunities, poverty is reinforced and deepens unequal gender relations as well as impacting opportunities for future generations. There are also adverse health outcomes for victims including unwanted pregnancies, sexually transmitted diseases and acquisition of HIV (UNFPA 2015).

Studies in the Global North have shown that forced marriage can be a precursor to self-harming and/or attempted suicide and other mental health problems (Chantler et al. 2003; Chantler and McCarry 2020; Hester et al. 2007). Kazimirski et al. (2009) also point out that forced marriage may lie behind other presenting problems such as eating disorders.

On a more positive note, many victims of forced marriage who have escaped or exited their forced marriage report that they have advocated for their siblings to ensure that they do not get forced into marriage and also say that they would offer greater freedoms to their own children regarding relationships and marriage (Chantler and McCarry 2020; Chantler 2020).

Gender and Forced Marriage

Whilst most forced marriage victims are women, men can also be victims. Chantler's work (2020), based on interviews with male survivors of forced marriage, found that as with women, emotional/psychological pressure was widely used via religious-cultural frameworks to extract consent from men. Studies also indicate that gay men are more likely to be forced to marry as homosexuality is seen as unacceptable, particularly in religious communities (Janssen and Scheepers 2018; Jaspal 2014). Of note, there is limited research on forced marriage and lesbians. The lack of attention to women's sexuality is perhaps linked to the construction of women as lacking sexuality and/or it being seen as unacceptable for women to express sexuality.

In Chanter's (2020) study, the role of physical violence in men's experiences of forced marriage was limited in comparison to women's experiences where the threat of violence as well as actual violence is much greater. However, the major difference between men's and women's accounts of forced marriage relates to what takes place post-marriage. Women often saw sex within such relationships as rape as they had not consented to the marriage. Men interviewed took a different stand in that they attempted not to consummate the marriage in the knowledge that they were planning a divorce. However, they also described the double standards related to forced marriage. They reported being aware of many of their (male) peers who had been forced into marriage despite being in relationships with someone else. They entered the marriage in the full knowledge that continuing their 'love' relationship with their partner would be sanctioned by their families if they married the person chosen for them. These 'sexual permissions' are highly gendered and women found to be behaving in such a manner would be chastised and punished. Furthermore, little consideration is given to the feelings of either the wife or the partner, thus both demonstrating and embedding male entitlement and privilege.

The other key difference between men's and women's experiences of forced marriage relates to the potential for domestic abuse post-marriage. Many women survivors of forced marriage also experience domestic abuse in their marital relationships, thus compounding their abusive experiences. This is less likely to happen to men as the prevalence of domestic abuse in men is much lower, with less serious impacts than women's experiences (ONS 2020). Importantly, Gangoli et al. (2006) found that there was no elevated risk of domestic abuse in forced marriages in South Asian communities in the north-east of England, notwithstanding that forced marriage is itself a form of domestic abuse.

Key Policy, Practice and Research Recommendations

At a global level, the eradication of poverty and unequal gender relations as well as creating opportunities for education are key to ending forced marriage. These form a central plank of the UN sustainable goals, with ambitions to reach them or make good progress towards them by 2030. As has been illustrated above, despite many countries ratifying various international instruments to protect women and girls from forced marriage, the custom and practice of early marriage persists. This indicates that prevention initiatives need to be undertaken at multiple levels: both at state-level and community levels to ensure that the messages relating to the harms of early and forced marriage are clearly conveyed in accessible and meaningful ways, taking account of local contexts. However, even with excellent messaging and prevention initiatives, structural arrangements which drive forced marriage need to be tackled to help eradicate forced marriage. There also needs to be an infrastructure of relevant support services available that those experiencing forced marriage can turn to. Low-income countries generally lack resources to plan and deliver a comprehensive approach to combating forced marriage, and this is a further barrier to forced marriage prevention and support.

Both men and women can be victims of forced marriage, but women form most victims. Services need to be attuned to both the similarities and crucially the different experiences and outcomes for men and women in forced marriages. Research within the UK and in Europe needs to be conducted with victims who have used available legal remedies to understand more about the facilitators and barriers to using such measures. There is also very little known about lesbian women's experiences of being forced into marriage. Mental health impacts of forced marriage are also under-researched. The effectiveness of prevention activities would be useful to evaluate, although measuring outcomes of prevention activities is complex.

Realising the ambition of combatting forced marriage is complex, and as this chapter has shown, relying on legal measures is only part of the story. A multi-modal method of responding to forced marriage is required in both the Global South and Global North. Importantly, progress has been made. A total of 25,000,000 child marriages have been prevented globally due to changes (UNICEF 2020), but this impetus needs to be sustained.

Summary

- Forced marriage and child and early marriage are most prevalent in a number of African countries and in India and Bangladesh, although it also occurs in the global North.
- Poverty and unequal gender relations drive forced and early marriage.
- Girls and women form the majority of victims of forced marriage; men and boys form the minority.
- Legal frameworks and legislations are not sufficient to prevent forced marriage but send clear messages about the unacceptability of this form of gender-based violence.
- Despite many countries ratifying various international instruments to protect women and girls from forced marriage, the custom and practice of early marriage persist.
- The role of Black and minoritized women's organisations in the UK has been central to providing support to victims of forced marriage.
- The impact of forced marriage can be devastating for both physical and mental health.
- Prevention initiatives need to be undertaken at multiple levels: both at state-level and community levels to ensure that the messages relating to the harms of forced/early marriage are clearly conveyed in accessible and meaningful ways, taking account of local contexts.

References

Anitha S, Gill A (2009) Coercion, consent and the forced marriage debate in the UK. Fem Leg Stud 17:165–184

Barter C, Bracewell K, Stanley N, Chantler K (2018) Scoping study: violence against women and girls services. Connect Centre, UCLan and Comic Relief, Preston. http://clok.uclan.ac.uk/24762/

Chantler K (2012) Recognition of and intervention in forced marriage as a form of violence and abuse. Trauma Violence Abuse 13:176–183

Chantler K (2020) Men's experiences of forced marriage: Ain't I a man? In: Idriss M (ed) Men, masculinities and honour-based violence. Routledge, Abingdon

Chantler K, McCarry M (2020) Forced marriage, coercive control, and conducive contexts: the experiences of women in Scotland. Violence Against Women 26(1):89–109

Chantler K, Thiara R (2017) We are still here: re-centering the quintessential subject of intersectionality. Atlantis 38(12):82–94

Chantler K, Burman E, Batsleer J (2003) South Asian women: exploring systemic service inequalities around attempted suicide and self-harm. Eur J Soc Work 6(1):33–48

Chantler K, Baker V, MacKenzie M, McCarry M, Mirza N (2017) Understanding forced marriage in Scotland, Edinburgh, Scottish Government. http://www.gov.scot/Resource/0051/00513514.pdf. Accessed 5 Nov 2021
Chantler K, Mirza N, McKenzie M (2021) Policy and professional responses to forced marriage in Scotland. Br J Soc Work 52:833–849. https://doi.org/10.1093/bjsw/bcab068
Committee on the Elimination of Discrimination Against Women (1994) UN Committee on the Elimination of Discrimination Against Women (CEDAW), CEDAW General Recommendation No. 21: Equality in marriage and family relations, 1994. http://www.refworld.org/docid/48abd52c0.html
Family Court Data (2021) Family Court. https://data.justice.gov.uk/courts/family-courts/. Accessed 28 Jul 2021
Gangoli G, Razak A, McCarry M (2006) Forced marriage and domestic violence among South Asian Communities in North East England. University of Bristol, Bristol. https://research-information.bris.ac.uk/ws/portalfiles/portal/188679401/Final_report.pdf. Accessed 30 Jul 2021
Hester M, Chantler K, Gangoli G, Devgon J, Sharma S, Singleton A (2007) Forced marriage: the risk factors and the effect of raising the minimum age for a sponsor, and of leave to enter the UK as a spouse or fiancé(e). University of Bristol and Manchester, University of Manchester, Bristol. http://www.bristol.ac.uk/sps/research/projects/completed/2007/rk6612/rk6612finalreport.pdf
Janssen D, Scheepers P (2018) How religiosity shapes rejection of homosexuality across the globe. J Homosex 66(14):1974–2001
Jaspal R (2014) Arranged marriage, identity, and well-being among British Asian Gay Men. J GLBT Fam Stud 10(5):425–448
Kazimirski A, Keogh P, Kumari V, Smith R, Gowland S, Purdon S, Khanum N (2009) Forced marriage prevalence and service response, NatCen. https://natcen.ac.uk/media/23519/forced-marriage-prevalence-service.pdf. Accessed 30 Jul 2021
ONS (2020) Domestic abuse victim characteristics, England and Wales: year ending March 2020. https://www.ons.gov.uk/peoplepopulationandcommunity/crimeandjustice/articles/domesticabusevictimcharacteristicsenglandandwales/yearendingmarch2020. Accessed 30 Jul 2021
Pew Research Center (2016) Many countries allow child marriage. https://www.pewresearch.org/fact-tank/2016/09/12/many-countries-allow-child-marriage/. Accessed 19 Jul 2021
Statista (2021) Countries with the highest child marriage rate as of 2021. https://www.statista.com/statistics/1226532/countries-with-the-highest-child-marriage-rate/. Accessed 2 Nov 2021
UNFPA (2015) Girlhood, not motherhood: preventing adolescent pregnancy. UNFPA, New York. https://www.unfpa.org/sites/default/files/pub-pdf/Girlhood_not_motherhood_final_web.pdf. Accessed 17 Aug 2021
UNICEF (2020) Child Marriages around the world. https://www.unicef.org/stories/child-marriage-around-world. Accessed 19 Jul 2021
UNICEF (2021) 10 million additional girls at risk of child marriage due to COVID-19. https://www.unicef.org/press-releases/10-million-additional-girlsrisk-child-marriage-due-covid-19. Accessed 5 Nov 2021
WHO (2016) Global health estimates 2015: deaths by cause, age, sex, by country and by region, 2000–2015. WHO, Geneva

Khatidja Chantler, PhD is Professor of Gender, Equalities and Communities in the Department of Nursing at Manchester Metropolitan University and leads the Global Perspectives, Marginalisation and Thriving Communities Research Cluster. Her key areas of research expertise are gender-based violence, particularly within minoritised communities, self-harm, gender and ethnicity.

Intimate Partner Violence

Julie McGarry and Kathryn Hinsliff-Smith

Learning Objectives
Having read this chapter, you should be able to understand

- What is meant by the term intimate partner violence.
- How intimate partner violence differs and is distinct from other forms of violence and abuse.
- The complexity and impact of intimate partner violence.
- The implications of intimate partner violence for policy and practice.

Introduction

The aim of this chapter is to introduce the reader to the concept of intimate partner violence (IPV). The term IPV can be found within the global literature alongside terms such as domestic abuse and family violence. IPV may also be included within more inclusive and extensive legislative definitions of abuse. In the United Kingdom (UK), for example, the 2021 statutory definition of domestic abuse encompasses IPV within the following detailed statement:

J. McGarry (✉)
Health Sciences School, University of Sheffield and Sheffield Teaching Hospitals NHS Foundation Trust, Sheffield, UK
e-mail: j.h.mcgarry@sheffield.ac.uk

K. Hinsliff-Smith
Faculty of Health and Life Sciences, Leicester School of Nursing and Midwifery, De Montfort University, Leicester, UK
e-mail: kathryn.hinsliff-smith@dmu.ac.uk

P. Ali, M. M. Rogers (eds.), *Gender-Based Violence: A Comprehensive Guide*, https://doi.org/10.1007/978-3-031-05640-6_6

Definition of 'domestic abuse'

This section defines 'domestic abuse' for the purposes of this Act. Behaviour of a person ('A') towards another person ('B') is 'domestic abuse' if—A and B are each aged 16 or over and are personally connected to each other, and the behaviour is abusive. Behaviour is 'abusive' if it consists of any of the following—physical or sexual abuse; violent or threatening behaviour; controlling or coercive behaviour; economic abuse (see subsection (4)); psychological, emotional or other abuse; and it does not matter whether the behaviour consists of a single incident or a course of conduct. 'Economic abuse' means any behaviour that has a substantial adverse effect on B's ability to— acquire, use or maintain money or other property, or obtain goods or services.

For the purposes of this Act A's behaviour may be behaviour 'towards' B despite the fact that it consists of conduct directed at another person (for example, B's child). References in this Act to being abusive towards another person are to be read in accordance with this section. For the meaning of 'personally connected', see section 2.

Definition of 'personally connected'

For the purposes of this Act, two people are 'personally connected' to each other if any of the following applies—.

(a) they are, or have been, married to each other;

(b) they are, or have been, civil partners of each other;

(c) they have agreed to marry one another (whether or not the agreement has been terminated);

(d) they have entered into a civil partnership agreement (whether or not the agreement has been terminated);

(e) they are, or have been, in an intimate personal relationship with each other;

(f) they each have, or there has been a time when they each have had, a parental relationship in relation to the same child (see subsection (2));

(g) they are relatives. (UK Home Office 2021)

However, while there may be overlaps with other forms of violence and abuse—indeed the UK definition has been developed with the explicit recognition that abuse can occur within different relationships and can be direct or indirect as in the case of children (although children are recognised as victim/survivors in their own right within the 2021 Act)—IPV is distinct and clearly characterised by the relationships within which it exists and has been defined by the World Health Organisation (WHO) as follows:

> ***Intimate partner violence*** *refers to behaviour by an intimate partner or ex-partner that causes physical, sexual or psychological harm, including physical aggression, sexual coercion, psychological abuse and controlling behaviours.* (WHO 2021)

IPV impacts a significant number of individuals and occurs amongst people of all gender identities, sexualities, and cultural, religious and ethnic groups. It is present in marital, cohabiting, heterosexual and same-sex relationships. However, the majority of those who experience IPV are women, with global estimates that 1 in 3 women experience IPV during their lifetime (WHO 2021). Of concern—and despite a growing awareness of IPV—is that this figure has remained largely unchanged over the last decade or so. The consequences of IPV are more serious for women in terms of severity and more likely to end in death, some of which have occurred within a workplace setting (Tiesman et al. 2012). Alarmingly, the United Nations Report states that 137 women are killed by a member of their family every day (UN 2021). IPV is also experienced across the lifespan: for example, as well as adulthood, IPV is present during adolescence (Kameg and Constantino 2020) and older age (McGarry et al. 2011).

As we have noted earlier, IPV is a global phenomenon and it is the intention of this chapter to explore IPV from an international perspective. This chapter will also highlight the range and scope of IPV and its implications for health and well-being. Finally, the chapter will conclude with a case study that highlights the complexity of IPV presentations and illuminates the challenges faced in identifying, reporting, and supporting those who have or who are experiencing IPV.

Types of IPV

In this section, the infographic indicates the main types or categories of IPV with examples of how these may manifest or be experienced. However, it is really important to make clear at the onset of this section that this list is not meant to be exhaustive, and the ways and means by which IPV is perpetrated continue to change over time and are inherently complex in nature. This, to some extent, reflects wider societal influences. A clear example might include the growth of technological devices in everyday life and therefore the emergence of 'tech abuse,' which, for instance, could include the use of 'smart' devices to exert coercion and control through their use to monitor a partner or ex-partner both within and outside of the home (Rogers et al. 2022; Slupska and Tanczer 2021). There is also the growth in 'sexting' and cyberbullying, which may also occur within IPV (Mori et al. 2020). Sexting refers 'to the practice of sending sexually explicit material including language or images to another person's cell phone' and cyberbullying refers to the 'use of this technology to socially exclude, threaten, insult or shame another person' (Korenis and Billick 2014, p. 97).

These are just two examples among many but again highlight the need to be mindful when considering the possible extent of IPV in contemporary contexts. It is also important to recognize that a victim/survivor of IPV may experience multiple types of abuse and that these may occur at different times or at different points during a relationship or after a relationship has ended (McGarry et al. 2011). This may also include post-relationship stalking (Senkans et al. 2021). An act of physical violence from a perpetrator to a partner or ex-partner can also be aligned with emotional, psychological or financial abuse, which may follow each other or can form separate longer-term abuse, often classed as historical abuse, which is often hidden or not considered by the perpetrator or survivor as abuse (McGarry et al. 2014).

Examples of Different Types of IPV

Physical IPV may include any act of physical violence including hitting, beating, burning, strangulation, kicking and cutting.

Examples of **sexual IPV** may include rape, forced watching of pornography and forcing someone to engage in sexual intercourse without protection.

Economic IPV may include preventing someone from working and earning money, restricting access to finances, monitoring spending or taking money or resources that belong to the victim/survivor without their permission.

Examples of **psychological IPV** include verbal abuse, monitoring and restricting movements, restricting access to friends and family and restricting economic independence.

In the UK, **coercive and controlling behaviour** is defined as 'a purposeful pattern of behaviour which takes place over time in order for one individual to exert power, control or coercion over another' (UK Home Office 2021). It is often a pattern of abusive and controlling behaviour used by one person against the other over a long period of time. It is often difficult to identify.

Box 1 Defining IPV

Definition

Intimate partner violence *refers to behaviour by an intimate partner or ex-partner that causes physical, sexual or psychological harm, including physical aggression, sexual coercion, psychological abuse and controlling behaviours.* (WHO 2021)

Alternative terminology

Battering, conjugal abuse, domestic abuse, domestic violence and abuse, femicide, intimate partner abuse, intimate partner violence, marital rape, marital violence, partner abuse, partner violence, spouse abuse, spouse assault, wife abuse.

Prevalence of IPV

As we have highlighted in the introduction to this chapter, IPV is a global phenomenon that predominantly involves women as the victim/survivor. Data gathering on the prevalence of IPV continues to improve: for example, in England and Wales, the Office for National Statistics (ONS) has, since 2018, started to record domestic abuse-related crimes for individuals over the age of 59 years (ONS 2021). Previous to this, records were not maintained for any forms of abuse, regardless of gender, for anyone over the age of 59 in England and Wales. The reporting of IPV is often difficult for the victim/survivor to accept, and a recent UN report revealed that a woman is assaulted an average of 35 times before she reports it, and 85% of rapes are never reported at all (SafeLives 2015).

Accurate estimates of IPV remain challenging for a number of reasons: for example, the hiddenness of IPV and the absence of recognition and/or reporting. An example of the global prevalence of IPV is in the USA, and from 2016 to 2018, there was an increase in IPV victimisations by 42% and during this time, on a typical day over 19,000 calls are made to a nationwide IPV helpline (Black et al. 2011). Furthermore, 20% of all violent crime reported in the USA relates to IPV (Black et al. 2011). The enormity of the reported and often hidden instances of IPV cannot be underestimated as they can have an economic legacy as well as a societal cost not least to the victims of the abuse. For example, WHO estimates that victims of IPV lose a total of 8,000,000 days of paid work each year—which is the equivalent of 32,000 full-time jobs—as a consequence of the abuse (WHO 2004).

IPV is not just confined to Western countries or high-income countries, but it is also present in low- and middle-income countries (LMIC), which may not have the infrastructure to offer support, referral services or educational tools to bring about change (Keynejad et al. 2021). It would also be remiss not to include the impact of the global pandemic (2020 onwards) on IPV reporting (Lyons and Brewer 2021; Moreira and da Costa 2020). Recognising that the closure of international borders, restrictions on travel and confinement at home provided a perfect storm for IPV perpetrators to operate and posed a serious risk to women (Thorne et al. 2020) and their families (Heward-Belle et al. 2021).

Health Impact of IPV

The detrimental impact of IPV is now well documented and may be experienced as physical injuries such as gynaecological problems (Campbell 2002), bone fractures or sensory injuries such as damage to hearing or sight (Sedziafa et al. 2016). IPV also impacts detrimentally mental health and well-being, and this may include anxiety and depression, post-traumatic stress disorder (PTSD), substance use and self-harm. Ultimately, IPV may result in death for which many cases have been reported and in some cases criminal procedures have been pursued with convictions for the perpetrator. It is also important to recognise that the health impacts of IPV may not be immediate but experienced in longer-term conditions that can manifest themselves months or years afterwards. The effects of IPV abuse may not be immediately identifiable or recognised as a consequence of IPV and can often be contained for a considerable period of time (McGarry et al. 2011).

Often a major consequence for survivors of IPV is the longer-term physical, mental and emotional impact of any form of IPV they may experience. The longer-term impacts, not to negate any immediate safety and welfare of the survivor and potentially any children, are paramount, but they can appear easier to address. For example, a victim/survivor who presents to an emergency department will be assessed, seen by a clinician and medical attention provided. However, as the evidence shows us, it can take up to and beyond five occasions before a victim will seek professional help and obtain medical attention, and getting that immediate care is only half of the story for IPV survivors (SafeLives 2015). Whilst procedures are in place in many emergency and community-based clinical settings in the most extreme cases, victims report that they attended emergency departments 15 times with various injuries (SafeLives 2015).

IPV covers a raft of behaviours that do not just relate to physical harm and may or may not require some form of medical attention. In addition to the possible delay for a victim to seek help, often any IPV abuse has a lasting impact on their mental health and well-being as well as their continual or delayed longer-term health consequences (McGarry and Ali 2019). It is not unusual to find that survivors have underlying health concerns such as depression, anxiety, sexual dysfunction, post-traumatic stress disorder (PTSD) or longer-term psychological issues. Effects on women's menopausal symptoms have also been reported as a consequence of IPV (Ali and McGarry 2019; Gibson et al. 2019).

A much more nuanced form of IPV is that of coercive controlling behaviours, which are often much more difficult to detect but can have a staggering and debilitating effect on a victim/survivor. This is often because the abuse is often much more subtle and can permeate all aspects of a relationship from how one dresses, who one speaks to or can socialise with to controlling someone's habits, routines and life functions—our case study later in this chapter illustrates the complexity of coercive control in greater detail. The dimension of coercive control is little understood (Havard et al. 2021), often due to the different ways of control, which can be verbal or physical as well as more recently via the use of technology, which can last for many years and is often hidden and subtle as viewed by outsiders, for example, by other family members. Connections between IPV, human trafficking, girls in gangs and the policing of these forms of violence against women and girls (VAWG) have yet to be extensively explored in the literature, as concepts of coercion have been developing separately in relation to each dimension (Verhoeven et al. 2015). What is now widely recognised is that forming an intimate relationship is often the starting point for abuse to commence (Havard et al. 2021).

Implications for Policy, Practice and Research

Numerous high-profile IPV cases have been cited in the global media over the years. In this section, a fictitious case study is presented, which illustrates the complexity of IPV and how this might appear or be experienced both within and outside of the relationship.

Box 2 Case Study

Sue was married to Nick for 10 years and they have two children—both boys—now aged 10 and 9 years of age. Nick owns a successful company and during the marriage Sue and Nick lived in a prosperous suburb of a large city in the UK. After Sue and Nick were married, although she had enjoyed working as a registered nurse previously, Sue didn't continue to work as she said that Nick wanted to look after her. Within the first year of marriage their first son Jamie was born and this was followed a year later by their second son Max. Sue has recently disclosed that she was so tired after the babies were born that she hadn't wanted to have sex with Nick but that she had felt under pressure to do so as avoiding sex just led to arguments—sex was painful although Nick didn't seem to notice. Sue says with two small children to care for she couldn't exercise or go to the gym or hairdressers as often as she had previously and that Nick said she was 'letting herself go', that she was an embarrassment to him and 'no one would look at you'. Sue says she tried harder but there was no one to help as Nick hadn't got on with her Mum and didn't feel comfortable around her old friends—so she had lost touch with them. Sue says that Nick has always been very 'house proud' and 'liked everything to be tidy and in its place'. He could become very cross if she didn't look after things properly and called her 'clumsy and stupid' when things were accidentally broken or out of place. Sue says she always felt that she didn't deserve to be married to Nick—he bought her expensive clothes and gifts and they enjoyed meals out and holidays. Sue was frightened that he would leave her. Sue often felt sad. Sue found it difficult to make decisions as these were often wrong and when things went wrong it was her fault. Over the past year or so Sue had started to forget things. She missed two school open evenings as she had muddled the dates—although she was sure that she had spoken to Nick and confirmed the dates—and on one occasion she hadn't collected the boys from school as she had thought it was Nick's turn—although he had been cross when she raised this and was clear that they had agreed otherwise the previous day. Sue could barely forgive herself. Sue also started to misplace things—although things were always so tidy in the house—such as her car keys or the boy's lunch boxes—the boys were sometimes late for school. Nick said she wasn't looking after the boys properly and Sue felt that she was not a 'good mother'. Sue was so worried about her lapses of memory that she made an appointment to see her general practitioner. At the appointment, gentle prompting by the doctor helped Sue to tell her that she felt sad a lot of the time and found it difficult to find the energy to do anything. At a subsequent appointment, Sue was also able to talk about some of the things that she had been experiencing within the marriage. Since her initial disclosure Sue has been supported to access specialist support.

As discussed earlier, IPV is inherently complex (as shown in the case study) and does not necessarily subscribe to the stereotypical images that have often been used to portray IPV or the taken-for-granted assumptions that have historically pervaded notions of abuse. It is now recognised, through work with older women (McGarry et al. 2014), that historically IPV was largely hidden and considered by some to be a private matter which was not talked about and where specialist services and support did not exist. It is also now documented, through research with women who have accessed emergency care as a result of IPV (McGarry and Hinsliff-Smith 2021), that women feel ashamed and embarrassed about experiencing IPV and feel that their accounts won't be believed. However, we have also seen positive developments in the visibility, understanding and responses to IPV both nationally and globally. In the UK, for example, national policy and legislation are cognisant of the breadth of IPV and now recognise coercive control within the wider definition of IPV. However, internationally, the World Health Organisation, among many other agencies, continues to work across a range of sustained and emergent IPV themes and programmes.

As we continue to develop our understanding of IPV, we can also identify gaps in our current knowledge. There are many areas where research is still needed and these include primary prevention and working with hard-to-reach communities in terms of experiences of IPV and access to services that meet individual needs. It is also important to note that while many of the issues surrounding IPV are generic across all areas, there are some issues that are region specific and readers of this chapter may be able to consider these from their particular perspective.

IPV is now widely recognised as a significant public health issue. Health care professionals, alongside other professionals, are well placed to recognise and respond to disclosure of IPV or to enquire where IPV may be in evidence and for some professions, for example, in the UK midwives, routine enquiry forms part of their core role. It is important therefore that professionals are alert to possible IPV and able to respond appropriately to disclosure. Many resources are now available to support professionals around IPV, and we would encourage readers to familiarise themselves with those available locally, nationally and internationally.

Summary

- In this chapter,
- We have provided an overview of IPV, the different types and forms of IPV.
- We have presented some context around the prevalence of IPV and its impact on health and well-being.
- We have highlighted the important points about IPV and how it is a significant social and public health issue for millions of women regardless of income, education, age or other characteristics.
- We have demonstrated that IPV has serious consequences for victims in the short and long term, impacting their physical, mental and emotional health.
- Finally, we have illustrated the complexity surrounding IPV presentations and some of the implications for policy makers, research and practice.

References

Ali P, McGarry J (2019) Intimate partner violence, post-traumatic disorders and menopausal symptoms. BMJ Evid Based Nurs 22:90

Black MC, Basile KC, Breiding MJ, Smith SG, Walters ML, Merrick MT, Chen J, Stevens M (2011) The national intimate partner and sexual violence survey: 2010 summary report. http://www.cdc.gov/violenceprevention/pdf/nisvs_report2010-a.pdf

Campbell JC (2002) Health consequences of intimate partner violence. Lancet 359(9314):1331–1336. https://doi.org/10.1016/S0140-6736(02)08336-8

Domestic Abuse Act (2021) https://www.gov.uk/government/publications/domestic-abuse-act-2021

Gibson CJ, Huang AJ, McCaw B et al (2019) Associations of intimate partner violence, sexual assault, and posttraumatic stress disorder with menopause symptoms among midlife and older women. JAMA Intern Med 179(1):80–87

Havard TE, Densley JA, Whittaker A, Wills J (2021) Street gangs and coercive control: the gendered exploitation of young women and girls in county lines. Criminol Crim Just: 17488958211051513

Heward-Belle S, Lovell RC, Jones J, Tucker H, Melander N (2021) Practice in a time of uncertainty: practitioner reflections on working with families experiencing intimate partner violence during the COVID-19 global pandemic. Feminist Inq Social Work:1–19. https://doi.org/10.1177/08861099211055519

Kameg BN, Constantino R (2020) Intimate partner violence in adolescents: preventive strategies for psychiatric-mental health nurse practitioners. J Child Adolesc Psychiatr Nurs 33(3):163–168

Keynejad RC, Bentley A, Bhatia U et al (2021) Research, education and capacity building priorities for violence, abuse and mental health in low- and middle-income countries: an international qualitative survey. Soc Psychiatry Psychiatr Epidemiol. https://doi.org/10.1007/s00127-021-02061-5

Korenis P, Billick SB (2014) Forensic implications: adolescent sexting and cyberbullying. Psychiatry Q 85:97–101. https://doi.org/10.1007/s11126-013-9277-z

Lyons M, Brewer G (2021) Experiences of intimate partner violence during lockdown and the COVID-19 pandemic. J Fam Violence 37:969–977. https://doi.org/10.1007/s10896-021-00260-x

McGarry J, Ali P (2019) The invisibility of older women as survivors of intimate partner violence. In: Bows H (ed) Violence against older women. Palgrave studies in victims and victimology, vol 1. Palgrave Macmillan, Cham. https://doi.org/10.1007/978-3-030-16601-4_3

McGarry J, Hinsliff-Smith K (2021) Silent voices: exploring narratives of women's experiences of health care professional responses to domestic violence and abuse. J Med Humanit 42(2):245–252

McGarry J, Simpson C, Hinchliff-Smith K (2011) The impact of domestic abuse for older women: a review of the literature. Health Soc Care Community 19(1):3–14

McGarry J, Simpson C, Hinsliff-Smith K (2014) An exploration of service responses to domestic abuse among older people: findings from one region of the UK. J Adult Protect 16(4):202–212. https://doi.org/10.1108/JAP-08-2013-0036

Moreira DN, da Costa P (2020) The impact of the Covid-19 pandemic in the precipitation of intimate partner violence. Int J Law Psychiatry 71:101606. https://doi.org/10.1016/j.ijlp.2020.101606

Mori C, Cooke JE, Temple JR et al (2020) The prevalence of sexting Behaviors among emerging adults: a meta-analysis. Arch Sex Behav 49:1103–1119

ONS (2021) Domestic abuse in England and Wales overview: November 2021 https://www.ons.gov.uk/peoplepopulationandcommunity/crimeandjustice/bulletins/domesticabuseinenglandandwalesoverview/november2021

Rogers M, Fisher C, Ali P, Allmark P, Fontes L (2022) Technology-facilitated abuse in intimate relationships: a scoping review. Trauma Violence Abuse. https://doi.org/10.1177/152483802210902

SafeLives (2015) Getting it right first time. https://safelives.org.uk/sites/default/files/resources/Getting%20it%20right%20first%20time%20-%20complete%20report.pdf

Sedziafa AP, Tenkorang EY, Owusu AY (2016) "… he always slaps me on my ears": the health consequences of intimate partner violence among a group of patrilineal women in Ghana. Cult Health Sex 18(12):1379–1392. https://doi.org/10.1080/13691058.2016.1187291

Senkans S, McEwan TE, Ogloff JR (2021) Assessing the link between intimate partner violence and post relationship stalking: a gender-inclusive study. J Interpers Violence 36(1–2):NP772–NP802

Slupska J, Tanczer LM (2021) Threat modelling intimate partner violence: tech abuse as cybersecurity challenge in the internet of things. In: The Emerald International Handbook of technology facilitated violence and abuse. Emerald, London

Thorne J, Buitendyk M, Wawuda R, Lewis B, Bernard C, Spitzer RF (2020) The reproductive health fall-out of a global pandemic. Sex Reprod Health Matters 28:1. https://doi.org/10.1080/26410397.2020.1763577

Tiesman HM, Gurka KK, Konda S, Coben JH, Amandus HE (2012) Workplace homicides among U.S. women: the role of intimate partner violence. Ann Epidemiol 22(4):277–284. https://doi.org/10.1016/j.annepidem.2012.02.009

United Nations (UN) (2021). https://www.un.org/en/observances/ending-violence-against-women-day

Verhoeven M, Van Gestel B, De Jong D, Kleemans E (2015) Relationships between suspects and victims of sex trafficking. Exploitation of prostitutes and domestic violence parallels in Dutch trafficking cases. European Journal on Criminal Policy and Research 21:49–64.

World Health Organisation (2004) The economic dimensions of intimate partner violence. http://apps.who.int/iris/bitstream/10665/42944/1/9241591609.pdf

World Health Organisation (2021) Violence against women (who.int)

Economic Abuse

Punita Chowbey and Nicola Sharp-Jeffs

Learning Objectives
Having read this chapter, you should be able to understand:

- The definition and patterns of economic abuse.
- Economic abuse does not stop at separation but continues post-separation, especially where children are involved.
- There are both short-term and long-term impacts of economic abuse on survivors and children.
- There are multifaceted barriers to economic abuse help-seeking, including social, cultural, financial and practical barriers, and they operate at many levels.

Introduction

This chapter introduces the phenomenon of economic abuse as a unique form of abuse (also encompassing financial abuse) that has recently drawn the attention of policy makers, scholars and domestic violence practitioners across the world. The chapter begins with defining economic abuse including post-separation economic abuse and provides a background on the development of scales for the measurement of economic abuse. The chapter then examines the historical context and short-term and long-term impacts of economic abuse on survivors including children. The

P. Chowbey (✉)
College of Health, Wellbeing and Life Sciences at Sheffield Hallam University, Sheffield, UK
e-mail: p.chowbey@shu.ac.uk

N. Sharp-Jeffs
Surviving Economic Abuse, London, UK
e-mail: nicola.sharp@survivingeconomicabuse.org

P. Ali, M. M. Rogers (eds.), *Gender-Based Violence: A Comprehensive Guide*,
https://doi.org/10.1007/978-3-031-05640-6_7

chapter explores various individual and institutions level barriers in responding to economic abuse and finally reflects on policy and practice to identify economic abuse and support survivors.

Economic Abuse: Conceptualisation, Forms and Prevalence

Some of the ways in which economic abuse has been recently described highlight its distinct and unique nature as compared to other forms of abuse. The scholarship on economic abuse reveals its invisible, hidden and subtle form, which can make it difficult to recognise and redress (Christy et al. 2020; Postmus et al. 2018). Only recently recognised in policy and research, it is considered in its infancy (Postmus et al. 2018).

The terms economic abuse and financial abuse are used interchangeably; however, financial abuse is a feature of economic abuse and is concerned with money, whereas economic abuse is broader and involves tactics or behaviours that can make an individual completely economically dependent on others and/or create economic insecurity—for example, through interfering with housing, transportation and employment opportunities (Sharp-Jeffs 2015). According to Adams et al. (2008), 'Economic abuse involves behaviours that control a woman's ability to acquire, use, and maintain economic resources, thus threatening her economic security and potential for self-sufficiency' (p. 564). This definition is widely used. Although there is recognition that men can be subjected to economic abuse too, less is understood about the context in which this happens. Postmus et al. (2016) identify three forms of economic abuse: economic control involving restricting women's ability to use resources, employment sabotage which is concerned with controlling women's access to employment and economic exploitation which entails generating costs and depleting funds and resources. However, later attempts at measuring economic abuse found the above categorisations of economic abuse do not sufficiently ground economic abuse tactics in control mechanisms (Adams and Beeble 2019). This reconsideration of economic abuse tactics takes cognisance of control as the underlying mechanism behind all abusive behaviour (Adams and Beeble 2019). To foreground the mechanism of control, Adams and Beeble (2019) postulated two distinct and broad dimensions of economic abuse: *economic restriction* which limits the access to and use of economic resources such as denying/controlling access to bank accounts and properties and *economic exploitation* which involves exploiting resources for abusers' benefit such as not contributing to the household expenses or stealing women's money (Adams and Beeble 2019). However, Sharp-Jeffs (2022), although concurring with the above construct, argues that it does not fully capture all forms of economic control. Building on Postmus et al.'s (2016) employment sabotage, Sharp-Jeffs suggests using *economic sabotage* to capture tactics that are aimed at generating costs through destruction of resources which will incur expenses replacing items or reconnecting, for example, utilities. This incremental progress in conceptualising and measuring economic abuse has firmly established controlling and coercive behaviour as the cornerstone of economic abuse.

Whilst control underlies all form of economic abuse, recent work on economic abuse with migrant and minority populations have revealed unique forms of abuse that are embedded in specific socio-cultural practices, transnationalism and migration backgrounds (Anitha 2019; Chowbey 2017; Singh 2020). For example, exploitation of customary marriage gifts such as *streedhan*[1] and dowry practices have been identified as economic abuse unique to South Asian women (Chowbey 2017). Economic abuse by in-laws and extended members is grounded in specific family practices such as joint family financial practices and both ways money flow practices between generations (Chowbey 2017; Singh 2020).

Economic abuse has been shown to continue post-separation (Kelly et al. 2014; Natalier 2018), often called post-separation economic abuse. Post-separation economic abuse involves coercive and controlling behaviour that continues to control women's resources using mediums such as previously shared financial services and products, family courts and child maintenance (Glinski 2021; Natalier 2018) for years after individuals have separated from their abusive partners.

The evidence on the prevalence of economic abuse is very limited. Considering that research on economic abuse is still in its infancy, there are several areas that need conceptual clarity and focus to be able to properly estimate the prevalence of economic abuse. For example, differentiating economic abuse patterns from economic insecurity experienced as a woman, especially from low-income background, may not be straightforward (Corrie and McGuire 2013). Furthermore, the evidence on prevalence based on gender, race, sexual orientation, migration status and other diverse social and economic locations is extremely limited. Much of the evidence on the prevalence of economic abuse comes from studies conducted with the survivors of domestic violence, often recruited through support services in the global north. These studies show a very high prevalence rate of over 90% (for example, see Adams et al. 2008; Postmus et al. 2012). However, there is limited evidence of the prevalence of economic abuse in the general population or individuals recruited through community networks. The existing evidence from multiple countries suggests that economic abuse is common among women recruited community networks (for example, see Chowbey 2017; Sharp-Jeffs 2015; Voth Schrag 2015). Considering the above, studies with bigger samples based on diverse populations and in multiple geographic locations are needed to provide a baseline to build evidence on prevalence.

Box 1

Definition

Economic abuse is a unique form of abuse that involves controlling a person's ability to acquire, use and maintain economic and financial resources to create dependency (Adams et al. 2008). Economic abuse often manifests in three forms: economic control, employment sabotage and economic exploitation (Postmus et al. 2016).

Alternative terminology:

Financial abuse, economic coercion, domestic violence, post-separation economic abuse, coercive control, intimate partner violence (IPV).

---

[1] *Streedhan* involves both movable and immovable assets given to women at the time of their wedding. Legally recognised in Indian context it is voluntary, and women have exclusive ownership of it.

Historical Context

Control over economic resources was first identified as a tactic used by perpetrators of domestic abuse in the 1980s, introducing the term 'economic abuse' into discourse through the Duluth Power and Control Wheel (DAIP 1984). However, and as noted above, the issue has received little attention in international research, policy, or practice (Sharp-Jeffs 2022). This is because domestic abuse continues to be predominantly associated with physical abuse. There is less recognition of 'non-physical' forms of abuse. A multi-country study in 2018 identified just 46 peer-reviewed articles with a full or partial quantitative focus on economic abuse, leading the authors to observe that this was 'considerably small in comparison to the number of articles that would likely be identified in a global review focused on physical or sexual violence' (Postmus et al. 2018, p. 277).

At the same time, economic abuse has historically been conceptualised as a form of emotional abuse within research studies (Loring 1994). It is only recently that researchers such as Adams et al. (2008) and Adams and Beeble (2019) and Postmus et al. (2016) have been able to 'measure' economic abuse and prove it as a distinct construct. Outlaw (2009) states that disaggregating forms of 'non-physical' abuse in this way is important since they may have different trajectories and vary both in prevalence and their relationship to physical violence.

Reflecting on the development of research literature on the different aspects of domestic abuse, Sharp-Jeffs (2016) suggests that economic (including financial) abuse has come last on a continuum of intervention—leading on from practice responses which initially focused on physical abuse and then sexual and emotional abuse. A UK study on economic abuse across three London Boroughs in 2017, for example, found that few professionals working in the domestic abuse sector had received training on economic abuse and there was no proactive screening for economic abuse. In many ways, economic abuse has been viewed as a 'lesser' form of violence or at the bottom of a hierarchy of harm (Sharp-Jeffs 2020). Domestic abuse services have focused on reducing the immediate risk of physical harm, with less attention given to the role economic security plays in preventative work and long-term safety (SEA 2020).

This is important since lack of control over income and other economic resources has a profound impact on survivors of domestic abuse. It is commonly given as the reason why they are unable to leave an abuser (Lyon 2002), forcing many to stay for longer than they want and so experiencing more injuries as a result (Earlywhite and Stohl 2005). Economic insecurity and/or economic abuse post-separation is also one of the reasons why many survivors say they have no option but to return to an abuser (Aguirre 1985; Davis 1999; Lyon 2002; Wilcox 2006). Additional impacts are outlined below.

Impact of Economic Abuse

Although the impacts of domestic violence on survivors and children are widely documented, we are just beginning to understand the specific impact of economic abuse on survivors, children and households as a whole. The scholars examining the impacts of economic abuse have identified not only economic impacts but also impacts on mental health, parenting style and children's behaviour (Stylianou 2018). The impact on women's economic self-sufficiency is well documented (Postmus et al. 2012; Sanders 2015; Stylianou 2018; Voth Schrag 2015). Another major area to be impacted by economic abuse is the mental and emotional well-being of the survivors. Several studies have attempted to understand the association between economic abuse and mental health of survivors. These studies have focussed on depression, anxiety, post-traumatic stress disorder (PTSD) and general psychological well-being (Adams and Beeble 2019; Stylianou 2018; Voth Schrag et al. 2019; Voth Schrag 2015). Studies suggest a varying degree of impact of economic abuse on psychological well-being (Adams and Beeble 2019; Davila et al. 2021; Postmus et al. 2012). For example, Adams and Beeble (2019), based on interviews with 94 women who were receiving IPV services, found an immediate effect of economic abuse was on the psychological well-being of survivors. Postmus et al. (2012), taking a longer-term view and using the first four waves of the Fragile Families and Child Wellbeing Study (FFCWS) found significant effects of psychological and economic abuse on maternal depression. In contrast, a more recent study by Davila et al. (2021), which examined the relationship between economic abuse and mental health among 254 Latina IPV survivors in the USA, found that when sociodemographic and other forms of IPV are taken into consideration, the impact of economic abuse may not be significant on symptoms of depression, anxiety or PTSD. The majority of these studies have been conducted with survivors of economic abuse, and as Davila et al. (2021) postulated, economic abuse may have more of an adverse impact on those who are not being supported by domestic violence services. In addition, economic abuse has been shown to impact parenting practices and children's behaviour (Stylianou 2018). For example, Postmus et al. (2012), based on the first four waves of the Fragile Families and Child Wellbeing Study (FFCWS), found that psychological and economic abuse also increased the use of spanking in children. They reported that the abuse at Year 1 had significant effects on mothers spanking their children at Year 5.

The literature suggests both long-term and short-term impacts of economic abuse on economic, health, parenting and other aspects of survivors' and children's lives. However, most of the studies that have attempted to understand the impact of economic abuse have focussed on women recruited through domestic services, and therefore, understanding of the impact of economic abuse may be limited, particularly in the context of abuse where women are living with their partners and have not reported violence (Chowbey 2017). An intersectional approach that considers multiple disadvantages grounded in race/ethnicity, social class, sexual orientation and other forms of disadvantages is key to understanding specific impacts on individuals and groups from diverse backgrounds. Although some recent studies have begun to fill this gap by engaging with women from diverse migration, ethnic and socioeconomic backgrounds (for example see Davila et al. 2021; Singh 2020), this remains a neglected area in economic abuse scholarship.

Barriers to Help-Seeking and Achieving Financial Security

Barriers to domestic abuse help-seeking are well documented; however, few studies have focussed specifically on barriers to help-seeking and building financial security for those experiencing economic abuse. The existing research identifies barriers to be operating at several levels: individual, community and institutional levels (Chowbey 2020). For example, individual-level barriers include a lack of awareness of economic abuse and a lack of financial literacy and linguistic skills. Community-level barriers include taboos around household finance and gender norms around money. Institutional-level barriers include state facilitation of economic abuse through inadequate service provision to victims of domestic violence and racial, gendered and classed assumptions in policy (Chowbey 2020). Economic barriers, which can take the form of not having enough resources for transportation, communication, food and housing, have been identified as one of the most significant barriers that survivors face in fighting economic abuse (Boyce et al. 2014; Sanders 2007; SEA 2018). Economic dependence can act as a barrier not only for essential items such as food and clothing but in other ways that are crucial to resist the abuse. For example, controlling the payment of a person's mobile phones can limit their ability to seek not only formal help but also informal help through family and friends (Sharp 2008; Havard and Lefevre 2020; Chowbey 2020).

Furthermore, arguing the role of the state and financial institutions in facilitating economic abuse post-separation, Natalier (2018) has demonstrated that the gendered nature of state institutions can lead to women's claims implicitly treated as illegitimate, discouraging women's engagement with services to seek financial redressal. Survivors of economic abuse may struggle with issues of address verification if they decide to leave their partners and prior negative ratings on their account caused by their abusers both of which are required for opening a new account (Boyce et al. 2014). These issues become even more complex in the case of *minoritised* and migrant populations due to visa status and restricted access to services (Chowbey 2020). Lack of awareness and training on economic factors in policy and practices can also act as a barrier. For example, Hageman and St. George (2018) examining the frequency of questions related to financial concerns asked by social workers to IPV survivors reported that less than 30% of social workers always asked questions regarding financial concerns and concluded that there's a potential gap in the training of social workers required for education and intervention. There are other missed opportunities to support survivors of economic abuse through services available to other vulnerable populations such as financial services (Boyce et al. 2014).

Policy and Practice

Following the ‘rediscovery’ of economic abuse, it is increasingly being recognised in policy and legislation, for example, in India, some provinces of Pakistan, in the UK and New Zealand and in some Australian and American states. This is consistent with the United Nations (UN) General Assembly’s (2002) Resolution on the Elimination of Violence against Women, which recognises that ‘domestic violence can include economic deprivation’[2] and the UN Secretary-General’s (2006) in-depth study on violence against women which states that economic abuse and exploitation are manifestations of violence ‘that require greater visibility and attention’ (United Nations 2006, p. 47).

Similarly, the 2011 Council of Europe Convention on preventing and combatting violence against women and domestic violence (the Istanbul Convention) recognises that all acts of gender-based violence result in, or are likely to result in, physical, sexual, psychological or economic harm or suffering to women (Article 3b). More specifically, the Convention’s definition of domestic violence is understood to mean all acts of physical, sexual, psychological or economic violence that occur within the family or domestic unit (Article 3c; Council of Europe 2011).

The case for ‘naming’ and defining economic abuse in policy and legislation is strong, not least because it provides a framework within which to report on the prevalence, hold perpetrators accountable and for services (both statutory and voluntary) to respond. For instance, in the UK, the Westminster Government announced its intention to bring forward new domestic abuse legislation in 2017, which would introduce a statutory definition of domestic abuse. The call for the inclusion of economic abuse within the statutory definition was led by the charity Surviving Economic Abuse (SEA), supported by victim-survivors and the women’s sector (Sharp-Jeffs 2022). In late January 2019, it was announced that economic abuse would be both named and defined within the Domestic Abuse Act. The Westminster Government explicitly recognised that economic abuse ‘encompasses a wider range of behaviours than financial abuse’ (Home Office 2019, p. 6) and the definition of economic abuse within the Domestic Act (2021) clearly draws on the academic definition developed by Adams et al. (2008):

> ‘Economic abuse’ means any behaviour that has a substantial adverse effect on B’s ability to (a) acquire, use or maintain money or other property, or (b) obtain goods or services.

In the same year, UK Finance, which represents the banking and finance industry, responded to calls from domestic abuse charities as well as a recommendation from the Financial Services Vulnerability Task Force to provide further support to victims of financial abuse (BBA 2016). This led to the development of a voluntary Financial Abuse Code of Practice in October 2018, which outlined a number of principles detailing how financial services firms should respond.

---

[2] OHCHR | Declaration on the Elimination of Violence against Women.

These included raising awareness and encouraging disclosure; training colleagues; identification and appropriate response; minimising the need to repeat what happened; helping to regain control of finances; and signposting and referrals.[3] The Code was updated in late 2021 (2021 Financial Abuse Code) to address coerced debt.

In Australia, a banking industry guideline has also been developed to respond to family and domestic violence. The Family Violence Protection Act (2008) in Victoria, Australia, recognises economically abusive behaviour. It is described in part 2(6) as:

> Behaviour by a person that is coercive, deceptive or which unreasonably controls another person without the second person's consent: (a) in a way that denies the second person the economic or financial autonomy the second person would have had but for that behaviour; or (b) by withholding or threatening to withhold the financial support necessary for meeting the reasonable living expenses of the second person or the second person's child, if the second person is entirely or predominantly dependent on the first person for financial support to meet those living expenses.

When, in February 2015, the Victorian Government convened a Royal Commission Inquiry into Family Violence, specific attention was paid to women's financial stability and independence. The Commission reported that:

> Women who have lived with a violent partner are more likely than other women to experience financial difficulty, and many women experience poverty as a result of family violence. The associated abuse can be financial in nature (defined by law as economic abuse) or can be characterised by other forms of family violence that affect a victim's financial well-being. A range of factors can exacerbate victims' experience of financial insecurity – among them difficulty obtaining child support payments, tenancy problems, a lack of control over household finances, and credit, utility and car-related debt incurred by the perpetrator (Royal Commission into Family Violence 2016: 30).

It also acknowledged that women's lack of financial independence and stability more generally contributes to them being at risk of being controlled or coerced by their male partners. Three 'pillars' were identified by the Commission as essential for rebuilding lives after family violence, with financial security sitting alongside secure and affordable housing and health and well-being. Fifteen recommendations were made that address economic abuse through initiatives that promote economic independence. They fall into four categories: debt, personal property, residential tenancies and economic recovery.

Clearly, responses will need to reflect different contexts. Industry initiatives do not support all survivors, for example, in societies where women do not use financial services. At the same time, survivors who are migrants may not be able to access the same levels of support as resident survivors. Recognition of the importance of economic resources for physical safety must be reflected across all policies and must be applied without discrimination.

[3] Financial-Abuse-Code-of-Practice.pdf (ukfinance.org.uk).

Implications for Policy, Practice and Research

Economic security must be put at the centre of efforts to develop an integrated approach to tackling the issue of domestic abuse. Policies need to consider how immigration status can make both women and men vulnerable to economic abuse, for example, due to reliance on partners for information or not having linguistic skills (Howard and Skipp 2015). Policies aimed at providing welfare support and child maintenance need to consider how an abuser may manipulate professionals and use policies to perpetuate abuse against their partners, for example, in the case of child maintenance (Howard 2018; Natalier 2018).

Evolving understandings of economic abuse need to be translated into practice responses. Economic abuse has been viewed as a 'lesser' form of violence or at the bottom of a hierarchy of harm. Control over economic resources enables a victim-survivor to leave and rebuild their life safely. This work can be done by domestic abuse services, as well as financial services. This highlights the need for collaboration between the public and private sector (Sharp-Jeffs 2022). An ideal response would also coordinate responses with statutory agencies, as well as legal systems—enabling a survivor to be able to move seamlessly between services, so that they are able to access justice and the abuser is held accountable for their actions.

Economic abuse is still an evolving concept that continues to be redefined and expanded. As indicated above, there is a need for more research that explores how economic abuse is experienced by men, individuals who are subject to multiple oppressions and those who are abused by both intimate partners and family members. The development of an accurate measure for economic abuse must be a priority for national governments. Economic abuse measures must be objective and capture the multifaceted nature of economic abuse.

Box 2 Case Study:

Zooni, a second-generation woman from Pakistani background, is married to Ahmed, a first-generation Pakistani who migrated to the UK after marriage for over 10 years. She was the sole earner for a couple of years whilst Ahmed settled in the UK. Ahmed learnt driving and soon started earning. Zooni kept paying for all the house expenses whilst Ahmed saved his to build properties in the UK and Pakistan. If there was some money left from Zooni's salary, it was being invested in the property. After the birth of her second son, Zooni wanted to take maternity leave for a year and asked her husband to pay for household expenses. Her husband refused to pay for anything in the house. Zooni had regarded the properties being built as jointly owned; however, she soon realised that she not only had no money, but she was also not included in any of the three properties that were built using her husband and her income. She was forced to cut short her maternity leave to be able to pay for her and children's expenses. She tried to get her parents and in-laws involved, who thought she was making a big deal out of nothing. She continues to live together with her husband, but she now feels vulnerable and trying to get a mortgage in her name so that she is not completely dependent on her husband should things go wrong.

Summary

- Economic abuse is a unique form of abuse that has recently been recognised in policy and practice focussed on domestic violence.
- Economic abuse often continues post-separation in many forms, for example, not paying child support and ongoing economic exploitation through previously jointly owned assets and savings.
- Economic abuse has been recently recognised legally in several countries, for example, in India, New Zealand and some provinces of Pakistan.
- Economic abuse can have multifaceted impacts on survivors and children, including on their economic self-sufficiency, psychological well-being, children's behaviour and parenting practices.
- There are many barriers that individuals experiencing economic abuse face, which need to be recognised by policy and practice aimed at supporting victims-survivors.
- There is a need for more research to understand how economic abuse is experienced by individuals who are subject to multiple oppressions and those who are abused by both intimate partners and family members.

References

Adams AE, Beeble ML (2019) Intimate partner violence and psychological well-being: examining the effect of economic abuse on women's quality of life. Psychol Violence 9(5):517

Adams AE, Sullivan CM, Bybee D, Greeson MR (2008) Development of the scale of economic abuse

Aguirre, B. E. (1985) Why Do They Return? Abused Wives in Shelters. National Association of Social Workers. https://doi.org/10.1093/sw/30.4.350

Anitha S (2019). Understanding economic abuse through an intersectional lens: Financial abuse, control, and exploitation of women's productive and reproductive labor. Violence against women 25(15);1854–1877

BBA (2016). Improving outcomes for customers in vulnerable circumstances. British Bankers Association: London

Boyce C, Koliner S, Koplin L, Trifone D, Wong J (2014) Barriers to building financial security for survivors of domestic violence. In: Workshop in Public Affairs

Chowbey P (2017) Women's narratives of economic abuse and financial strategies in Britain and South Asia. Psychol Violence 7(3):459

Chowbey P (2020) Economic justice, economic abuse and household resources among South Asian Women. PhD thesis, Sheffield Hallam University

Christy K, Welter T, Dundon K, Valandra, Bruce A (2020) Economic abuse: a subtle but common form of power and control. J Interpers Violence 37:NP473–NP499

Corrie T, McGuire M, Deakin K, Fraser S, Hucks K, Jackson E, Landvogt K (2013). Economic abuse: Searching for solutions. A Spotlight on Economic Abuse Research Report Melbourne: Good Shepherd Youth & Family Service i Kildonan Uniting Care, 9, 2018

DAIP (1984). Retrieved from http://www.theduluthmodel.org/training/wheels.html

Davila AL, Johnson L, Postmus JL (2021) Examining the relationship between economic abuse and mental health among Latina intimate partner violence survivors in the United States. J Interpers Violence 36(1–2):NP287–NP310

Davis MF (1999) The Economics of Abuse: How Violence Perpetuates Women's Poverty. Brandwein, R.A. (1999). Battered Women, Children and Welfare Reform, California: Sage Publications
Earlywhite M, Stohl I (2005) In Our Shoes: The Next Steps. Washington: State Coalition Against Domestic Violence
Glinski J (2021). Post-Separation economic power and control. glasgow: university of glasgow. Available at: https://www.theduluthmodel.org/wp-content/uploads/2021/07/Post-Separation-Economic-P-and-C-Univesity-of-Glasgow.pdf
Hageman SA, St. George DMM (2018) Social workers, intimate partner violence (IPV), and client financial concerns. J Soc Serv Res 44(3):391–399
Havard TE, Lefevre M (2020) Beyond the power and control wheel: how abusive men manipulate mobile phone technologies to facilitate coercive control. J Gender Based Violence 4(2):223–239
HM Government (2019) Transforming the response to domestic abuse: consultation response and draft bill, https://assets.publishing.service.gov.uk/government/uploads/system/uploads/attachment_data/file/772202/CCS1218158068-Web_Accessible.pdf
Howard M, Skipp A (2015). UneqUal, trapped & controlled. Women's experience of financial abuse and universal credit. London: Women's Aid and TUC.
Kelly L, Sharp N, Klein R (2014) Finding the costs of freedom: how women and children rebuild their lives after domestic violence. Solace Women's Aid and Child and Woman Abuse Studies Unit, London
Loring MT (1994) Emotional abuse. New York: Lexington Books
Lyon E (2002) Welfare and Domestic violence Against Women. Pennsylvania: National Research Center on Domestic Violence
Natalier K (2018) State facilitated economic abuse: a structural analysis of men deliberately withholding child support. Fem Leg Stud 26(2):121–140
Outlaw M (2009), No One Type of Intimate Partner Abuse: Exploring Physical and Non- Physical Abuse Among Intimate Partners. Journal of Family Violence 24;263–272. https://doi.org/10.1007/s10896-009-9228-5
Postmus JL, Huang CC, Mathisen-Stylianou A (2012) The impact of physical and economic abuse on maternal mental health and parenting. Child Youth Serv Rev 34(9):1922–1928
Postmus JL, Plummer SB, Stylianou AM (2016) Measuring economic abuse in the lives of survivors: revising the scale of economic abuse. Violence Against Women 22(6):692–703
Postmus JL, Hoge GL, Breckenridge J, Sharp-Jeffs N, Chung D (2018) Economic abuse as an invisible form of domestic violence: a multicountry review. Trauma Violence Abuse 21(2):261–283
Royal Commission into Family Violence (2016) Royal Commission into Family Violence: final report, Summary and recommendations, available at https://apo.org.au/node/62334
Sanders CK (2007) Domestic violence, economic abuse, and implications of a program for building economic resources for low-income women findings from interviews with participants in a Women's Economic Action Program. Washington University, St. Louis. https://openscholarship.wustl.edu/cgi/viewcontent.cgi?article=1183&context=csd_research
Sanders CK (2015) Economic abuse in the lives of women abused by an intimate partner: A qualitative study. Violence against women, 21(1);3–29
SEA (2018) 'Economic abuse is your past, present and future'. A report on the practical barriers women face in rebuilding their lives after domestic violence. https://survivingeconomicabuse.org/wp-content/uploads/2020/11/SEA-Roundtable-Report-2018-1.pdf
Sharp N (2008) What's yours is mine': The different forms of economic abuse and its impact on women and children experiencing domestic violence. London: Refuge
Sharp-Jeffs N (2015) Money Matters: Research into the extent and nature of financial abuse within intimate relationships in the UK. Project Report. London Metropolitan University, London
Sharp-Jeffs N (2016) Supporting Survivors of Financial Abuse: Learning for the UK
Sharp-Jeffs N (2022) Understanding and responding to economic abuse. Emerald, London
Singh S (2020) Economic abuse and family violence across cultures: gendering money and assets through coercive control. In: Criminalising coercive control: family violence and the criminal law, pp 51–72

Stylianou AM (2018) Economic abuse within intimate partner violence: a review of the literature. Violence Vict 33(1):3–22

Surviving Economic Abuse (2020) Recognising and responding to the scale of coerced debt: Final evaluation of the Economic Justice Project

United Nations Secretary General (2006) In-Depth Study on all Forms of Violence Against Women, New York: United National General Assembly

Voth Schrag RJ (2015) Economic abuse and later material hardship: is depression a mediator? Affilia 30(3):341–351

Voth Schrag RJ, Robinson SR, Ravi K (2019) Understanding pathways within intimate partner violence: economic abuse, economic hardship, and mental health. J Aggress Maltreat Trauma 28(2):222–242

Wilcox P (2006) Surviving Domestic Violence: Gender, Poverty and Agency. London: Palgrave Macmillan

Punita Chowbey is a Senior Research Fellow at the College of Health, Wellbeing and Life Sciences at Sheffield Hallam University. Taking a social justice and intersectional approach, her research is concerned with gender and ethnic inequalities in health, household economies, economic abuse, women's employment and food practices in the UK and South Asia.

Nicola Sharp-Jeffs is the CEO of Surviving Economic Abuse.

The Intersection Between Domestic Abuse, Substance Misuse and Mental Health Problems

Susan Heward-Belle

Learning Objectives

Having read this chapter, you should be able to understand:

- The intersections between domestic abuse, mental distress and substance misuse.
- The characteristics of substance use coercion and mental health coercion.
- Problematic service system responses.
- Priorities for domestic abuse-centred and woman-centred practice.

Introduction

Domestic abuse, substance misuse and mental health problems commonly co-occur within families and frequently feature as presenting problems within legal, health and social services (Gilchrist et al. 2010; Oram et al. 2013). Professionals working in the fields of domestic abuse, statutory child protection, mental health, and alcohol and other drugs frequently work with individuals experiencing these co-occurring and complex problems (Oram et al. 2013). This chapter introduces the reader to the phenomenon of mental health and/or substance use coercion, both of which are commonly overlooked manifestations of coercive control deployed by perpetrators of domestic abuse. Understanding the complex interplay between domestic abuse, substance misuse and mental health will enable professionals to better meet the needs of victims/survivors and perpetrators. The chapter considers common

S. Heward-Belle (✉)
Sydney School of Education and Social Work at the University of Sydney, Sydney, NSW, Australia
e-mail: susan.hewardbelle@sydney.edu.au

P. Ali, M. M. Rogers (eds.), *Gender-Based Violence: A Comprehensive Guide*,
https://doi.org/10.1007/978-3-031-05640-6_8

problematic service system responses and ends with a case study illustrating the ingredients of domestic abuse-centred and woman-centred practice.

Definition and Types

A growing body of work identifies mental health and/or substance use coercion as two instrumental tactics deployed by perpetrators of domestic abuse who are overwhelmingly, but not only, men who perpetrate abuse against victims/survivors who are overwhelmingly, but not only, women and children (Cox 2015). In Stark's (2007) influential book, *Coercive Control: How Men Entrap Women in Everyday Life*, he defined coercive control as a 'strategic course of oppressive behaviour to secure and expand gender, race and class privileges by depriving women of their autonomy and liberty, and establishing them in a position of subordination through psychological terror and the use or threat of physical violence' (p. 7). Stark argued that the narrow focus on acts of physical violence in relation to understanding and responding to domestic abuse had catastrophic consequences for survivors. This narrow focus has led to responses that render victims'/survivors' common experience of living under a regime of coercive control invisible. Other terms for mental health coercion include emotional or psychological abuse, and there are no other commonly used terms used to describe substance use coercion.

Two forms of coercive control that have received limited attention and are undertheorized are 'mental health coercion' and 'substance use coercion'. See Box 1 below for definitions of each, developed by Warshaw et al. (2014).

Box 1 Definitions: Mental Health Coercion and Substance Use Coercion

Mental health coercion

Abusive tactics targeted towards a partner's mental health as part of a broader pattern of abuse and control. This often involves the use of force, threats, or manipulation and can include deliberately attempting to undermine a survivor's sanity, preventing a survivor from accessing treatment, controlling a survivor's medication, using a survivor's mental health to discredit them with sources of protection and support, leveraging a survivor's mental health to manipulate police or influence child custody decisions, and/or engaging mental health stigma to make a survivor think no one will believe them, among many other tactics.

Substance use coercion

Abusive tactics targeted towards a partner's substance use as part of a broader pattern of abuse and control. This often involves the use of force, threats, or manipulation and can include forcing a survivor to use substances or to use more than they want, using a survivor's substance use to undermine and discredit them with sources of protection and support, leveraging a survivor's substances use to manipulate police or influence child custody decisions, deliberately sabotaging a survivor's recovery efforts or access to treatment, and/or engaging substance use stigma to make a survivor think that no one will believe them, forcing a partner into withdrawal.

A growing body of evidence, which draws upon the perspectives of both victims/survivors and domestically violent men, has illuminated examples of both forms of coercive control. For example, Warshaw and colleagues' study of American survivors of domestic abuse found that 89% of 2741 respondents had experienced at least one type of mental health coercion and 43% of 3248 respondents had experienced one form of substance use coercion. Women who experienced mental health coercion identified that their abusive (ex)partners had used the following tactics to destabilize their mental health and leverage their mental distress against them:
Called them 'crazy' or accused them of being 'crazy' (85.6%).
Deliberately done things to make women feel like they were going 'crazy' or losing their mind.
Discouraged or prevented women from taking medication or receiving professional health/welfare services (53.5%).
Threatened to report women as 'crazy' to authorities to gain child custody and protection orders and have them medicated and/or treated.

Women who experienced substance use coercion identified that abusive (ex)partners had used the following tactics to leverage their current or previous struggles with substance misuse:

- Inflicted painful injuries on women that led to women using addictive pain relief medications (26%).
- Forced or pressured women into using alcohol and/or other drugs and/or using more than they wanted (27%).
- Discouraging women who sought treatment for substance misuse from obtaining it (60%).
- Threatening to report women's alcohol and/or other drug use to authorities such as police and child protection services to control women (37.5%).

Women also described how perpetrators controlled their medication, treatment regimes, alcohol and/or other drug supply, coerced them into overdosing, forced them to engage in illegal activities, and undermined their sanity, credibility, parenting and recovery. Many women who experienced either mental health coercion or substance use coercion indicated that these tactics made them fearful of reaching out to police or professionals for assistance because they feared that they would not be believed.

Research with perpetrators of domestic abuse found that many targeted and exploited aspects of women's lives that they considered to be 'weaknesses', including women's experiences of depression and/or substance use. The following quotes from domestically violent men (pseudonyms have been used) from original research conducted by the author (Heward-Belle 2016) provide men's accounts of using such tactics, including how they manipulated professionals:

> I reported her to child protection because she went crazy … she placed our baby down on the floor (after being physically cornered and restrained by him) and after that she jumped out the window and when I looked out the window there was blood everywhere. (Todd)

> I called the police and reported her and child protection came and removed her kid after an incident. I walked in and I wanted beer and she stood in front of the fridge and said you're not having any more to drink. I said, 'If I want a beer, get out of the road' and she wouldn't, so I grabbed her by the throat and I've basically thrown her across the kitchen. (Augustus)

> I've tried to tell the professionals but they don't believe me. She's got a long history of, in my unprofessional opinion, BiPolar and Schizophrenia and um in full active addiction with any drugs known to mankind … she's a very intelligent sick person. She's not been diagnosed like she's been in and out of psychiatric wards and they all say she's fine. (George)

Men in the study did not perceive their abuse as something that was directly creating and sustaining an oppressive environment conducive to developing and promoting mental health problems and/or substance misuse. Men conveniently decoupled their violence and coercive control from their (ex)partners' struggles.

The Intersection of Domestic Abuse, Substance Misuse and/or Mental Health Problems

Given the commonality of these interfacing issues, it is highly likely that professionals from a range of disciplines will work with individuals and/or families experiencing co-occurrence. It is important for professionals to untangle and connect the dots on the complex relationship between domestic abuse, substance misuse and/or mental distress. Failing to understand how survivors' struggles with alcohol and/or other drugs and/or mental distress originated and are sustained can lead to disastrous consequences for women and children. Failing to understand the perpetrator's full pattern of violence and coercive control, including their potential use of substance use and/or mental health coercion, can lead to practices that decontextualize survivors' mental distress and/or substance misuse.

Women who have problematic relationships with alcohol and/or other drugs are more likely to have experienced domestic abuse than women who do not misuse substances (McPherson et al. 2007) and many women's substance misuse commences after experiencing male violence whereas men frequently misuse substances before their perpetration pattern begins (Humphreys et al. 2005). Substance misuse in women is influenced by the frequency and severity of domestic abuse they experience (Martin et al. 2003).

There is general agreement in the literature that the relationship between domestic abuse and men's use of alcohol and other drugs is complex and multi-faceted. There is a large body of evidence that shows a high incidence of substance misuse amongst male perpetrators of domestic abuse. When compared to men who do not use violence and coercive control against partners and children, perpetrators exhibit higher levels of chronic alcohol abuse and numerous studies have found a correlation between substance misuse and perpetration (Hamberger and Hastings 1991). Yet, other research has found that perpetrators are equally violent and controlling when sober and that they are likely to use alcohol and other drug use to justify, excuse and minimise abusive behaviour (Bancroft et al. 2012).

The deleterious physical and mental health impact of domestic abuse on victims/survivors is well established. Victims/survivors living with perpetrators who misuse substances and/or have mental health issues are at increased risk of experiencing more frequent abuse, sustaining more severe injuries, resulting in death, disability and mental health problems. Termed a 'toxic trio' by Radcliffe and Gilchrist (2016), the presence of these co-occurring risk factors has been repeatedly identified in formal child death reviews, child serious injury reviews and domestic homicide reviews.

The deleterious mental health consequences of domestic abuse on victims/survivors are unequivocal. Victims/survivors are more likely to experience psychological and emotional distress. They are more likely to be diagnosed with mood disorders including depression and/or anxiety and are more likely to commit suicide than women who are not domestically abused. Kessler et al. (2001) found that many victims/survivors were found to have no pre-existing mental disorders, suggesting that psychological symptoms resulted directly from domestic abuse. Perpetrators of domestic abuse are more likely to be diagnosed with personality disorders, including anti-social, borderline, narcissistic and dependent personality disorders, as well as mood disorders including depression and/or anxiety than are non-abusive men (Hamberger and Hastings 1991). However, concerns exist over labelling perpetrators as mentally ill as this construction can be used to obfuscate their responsibility for their use of violence and coercive control.

Policy and Practice

In the last three decades, the risks posed by the interface of domestic abuse with mental health issues and substance misuse have received increasing attention, particularly within the child protection and domestic abuse fields. Despite the recognition of the potential for harm, serious concerns exist about the service system's response to families (Featherstone et al. 2014; Heward-Belle et al. 2018). Critiques of the service system's response stress the fragmented, inconsistent and siloed nature of service delivery (Hester 2011), the lack of a domestic violence-informed approach (Mandel 2014), sexist institutional practices that render perpetrators of domestic abuse invisible and unaccountable (Heward-Belle 2017; Douglas and Walsh 2010), de-gendered analyses that foreground survivors' mental health and/or substance misuse issues reified from the abusive regime established by perpetrators (Humphreys and Thiara 2003) and the lack of attention to children who are frequently the forgotten victims (Frederico et al. 2014).

There is a growing body of evidence that demonstrates poor service responses in the mental health and alcohol and other drugs fields in particular. Numerous studies point to the failure of agencies and practitioners in these fields to identify the presence of domestic abuse, assess danger and risk and intervene safely to address domestic abuse despite the fact that substance misuse and mental ill-health are commonly the symptoms of abuse (Humphreys and Thiara 2003).

Children and Young People

When children are involved, services often focus their gaze on mothers and mothering, rather than fathers and fathering, and attempt to enforce women's compliance with drug screening rather than providing support for dealing with the effects of domestic abuse on mental health (Tsantefski et al. 2015; Frederico et al. 2014). Moreover, health and welfare services are frequently inadequately designed to attend to intersecting complex problems (Humphreys and Absler 2011). A scoping review summarised the systemic problems thus:

> (w)omen who experience co-occurring problems are required to parse out the complexities to identify a single priority issue in order to access services. Should intimate partner violence first be addressed, or depression and low self-esteem? Should dependence on painkillers or alcohol be the primary focus or the violence and abuse? (Mason and O'Rinn 2014, p. 13)

Concerns about poor service system responses are compounded for families from underserved communities. For example, women and children from poor socio-economic backgrounds, who are Indigenous, from culturally and linguistically diverse communities, and/or live in rural and remote locations are not only at increased risk of experiencing co-occurring domestic abuse, mental health issues and substance misuse, but they are also more likely to experience poor service responses.

The predictable problems resulting from poor service system responses pose particularly pernicious problems for survivors of domestic abuse and their children. Poor responses can compound their trauma, increase the danger they experience, exacerbate mental illness symptoms and result in a sense of diminished confidence in the system. As a result, women survivors may feel understandably reluctant to engage with practitioners, particularly if they feel that they do not understand domestic abuse and/or that their involvement with services may lead to the removal of their children (Macy et al. 2013). This is becoming more common in Australia where in 2015–2016, 55,600 children were placed in out-of-home care for reasons directly connected with domestic abuse (Australian Institute of Health and Welfare 2017).

These concerns are particularly salient for Aboriginal and Torres Strait Islander families whose children are disproportionately reported to statutory child protection services, removed and placed in out-of-home care. A significant proportion of all children and First Nations children in particular experienced cumulative harm associated with living with domestic abuse, parental substance misuse and/or mental health issues. Aboriginal and/or Torres Strait Islander peoples also experience disproportionate rates of socioeconomic disadvantage and poverty linked directly with the ongoing impact of colonisation, forced child removal, dispossession from land and racism (Family Matters 2021). The disproportionate representation of Indigenous children due to intersecting forms of oppression including exposure to domestic abuse, parental substance misuse and/or parental mental health problems within a context of colonization is also seen in other colonized countries including Canada, New Zealand, and the United States.

Domestic Abuse and Survivor-Centred Practices

Effective practice at the interface of domestic abuse, substance misuse and/or mental distress requires professionals to be both domestic-abuse-centred and survivor-centred in their approach. Being domestic abuse-centred involves understanding the aetiology and dynamics of gender-based violence and designing interventions and systems that aim to disrupt the patriarchal structures and systems that embed violence against women. Moreover, it involves understanding and being cognisant of how gender-based power relations are expressed in both the private and public spheres. For professionals, developing interventions that distribute power differentials is critical to survivor-centred practice (Hunnicutt 2009). To be survivor-centred in this context is to ensure that survivors' lived experiences, perspectives, agency, needs, desires and plans for their safety and well-being are at the core of service provision, policy and system design. Survivor-centred practice also requires professionals to assess, document and build upon survivors' strengths. This is an aspect of practice that is often neglected, particularly within agencies that are laden with deficit-informed policies and practices. As Wade (1997) argues, it is imperative that the myriad ways that survivors engage in small daily acts of resistance are noticed, honoured, documented and built upon in all interventions.

Box 2 below provides an example of how lived experience experts and professionals in Australia work collaboratively with pregnant women struggling with domestic abuse, substance misuse and mental health issues to create safe futures for their unborn children.

Box 2 Case Study

Pregnancy Family Conferencing is a program in New South Wales, Australia, that works with women during pregnancy to address child protection issues that are identified during the prenatal period. The child protection legislation in this state enables people to make 'pre-natal reports' and allows statutory child protection services to investigate such reports. The decision to accept intervention from child protection workers during pregnancy, however, is a voluntary one and women can refuse services. Many women who choose to accept support during this time are referred to participate in a Pregnancy Family Conference in which a comprehensive plan is developed through a multi-disciplinary process, the purpose of which is to identify key child protection risk factors, strengths and protective factors within families. Women who access this service are referred by statutory child protection workers and many have complex issues including living with domestic abuse, mental health challenges and substance misuse. Staff within the program include professionals and paid lived experience experts, who are women who were previously clients of the program. Lived experience experts are strong women who have faced significant challenges in their lives—including journeying away from domestic abuse, overcoming substance dependency and addressing mental health problems. All women who participate in the program are at significant risk of having their babies removed from their care at birth if risk factors are not sufficiently addressed during pregnancy. Professionals and lived experience experts in the program help women see the interface between their experiences of domestic abuse, substance use and mental distress. Addressing violence and its impact are central features of casework practice that enable women to move more harm minimization strategies that address substance misuse and/or mental distress. Whereas other programs may see domestic abuse as a by-product of 'mental illness' or 'addiction', workers within this program centre domestic abuse as the root cause of other problems. As a result, casework practice and program policy pivot on working in a violence-informed and woman-centred way. This involves understanding the part that violence has played in directly shaping current life challenges and choices. Walking alongside women to support and strengthen their ability to journey away from violence is a key aspect of women-centred practice. Rather than blaming women for drug use in pregnancy, workers support women in understanding the context in which they are using. Helping women journey away from domestic abuse has enabled many women to experience better mental health and feel less inclined to misuse substances.

Summary

- Substance abuse and/or mental health coercion are common tactics used by domestically violent men to exert power and control over victims/survivors.
- Current practice and policy approaches are often ineffective as they tend to silo domestic abuse, mental health problems and substance misuse.
- Effective practices with victims/survivors and/or perpetrators require a conceptual shift that enables professionals to understand the interface between these issues.
- Further research is needed that explores the impact of living with these forms of coercive control from the perspective of victims/survivors and that explores how perpetrators deploy substance use and/or mental health coercion.

References

Australian Institute of Health and Welfare (2017) Child protection Australia 2015–16. Child welfare series no. 66. Cat. no. CWS 60. AIHW, Canberra

Bancroft L, Silverman L, Ritchie D (2012) The batterer as parent: addressing the impact of domestic violence on family dynamics, 2nd edn. Sage, Thousand Oaks

Cox P (2015) Violence against women: additional analysis of the Australian Bureau of Statistics' Personal Safety Survey. (Horizons. Research Paper No. 1). Australia's National Research Organisation for Women's Safety Limited (ANROWS), Sydney. anrows.org.au/publications/horizons/PSS

Douglas H, Walsh T (2010) Mothers, domestic violence, and child protection. Violence Against Women 16(3):489–508

Family Matters (2021) The family matters report. https://www.familymatters.org.au/the-family-matters-report-2021

Featherstone B, White S, Morris K (2014) Re-imagining child protection: towards human social work with families. Policy Press, London

Frederico M, Jackson A, Dwyer J (2014) Child protection and cross-sector practice: an analysis of child death reviews to inform practice when multiple parental risk factors are present. Child Abuse Rev 23(2):104–115. https://doi.org/10.1002/car.2321

Gilchrist G, Hegarty K, Chondros P, Herman H, Gunn J (2010) The association between intimate partner violence, alcohol and depression in family practice. BMC Fam Pract 11:72. https://doi.org/10.1186/1471-2296-11-72

Hamberger L, Hastings J (1991) Personality correlates of men who batter and non-violent men: Some continuities and discontinuities. J Fam Violence 1(4):323–341

Hester M (2011) The three planet model: towards an understanding of contradictions and approaches to women and children's safety in contexts of domestic violence. Br J Soc Work 41:837–853

Heward-Belle S (2016) The diverse fathering practices of men who perpetrate domestic violence. Aust Social Work 69(3):323–337

Heward-Belle S (2017) Exploiting the "good mother" as a tactic of coercive control: domestically violent men's assaults on women as mothers. Affilia 32(3):374–389

Heward-Belle S, Humphreys C, Laing L, Toivonen C (2018) Intervening with children living with domestic violence: is the system safe? Aust Social Work 71:135–147

Humphreys C, Absler D (2011) History repeating: child protection responses to domestic violence. Child Fam Soc Work 16(4):1–10

Humphreys C, Thiara R (2003) Mental health and domestic violence: 'I Call it Symptoms of Abuse'. Br J Soc Work 33(2):209–226. https://doi.org/10.1093/bjsw/33.2.209

Humphreys C, Regan L, River D, Thiara R (2005) Domestic violence and substance use: tackling complexity. Br J Soc Work 35:1303–1320

Hunnicutt G (2009) Varieties of patriarchy and violence against women: resurrecting patriarchy as a theoretical tool. Violence Against Women 15(5):553–573

Kessler R, Molar B, Feurer I, Appelbaum M (2001) Patterns and mental health predictors of domestic violence in the United States: results from the National Comorbidity Survey. Int J Law Psychiatry 24:487–508

Macy RJ, Renz C, Pelino E (2013) Partner violence and substance abuse are intertwined: women's perceptions of violence-substance connections. Violence Against Women 7:881–902. https://doi.org/10.1177/1077801213498208

Martin SL, Beaumont JL, Kupper LL (2003) Substance use before and during pregnancy: links to intimate partner violence. Am J Drug Alcohol Abuse 29(3):599–617

McPherson L, Gopalan G, Chugh R, & Monahan J (2007) Substance abuse coercion. Journal of Addictive Diseases 26(3):31–40. https://doi.org/10.1300/JO69v26n03_04

Mandel D (2014) Beyond domestic violence perpetrator accountability in child welfare systems. No To Violence J Spring:50–85

Mason R, O'Rinn SE (2014) Co-occurring intimate partner violence, mental health, and substance use problems: a scoping review. Glob Health Action 7:24815. https://doi.org/10.3402/gha.v7.24815

Oram S, Trevillion K, Feder G, Howard L (2013) Prevalence of experiences of domestic violence among psychiatric patients: systematic review. Br J Psychiatry 202:94–99

Radcliffe P, Gilchrist G (2016) "You can never work with addictions in isolation": addressing intimate partner violence perpetration by men in substance misuse treatment. Int J Drug Policy 36:130–140. https://doi.org/10.1016/j.drugpo.2016.03.010

Stark E (2007) Coercive control: how men entrap women in personal life. Oxford University Press, Oxford

Tsantefski M, Jackson AC, Humphreys C (2015) A delicate balance: intervention with mothers with dual diagnosis and their infants. Adv Dual Diagn 8(2):78–89. https://doi.org/10.1108/ADD-09-2014-0027

Wade A (1997) Small acts of living: everyday resistance to violence and other forms of oppression. Contemp Fam Ther 19:23–39

Warshaw C, Lyon E, Bland P, Phillips H, Hooper M (2014) Mental health and substance use coercion surveys: report from the National Center on Domestic Violence, Trauma and Mental Health and the National Domestic Violence Hotline

Susan Heward-Belle, PhD is a Professor in Social Work in the Sydney School of Education and Social Work at the University of Sydney. Her research is concerned with promoting socially just and gender-equitable approaches to social work and social policy.

Post-Separation and Divorce-Related Abuse

Ikenna Fernandez Nnoli, Michaela M. Rogers, and Parveen Ali

Learning Objectives

At the end of this chapter, you should be able to:

- Understand post-separation and divorce-related abuse (DRA).
- Identify the different forms and elements of post-separation and DRA.
- Identify risk factors of post-separation and DRA.
- Understand the impact of DRA on health and economy.
- Articulate recommendations for policy and practice.

Introduction

Initiation of a relationship or marriage is often celebrated and is an exciting life event. It is celebrated not only by the individuals involved but their family members and friends too. Contrary to this, leaving a relationship is generally not easy or straightforward for any partner. It often involves conflicts, stress, and other complications. Post-separation and divorce-related abuse (DRA) is a global concern affecting both developing and developed nations across the globe with devastating impacts

I. F. Nnoli (✉)
Department of Nursing Science, University of Benin, Benin, Edo State, Nigeria

M. M. Rogers
Department of Sociological Studies, University of Sheffield, Sheffield, UK
e-mail: m.rogers@sheffield.ac.uk

P. Ali
The Health Sciences School, University of Sheffield, Sheffield, UK
e-mail: parveen.ali@sheffield.ac.uk

P. Ali, M. M. Rogers (eds.), *Gender-Based Violence: A Comprehensive Guide*,
https://doi.org/10.1007/978-3-031-05640-6_9

on individuals and communities, as well as socio-economic systems. Since the 1990s, many countries across the world have responded to the presence of abuse after parents separate or divorce through policy and legislative change (Radford 2013). This work continues as policymakers learn more about the links between divorce and abuse and its impact on women and children. Understanding these links is critical as separating parents and divorce alone, without associated abuse, can have damaging effects on individuals as well as the society at large with considerably more implications where there is maltreatment.

While there is evidence showing that at least one form of abuse might play a role in the dissolution of many statutory marriages, and that post-separation abuse often occurs in the context of a prior history of domestic abuse (Holt 2015), there is still surprisingly too little attention paid in research to the abuse men and women experience during and after their separation and/or divorce. This is a complex issue, and perpetrators can be partners, a family member or friend of either partners, or members of institutions like the church, a law firm or the judiciary. For such an issue that has serious impacts, there is still inadequate global data about the extent of the impact that post-separation and DRA have on individuals and families, especially children. This is why understanding post-separation and DRA is important within the field of gender-based violence. Post-separation and DRA might not be considered a universal phenomenon because what constitutes abuse in one culture might be a normal way of life in another culture. According to Burrill et al. (2010), these terms have the merit of drawing our attention to the gendered nature of DRA and of challenging characterizations of such violence as a private matter rather than a public concern.

Definition of Terms

In contemporary society, it is common in many countries for adults to live as couples and raise families outside marriage. Ending such a relationship is similar to divorce for married couples because property, child welfare, custody and child contact still have to be negotiated. These negotiations put a strain on separation and can result in any form of abuse categorized as post-separation and DRA (several alternate terms are used—see Box 1). Divorce is also known as dissolution of marriage as it is the formal end of a marital union. Divorce is an official or legal process to end a marriage (Cambridge Dictionary 2021b). Divorce can involve a legal proceeding in the case of a statutory marriage, or a recognized customary rule in the case of non-statutory marriages. A statutory marriage refers to marriage in accordance with the law.

In the context of this chapter, abuse refers to any harmful or morally wrong act or incident that adversely affects a person's sense of well-being and safety (Cambridge Dictionary 2021a). Therefore, post-separation and DRA can be broadly defined as any violent or abusive incident, or pattern of incidents, that adversely affects a person's sense of well-being, either physically, sexually, mentally or psychosocially, which are often endured or inflicted by those in marriage, or regulating its dissolution, or in separating partners. By using this definition, it should be emphasized that the perpetrators of post-separation and DRA are not limited to the involved couples but extends to their families, communities and institutions that justify or practice any kind of ideology that harms those affected.

Box 1
Alternative terminology: Abuse during divorce, abuse after divorce, divorce-related violence, ex-partner abuse, ex-partner violence, ex-related abuse, ex-abuse, post-separation abuse, post-separation violence.

Comparing Grounds for Divorce

The grounds for a divorce vary considerably from country to country, with specific differences influenced by ethno-religious factors and the status of marriage as statutory or non-statutory. In many countries around the world, divorce is fault-based, which means that any partner seeking divorce has to prove that the marriage has broken down irretrievably. The UK provides an example: according to the Matrimonial Causes Act 1973 for England and Wales, the only grounds for divorce is evidence that the marriage has broken down 'irretrievably'. Evidence of at least one of the following is required for the dissolution of a marriage:

- Adultery.
- Desertion.
- Five years of separation without consent.
- Two years of separation with consent.
- Unreasonable behaviour.

In some countries, the grounds for a divorce can be complicated, especially where other marriage practices are recognised such as customary marriage (that which is undertaken in accordance with traditional custom) or religious marriage (a marriage celebrated by a cleric in accordance with the recognised rites of a religion, religious body, denomination or sect to which one or both parties to the marriage belong). The following section describes some of the nuances pertaining to divorce to be found across the world.

Islamic Law and Divorce

Under Islamic law, the basis of divorce is the inability of the spouses to live together rather than any specific cause, on account of which the parties cannot live together. A divorce may be either by the act of the husband or by the act of the wife. A man can divorce his wife without the involvement of religious authorities; he is not questioned or challenged about his grounds for divorce. However, women have to involve a religious authority and need to provide grounds for divorce. The example of such grounds includes unreasonable behaviour (e.g., emotional/physical abuse, habits such as gambling, drug-taking), financial irresponsibility, unreasonable sexual behaviour (e.g., sodomy, rape, demanding too much sex, refusal to have sex, not satisfying sexual needs), or cohabiting with another spouse. Other reasons could be adultery, failure of the husband to provide, incompatibility, impotence, long imprisonment of the husband, insanity or any incurable disease. Divorce is allowed in Islam, and both the husband and the wife have the right to initiate a divorce; however, it is often frowned upon in communities on cultural grounds. The husband or father of the children remains responsible for providing for his children from an Islamic perspective.

Christianity and Divorce

In Christianity, there are various denominations, each with a set of doctrines that determines how divorce is treated. Many Christian denominations allow divorce, but the largest Christian denomination – Catholicism – views divorce differently. In Catholicism, matrimony is a sacrament, which means it is ordained by God and no man can put asunder what God has joined together. Canon 1012 of the Codex Juris Canonici states that Christ elevated the very contract of marriage between two baptized persons to the dignity of a sacrament. It would be impossible, therefore, for a valid contract of marriage to exist between two baptized persons without being a sacrament. It is not so much the divorce that the Roman Catholic Church objects to as the remarriage after divorce. In contemporary society, sometimes the interpretation of the Canon law regarding divorce can be ambiguous even for practicing Catholics and their clerics—highlighted in the case study in Box 2 below.

Box 2 Case Study: Boris Johnson to Remarry

Following the matrimony of the British Prime Minister Boris Johnson to Carrie Symonds in May 2021, Father Mark Drew, an assistant priest in Warrington, tweeted in response to the news: ‘Can anyone explain to me how “Boris” Johnson, who left the Catholic church while at Eaton and is twice divorced, can be married at Westminster Cathedral, while I have to tell practising Catholics in good faith who want a second marriage in Church that it’s not possible?’

The papal biographer Austen Ivereigh responded with the following tweet, ‘Boris’s two previous marriages (probably) lacked canonical form, that is, are not recognised in Catholic law. So he (probably) didn’t need an annulment. When the canonical form of marriage has not been observed and the marriage was not later validated in the Church, a simple administrative process is used to declare such marriages invalid in church’.

Source: Wolfe-Robinson 2021, for The Guardian.

Prevalence

While it is highly problematic to determine the rates of post-separation and DRA (due to varied definitions, under-reporting, a lack of and mis-recording), it is possible to establish the rates of divorce by country. For example, according to the National Center for Health Statistics (2022) in the United States, approximately 4–5 million people get married every year in the United States and approximately 42–53% of those marriages eventually end in divorce. According to data from the United Nations and other sources, in 2020 the country with the highest divorce rate in the world was the Maldives, which recorded 2984 divorces against a population of 540,544, resulting in a divorce rate of 5.52 per 1000 people. Information collated by the World Population Review demonstrates that the global divorce rate average is 1.7 per 1000 people and Table 1 shows the top 13 countries with the highest divorce rates.

Table 1 Top 10 countries with the highest divorce rates

Rank	Country	Annual divorce rate per 1000 people
1	Maldives	5.52
2	Kazakhstan	4.6
3	Russia	3.9
4	Belarus (tie)	3.7
5	Belgium (tie)	3.7
6	Moldova	3.3
7	China	3.2
8	Cuba	2.9
9	Ukraine	2.88
10	Denmark (tie)	2.7
11	Latvia (tie)	2.7
12	Lithuania (tie)	2.7
13	USA (tie)	2.7

Source: World Population Review (2022)

Forms of Post-Separation and Divorce-Related Abuse

Post-separation and DRA is not a single act or incident. It is a pattern of behaviour perpetrated during separation or post-divorce. In addition, there is no evidence to suggest that finalising a separation or divorce brings an end to the abuse. In many cases, the duration of post-separation or DRA may be much longer than the entire length of the separation or divorce process. Unfortunately, abuse might continue for years post-separation.

Post-separation and DRA can take various forms and can include verbal abuse, sexual abuse and harassment, violence and physical threat, emotional/psychological abuse, economic abuse and financial exploitation, defamation and character assassination. Often separating or divorcing partners are involved in a legal battle, especially when something valuable is at stake, whether it is child custody and support, alimony or possession of the shared home.

In addition to the multiple forms of abuse that can be experienced by partners in a relationship or marriage and that are perpetrated in private, public (especially in family courts) and virtual environments, there are specific forms that occur in separating couples including post-separation economic abuse, use of child contact as a weapon of abuse and post-separation domestic homicide. A brief overview of each of these is given below.

Post-Separation Economic Abuse

While economic abuse rarely happens in isolation (more likely it is found co-occurring with other forms of violence), in the case of post-separation and DRA, these are intrinsically linked with economic abuse. The economic impact of separating or divorcing a partner can be life changing. One of the major issues debated and negotiated for during separation and divorce relates to splitting material resources, domestic arrangements, payment of maintenance and child support. The evidence of economic abuse and its negative impact on divorce is well documented. In the short term, a majority of divorces put an economic burden on men, who often lose their homes and are required to split assets with ex-spouses and pay child support and alimony (Leopold 2018). Post-separation economic abuse can be severe and even result in self-injurious behaviour in a desperate attempt to provide evidence or put their ex-partner at a disadvantage as some people have been reported to destroy their own property to deny their partner certain possessions and benefits (Surviving Economic Abuse 2022). For example, in June 2021, a 75-year-old British man burned down his £550,000 cottage to stop his estranged wife from getting her half-share in their divorce (Ridler 2021).

Child Contact as a Weapon of Abuse and Control

The rights of women in relation to the residence of and contact with their children following separation and divorce differ across the world. In some countries, the rights of fathers have been subject to considerable campaigning. For example, in the UK, the rights of mothers were only recently enshrined in the Guardianship Act 1973 as previously children were subject to the will of the husband and father (Mackay 2018). Yet immediately following, there was a barrage of activity with the founding of the group 'Families Need Fathers'. Such activism has influenced the developing of domestic policy in the UK, and it is now the case that fathers in the UK benefit from automatic parental rights in respect of their children so long as they are named on the child's birth certificate. However, that children are weaponised in cases before the courts in separated or divorcing couples, and in the negotiation of parental rights, is not new, and there is a body of evidence to support such claims. For example, research by Holt (2015) produced clear evidence of post-separation contact facilitating the continued abuse of women and children.

Taking legal action for contact with children is one method for a man to gain access to an ex-partner and/or children (Harne 2011). Evidence in this area draws into question the assumption that contact between an abusive father and a child promotes the welfare of the child and the woman. However, scholarship shows that abusive men often lack insight into how their behaviour impacts their child in post-separation conflict (Holt 2015). In a mixed-methods study of court cases, Mackay (2018) surmised that there are three means of re(asserting) control over a former partner in child contact cases, including documentary harms (e.g., through court papers which contain slurs on mother's parenting ability), formal hearing harms (e.g., the requirement for victim/survivors to be in the court space as the abusive former partners) and contact harms (e.g., mother's fear of abduction, or fear of abuse at contact handover points).

Domestic Homicide in Separating or Separated Couples

Separation is a time of high risk for violence, including fatal violence, for both women and children (Women's Aid 2016). In the UK, over the three-year period April 2016 to March 2019, a total of 222 women were killed by a partner or ex-partner. The majority of suspects were male (n = 218, 98%) (ONS 2020). This means that during this time period, an average of three women every fortnight were murdered by their male partner or ex-partner (ONS 2020). In Jamaica, a study by Bourne et al. (2014: 298) examined secondary data analysis to understand the 'murder pandemic'. The study reported that marriage and divorce rates accounted for 82.2% of the variability in the murder rate. Both factors were positively correlated with the murder rate, with the divorce rate accounting for most of the variance in the murder rate of 79.2% (Bourne et al. 2014). This finding demonstrated that many women experienced violence from their partners both during and after the ending of their marital relationships, that violence caused some women to leave their marriages and caused others difficulty in negotiating their share of marital resources (Kurz 1996). Divorce-related homicides are well documented in other countries too. For instance, a study of murder victims in the Eskişehir Province of Turkey found that of a total of 141 murdered women 48.2% (n = 68) had been killed by the husband and 7.8% (n = 11) by the ex-husband.

Murderers generally stated that the reason for killing was the woman's request for a divorce or for taking action to separate from their husbands ($n = 40$, 28.4%) (Karbeyaz et al. 2013).

Risk Factors

Some important risk factors associated with post-separation and DRA include historic domestic violence and abuse, especially coercive control; perpetrator's psychological instability, drug or substance abuse; actual or threatened character assassination and defamation during separation or divorce; and fear of losing one's assets, valuable property and hard-earned savings following divorce; (Brownridge et al. 2008; Holt 2015; James-Hanman and Holt 2021). Research also shows that the existence of children in the family is a risk factor for continued abuse, with the fear of losing contact or residence of one's own children to violent ex-partners representing another vulnerability (Brownridge et al. 2008; Holt 2015; Morrison 2015).

In many communities, on a structural level, patriarchy plays a significant role in the risk of violence in both marriage and post-separation (Hunnicutt 2009). Post-separation and post-divorce, men may use violence and abuse to reassert their position of dominance over their partner, perpetuating the notion that men are entitled to the ongoing expectation of female obedience, loyalty and dependence (Brownridge et al. 2008). In many cases, women are regarded as their husband's property and separation is thus seen as a challenge to their patriarchal authority. A contemporary example of patriarchy can be found in Southern India where a court recently ruled that a woman divorced for being adulterous could not claim maintenance from her ex-husband (Pandey 2015). The ruling by Justice S Nagamuthu of the Madras high court may be legally sound, but the language of the judgement has raised concerns from women's activists (Pandey 2015).

Impact of Post-Separation and Divorce-Related Abuse

The negative consequences and effects of divorce on couples, children and their future can be overwhelming, with increased risk to mental and emotional health. As noted above, there are physical risks, including fatality, for separating or separated partners. Victims of post-separation and DRA might have difficulty coping, particularly if engaged in stressful court proceedings, and can find themselves engaging in harmful behaviours such as alcohol and substance abuse. There are also negative impacts for many children over the course of childhood and young adulthood (Cherlin 2010), with consequences for emotional, behavioural, social, and academic aspects of everyday life (Amato et al. 2010). Separation and divorce might lead to different outcomes for children based on culture, ethnicity, family structure, and special needs; for instance, children with special needs might experience more heightened impacts on their later life outcomes due to separated families

(Demir-Dagdas et al. 2018). It is important to note that poor outcomes can be moderated by positive parenting, counselling and quality contact post-separation/post-divorce (Holt 2016; Demir-Dagdas et al. 2018).

Post-separation and DRA can be intensely painful and impactful for the victim/survivor to process. While both a husband and wife are involved in the divorce process, women seem to be worse off materially and financially following a divorce and are often subjected to various forms of abuse. This is certainly the case if there was previously no maltreatment as the reluctance to admit that one's previously agreeable partner/spouse can be abusive following a dissolution could be one of the causes of delays in confronting the abuse or seeking help.

Inevitably, there are economic impacts for separating or divorcing partners. There is increased welfare dependency on the state, especially for those who are unable to earn a living due to the age of children. The cost of a legal battle in family courts to prove certain types of abuse or vindicate a falsely accused ex-partner often leaves the affected in an economic disadvantage. Post-separation and DRA can result in employment loss, loss of income or means of livelihood, thereby reducing the victim/survivor's quality of life. Victim/survivors might have undergone extensive surgeries and prolonged hospitalizations from injuries inflicted by their abusive ex-partners causing economic hardship for those unable to work as a result. These factors can result in women's disproportionate losses in household income and increase their risk of poverty and single parenting (Leopold 2018). There is a structural impact via the impact on health services as well as the increased economic burden on the state for the provision and maintenance of social security and welfare benefits.

Implications for Research, Policy and Practice

There has been a surge of interest in post-separation and DRA illustrated in recent policy changes in developed countries. For example, the new Divorce Act in Canada 2021 is an attempt to build the legislative framework to help parents, judges and others make safe and appropriate arrangements when there has been family violence. In the UK, post-separation abuse is recognised in the new Domestic Abuse Act 2021 (Surviving Economic Abuse 2021). However, legal remedies are not universally available, and on a global level, there are implications for future policy and practice including the need for

1. A global public health campaign to raise awareness of the prevalence and impact of post-separation and DRA at national and international levels.
2. Strategies to strengthen partnerships and marriages through freely available relationship education and counselling that equips adults with relationship and conflict resolution skills.
3. Accessible and accurate statistics on post-separation and DRA for better understanding of the causes and implications for individuals, families and communities.

4. Welfare funds for safeguarding victims/survivors of post-separation and DRA and their children.
5. Policy, such as that in Canada, to promote equality in family courts with regard to alimony, child custody and contact after divorce.
6. The understanding of the judiciary in terms of post-separation and DRA.
7. Accessible systems for raising concerns, reporting and investigating post-separation DRA.

There is also a continuing need for stronger linkages and relationships between research, policy and practice (James-Hanman and Holt 2021) and more activity in least developed countries. Emphasising the need to recognise that post-separation and DRA are gendered, Holt's (2015) research offers further implications. Holt (2015: 210) argued that her research findings highlight a lack of attention to 'the parenting of abusive men who were identified as struggling to realise their fathering aspirations and take responsibility for the impact of their abusive behaviour on their children and ex-partners'. She went on to observe that some constructions of family life were found to sustain the frequently unregulated presence of abusive men in post-separation family life. To remedy this, Holt concluded that a priority for legal and safeguarding policy and practice should be the integration of the construction of fathers as 'risk' in the context of post-separation father–child contact. This, Holt argued, was not a means of excluding fathers from children's lives; instead, it is intended to find ways to ensure that abusive men can be 'good enough' fathers.

Summary

- The irregularities in marriage and divorce practices across the globe make post-separation and DRA a challenging issue to tackle and pose a greater risk to certain demographics.
- The health and economic impact of DRA on victims can be devastating and long lasting.
- Post-separation and DRA are a gendered issue with impacts for men and women that are different in the short, medium and long term.
- There are research, policy and practice implications in relation to post-separation and DRA in terms of prevention, identification and existing responses.

References

Amato PR, Deboer DD, Cavanagh SE, Schiller KS, Riegle-Crumb C, Herd P, Ingersoll-Dayton B et al (2010) The future of historical family demography. J Health Soc Behav 46:848–861

Bourne PA, Hudson-Davis A, Sharpe-Pryce C, Clarke J, Solan I, Rhule J, Francis C, Watson-Coleman O, Sharma A, Campbell-Smith J (2014) Does marriage explain murders in a society? In what way is divorce a public health concern? Int J Emerg Ment Health 16(2):298–307

Burrill E, Roberts R, Thornberry E (2010) Domestic violence and the laws in Africa. Ohio University Press, Ohio

Cambridge International Dictionary of English (2021a) Abuse. Cambridge University Press. https://dictionary.cambridge.org/dictionary/english/abuse

Cambridge International Dictionary of English (2021b) Divorce. Cambridge University Press. https://dictionary.cambridge.org/dictionary/english/divorce

Cherlin AJ (2010) Demographic trends in the United States: a review of research in the 2000s. J Marriage Fam 72:403–419

Demir-Dagdas T, Isik-Ercan Z, Intepe-Tingir S, CavaTadik Y (2018) Parental divorce and children from diverse backgrounds: multidisciplinary perspectives on mental health, parent-child relationships, and educational experiences. J Divorce Remarriage 59(6):469–485

Harne L (2011) Violent fathering and the risks to children: the need for change. Policy Press, London

Holt S (2015) Post-separating fathering and domestic abuse: challenges and contradictions. Child Abuse Rev 24:210–222

Holt S (2016) 'Quality' contact post-separation/divorce: a review of the literature. Child Youth Serv Rev 68:92–99

Hunnicutt G (2009) Varieties of patriarchy and violence against women. Violence Against Women 15(5):553–573. https://doi.org/10.1177/1077801208331246

James-Hanman D, Holt S (2021) Post-separation contact and domestic violence: our 7-point plan for safe[r] contact for children. J Fam Violence 36(8):991–1001

Karbeyaz K, Akkaya H, Balci Y (2013) An analysis of the murder of women in a 10-year period in Eskişehir Province located in western Anatolia in Turkey. J Forensic Leg Med 20(6):736–739

Kurz D (1996) Separation, divorce, and woman abuse. Violence Against Women 2(1):63–81

Leopold T (2018) Gender differences in the consequences of divorce: a study of multiple outcomes. Demography 55(3):769–797

Mackay K (2018) Child contact as a weapon of control. In: Lombard N (ed) The Routledge of handbook of gender and violence. Routledge, Abingdon

Morrison F (2015) 'All Over Now?' The ongoing relational consequences of domestic abuse through children's contact arrangements. Child Abuse Rev 24(4):274–284

National Center for Health Statistics (2022) Stats of the States. https://nchstats.com/category/divorce-rate/. Accessed 26 Apr 2022

Office for National Statistics (2020) Appendix tables: Homicide in England and Wales. ONS. https://www.ons.gov.uk/peoplepopulationandcommunity/crimeandjustice/datasets/appendixtableshomicideinenglandandwales

Pandey G (2015) Why Indian women must shun sex to claim alimony. BBC News. https://www.bbc.co.uk/news/world-asia-india-34019457

Radford L (2013) Domestic violence, safety and child contact in England; Hiding violent men in the shadows of parenting. In: Lombard N, McMillan N (eds) Violence against women: current theory and practice in domestic abuse, sexual violence and exploitation. Jessica Kingsley, London

Ridler F (2021) Mail online. Published June 2021. Dailymail. https://www.dailymail.co.uk/news/article-9725967/Husband-75-burned-550k-cottage-blowtorch.html. Accessed Aug 2021

Surviving Economic Abuse (2021) Criminalising post separation (economic) abuse. https://survivingeconomicabuse.org/wp-content/uploads/2021/03/SEA-briefing_post-separation-abuse_Final.pdf. Accessed Jan 2022

Surviving Economic abuse (2022) What is economic abuse? Surviving economic abuse. https://survivingeconomicabuse.org/what-is-economic-abuse/. Accessed Apr 2022

Wolfe-Robinson M (2021) Catholics question why Boris Johnson was able to marry in church. The Guardian. Published May 2021. https://www.theguardian.com/politics/2021/may/30/boris-johnson-carrie-symmonds-married-catcholic-church. Accessed Dec 2021

Women's Aid (2016) Nineteen child homicides. Women's Aid, Bristol

World Population Review (2022) Divorce rates by country 2022. https://worldpopulationreview.com/country-rankings/divorce-rates-by-country. Accessed 26 Apr 2022

Michaela M. Rogers, PhD is a Senior Lecturer in Social Work in the Department of Sociological Studies at the University of Sheffield. Her research examines interpersonal violence with a focus on marginalised groups, impacts, help-seeking, service access and service responses.

Parveen Ali, PhD Professor of Gender Based Violence and Professor of Nursing in the Health Sciences School, the University of Sheffield and Doncaster and Bassetlaw Teaching Hospitals. Her research examines gender-based violence, inequalities in health related to gender and ethnicity, and nursing as a profession.

Stalking

Abby Hare, Jennifer E. Storey, and Afroditi Pina

Learning Objectives

Having read this chapter, you should be able to understand

- The key findings from the adult and adolescent stalking literature.
- The features of stalking that are gendered.
- The merits of using a gendered approach as a framework for understanding the gender differences within stalking.

Introduction

Our understanding of stalking as a significant social problem has increased substantially over the past four decades. Stalking was first recognised as an issue during the 1980s when the media began to document cases of 'obsessional following' and 'psychological rape' (Coleman 1997; Lowney and Best 1995). These cases typically involved women subjected to harassment (such as unwanted

A. Hare (✉)
Forensic Psychology, University of Kent, Kent, UK
e-mail: alh57@kent.ac.uk

J. E. Storey
Forensic Psychology in the School of Psychology, University of Kent, Kent, UK
e-mail: j.storey@kent.ac.uk

A. Pina
Centre for Research and Education in Forensic Psychology (CORE-FP), University of Kent, Kent, UK
e-mail: a.pina@kent.ac.uk

P. Ali, M. M. Rogers (eds.), *Gender-Based Violence: A Comprehensive Guide*,
https://doi.org/10.1007/978-3-031-05640-6_10

letters and calls) and pursuit behaviours. While obsessional following and psychological rape were considered to be problematic and uncomfortable for targets, the media portrayal of these cases did not demand public or legal attention (Lowney and Best 1995; Mullen et al. 2009). Towards the end of the 1980s, there was a substantial shift in public interest in stalking due to the high-profile victimisation of several celebrities, most notably the actress Rebecca Schaeffer who was murdered in 1989 by an 'obsessed' fan (Coleman 1997; Lowney and Best 1995). Following Rebecca Schaeffer's murder, the term 'stalking' emerged and was used to describe the harassment and pursuit of celebrities (Coleman 1997; Melton 2000).

Celebrity or 'star' stalking gained significant public and media attention and prompted the criminalisation of stalking across North America, Australia, and the United Kingdom (UK) throughout the 1990s (Miller 2012; Mullen et al. 2009). Concurrent to the introduction of anti-stalking legislation was an increased research interest in stalking (Melton 2000; Mullen et al. 2009). This research identified large numbers of cases involving non-celebrity targets, and stalking became understood as a problem experienced primarily by women within the context of a current or former intimate relationship (Coleman 1997; Mullen et al. 2009). Today, our understanding of stalking has developed further, and it is acknowledged that stalking can also be targeted towards men and can occur across a range of relationship types, including between friends, co-workers, and strangers (Miller 2012; Smith et al. 2017). However, women and individuals within an intimate relationship remain at the highest risk of stalking.

This chapter will provide an overview of the stalking literature to date and discusses prevalence rates, target and perpetrator characteristics, stalking behaviours, and the impacts of stalking. As stalking research has almost exclusively focused on stalking amongst adults (aged 18 years plus), most of the research described in this chapter is in reference to adults. Findings from research investigating stalking amongst adolescents (aged 13–17 years) is discussed where available. There is also limited research examining stalking across different countries and cultures, so the research reviewed within this chapter has primarily been conducted in Western countries. The chapter begins with a brief discussion of stalking definitions and definitional issues. Research from the adult and adolescent stalking literature is then described in turn before a discussion of the implications for research and practice. Throughout this chapter, gender is used as a focal point and the utility of framing stalking as a form of gender-based violence is discussed.

Defining Stalking

Currently, there is no universally agreed definition of stalking. Legal definitions vary considerably between countries (and even between jurisdictions) and different definitions have been adopted within research (Mullen et al. 2009; Owens 2016). Furthermore, various terms have been used to describe stalking behaviours (see Box 1).

Individual definitions can differ on several factors including the type of threat posed by the perpetrator, the intentions of the perpetrator, the behaviours that constitute stalking, and the level of fear the stalking causes the target (Melton 2007; Owens 2016). Most definitions, however, share three key features: (1) a pattern of behaviour that is (2) unwanted by the target and (3) causes the target fear or distress (Miller 2012; Mullen et al. 2009).

While in-depth discussions of the issues associated with stalking definitions are beyond the scope of this chapter, it is important to note the impact definitions have on our understanding of stalking. For example, the 2006 Supplemental Victimization Survey, a stalking questionnaire included with the annual National Crime Victimization Survey in the United States, estimated the prevalence of stalking in the past year. Participants (aged 18 years plus) were identified as stalking targets if they had experienced at least one stalking behaviour (e.g., unwanted telephone calls and letters) more than once in the previous 12 months. This broad definition identified approximately 5.3 million targets of stalking. When the definition was amended to include a fear requirement (e.g., the respondent stated they were afraid because of the stalking behaviour), approximately 3.4 million targets were identified (Baum et al. 2009). Definitions are therefore fundamental to our understanding of the extent of stalking.

Definitions can also have practical implications for targets, as some definitions may prevent certain targets from receiving legal protection and support because they do not meet the 'victim' criteria in a given definition. For example, California Law (under Penal Code 646.9 PC) requires the stalking perpetrator to make a credible threat towards the target (Mullen et al. 2009). Given that studies of stalking have found that threats are made in approximately 40–50% of cases (Baum et al. 2009; Budd et al. 2000; Pathé and Mullen 1997), definitions requiring threats (such as the California stalking law) may ignore substantial numbers of targets.

Evidently, the lack of a single, unified stalking definition has important implications for our understanding of the nature and extent of the issue and the provisions made available to targets (Lyndon et al. 2012; Owens 2016). As we will see further in this chapter, definitions may also have implications for gender and research.

Box 1

Definition

Stalking is a 'course of conduct in which one individual inflicts on another repeated unwanted intrusions and communications to such an extent that the victim fears for his or her safety' (Pathé and Mullen 1997).

Alternative terminology

Criminal harassment, Harassment, Intrusive contact, Obsessional following, Obsessional relational intrusion, Obsessive pursuit, Psychological rape, Unwanted pursuit behaviours.

Prevalence Rates

Estimates of stalking prevalence rates vary widely due to differences in the definitions, samples, and research methods used across studies (Dressing et al. 2020; Lyndon et al. 2012). However, there is agreement amongst researchers, governments, and practitioners that stalking is a prevalent social issue. For example, in the United States, stalking is estimated to affect 1.4–1.5% of adults (aged 18 years plus) each year, which equates to approximately 4.5–4.9 million targets annually (Baum et al. 2009). In the UK, the Crime Survey for England and Wales indicated that 25,254 people (aged 16–74 years) were targets in the year ending March 2020 (Office for National Statistics 2020). The lifetime prevalence of stalking has been estimated to be between 2% and 15% in Western populations (Whyte et al. 2011).

Despite variations in prevalence rates across studies, research has consistently found that females are more at risk of being stalked than males. In the United States, the 2006 Supplemental Victimization Survey estimated that 2% of women experience stalking each year compared to 0.7% of men (Baum et al. 2009). Results from the 2010 National Intimate Partner and Sexual Violence Survey estimated the lifetime prevalence of stalking to be 15.8% for women (1 in 6) and 5.3% for men (1 in 19) (Smith et al. 2017). Similar results have been found across several countries, including the UK (Budd et al. 2000), Germany (Dressing et al. 2020), and Australia (Purcell et al. 2002).

Owing to a lack of research, our understanding of the prevalence of stalking amongst adolescents (aged 13–17 years) is limited. Studies of adult stalking prevalence rates can provide retrospective estimates of adolescent stalking: for example, the 2010 National Intimate Partner and Sexual Violence Survey found that among 18.3% of female and 7% of male adult targets, the stalking had occurred before age 18 (Black et al. 2011). Fisher et al. (2014) have conducted the only representative population-based assessment of adolescent stalking to date, surveying 18,013 adolescents (aged 14–18 years) in Kentucky. Results showed that 16.5% of adolescents had been targets in the previous 12 months, which suggests that stalking may be more prevalent amongst adolescents than adults. Much like adult stalking, adolescent stalking is more prevalent amongst females (18.8%) than males (13.9%). Fisher et al. (2014) also measured self-reported stalking perpetration amongst adolescents. Findings indicated that 5.3% of adolescents had engaged in stalking in the past 12 months, 6.5% of males and 4.2% of females.

While gender differences in adolescent stalking prevalence rates are yet to be explored, the observed gender differences in adult stalking prevalence rates could be attributed to how stalking has been defined within research. As discussed previously, there is little agreement on how best to define stalking and it has been argued that some definitions alienate male targets (Lyndon et al. 2012). For example, men are significantly less likely to admit feeling afraid of stalking behaviours (Owens 2017), so stalking definitions requiring fear may exclude many male targets. Indeed, Owens (2016) examined the 2006 Supplemental Victimization Survey and found that the proportion of male targets increased from 13.8% to 33.1% when fear was removed from the definition. Consequently, gender differences in adult stalking prevalence rates may be exacerbated by the definitions used in individual studies.

The type of relationship between the target and perpetrator may also contribute to gender differences in stalking prevalence rates. For example, results from the 2010 National Intimate Partner and Sexual Violence Survey indicate that 61.5% of female targets were stalked by a current or former intimate partner compared to 42.4% of male targets. In contrast, 26.1% of female targets were stalked by an acquaintance (such as a friend or neighbour) compared to 37.2% of male targets (Smith et al. 2017). Given that approximately 50% of stalking cases involve a current or former intimate partner (Logan 2010), it is unsurprising that women are significantly more likely to be targets of adult stalking.

Target and Perpetrator Characteristics

Amongst adults, targets of stalking are significantly more likely to be female than male (Smith et al. 2017). Female targets are most likely to be stalked by a male perpetrator, whereas male targets are equally likely to be stalked by a male or female perpetrator (Baum et al. 2009; Smith et al. 2017). Stalking victimisation rates are highest amongst young adults (aged 18–30 years), with the risk of stalking decreasing with age (Baum et al. 2009; Budd et al. 2000; Purcell et al. 2002). Marital status is a risk factor for stalking as individuals who are divorced or separated are at the highest risk of stalking (Baum et al. 2009), which accounts for why stalking by intimate and ex-intimate partners comprises approximately half of all adult stalking cases. The relationship between ethnicity and stalking victimisation is less clear, with consistent patterns yet to be identified. Some national studies in the United States have found no significant differences between victimisation rates amongst black and white individuals, but individuals who are Native American, Hispanic, or multi-racial may be at an increased risk (Baum et al. 2009; Smith et al. 2017).

Most adult stalking perpetrators are male, with research finding that approximately two-thirds are men (Baum et al. 2009; Budd et al. 2000; Purcell et al. 2002). Perpetrators are most likely to be aged between 30 and 40 years (Mullen et al. 1999; Purcell et al. 2002), which means that adult perpetrators are older on average than perpetrators of other types of interpersonal violence. Perpetrators are most likely to target individuals of the same ethnicity (Baum et al. 2009). Female perpetrators are significantly more likely than male perpetrators to stalk targets of the same gender (Mullen et al. 2009).

Findings relating to the characteristics of adolescent stalking targets and perpetrators typically parallel the findings from the adult stalking literature. For example, Fisher et al. (2014) found that adolescent targets are most likely to be female and adolescent perpetrators are most likely to be male. In Australia, Purcell et al. (2009) examined 299 applications for a restraining order against an adolescent perpetrator and found that 69% of applications involved a female target and 64% a male perpetrator. Adolescents who have had a relationship may be at an increased risk of stalking, especially if the adolescent is in multiple relationships simultaneously (Fisher et al. 2014). Adolescent perpetrators tend to target other adolescents (Fisher et al. 2014; Purcell et al. 2009). Non-white adolescents may be at a greater risk of stalking victimisation and perpetration than white adolescents, but to date only Fisher et al. (2014) have examined the relationship between ethnicity and stalking amongst adolescents. Unlike adult stalking, a majority of adolescent stalking cases involve same-gender stalking (Purcell et al. 2009, 2010), with female adolescent perpetrators being more likely than male adolescent perpetrators to engage in same-gender stalking (Purcell et al. 2010).

Several attempts have been made in the literature to develop a typology of adult stalking perpetrators. The most referenced typology was proposed by Mullen et al. (1999) who, based on their examination of 145 perpetrators (115 males) referred for treatment at a forensic psychiatry centre, developed five sub-types of stalking perpetrators. The *rejected stalker* typically engages in stalking following the breakdown of their relationship with the target and is motivated by a desire to reconcile the relationship and/or enact revenge. The *intimacy seeker* wants to develop an intimate and loving relationship with the target, despite the target not reciprocating this desire. The *incompetent suitor* typically wants to develop a short-term sexual relationship but is unable to achieve this due to intellectual limitations and limited social skills. The *resentful stalker* pursues their target following a perceived wrongdoing and aims to scare the target, and the *predatory stalker* stalks their target in preparation for a physical and/or sexual attack.

Prior Relationship

Most perpetrators are previously known to the target, with stranger stalking accounting for only 9–17% of adult stalking cases (Baum et al. 2009; Smith et al. 2017). In cases of stranger stalking, the perpetrator is more likely to be male (Meloy and Boyd 2003; Purcell et al. 2001). Irrespective of gender, targets are most likely to be stalked by a current or former intimate partner, followed by an acquaintance (e.g., co-worker, neighbour), a stranger, a family member, and finally an authoritative figure (e.g., manager, doctor; Smith et al. 2017). Female targets are significantly more likely than male targets to be stalked by a current or former intimate partner. Conversely, male targets are significantly more likely than female targets to be stalked by an acquaintance (Smith et al. 2017).

In most cases of adolescent stalking, the target and perpetrator are known to one another; only 2% of the restraining order applications in Purcell et al.'s (2009) study involved a stranger. Irrespective of gender, adolescent targets are more likely to be stalked by a friend or acquaintance rather than a current or former intimate partner (Fisher et al. 2014; Purcell et al. 2009), the latter being the most likely prior relationship amongst adult targets and perpetrators. This finding most likely reflects differences between adult and adolescent intimate relationships, as adolescents tend to engage in multiple casual relationships and, by virtue of their age, have had limited opportunities to develop long-term romantic relationships (Collins et al. 2008). In adolescent cases involving an ex-intimate partner, the perpetrator is more likely to be male (Purcell et al. 2010).

Stalking Behaviours

Perpetrators engage in a range of behaviours when stalking their target. It is noteworthy that many of those behaviours, when considered in isolation, are not illegal. For example, sending gifts to an individual you are romantically interested in or sending messages to a recent ex-intimate partner can be considered normative relationship pursuit and break-up resolution behaviours. However, it is the repetition and persistence of the behaviour against the will of the target, which causes fear, that transforms the conduct from socially acceptable to criminal.

For both male and female adult perpetrators, the most used stalking behaviour is unwanted communication via methods such as telephone calls, letters, emails, and gifts (Baum et al. 2009) and more recently social media (Dressing et al. 2014). Surveillance tactics are also frequently used, which can involve the perpetrator following or spying on the target and loitering outside of the target's home or work address (Baum et al. 2009; Smith et al. 2017). Other behaviours that may be used are threats, property damage, and physical or sexual violence. For example, Baum et al. (2009) found that 43.3% of stalking targets were threatened by the perpetrator, 24.4% had their property damaged, and 21% were physically attacked. Perpetrators may also engage in stalking by proxy, which occurs when the perpetrator uses another person (who may or may not be aware of the stalking) to contact or follow the target (Mullen et al. 2009). Approximately 50% of cases involving an intimate or ex-intimate partner include stalking by proxy (Logan 2010). Many of the behaviours described above are now occurring online: for example, perpetrators can contact their target privately and publicly on social media; post information, images, or defamatory comments about the targets online; and hack the target's devices (Dressing et al. 2014).

While the stalking behaviours outlined above are used by both male and female perpetrators, research suggests that female perpetrators prefer more indirect stalking behaviours (e.g., telephone calls and letters) whereas male perpetrators engage in more direct behaviours such as in-person contact and following (Meloy et al. 2011; Purcell et al. 2001). Arguably, the direct tactics favoured by male perpetrators are more frightening, which may account for why female targets (whose perpetrators are overwhelmingly male) report more fear (Lyndon et al. 2012).

Adolescent perpetrators typically engage in the same stalking behaviours as adult perpetrators, with research identifying unwanted communication, surveillance tactics, and cyberstalking behaviours in cases of adolescent stalking (Fisher et al. 2014; Purcell et al. 2009, 2010). Adolescent perpetrators commonly use threats and physical violence; Purcell et al. (2009) found that, of the 299 restraining order application cases, 75% involved a threat to the target, 15% a threat to another person (e.g., a family member), and approximately 50% physical violence. While the findings of Purcell et al. (2009) initially indicate that adolescent stalking involves higher rates of threats and violence compared to adults, the findings may reflect the sample examined, as all 299 cases of adolescent stalking were deemed 'serious' enough to warrant court involvement. Stalking by proxy was identified in 30% of the adolescent stalking cases examined by Purcell et al. (2009).

Male adolescent perpetrators are significantly more likely than female perpetrators to attend and loiter outside of the target's home, school, or workplace, whereas female adolescent perpetrators are more likely to use telephone calls and to spread malicious rumours (Fisher et al. 2014; Purcell et al. 2009, 2010). This gender difference in stalking behaviours amongst adolescent perpetrators mirrors research from the adult stalking literature as, amongst adult perpetrators, males tend to engage in direct stalking behaviours and females favour more indirect behaviours. Female adolescent perpetrators are significantly more likely to use stalking by proxy (Purcell et al. 2010), which may reflect female adolescent perpetrator's preferences for indirect stalking behaviours. Purcell et al. (2010) found no significant differences between male and female adolescent perpetrators' use of threats and violence, but male adolescents were more likely to inflict property damage.

Impacts of Stalking

Stalking can have profound consequences for targets. *Psychologically*, targets are at an increased risk of developing anxiety, depression, and post-traumatic stress symptoms; *physically*, targets can develop somatic symptoms, such as digestive problems and extreme tiredness, and are also at an increased risk of violence resulting in injury or death; *socially*, targets may become isolated from their family and friends, and interpersonal relationships may be disrupted; and *financially*, targets may lose money due to time taken off work (e.g., to attend court) or because of costs incurred when attempting to escape the perpetrator (Diette et al. 2014; Dressing et al. 2005; Pathé and Mullen 1997; Purcell et al. 2002). Stalking can also have significant personal impacts on targets, with many targets having to make lifestyle changes in an attempt to deter the perpetrator (Dressing et al. 2005; Pathé and Mullen 1997). For example, targets may move home, workplace, or school and may change their telephone number. Targets often report that they modify their routines and avoid places where the perpetrator is likely to be present; some targets even report taking circuitous routes when driving to minimise the risk of being followed (Pathé and Mullen 1997). Beyond making lifestyle changes, targets may implement additional safety measures, such as alarm systems and self-defence training (Purcell et al. 2002). Stalking can also impact the families of targets, as family members may be threatened or targeted by the perpetrator themselves or may experience emotional and psychological trauma due to concern for their loved one (Morewitz 2003; see Box 2 for an example of the significant impact of stalking on targets and their families).

Both male and female targets are significantly and adversely affected by their experiences of stalking, but the consequences for women may be greater. Female targets typically report greater psychological disturbance and post-traumatic stress symptoms compared to male targets and are also more likely to be assaulted by their perpetrator (Logan and Walker 2019). Women report greater levels of fear resulting from stalking and are more likely than men to make lifestyle changes (Logan and Walker 2019). Most importantly, women are at a greater risk of homicide following stalking than men, particularly in cases where the perpetrator is a current or former intimate partner (Logan and Walker 2010).

Our understanding of the impacts of stalking on adolescent targets is limited. In their study of restraining order applications, Purcell et al. (2009) examined victim impact statements and identified several significant consequences of stalking. Adolescent targets frequently reported experiencing pervasive anxiety and fear of the perpetrator, and 11% of targets reported severe depression and suicide ideation. Stalking impacted adolescents' education, with targets reporting difficulties concentrating in lessons, especially if the perpetrator was another student, and would miss days of school to avoid the perpetrator. Difficulties with concentration and absenteeism likely contributed to the decline in school performance reported by some targets. Parents of targets were also impacted by the stalking, with some parents reporting that they had begun accompanying their child to and from school out of concern for their child's safety. Parents also reported that they had changed their child's school and home address at a substantial financial cost in 5% of cases.

Box 2 Case Study: Hollie's Story

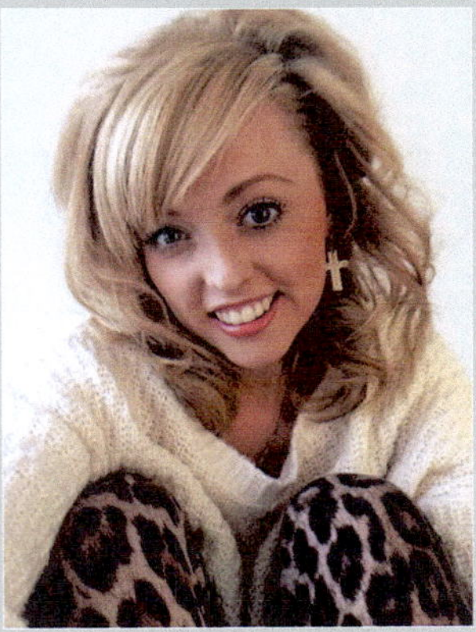

Hollie Gazzard was 19 years old when she began dating Asher Maslin, a confident and charming 21-year-old she had met at a bar in Gloucester, UK in early 2013. The relationship started strong, and Hollie seemed happy with Maslin. He initially appeared to be polite and respectful towards Hollie, but his behaviour soon changed and became increasingly controlling and abusive. Maslin would bombard Hollie with calls and texts and would want to know where Hollie was at all times. He would turn up unexpectedly when Hollie was with her friends and would make negative comments to Hollie in public, including in front of Hollie's family. When Hollie and Maslin moved to London in May 2013 to pursue a hairdressing job, Maslin continued to control Hollie and tried to isolate her from friends and family. His behaviour escalated to physical violence and in August he assaulted Hollie publicly at the Notting Hill Carnival because she did not answer his call when they had become separated in the crowd. After this incident, Hollie left the job she loved to return home and escape Maslin, but he quickly followed Hollie back to Gloucester to resume their relationship. He frequently messaged and called Hollie and would show up at Hollie's home and workplace. Hollie became quiet and withdrawn. In late 2013, after almost a year of physical abuse and coercive and controlling behaviour, Hollie decided she no longer wanted to be with Maslin. On 14 February 2014, Hollie ended their relationship. Maslin was furious and inundated Hollie with messages threatening her and her family and stole money from Hollie's bank account. Maslin's behaviour prompted Hollie to report him to the police. Several days later, on 18 February 2014, Maslin violently attacked Hollie while she was at work with a knife, stabbing her 14 times. Hollie sadly died from her injuries.

The impact of Hollie's death has been profound, but Hollie's family and friends have been determined to create something positive out of their loss. Hollie's family have started a charity in her memory, The Hollie Gazzard Trust. Through the Trust, Hollie's family aim to reduce domestic violence and raise awareness of stalking through a number of projects in the community.

Target Help-Seeking

Targets can seek support from various sources, including their friends and family, the police, and medical or legal professionals (Baum et al. 2009; Purcell et al. 2002). Female targets are more likely to seek support from informal sources (e.g., friends and family) than male targets (Purcell et al. 2002; Reyns and Englebrecht 2014). This could be because female targets typically experience more stalking-related fear, which is a significant predictor of informal help-seeking amongst stalking targets (Reyns and Englebrecht 2014). Male and female targets are equally likely to report their victimisation to the police (Baum et al. 2009; Reyns and Englebrecht 2014). Adolescent target help-seeking is yet to be explored.

Implications and Future Directions

Throughout this chapter, research from the adult and adolescent stalking literature has been discussed and several notable gender differences have been identified. Although both men and women can be targets and perpetrators of stalking, it is clear that the risk of victimisation is significantly higher for women and that men are significantly more likely to be perpetrators. Female targets experience more stalking-related fear than male targets and also report greater levels of anxiety, depression, and post-traumatic stress symptoms. Female targets are more likely to make lifestyle changes and to take safety precautions following victimisation. Furthermore, female targets are more likely to be assaulted by perpetrators and are at a higher risk of homicide than male targets. For these reasons, it is argued that stalking can and should be considered a form of gender-based violence.

The identification of stalking as a form of gender-based violence does not minimise male victimisation and female perpetration or the experiences of male targets; it simply acknowledges the gendered nature of stalking. By taking a gendered approach within research, an understanding of the similarities and differences between male and female targets can be increased and subsequently our responses to targets can be enhanced. For example, a greater understanding of the detrimental impacts that stalking can have on male and female targets, as well as gender differences in help-seeking, can contribute to the development of appropriate risk assessments, safety plans, and support services for both men and women. Professionals who work with stalking perpetrators should also consider gender when conducting risk assessments to ensure that the different risk factors for male and female perpetrators are understood and managed appropriately. Future research must therefore consider taking a gendered approach when examining stalking.

Additionally, future research should examine existing stalking definitions and attempts should be made to reconcile the different definitions used across studies. The development of a single, unified stalking definition will enable researchers to better capture the nature and extent of the issue. Research should also examine measures of stalking victimisation, particularly amongst male targets. As men are less likely than women to report feeling afraid of stalking behaviours, research should consider reframing how men are asked about fear. For example, men may need to be asked if the stalking behaviours have caused them concern instead.

Finally, it is evident from this chapter that our understanding of adolescent stalking is limited. Future research should therefore further examine adolescent stalking, such as the prevalence rates and risk factors for adolescent stalking perpetration. An increased understanding of adolescent stalking perpetration, as well as the similarities and differences between adolescent and adult perpetrators, would contribute to the development of risk assessments and interventions for use with adolescents. It is vital that future research also considers the impacts of stalking on adolescent targets, particularly its long-term impacts. Given that adolescence is a critical stage of psychosocial and physical development (Christie and Viner 2005), it is possible that stalking during adolescence could have greater and longer-lasting consequences than stalking during adulthood. By examining the short- and long-term effects of stalking on adolescent targets, interventions and support services can be developed and tailored appropriately.

Summary

- There is no universally agreed definition of stalking, but most definitions include a persistent pattern of unwanted behaviours that causes fear of distress for targets.
- Different stalking definitions have implications for our understanding of the extent of stalking, as well as practical implications for targets.

- Stalking is a prevalent social issue affecting both men and women and occurs across a range of relationship types.
- Women are significantly more likely to be targets of stalking than men, and the impact is found to be greater.
- Men are significantly more likely to be perpetrators of stalking, and there are some gender differences in the stalking behaviours used by male and female perpetrators.
- Adolescent stalking may be more prevalent than stalking amongst adults, and there are similarities and differences between the adolescent and adult stalking literature.
- Stalking should be considered a form of gender-based violence, and a gendered approach should be considered in future research.

References

Baum K, Catalano S, Rand M, Rose K (2009) Stalking victimization in the United States. Bureau of Justice Statistics. https://www.justice.gov/sites/default/files/ovw/legacy/2012/08/15/bjs-stalking-rpt.pdf. Accessed 25 Feb 2021

Black MC, Basile KC, Breidig MJ, Smith SG, Walters ML, Merrick MT, Chen J, Stevens MR (2011) The National Intimate Partner and sexual violence survey (NISVS): 2010 summary report. National Center for Injury Prevention and Control, Centers for Disease Control and Prevention. https://www.cdc.gov/violenceprevention/pdf/nisvs_report2010-a.pdf. Accessed 15 Mar 2021

Budd T, Mattison J, Myhill A (2000) The extent and nature of stalking: findings from the 1998 British crime survey. Home Office Research, Development and Statistics Directorate. https://citeseerx.ist.psu.edu/viewdoc/download?doi=10.1.1.192.5164&rep=rep1&type=pdf. Accessed 28 Feb 2021

Christie D, Viner R (2005) Adolescent development. BMJ 330(7486):301–304. https://doi.org/10.1136/bmj.330.7486.301

Coleman FL (1997) Stalking behaviour and the cycle of domestic violence. J Interpers Violence 12(3):420–432. https://doi.org/10.1177/088626097012003007

Collins WA, Welsh DP, Furman W (2008) Adolescent romantic relationships. Annu Rev Psychol 60:631–652. https://doi.org/10.1146/annurev.psych.60.110707.163459

Diette TM, Goldsmith AH, Hamilton D, Darity W Jr, McFarland K (2014) Stalking: does it leave a psychological footprint? Soc Sci Q 95(2):563–580. https://doi.org/10.1111/ssqu.12058

Dressing H, Kuehner C, Gass P (2005) Lifetime prevalence and impact of stalking in a European population: epidemiological data from a middle-sized German city. Br J Psychiatry 187(2):168–172. https://doi.org/10.1192/bjp.187.2.186

Dressing H, Bailer J, Anders A, Wagner H, Gallas C (2014) Cyberstalking in a large sample of social network users: prevalence, characteristics, and impact upon victims. Cyberpsychol Behav Soc Netw 17(2):61–67. https://doi.org/10.1089/cyber.2012.0231

Dressing H, Gass P, Schultz K, Kuehner C (2020) The prevalence and effects of stalking: a replication study. Deutsch Arzteballt Int 117(20):347–353. https://doi.org/10.3238/arztebl.2020.0347

Fisher BS, Coker AL, Garcia LS, Williams CM, Clear ER, Cook-Craig PG (2014) Statewide estimates of stalking among high school students in Kentucky: demographic profile and sex differences. Violence Against Women 20(10):1258–1279. https://doi.org/10.1177/1077801214551574

Logan TK (2010) Research on partner stalking: putting the pieces together. https://www.ojp.gov/pdffiles1/nij/245387.pdf. Accessed 19 May 2021

Logan TK, Walker R (2010) Toward a deeper understanding of the harms caused by partner stalking. Violence Vict 25(4):440–455. https://doi.org/10.1891/0886-6708.25.4.440

Logan TK, Walker R (2019) The impact of stalking-related fear and gender on personal safety outcomes. J Interpers Violence 36:1–23. https://doi.org/10.1177/0886260519829280

Lowney KS, Best J (1995) Stalking strangers and lovers: changing media typifications of a new crime problem. In: Best J (ed) Images of issues: typifying contemporary social problems, 2nd edn. Routledge, New York, pp 33–58

Lyndon AE, Sinclair HC, Ratajack E (2012) An introduction to issues of gender in stalking research. Sex Roles 66(5–6):299–310. https://doi.org/10.1007/s11199-011-0106-2

Meloy JR, Boyd C (2003) Female stalkers and their victims. J Am Acad Psychiatry Law 31(2):211–219

Meloy JR, Mohandie K, Green M (2011) The female stalker. Behav Sci Law 31:211–219. https://doi.org/10.1002/bsl.976

Melton HC (2000) Stalking: a review of the literature and direction for the future. Crim Justice Rev 25(2):246–262. https://doi.org/10.1177/073401680002500206

Melton HC (2007) Closing in: stalking in the context of intimate partner abuse. Sociol Compass 1(2):520–535. https://doi.org/10.1111/j.1751-9020.2007.00046.X

Miller L (2012) Stalking: patterns, motives, and intervention strategies. Aggress Violent Behav 17(6):495–506. https://doi.org/10.1016/j.avb.2012.07.001

Morewitz SJ (2003) Stalking and violence: new patterns of trauma and obsession. Kluwer Academic, New York

Mullen PE, Pathé M, Purcell R, Stuart GW (1999) Study of stalkers. Am J Psychiatry 156(8):1244–1249. https://doi.org/10.1176/ajp.156.8.1244

Mullen PE, Pathé M, Purcell R (2009) Stalkers and their victims, 2nd edn. Cambridge University Press, Cambridge

Office for National Statistics (2020) Stalking: findings from the crime survey for England and Wales. Office for National Statistics. https://www.ons.gov.uk/peoplepopulationandcommunity/crimeandjustice/datasets/stalkingfindingsfromthecrimesurveyforenglandandwales. Accessed 16 Apr 2021

Owens JG (2016) Why definitions matter: stalking victimization in the United States. J Interpers Violence 31(12):2196–2226. https://doi.org/10.1177/0886260515573577

Owens JG (2017) A gender-biased definition: unintended impacts of the fear requirement in stalking victimization. Crime Delinq 63(11):1339–1362. https://doi.org/10.1177/0011128715615883

Pathé M, Mullen PE (1997) The impact of stalkers on their victims. Br J Psychiatry 170(1):12–17. https://doi.org/10.1192/bjp.170.1.12

Purcell R, Pathé M, Mullen PE (2001) A study of women who stalk. Am J Psychiatry 158:2056–2060. https://doi.org/10.1176/appi.ajp.158.12.2056

Purcell R, Pathe M, Mullen PE (2002) The prevalence and nature of stalking in the Australian community. Aust N Z J Psychiatry 36(1):114–120. https://doi.org/10.1046/j.1440-1614.2002.00985.x

Purcell R, Moller B, Flower T, Mullen PE (2009) Stalking among juveniles. Br J Psychiatry 194:451–455. https://doi.org/10.1192/bjp.bp.108.054833

Purcell R, Pathé M, Mullen P (2010) Gender differences in stalking behaviour among juveniles. J Forensic Psychiatry Psychol 21(4):555–568. https://doi.org/10.1080/14789940903572035

Reyns BW, Englebrecht CM (2014) Informal and formal help-seeking decisions of stalking victims in the United States. Crim Justice Behav 41(10):1178–1194. https://doi.org/10.1177/0093854814541441

Smith SG, Chen J, Basile KC, Gilbert LK, Merrick MT, Patel N, Walling M, Jain A (2017) The National Intimate Partner and sexual violence survey (NISVS): 2010-2012 state report. National Center for Injury Prevention and Control, Centers for Disease Control and Prevention. https://www.cdc.gov/violenceprevention/pdf/nisvs-statereportbook.pdf. Accessed 25 Feb 2021

Whyte S, Penny C, Christopherson S, Reiss D, Petch E (2011) The stalking of psychiatrists. Int J Forensic Ment Health 10(3):254–260. https://doi.org/10.1080/14999013.2011.599097

Abby Hare is a Forensic Psychology PhD student at the University of Kent. Her research focuses on stalking and harassment behaviours amongst young people, with a particular focus on stalking amongst adolescents.

Jennifer E. Storey, PhD, and HCPC Registered Forensic Psychologist, is a Lecturer in Forensic Psychology in the School of Psychology at the University of Kent. Her research examines interpersonal violence with a focus on older adult abuse (or elder abuse), stalking and intimate partner violence.

Afroditi Pina, PhD, (University of Kent) is a Senior Lecturer in Forensic Psychology and a member of the Centre for Research and Education in Forensic Psychology (CORE-FP) at Kent. She is also the Chair of the University of Kent Harassment Contacts Network. Her research focuses on sexual violence, victimisation and gender equality more broadly. Specifically she conducts and supervises research on sexual and intimate partner abuse and harassment and stalking. Of particular interest to Afroditi is the intersection of the internet and technology with abuse such as Image Based Abuse and Technology-facilitated Intimate Partner Abuse, online hate speech and Trolling.

Femicide

Parveen Ali and Michaela M. Rogers

Learning Objectives
Having read this chapter, you should be able to understand:

- What is femicide and where is it practiced.
- The impact of femicide on victims and others.
- The complexity of femicide and its impact on children whose mothers are murdered.
- Risk factors associated with femicide.
- The Implications for future research, policy and practice.

Introduction

Every day hundreds of women become victims of femicide in many different scenarios and circumstances across the globe. They may be killed by their intimate partners, family members or others in the context of domestic violence and abuse (DVA), intimate partner violence (IPV), family violence, honour-based violence, dowry-related violence and or any other form of violence against women. Women are also killed in armed conflicts and wars because they belong to the opposite group and because they are women. Every day, thousands of girls and women also become victims of female infanticide, sex-selected foeticide, genital mutilation-related

P. Ali (✉)
The Health Sciences School, University of Sheffield, Sheffield, UK
e-mail: parveen.ali@sheffield.ac.uk

M. M. Rogers
Department of Sociological Studies, University of Sheffield, Sheffield, UK
e-mail: m.rogers@sheffield.ac.uk

P. Ali, M. M. Rogers (eds.), *Gender-Based Violence: A Comprehensive Guide*,
https://doi.org/10.1007/978-3-031-05640-6_11

femicide, femicide connected with gangs, organized crime, drug dealing, human trafficking and the proliferation of small arms (Laurent et al. 2013; Eklund and Purewal 2017).

This chapter provides an overview of femicide, starting with a critical discussion of the contested nature of definitions and terminology. It also highlights the diversity of practices that can be classed as femicide. Although rates of femicide are notoriously difficult to establish due to variations in definitions, methodologies, reporting and recording, some data on prevalence is offered to illustrate the widespread nature of this pernicious crime. While the range of diverse acts considered to be femicide is under-researched, so are the impacts on children; the *hidden victims of femicide*. Therefore, attention is paid to the intersection of femicide and children's experiences to highlight the extensive and long-term consequences when mothers are murdered. The chapter ends with some discussion of risk factors and risk management before advocating for future research into femicide, which is needed to inform policy and practice.

Definitions and Terminology

Killing or murdering women and/or girls simply because of their gender is termed as femicide (Weil and Kouta 2017). Russell (2011) extended this understanding to include the distinction that in cases of femicide it is primarily men who are killing women and girls. However, femicide can be perpetrated by anyone including strangers or family members such as father, brothers, mother, sisters and other family members albeit a large majority of murdered women are killed by their current or former intimate partner. Regardless of the context, women are killed in various situations because of hate against women (misogyny), because women are considered less valuable in a patriarchal world and because they are less able to defend themselves. In this way, femicide is a misogynistic practice that can be understood within a broader feminist political framework (Grzyb and Hernandez 2015). There are serval definitions provided for various terms related to femicide and these are shown in Box 1.

Box 1 Definitions and Alternative Terminology

Definitions

Femicide: The intentional killing or murdering women and/or girls simply because they are female.

Femicide: The killing of females by males because they are female.

Femicide: The intentional killing of females by men and of females by other females in the interests of men.

Racist femicide: The racially motivated killing of women by men of a different race.

Serial femicide: The sexually sadistic killing of women.

Female infanticide: The killing of female infants.

Alternative terms

Feminicide, lethal killing of women, female homicide, female homicide victimization, gendercide, manslaughter, honour killings, wife murder, uxoricide.

Associated terms

Intimate femicide, intimate partner femicide, intimate partner homicide, romantic femicide.

Femicide has been defined using gender neutral or male-centred terminology, including 'lethal killings of women', 'female homicide', 'female homicide victimization' and 'manslaughter'. When conducted in the context of DVA, femicide is described as 'honour killings', 'wife murders' or 'uxoricide'. Use of gender-neutral terms takes the attention away from the gendered nature of this crime (Weil 2018). Box 2 provides a summary of various acts classed as femicide, which are described in the existing literature.

Box 2 Different Types of and Contexts for Femicide

- Killing of women because of DVA/ IPV.
- Torture and misogynist slaying of women.
- Killing of girls and women in the name of 'honour'.
- Killing of women and girls in the context of armed conflict.
- Dowry-related killings.
- Killing of women and girls because of their sexual orientation and gender identity.
- Killing of aboriginal and indigenous women and girls.
- Female infanticide.
- Sex selection foeticide.
- Genital mutilation-related femicide.
- Accusations of witchcraft.
- Femicide connected with gangs, organized crime, drug dealers, human trafficking and the proliferation of small arms.

Prevalence

Available evidence suggests that perpetrators of most women murdered are someone they know, often their husband or intimate partner. This is exemplified by the fact that 58% of the 87,000 women killed intentionally in 2017 were killed by their intimate partners or family members. This means that 137 women across the world are killed by a member of their own family every day. Among these, more than a third (30,000) were killed by their current or former intimate partner

(United Nations Office on Drugs and Crime 2019). An examination from media and Internet sources of every single murder of an elderly woman committed between 2006 and 2015 revealed that all the cases in Israel were exclusively intimate partner femicides (Campbell et al. 2003). About 67% of the women killed by their partners are killed with a gun, which suggests that access to guns plays an important role (Campbell et al. 2003). It recognised that women could also be perpetrators of femicide, either as lesbian partners or kin; however, the phenomenon is rare. According to available data, the largest number (20,000) of all women killed worldwide was in Asia, followed by Africa (19,000), the Americas (8000), Europe (3000) and Oceania (300). Evidence from Europe suggests an average annual rate of 0.4 victims of femicide for every 100,000 women. Countries including Montenegro, Lithuania and Latvia appear to be worst in this regard. The perpetrator usually is a partner; however, in some countries such as Lithuania and Bosnia and Herzegovina, most femicides are committed by family members. From 2013 to 2017, 30 European countries joined a COST (Cooperation on Science and Technology) project called 'Femicide across Europe' (see Fig. 1, which depicts femicide rates across Europe).

While research on DVA and other forms of gender-based violence is increasing, evidence related to femicide is still scarce. However, femicide appears to affect women in all parts of the world. In particular, during the COVID-19 pandemic, the

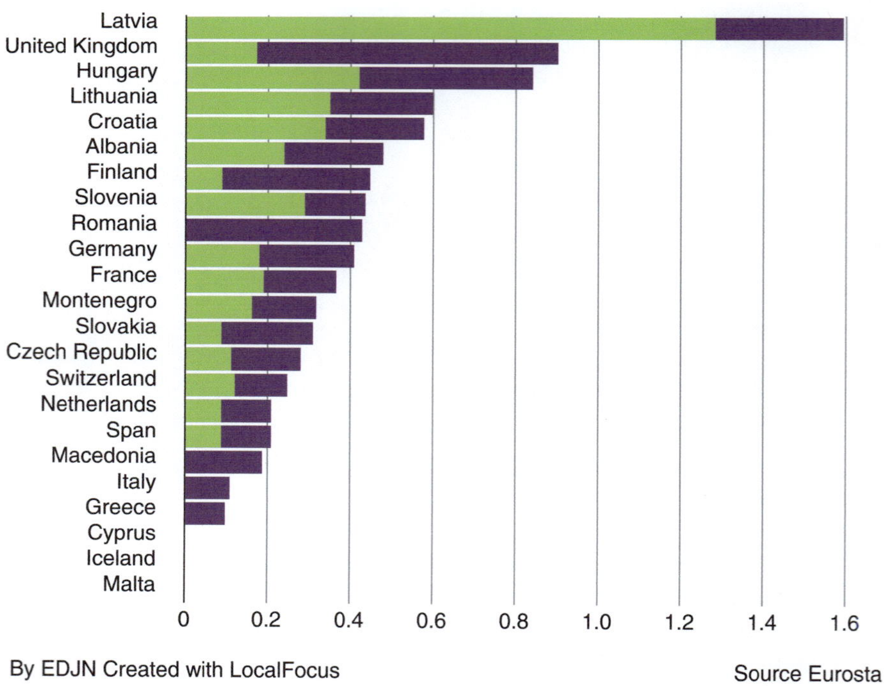

Fig. 1 Femicide in Europe (2019) 2 years later. (Adapted from https://www.balcanicaucaso.org/aree/Europa/Femminicidio-in-Europa-due-anni-dopo)

rate of femicides has drastically increased and around 50,000 women are being murdered every year (Weil 2020). This is because the stay-at-home measures increased the levels of isolation for women and girls. While there is no systematic data gathered on femicide during COVID-19, there are a few empirical reports available. For instance, in Spain, there were 18 femicide fatalities from the beginning of 2020 till mid-March 2020 (Weil 2020). In Argentina, 86 femicides have been perpetrated since the beginning of 2020. In Turkey, 18 women have been killed since the lockdown. In the United Kingdom, nearly three times as many women were murdered in March 2020 by men.

Impacts on Families

Femicide not only results in the killing of a girl or a woman but also destroys the lives of their family members including parents. When femicide involves women with children, the impact on their children is considerable, as they lose their mother. In some instances, children are also killed by their father and other family members. If children survive, they not only lose their mother, but may also lose their father because of imprisonment or suicide. However, very little research is available on this most vulnerable, but overlooked population who experience the most drastic and lifelong impact of the loss of their prime caregiver (Weil 2018). A study conducted in Italy found 1600 children of women murdered between 2001 and 2016; among them, 84% were aged 18 or under, 40% of them had witnessed the killing and 44% saw their mother's dead body (Ferrara et al. 2018). Twenty percent of the children also lost their father who killed themselves after killing children's mother. The authors highlighted that research involving children who lost their mother through femicide is extremely limited (Weil 2018). Box 3 details the high-profile murder of Nicole Brown Simpson.

Another study conducted in the Netherlands identified all children bereaved by parental intimate partner homicide and described demographics and family circumstances and assessed their prior exposure to violence at home and to the homicide itself. Findings revealed that during 2003–2012, 256 children lost one of their parents (87.1% lost their mother) due to 137 cases of intimate partner homicide (Alisic et al. 2017). On average, the children were 7.4 years old at the time of the homicide (51.1% were boys) and most of them were immigrants (59.4%). The majority (84.4%) of children were exposed to previous violence at home. Most of these children had not received any social services or mental health care. Findings also suggest that most of the children (58.7%) were present at the location when the killing took place, with varying levels of exposure. Further research is essential to understand this important issue, so appropriate support mechanisms and services can be developed for orphan children of women victims of femicide to support them in overcoming the impact of witnessing/experiencing abuse in the family and the killing of their mother (Alisic et al. 2017; Ferrara et al. 2018).

Box 3 The Killing of Nicole Brown Simpson

On the evening of 12 June 1994, US professional football legend O.J. Simpson attended his daughter's dance recital as did his ex-wife, Nicole Brown Simpson. Afterwards, Brown Simpson had dinner with family and friends at Mezzaluna restaurant where waiter Ronald Goldman worked. While there, Brown Simpson's mother forgot her glasses. Goldman volunteered to drop them off at Brown Simpson's house.

Later that night, Brown Simpson's dog, a white Akita, was discovered by a neighbour walking in the neighbourhood by itself and with bloody paws. Just after midnight, the dog led to the discovery of the bloodied bodies of Brown Simpson and Goldman outside her home. The first police officer to arrive at the scene on 13 June 1994 described the master bathroom as being lit with candles. The bathtub was full, the television was on, a cup of half-melted ice cream was on the downstairs banister and her children were asleep in their rooms.

Brown Simpson, aged 34 years, was found brutally murdered on the sidewalk outside her home, stabbed 12 times, along with her friend, Ron Goldman, aged 25, who was stabbed 25 times. The story exploded quickly as Brown Simpson was identified as the ex-wife of legendary professional football player O.J. Simpson. On 13 June, police went to O.J.'s house while he was returning from Chicago and found a trail of blood from his vehicle to the front door and a bloody glove matching one found by Goldman's body. He had agreed to turn himself in but then fled on June 17. Millions of TV viewers watched as Simpson led police on a low-speed chase in his white Ford Bronco. According to anecdotal evidence, Simpson was carrying his passport, a disguise and $8750 in cash. Eventually, Simpson gave himself up. He was charged with two counts of murder.

O.J.'s preliminary hearing lasted 8 days, 30 June to 8 July. The municipal judge found there was enough evidence for him to be put on trial. There was extensive evidence linking Simpson to the crime: his blood was found at the murder scene; blood, hair and fibres from Brown Simpson and Goldman were found in Simpson's car and at his home; one of his gloves was also found in Brown's home, the other outside his own house; and bloody shoeprints found at the scene matched those of shoes owned by Simpson.

Simpson was defended at trial by infamous lawyers, Johnnie Cochran and F. Lee Bailey. They claimed Simpson was framed by racist police officers. After an 8-month trial and 3 hours of deliberation, Simpson was acquitted on 3 October 1995. In later years, the Brown and Goldman families sued Simpson. He was found liable for damages for the wrongful death of Goldman and battery of Brown. A $33.5 million civil judgment was lodged against O.J. On 3 October 2008, he was found guilty and sentenced to 33 years in prison. He was released from prison in 2017.

Following Brown Simpson's death, her children, Sydney and Justin, who were just 8 and 5 years old at the time of the killing, went to live with their maternal grandparents. However, 2 years later, a family court judge ended this temporary guardianship and restored O. J. Simpson's full custody of the young children despite his being on trial in the wrongful death suit.

The ruling was of no surprise as it reflected the overwhelming tendency in California's custody proceedings to award children to their biological parents. However, Sydney and Justin's grandparents were open about their concerns as their lawyer, Natasha Roit, released the following statement: 'we love Sydney and Justin and pray for their safety and well-being as they return to their father'. Asked whether she thought the children were being exposed to risk, Roit said, 'absolutely'. However, the judge refused to allow the consideration of allegations about the killing of Brown Simpson and Goldman to be considered. Roit had argued that Simpson's record of spousal abuse alone made him an unfit parent. The judge noted that there was no evidence O.J. Simpson had ever abused his children. The children grew up to live away from the glare of public scrutiny.

Children of Murdered Women: The Hidden Victims of Femicide

As noted, the children of murdered women are a neglected group and not much is known about their demographics; they are hidden victims in the context of femicide. The impact on children depends on their age, level of understanding, attachment with parents, experience of the situation (if they have seen domestic abuse or saw the murder of their mother) and availability of support by health and social care systems, family members and others. Children may develop post-traumatic stress disorder (PTSD) and other psychosomatic symptoms such as enuresis (involuntary urination at night), encopresis (soiling of underwear with stool by children who are past the age of toilet training), sleep disturbance, behaviour problems, anger, tantrums, passive and aggressive behaviours, flashbacks, dissociation, anxiety and depression. Box 4 offers a reflective account highlighting the impact on a child whose mother was killed by her partner in the presence of the child (Naas 2018).

Box 4 Reflections After Femicide: Coping

'When people ask me how I managed, I tell them there were times when I don't think I ever really managed at all. I dropped out of college, I lost my job, I moved around a lot. I tried medication, I tried therapy and, when nothing seemed to work in the way I needed it to, I became extremely desperate for peace. I stopped eating. Days would pass, but I would never feel hungry. Even drinking water became an impossible task. I was convinced that my grief had

a life of its own, that it was growing through my anguish, that it was stronger than the person underneath it all. I tried bargaining with God to bring my mother back. Late at night I would walk down to the alley where she was killed and replay the incident inside my head. I would drive my car around Vallejo every night for months until the sun came up because my grief made me delusional enough to believe that if I just looked hard enough, I would find her again.'

The impacts experienced by the children of a murdered mother with regard to trauma, anger and guilt, guardianship and fulfilment of needs, disruption in routine and environment, and expression of feelings are described below.

Experiencing Trauma

Losing one's mother at any age is traumatising; however, as a child, it is even more traumatic as a mother is a fundamental attachment figure in a child's life. Separation from a mother causes separation anxiety among young children who cannot understand the reason for their mother's absence. The trauma experienced can have a lasting impact on a child's personality and development (Ferrara et al. 2015). In addition, if a child/children witness intimate partner violence between parents or have seen their mother being killed, the impact becomes more dramatic. Surrounding events and stressors can further compound the issue and make coping difficult. For instance, soon after the death of their mother, children may be interviewed by police, social services and other organisations and may be subject to court interventions and welfare decisions (van Nijnatten and van Huizen 2004). They may or may not have an opportunity to understand the situation or ask questions. In fact, they may get discouraged from asking questions contributing to unresolved questions in their mind as voiced in the following quote by a woman who lost both her parents as a child: 'everyone believed they were protecting me, but what goes around in a child's head when they are bereaved needs to be voiced. Otherwise, it can grow into a world of fantasy that is often more terrible than the reality' (Naas 2018).

Anger and Guilt

Anger and guilt are normal emotions that most people experience through their life. However, these feelings and emotions can be more strongly felt by children of murdered women and especially if they have seen the murder of their mother. Such children may have witnessed conflict and abuse, the process of separation and disputes over child contact and residence (Ahmed and Montanez 2019). They may have tried to defend or protect their mother, find help, before and after her death, and may have been left with the dead body of their mother for some time. In addition, some may also witness the suicide of their father. Children exposed to such circumstances may blame themselves for the issues between their parents or for not being able to stop violence or murder as highlighted in Box 5.

Box 5 Reflections after Femicide: Guilt

'*After mama was killed, I was overtaken by guilt: guilt for leaving her that afternoon when perhaps the only thing that would have saved her was my continuing to stand in between her and my father, and guilt for not recognizing that my father could be capable of such extreme violence because his primary method of abuse had always been psychological.*' (Ferrara et al. 2018).

Fulfilment of Needs

Children may lose both parents, are left without a guardian or may end up with surrogate parents. They may be raised by their grandparents or family members, or foster parents who may or not be able to understand or fulfil all their needs depending on their financial condition and other responsibilities (Laurent et al. 2013). Children may be unable to articulate their needs effectively (Tucker 2012). In situations where the perpetrator is given a short-term prison sentence, he may still be able to reclaim access to his children. This then means that children and especially those who are aware of their mother's killing by their father must live with their mother's killer and this would have a considerable impact on their mental health. In the UK, a public discourse is emerging, however, to remove custody rights from femicide perpetrators to prevent them from reconnecting with their children following their release from prison. Argentina and Italy are among the first countries that have adopted laws to protect the rights of such children and remove custody rights from perpetrators. Italy has gone one step ahead and minors who share their family name with the parent convicted of killing the other parent can request to have it changed. When it comes to appointing guardians, the law gives priority to other relatives and family members (Laurent et al. 2013).

Disruption in the Everyday Environment

Losing parents and living with grandparents or other guardians means that children are displaced from their own home and familiar environment. They may be exposed to a different routine and regulations depending on their carers, and this means that children have to adapt to the situation. They may also have to change schools and lose touch with their usual social environment, further complicating the situation (Alisic et al. 2015). Such disruption may also have an impact on children's ability to articulate their needs and may lead to their assumptions about the availability and reliability of a 'new family' (Alisic et al. 2015).

Expressing Feelings

Orphaned children are often raised by their paternal or maternal grandparents and both parties may have very different motivations and factors affecting their ability to raise children (Laurent et al. 2013). For example, maternal grandparents and other family members may be going through grief and bereavement processes themselves and may not like to talk about the perpetrator or they may express hate towards the perpetrator. Likewise, paternal family may experience shame and guilt and a sense of responsibility towards the action of the perpetrator. They may also express a victim-blaming attitude by talking negatively about the victim (the children's mother). This may have an impact on children and their ability to communicate their own feelings about their parents. If living with a maternal family, they may not express love and affection towards their father and anger or resentment towards their mother. Similarly, when living with the father's family, they may not be able to express love and affection towards their mother and anger or resentment towards their father. In both scenarios, children may live with unresolved issues for a long time or for life.

Stigma

In almost every culture, women are often blamed for the abuse they experience. Similarly, murdered women are often blamed for their murder. For instance, in the case of honour killing, a woman is killed because she has done something to dishonour her family and community. Such victim-blaming attitudes also mean that children of the women killed in the name of honour are shunned, stigmatised and made to feel embarrassed and ashamed by the society. They may be taunted and bullied by other children and adults within and outside family or may have to hear negative comments and remarks about their mother. They may find themselves in situations where they must defend their mother. They may also have to experience negative remarks, comments and attitudes because of their father's action of killing their mother. In both ways, the impact on children's physical and mental health could be catastrophic.

Responding to Children Affected by Femicide

It may help them to talk about the issue and to ask questions in a supportive environment; however, they may not get an appropriate response from their carer. They may be pressured not to talk about it, or their version of events is negated, or their questions are ignored (Ferrara and Bernasconi 2017). Such approaches are often used with positive intentions by family members but effectively reduce the opportunities to mourn their loss.

Femicide Risk Factors and Risk Assessment

Risk assessment for femicide is, by necessity, targeted at prevention (Hart 2008). This is predicated on the notion that some femicides are preventable with an assessment and the management of risk factors such as previous history of violence, stalking and other known concerns. Risk assessment relies on the identification of vulnerabilities and dynamic risk factors within the context of the presenting situation, relationship and other relevant information. An assessment of the interactions of these factors and the level of risk can inform the management of risk. Effective risk management must take into account the dynamic nature of vulnerability and risk factors and tools have been developed for this purpose, e.g., SARA (Spousal Assault Risk Assessment) (Kropp and Hart 2000). Such models for assessment are rooted in evidence and empirical research, which have examined risk and risk factors and the correlates of repeat violence, the escalation of violence and killing. Risk factors can be identified using an ecological approach to explore risk at individual, interpersonal, community and social levels (see Table 1).

Table 1 An ecological approach to understanding risk factors for intimate partner femicide (adapted from Baldry and Magalhães 2018)

Category	Risk factor
Perpetrator (individual level)	Substance misuse Criminal history Previous IPV Possession of firearms Victims of child abuse/exposure to IPV Mental health problems Social disadvantage
Victim (individual level)	Substance misuse Mental health problems Previous IPV (same or different partner) Social disadvantage Social isolation
Victim–perpetrator relationship (interpersonal level)	Relationship status (separated or still cohabiting) IPV (previous or same relationship) Stalking Children from another relationship
Community	Insufficient social support network Insufficient community resources Lack of coordination between community resources Attitudes accepting of violence against women Lenient legislations
Lethality violence-related risk factors	Attempted strangulation Threats to kill with a firearm Extreme fear of being killed on the part of the victim

Future Research: Improving the Evidence Base

Despite some evidence of risk management and prevention strategies, the lack of appropriate reporting and systems to enable the identification of potential victims and perpetrators and an increased understanding of the dynamics and motives of murder, the evidence base is nascent in relation to various forms of femicide. While understanding is increasing, and reporting mechanisms are improving, significantly more knowledge thorough research is needed as well as changes to policy and practice. These are needed to develop robust mechanisms and systems to truly capture and understand the extent of femicide and its impact through better reporting and recording of the crime by criminal justice and other agencies.

It is also evident that not enough information is available about the children of murdered women and their experiences because of many different factors, including the age of children (affecting their ability to express), how children are perceived in the society with regard to their knowledge and understanding and lack of understanding about their needs. Further research is needed to understand the perspective of children, the placement of children, contact with the perpetrator (maybe the father) and the impact of their experiences on their health through longitudinal and multi-centre studies. Such research will help professionals in relevant fields and disciplines to understand the impact on children and, therefore, may help them to recognise the need of putting children's right to well-being and safety first (Birchall and Choudhry 2018).

Understanding and responding appropriately to children's needs at the time of their experience is also crucial. Such children should be placed in a familial environment with familial people. They should also be provided with appropriate services to ensure access to counselling and other social care and mental health services to minimise the social, health and mental health impacts of the experience. In addition, efforts are needed to highlight the issue of femicide and to develop appropriate measures and strategies to reduce/eliminate the prevalence of femicide internationally.

Summary

- Femicide is a diverse phenomenon and is known by various terms across the globe.
- Femicide leads to the killing of women, mostly by men, just because of their gender.
- Children are the hidden victims of femicide as there is a rather modest evidence base that describes their experiences post-femicide.
- A better understanding of femicide is needed to improve policy and practice responses across a number of sectors.

References

Ahmed S, Montanez R (2019) Father kills mother of their child at custody exchange in front of Hawthorne Police Station, Police Say. https://www.nbclosangeles.com/news/local/Shooting-Hawthrone-508246211.html

Alisic E, Groot A, Snetselaar H, Stroeken T, van de Putte E (2015) Parental intimate partner homicide and its consequences for children: protocol for a population-based study. BMC Psychiatry 15(1):177

Alisic E, Groot A, Snetselaar H, Stroeken T, Van De Putte E (2017) Children bereaved by fatal intimate partner violence: a population-based study into demographics, family characteristics and homicide exposure. PLoS one, 12(10):e0183466.

Baldry AC, Magalhães MJ (2018) Prevention of femicide. In: Weil S, Corradi C, Naudi M (eds) Femicide across Europe: theory, research and prevention. Policy Press Shorts, Bristol, pp 71–92

Birchall J, Choudhry S (2018) What about my right not to be abused? Domestic abuse, human rights and the family courts. Women's Aid, Bristol

Campbell JC, Webster D, Koziol-McLain J, Block C, Campbell D, Curry MA, Gary F, Glass N, McFarlane J, Sachs C, Sharps P, Ulrich Y, Wilt SA, Manganello J, Xu X, Schollenberger J, Frye V, Laughon K (2003) Risk factors for femicide in abusive relationships: results from a multisite case control study. Am J Public Health 93(7):1089–1097

Eklund L, Purewal N (2017) The bio-politics of population control and sex-selective abortion in China and India. Fem Psychol 27(1):34–55

Ferrara P, Bernasconi S (2017) From "classic" child abuse and neglect to the new era of maltreatment. Ital J Pediatr 43(1):16

Ferrara P, Caporale O, Cutrona C, Sbordone A, Amato M, Spina G, Ianniello F, Fabrizio GC, Guadagno C, Basile MC, Miconi F (2015) Femicide and murdered women's children: which future for these children orphans of a living parent? Ital J Pediatr 41(1):68

Ferrara P, Ianniello F, Semeraro L, Franceschini G, Lo Scalzo L, Giardino I, Corsello G (2018) Murdered women's children: a social emergency and gloomy reality. Signa Vitae 14(1):71–74

Grzyb M, Hernandez M (2015) "Still a long way ahead": criminalisation of femicide and addressing impunity in Latin America: recent developments. In: Dimitrijevic M, Filip A, Platzer M (eds) Femicide: a global issue that demands action (vol IV). ACUNS, Vienna, pp 84–93

Hart SD (2008) Preventing violence: the role of risk assessment and management. In: Baldry AC, Winkel FC (eds) Intimate partner violence prevention and intervention: the risk assessment and management approach. Hauppauge, NY, Nova Science, pp 7–18

Kropp PR, Hart SD (2000) The spousal assault risk assessment (SARA) guide: reliability and validity in adult male offenders. Law Hum Behav 24(1):101–118

Laurent C, Platzer M, Idomir M (2013) Feminicide: a global issue that demands action. Academic Council on the United Nations System (ACUNS). Vienna Liasson Office, Vienna

Naas N (2018) I watched my dad murder my mom. It changed everything i thought i knew about abuse. https://www.huffpost.com/entry/domestic-abuse-psychological_n_5bbf5299e4b0bd9ed5578fe6

Russell DEH (2011) The origin and importance of the term femicide. www.dianarussell.com/origin_of_femicide.html

Tucker J (2012) The pain of orphanhood: 'Things get neglected when parents aren't around'. https://www.telegraph.co.uk/women/mother-tongue/9550449/The-pain-of-orphanhood-Things-get-neglected-when-parents-arent-around.html

United Nations Office on Drugs and Crime (2019) Global study on homicide 2019. Vienna, Austria. https://www.unodc.org/documents/data-and-analysis/gsh/Booklet_5.pdf

van Nijnatten C, van Huizen R (2004) Children of uxoricide: the anti-therapeutic effects of the construction of parenthood pathology in cases of family trauma. J Social Welfare Fam Law 26(3):229–244

Weil S (2018) Research and prevention of femicide across Europe. In: Weil S, Corradi C, Naudi M (eds) Femicide across Europe: theory, research and prevention. Policy Press Shorts, Bristol, pp 1–16

Weil S (2020) Two global pandemics: femicide and COVID-19. Trauma Memory 8(2):110–112

Weil S, Kouta C (2017) Femicide: a glance through qualitative lenses. Qual Sociol Rev 13(3):6–12

Parveen Ali, PhD is a Professor of Gender Based Violence and Professor of Nursing in the Health Sciences School, the University of Sheffield and Doncaster and Bassetlaw Teaching Hospitals. Her research examines gender-based violence, inequalities in health related to gender and ethnicity, and nursing as a profession.

Michaela M. Rogers, PhD is a Senior Lecturer in Social Work in the Department of Sociological Studies at the University of Sheffield. Her research examines interpersonal violence with a focus on marginalised groups, impacts, help-seeking, service access and service responses.

Familicide as a Form of Abuse

Carolyn Harris Johnson

Learning Objectives

- Having read this chapter, the reader should be able to understand
- Different types of familicide offences and their antecedents.
- How in type 1 familicide offences, patriarchal suicidal men exercise ultimate control over their wives and children by killing them when facing a loss of social status (shaming).
- How in type 2 familicide offences, patriarchal suicidal men kill children to punish their wives for leaving the relationship (abandonment).
- Factors indicative of risk.

Introduction

This chapter presents information about familicide, a rare type of intra-familial homicide that almost always includes suicide of the perpetrator. Familicide breaks several societal taboos, murder, suicide and child killing and remains poorly understood. Although the term familicide can be used to describe homicide where there is a range of different configurations of perpetrator and victim relationship, offences appear to fall into two broad categories, and while there are similarities between them, there are also major differences. The first type of offence, 'Perpetrator's Crisis of Shame', appears to be the rarer of the two. The second type, 'Perpetrator's Crisis of Abandonment' is more common, although neither offence occurs frequently. The terms used here were developed by the author, after studying the literature on familicide and interviewing survivors of the offences, who were able to provide much

C. H. Johnson (✉)
University of Western Australia, Perth, WA, Australia

P. Ali, M. M. Rogers (eds.), *Gender-Based Violence: A Comprehensive Guide*, https://doi.org/10.1007/978-3-031-05640-6_12

needed insight into offence antecedents and who, willingly and courageously, shared their experience in the hope of contributing to better understanding of the offence, and ultimately to prevention.

Box 1 Defining Familicide

Definition

The term 'familicide' is imprecise and evolving and may be used to describe offences where the configuration of victims varies, whether or not the perpetrator dies as part of the incident. Some examples of this are:

- Murder-suicide within the nuclear family, where the spouse and children are killed (Alder and Polk 2001: 13).
- Murder-suicide within the nuclear family, where some/all of the children are killed but not the spouse (Johnson 2005: 256).
- Massacres, which include members of the extended family, whether or not the perpetrator suicides (Ewing 1997: 134).
- Murder of the spouse and children where the perpetrator does not necessarily attempt suicide (Daly and Wilson 1980).
- Murder of some/all of the children, and/or the spouse, but where the perpetrator's suicide attempt was unsuccessful (Johnson 2005: 126–127).

Alternative Terminology

Familicide; Filicide-suicide; Family murder; Child murder-suicide; Family Annihilation; Mass murder.

Key Theories and Concepts

The literature available on familicide emanates from a range of disciplines, and whilst there are different explanations proffered for the offence, even within disciplines, there are also some common threads amongst them, which will continue to guide the direction of future research. Whilst not attempting to encompass the full breadth of theoretical approaches, which may make a comment on this phenomenon. This chapter shall attempt to illustrate this variation in interpretation by providing relevant examples of the work of some significant researchers from different disciplines and theoretical orientations, who have all contributed to the literature on familicide. It should be noted here that variations in definitions of the offence, how and what data is collected, and the fact that not all researchers attempt to classify the offence into types often lead to contradictions in how offences are described and how causal factors are posited.

Wilson et al. (1995), taking a psycho-evolutionary approach, undertook a study on familicide in which 109 cases of familicide were examined across three countries, Canada, England and Wales. It was found that there were two types of familicide scenario, both of which were described as evidencing a 'masculine uxorial proprietariness' (Wilson et al. 1995: 287). The first type of familicide they describe is one where the perpetrator is depressed and despondent, and where it appears there was evidence of him thinking that the homicide was a protective act because his wife and children would be saved from a situation that would be unbearable to them (Wilson et al. 1995: 287–288). In this type of familicide, wives are almost always killed. Although there may be some evidence to support the psycho-evolutionary perspective on familicide, there are some serious contradictions and many questions that remain unanswered by this theoretical position, not the least of which is why do some perpetrators, as found by Johnson (2005), show evidence of both depression and retaliation?

The second type is characterised by anger expressed by the perpetrator towards his wife, as a result of paranoia, for real or imagined infidelity and/or for her intention to leave the relationship. Whilst this may very well explain why a man in this situation may kill his wife, it is not so apparent as to why he should kill his children in this circumstance. Wilson et al. (1995) hypothesise that one reason for this may be that there could be a higher incidence of non-paternity amongst the perpetrators' putative children, but there is no evidence tendered to support this. In fact, most studies, including theirs, note the somewhat lower incidence of step-children in familicide than in filicide (Johnson 2005; Wilson et al. 1995). Neither does the psycho-evolutionary approach explain why men in this situation rarely kill their wives.

Australian criminologists, Alder and Polk focus on Australian cases of filicide (the killing of a child by a parent), including filicide-suicide but also incorporating some useful comparative statistics, from both the United Kingdom and North America. They found that filicide differed quite markedly from the cases of filicide-suicide because amongst this cohort, with only one exception, all the fathers were the biological parent of the child. Unlike the fatal assault cohort, where the context was one of unemployment, economic hardship and arguments, often coloured by substance abuse, the filicide-suicide cases were more likely to occur against the background of marital separation and custody battles. A feature of this cohort was that the perpetrator tended to be older (in their 30s) and the children were also older than those in the filicide-only cohort (Alder and Polk 2001).

Charles Patrick Ewing found, as have others (Karlsson et al. 2021; Johnson 2005; Websdale 2010), that familicide is almost always committed by males and that there are common factors in their personalities that make it more likely that they will kill when confronted with impending loss of that control. He reminds us that the men who commit this offence are not only very controlling but are concomitantly emotionally dependent upon their families (Ewing 1997: 134). When they feel this control begin to dissipate, they feel threatened. Whilst acknowledging the propensity for men whose marital relationships are breaking up to commit this offence, Ewing makes the point that familicidal men are most often those who see themselves as losing control, not simply with respect to their intimate and familial relationships, but in all aspects of their lives which they deem as meaningful (Ewing 1997: 135).

Carl Malmquist, a psychiatrist, raises the issue of psychotic depression as being a factor in many familicide offences. He explains that the anger towards self, which usually inhibits the offender from acting out, becomes mobilised in these cases and the resultant homicidal impulse emanates from an externalisation of this anger. It is not clear from Malmquist's description of this process, as to how or why the anger becomes mobilised, or what sort of trigger he sees there may be to cause this shift (Malmquist 2006: 253). He warns that failing to make the important distinction between familicide and other mass killings may hinder understanding of the offence, as familicide is characterised by very different psychodynamic and psychiatric features than mass murder of strangers (Malmquist 2006: 44). He explains how perpetrators with psychiatric symptoms, who may also be manic, can have poor reality testing and compromised boundary formation, with the typical grandiosity and sense of righteousness, which occurs with mania. This may lead to the thought processes being contaminated, making it appear (to the perpetrator) that the action is not only justified but that he has the right to take such action (Malmquist 2006: 252).

Alternatively, a feminist approach might interpret the perpetrator's grandiosity and sense of righteousness as evidence of male privilege or proprietary, where the power and right to commit the offence is generated from a historical socio-political framework, where women and children are subordinate and men hold proprietary attitudes towards them, as a result of traditionally holding the more powerful position in society. This is not to espouse that mental illness, including mania, is never a factor in these offences but simply to reiterate that the wider view that can be accommodated in approaching the topic, the better understanding that will result, leading to more effective strategies to identify risk and to act preventatively.

Australian researchers, Johnson and Sachmann, propose an alternative theoretical formulation for type 2 familicide. Their formulation is based on a synergistic combination of attachment style, personality dysfunction and hypothesised psychodynamic factors, as an explanation for the failure of perpetrators to manage the trauma of separation. They offer explicit formulations and analyses of the various attachment themes, individual psychodynamics, defensive functioning and finally behavioural sequelae that represent risk factors for familicide. This formulation augments current theories of familicide by incorporating what is known about the psychological process of attachment, personality and the neurobiology of trauma. They propose, in familicide, it is the perpetrator's lack of individuation that makes it difficult to separate and increases the risk of lethality to the partner and to the self (Johnson and Sachmann 2014, 2018).

Box 2 Familicide-Suicide Internationally

Karlsson and colleagues conducted a systematic literature review of familicide across 18 countries. They found that familicide usually has a low incidence, and in some places, it is reducing. Perpetrators of familicide were found to be almost always male and problems with mental health, relationships, domestic violence and finances were common antecedents to the offence. They noted the difficulties in determining typologies, population base rates and risk factors (Karlsson et al. 2021).

International Comparisons

As familicide is such a rare occurrence and is often defined differently by researchers, it is difficult to provide international comparisons. Most countries do not keep separate statistics on the offence, so data is hidden amongst other homicidal events, and may prove difficult to retrieve. Current research in the area appears limited, primarily to Europe (Liem et al. 2013; O'Hagan 2014), North America (Websdale 2010; Wilson et al. 1995) and Australia (Johnson and Sachmann 2014; Johnson 2005), but this does not mean the offence does not occur elsewhere. A recent systematic literature review, which was limited to cases where the suicidal perpetrator killed a spouse and children, but did not include cases where the spouse was not killed, drew attention to the need for clearer definitions to gain a better understanding of the offence (Karlsson et al. 2021).

Categorising the Offence

Notwithstanding the paucity of research on familicide and the disparities between offences, after examining the literature on familicide and interviewing survivors, it appears offences may be categorised into two distinct types. Each of them appears to involve a crisis relating to the inner psychological self of the perpetrator, precipitating concurrent suicidal and homicidal ideation. The first appears to emanate from a crisis in the perpetrator's perception of the self, where he feels ashamed. Typically, this is caused by an impending loss of public status, which he is unable to accommodate. The second appears to emanate from a crisis in the perpetrator's perception of the self, where he feels abandoned. Typically, this is caused by the loss (or perceived loss) of an intimate partner where the perpetrator's lack of individuation leaves him feeling unable to survive on his own.

Type 1: Perpetrator's Crisis of Shame

Type 1 familicide is the less common type and typically appears to occur when the perpetrator.

- Faces a crisis in perception of self (shame).
- Is patriarchal in his attitude towards his family.
- Is well-respected, conservative and law abiding.
- Is highly controlled, constrained or obsessive.
- Fears loss of reputation or status in society.
- Faces an impending crisis, affecting his way of life (Websdale 2010: 167).

Websdale also found that due to the suicide of the perpetrator, there is often scant information about their early lives. Interestingly, where information was available, it indicated that many 'experienced attenuated or disrupted bonding with their parents; some experienced varying degrees of parental neglect' (Websdale 2010: 179). This type of early aversive life experience has been shown to have the potential to cause emotional damage, affecting personality development and the ability to cope with stress and adversity into adulthood (van der Kolk 2003; Nijenhuis et al. 2002; Perry et al. 1995; Sachmann 2001).

In contrast to type 2 offences, in type 1 familicide the woman is almost always killed by her husband at the same time as he kills the children, and just prior to his suicide. The offence is usually premeditated, well planned and finely executed, meaning few victims survive, which further adds to the lack of information available to assist those trying to unravel its antecedents and causal factors. The mode of homicide-suicide in type 1 offences is often shooting, with stabbing being a common alternative when a firearm is not available.

Type 2: Perpetrator's Crisis of Abandonment

Type 2 familicide occurs when there is a crisis in the perpetrator's perception of the existence of self, and appears to be precipitated by real or imagined loss of an intimate partner, and typically occurs when the perpetrator.

- Faces a crisis in perception of self (abandonment).
- Is consumed by rage towards his ex-partner for initiating the break-up.
- Has a history of family and domestic violence, not always reported or recognised.
- Faces an imagined, impending or actual separation from his partner.
- Experiences a deterioration in mental health following separation.
- Has a history of making homicidal and suicidal threats.
- Has a history of substance misuse.
- Is not recognised by decision-makers as posing a significant risk to children.

The major difference between this type of familicide and type 1 is that in this offence the woman is rarely killed, even though she may have been threatened many times with death. The children are most often killed when on access visits to their father, which have either been agreed to by the child's mother, and/or had been sanctioned by a court order (Johnson 2005). There is evidence to suggest that the reason women are not killed in these offences is that the perpetrator wants to inflict the most harm on her, as punishment for abandoning him, realising that it will be more painful for her to survive her children's death than to be killed alongside them. The psycho-social context in type 2 familicide appears remarkably consistent. Research indicates that commonly perpetrators have had a history of trauma, but also their partners and other family members had similar backgrounds. This should not be surprising, as it is recognised that trauma is transmitted inter-generationally, and those with trauma histories are likely to seek out, and to attract, partners with a similar psycho-social history (Johnson 2008).

In Australia, a common mode of homicide-suicide chosen by the perpetrator, where gun ownership laws restrict access to firearms, is carbon monoxide poisoning. These offences are committed after the perpetrator manufactures a device that will direct car fumes from the exhaust pipe into the vehicle, drives to a secluded location, sedates the children and then fixes the device and leaves the engine running until he and the children concurrently expire. Prior to killing them, fathers often sedate or restrain children in their seats to prevent their escape. In other jurisdictions, where a weapon may be chosen to murder, the murders are usually immediately followed by the perpetrator's suicide.

Themes in Familicide

There are three themes that have been identified by researchers as being common to both types of familicide. They are, first; depression or other mental illness in the perpetrator (Johnson; 2005; Polk 1994; Sachmann 2001; Karlsson et al. 2021); second, a male proprietary attitude, where a sense of ownership and a drive to obsessively control their partner, allows men to kill their partners and their children either, to 'protect' them from a loss of economic security and social status, or to avoid them leaving (Ewing 1997: 135; Polk 1994; Websdale 2010); and, third, premeditation. However, there are others that appear to occur in one type of offence but not the other. For example, a stable domestic situation typifies type 1 offences, whereas type 2 offences are typified by the volatility of actual or impending separation. Retaliation is not usually apparent in type 1 but is common in type 2 offences. This may explain why wives are usually killed in type 1 offences but rarely in type 2.

Depression or Other Mental Health Issues

Depression has often been linked to intra-familial homicide generally and particularly to parents killing their children. In times of financial adversity or ruin, depressed men have been known to kill their entire families in an apparently altruistic attempt to protect them from ensuing hardship (Ewing 1997: 139). Where familicide occurs as a result of a deep depression in the perpetrator, there are a number of different views about why this occurs. Easteal (1993: 97) saw the suicide component of familicide as possibly being remorse driven, following the homicide. Carcach and Grabosky explained the suicide component of these offences as originating in anger directed at the self as a response to a 'homicide induced frustration at the loss of the source of nurturance' (Carcach and Grabosky 1998: 4). The following case examples illustrate perpetrator depression prior to familicide in both types of offences.

Box 3 Type 1 and 2 Familicide

Type 1 Familicide:

'Motson donned a Halloween mask as he killed his family. Successful financier facing charges of embezzlement. Deeply depressed and anxious' (Websdale 2010: 179).

Kevin Wu was a respected businessman, who was involved in lawsuits and reportedly worried, depressed and anxious as a result. Kevin, 'killed his family while they slept … placed gold bullet shaped objects under the bodies' (Websdale 2010: 179).

Type 2 Familicide:

One survivor referring to the perpetrator said, 'He admitted being depressed but he couldn't talk about problems in the marriage. He never showed his feelings. He never saw a psychologist' (Johnson 2005: 65).

'In one case, though, a woman reported that she knew that her husband had been prescribed antidepressant medication, which he combined with excessive amounts of alcohol' (Johnson 2005: 45).

Male Proprietariness

There is considerable evidence to suggest that perpetrators in both type 1 and type 2 offences saw their wives and children as 'property' (Wilson et al. 1995: 286; Ewing 1997: 135; Polk 1994: 56; Websdale 2010). There is also evidence that they made statements and comments which indicated they viewed themselves as having the right of life and death over their families. 'Their solitude in this regard provided them with some semblance of control … Perpetrators appeared to have a sense of entitlement to kill' (Websdale 2010: 205–6). The following examples illustrate this perspective:

Type 1

(They) 'almost always made the decision to commit familicide on their own. Only in rare cases do we see them even broaching the topic with loved ones or others …' (Websdale 2010: 205).

Type 2

During a prison interview, one perpetrator, who had killed his wife and two children, but survived his suicide attempt, explained the reason for familicide in these words:

'We (men) think we own our wives and children, but we don't' (Johnson 2008: 168).

When asked to provide an explanation of her husband's offence, one survivor, Clare, reported, 'it's motivated by obsession and possession' (Johnson 2005).

Danni, an aunt of two children murdered by their father said, 'They were possessions, she and the kids belonged to him ... He told her 'you're always mine. I'll own you forever' (Johnson 2005: 67).

Premeditation

Previous research suggests the premeditation involved in the offences was concomitant to both the suicidal and homicidal components of the offence (Johnson 2005: 126–129; Karlsson et al. 2021). This and the obvious premeditation and careful planning that takes place prior to killing sometimes over days weeks, or even months, indicates these offences are not spontaneous and calls into serious question remorse as a motivator. There is also a consistent theme across both types of familicide, of lack of individuation, with perpetrators reportedly being unable to conceive a life separate from their partner and/or children.

Lack of Individuation

It appears likely from the case studies available in both types of familicide that the perpetrator's lack of individuation from his intimate partner may be a factor in the decision to kill self and others). In type 1 offences, the perpetrator's decision to kill all members of his family appears to demonstrate his sense of omnipotent control, coupled with an inability to conceive that his wife and children may have an ability and/or desire to withstand whatever disaster he sees as about to befall them. Therefore, he makes the homicidal-suicidal decision without discussion or negotiation and then carries it out in isolation and with brutal efficiency. Whereas in type 2 offences, a homicidal rage emanating from his perception of abandonment appears to cause the perpetrator to want to retaliate against his partner, causing the most hurt possible. Thus, he does not kill her but allows her to survive the loss of her children knowing this is a pain worse than death and arguably the worst form of abuse.

Retaliation

Research into familicide following separation repeatedly identifies retaliation as a motive (Johnson 2006; O'Hagan 2014), which challenges the notion of remorse-driven suicide in these offences. Evidence also points to the suicidal component of the offence as being very much a component of the premeditated homicidal act rather than a subsequent action. Whilst retaliation does not appear to be a factor in type 1 familicide, research has shown that in type 2 familicide, male perpetrated familicide often appears to be motivated by the offender's wish to retaliate against his wife for leaving the relationship to pay her back for her abandonment (Alder and Polk 2001: 83; Ewing 1997: 99; Johnson 2005:127–128). This motivation is sometimes referred to as 'spouse revenge' (Resnick 1969). This may explain why in cases that involve separation, the woman is often not killed, but allowed to survive so that she may experience the pain of living without her children. Whilst this may seem a very distorted and extreme form of revenge, research has found that the motive in this type of familicide 'most often appears to result from a desire to inflict harm on the child's other parent rather than from any underlying psychopathology' (Ewing 1997: 99). It also implies a complete lack of emotional attunement to their children, that they may murder them in cold blood to exact revenge on their mothers. The following familicide scenarios exemplify this:

Type 2

In one case, a survivor explained how the perpetrator had recorded their daughter's death in detail, with the intention that police would provide it to the child's mother when it was found. 'He left me a diary of the whole event. The police won't let me see it. He sat and watched until the last breath went out of her little face' (Johnson 2005).

In another, a member of the children's extended family explained, 'If he'd thought it would hurt her more to kill her, he would have. But it hurts more for her to live with the children gone. That's why he did it, to hurt her' (Johnson 2005: 85).

Familicide-Suicide as a Form of Abuse

Whilst in both types of familicide Ewing and others have captured the essence of the perpetrator's obsessive personality and need to control partner and family, there is little evidence of domestic violence in type 1, whilst in type 2 offences there is frequently a history of violence that increases after separation, although this often goes unreported or unrecognised and often comes to light after the offence (Johnson 2005). There remain questions about why the need to control is so strong in perpetrators. For example, how might any individual get to the point where killing those closest to him appears to be a valid solution to the stressors he currently experiences? And how does the homicidal-suicidal act achieve the desired control?

Whatever the answer to these questions, it is impossible to ignore that homicide is the most extreme form of violence and therefore when it occurs within a family must be considered the most extreme form of domestic violence. Additionally, in type 2 offences, where it appears that retaliation is at least part of the motivation for killing the children, the offence assumes an even more sinister nature.

Box 4 Type 1 Case Study

Ali Ibrahim

Suffocated his three children as they slept and shot dead his pregnant wife before committing suicide. The principal cause seems to have been his large gambling debts that pushed him towards bankruptcy (Websdale 2010: 178).

Box 5 Type 2 Case Study

The Aftermath

Murray and Theresa

Murray and Theresa had been separated for 6 weeks. Murray went to Theresa's home before the offence and seriously assaulted her, leaving her bound and gagged. He then went to their children's school where he lured them both away with the promise of gifts. Murray drove to an isolated spot and gassed the children by placing a hose from the exhaust to the inside of the car. He stabbed them to ensure their death. He then set fire to the car.

When he saw the police and ambulance arrive, Murray poured turpentine on himself and set himself alight. Both police and ambulance officers suffered burns as they tried to retrieve the children from the burning vehicle and douse the flames engulfing the children's father (Johnson 2005: 5).

Survivors reported extended families remaining in a state of acute shock for weeks after the offence. Some did not appear to have published obituaries or funeral notices. They also explained that their families were damaged permanently and irrevocably altered by familicide. There were reports of survivors being unable to work, sleep or eat properly for months and even years afterwards. Some resorted to alcohol or drugs to help them sleep (Johnson 2005: 74–88). As by definition, familicide is an offence committed against family members by another member of the family, it is likely that individuals who had a relationship with the perpetrator would also have had a relationship with the victims. This may cause conflict after the offence because although in some ways he might be viewed as a victim, by virtue of his suicide, the homicidal component of his act contradicts this perception and will be at variance from the perception of most other people. Irrespective of this, the murder of the children is likely to set them forever apart from the maternal family and from the remainder of the community and may hinder their ability to seek and gain support from the usual sources. Following the offence, it seems most families, once joined by an intimate relationship, became fractured and alienated by shock, anger, blame and loss, adding another layer of pain, to what is already a family tragedy of immense proportions, the trauma of which has been found to percolate across generations (Johnson 2005: 121–134).

One family member recalled that the extended family received news of the offence as they celebrated a birthday:

> We were at the party, having a great time. Halfway through … the police came. My brother went (to see what they wanted). When he came back, we knew by the look on his face that it was the end of our lives (Johnson 2005: 74).

The murders of two very young children in this family caused major trauma for the whole extended family, which persisted into the next generation. It was explained that two older male relatives died of heart attacks shortly afterwards. The family attributed these deaths to the shock of the murders. One of these men had suffered the additional shock of finding the bodies. The mother of the children who had not suffered mental illness previously would become psychotic on anniversaries, such as Christmas, or the children's birthdays, disappearing into bushland to try to find them and sparking intensive police searches. Across the extended family, adults became overly indulgent of children and women became over-protective. When marital relationships broke down, children were prevented from having unsupervised contact with their fathers.

Summary

- Internationally, across all jurisdictions, familicide is a rare offence.
- The gender of the perpetrator is predominantly male. The gender of children is equally male and female.
- There is an emerging sense of there being two separate categories to the offence.
- Future research should prioritise type 1 familicide to address the lack of information available about this offence.
- A careful appraisal of homicidal and/or suicidal threats should be undertaken when considering access to children.
- Family members may not perceive the risk to children or be suitable to supervise access.
- Prevention is dependent upon an integrated interagency approach. Prevention is also dependent on more research being undertaken.
- Judicial decisions should be informed by comprehensive psychological profiles, including adult attachment assessments, dynamic risk assessment and a clear appraisal of the long-term antecedents.

References

Alder C, Polk K (2001) Child victims of homicide. Cambridge University Press, Cambridge, Melbourne

Carcach C, Grabosky PN (1998) Murder-Suicide in Australia. In: Trends and issues in criminal justice. Australian Institute of Criminology Series. Australian Institute of Criminology, Canberra

Daly M, Wilson M (1980) Homicide. A. de Gruyter, New York

Easteal PW (1993) Killing the beloved homicide between adult sexual intimates. Australian Institute of Criminology, Canberra

Ewing CP (1997) Fatal families: the dynamics of intrafamilial homicide. SAGE, Thousand Oaks

Johnson CH (2005) Come with daddy: child murder-suicide after family breakdown. University of Western Australia Press, Crawley, WA

Johnson CH (2006) Familicide and family law: a study of filicide–suicide following separation*. Fam Court Rev 44:448–463

Johnson CH (2008) Killing the other-killing the self: a distorted strategy for survival. PhD, University of Western Australia, School of Social and Cultural Studies

Johnson CH, Sachmann M (2014) Familicide-suicide: from myth to hypothesis and toward understanding. Fam Court Rev 52:100–113

Johnson CH, Sachmann M (2018) Familicide-suicide. In: Brown T, Tyson D, Fernandez Arias P (eds) When parents kill children. Palgrave Macmillan, London

Karlsson LC, Antfolk J, Putkonen H, Amon S, da Silva Guerreiro J, de Vogel V, Flynn S, Weizmann-Henelius G (2021) Familicide: a systemic literature review. Trauma Violence Abuse 22:83–98
Liem M, Levin J, Holland C, Fox J (2013) The nature and prevalence of familicide in the United States, 2000-2009. J Fam Violence 28:351–358
Malmquist CP (2006) Homicide: a psychiatric perspective. American Psychiatric Publishing, Washington, DC
Nijenhuis ERS, Der Hart V, AL., E. (2002) The emerging psychobiology of trauma-related dissociation and dissociative disorders. Wiley, Chichester
O'Hagan K (2014) Filicide-suicide the killing of children in the context of separation, and divorce and custody disputes. Palgrave Macmillan, New York
Perry BD, Pollard RA, Blakley TL, Baker WL, Vigilante D (1995) Childhood trauma, the neurobiology of adaptation, and "use-dependent" development of the brain: how "states" become "traits". Infant Ment Health J 16:271–291
Polk K (1994) When men kill: scenarios of masculine violence. Cambridge University Press, Cambridge
Resnick PJ (1969) Child murder by parents: a psychiatric review of filicide. Am J Psychiatry 126:73–82
Sachmann MD (2001) The aetiological significance of early childhood trauma and temperament in the pathogenesis of borderline personality disorder. PhD thesis, University of Western Australia
Van Der Kolk BA (2003) The neurobiology of childhood trauma and abuse. Child Adolesc Psychiatr Clin N Am 12:293–317
Websdale N (2010) Familicidal hearts the emotional style of 211 killers. Oxford University Press, New York
Wilson M, Daly M, Daniele A (1995) Familicide: the killing of spouse and children. Aggress Behav 21:275–291

Carolyn Harris Johnson, PhD is a private clinician, consultant and adjunct senior lecturer at the University of Western Australia. Her research examines familicide, intimate partner homicide and intimate partner homicide followed by suicide.

Widowhood

Tazeen Saeed Ali, Anum S. Hussaini, Parveen Ali, and Michaela M. Rogers

Learning Objectives
Having read this chapter, you should be able to understand the following:

- The concept of widowhood as being gendered in varying emotional and physical aspects
- The extent to which instances of customary death and burial practices, in parts of Africa and Asia, can become extreme and negatively affect widows/widowers
- The perception of widowhood through a religious lens and how this can affect the treatment of widows/widowers
- The various amendments needed to respect the mourning and life of widows/widowers

T. S. Ali (✉)
School of Nursing and Midwifery, The Aga Khan University, Karachi, Pakistan

Department of Community Health Sciences, The Aga Khan University, Karachi, Pakistan
e-mail: tazeen.ali@aku.edu

A. S. Hussaini
Clinical Trials Unit at the Aga Khan University, Karachi, Pakistan

P. Ali
The Health Sciences School, University of Sheffield, Sheffield, UK
e-mail: parveen.ali@sheffield.ac.uk

M. M. Rogers
Department of Sociological Studies, University of Sheffield, Sheffield, UK
e-mail: m.rogers@sheffield.ac.uk

P. Ali, M. M. Rogers (eds.), *Gender-Based Violence: A Comprehensive Guide*,
https://doi.org/10.1007/978-3-031-05640-6_13

Introduction

> 'I always felt different because everywhere I go people either give me sympathetic looks or are scared that I will bring bad luck. But the first time I actually felt betrayed was when one of my sisters was getting married. I was treated like an outcast by my own family, all of whom thought that if I touched the bridal clothes or anything related to the nuptial ceremony something catastrophic would happen', narrated by Mahar whilst describing her experience as a widow in Pakistan (Mirza 2012).

Widowhood is stereotypically associated with old age. The proportion of widowhood is higher among older women than older men, specifically, those aged 65 years and above (Streeter 2020). However, death is inevitable, and therefore, young individuals can experience widowhood as well (Martikainen and Valkonen 1996; Moon et al. 2011). In this chapter we adopt the term widow to refer to women who have lost their spouse, whereas widower refers to men who have lost their spouse. The number of widows, around the globe, is much higher, perhaps because men die at an early age compared with women. Half of marriages tend to end with the husband's death, while only one-fifth are reported to end with the wife's death; therefore, widowhood is considered to be a gendered phenomenon. Women are also subjected to greater negative stereotypes, economic instability, stigma and negative experiences, while men experience a greater personal loss and mental health problems (Koren and Lowenstein 2008). The death of a spouse can cause severe emotional shock to the surviving partner/spouse (Nwadinobi 2014) with impacts including loneliness, financial instability psychological and emotional distress. However, research concerning widows and their experiences and status, especially in developing countries, is lacking.

In the initial phase of widowhood, widows and widowers undergo profound sorrow and grieving. Different cultures and religions deal with this grief in various ways including performing death and burial rites; surviving family members take the custody of the widow and her living children; and in some cases, communities ignore grief altogether by banishing the grieving spouses and family. As a universal experience, it is important to understand the diversity of rituals and norms in relation to widowhood and how they may affect the widow/widower. This chapter aims to explore widowhood as a gendered experience in different cultures and religions.

Gendered Differences in Widowhood Research

Low-income countries are where people tend to hold strong mythical beliefs related to widowhood, often causing the marginalisation of women. Indeed, one of the most orthodox findings in widowhood research is that pertaining to gender difference. Across the globe, it is more likely that women widows receive inadequate social support, emotional comfort and go through economic turmoil (Houston et al. 2016). African widows, for example, are among the most helpless and destitute women in the African region (Hashim et al. 2018). The rights of ownership and their husband's property are seized as the widow is demanded to meet the rituals of her late husband (Hashim et al. 2018; Mezieobi et al. 2011).

While it has been well-established that spousal death can have devastating consequences, research shows that the survival of the widow/widower after the spouse's hospitalisation and/or death varies (Elwert and Christakis 2006, 2008). Hence, the recently widowed are also at a relatively much greater risk of dying following the death of their spouse. When a spouse is hospitalised although there is no difference in men's and women's responses to this, the physical health of men is generally more adversely affected, in the long term, by spousal death than women, and they experience greater psychological and financial loss in the immediate term (Martikainen and Valkonen 1996; Elwert and Christakis 2006; Lillard and Waite 1995). Hence, men are prone to experience the *widower effect* which is linked with depressive moods, obsessive thought patterns, disturbed sleeping and eating behaviours and cognitive distortions (Wells and Browning 2002). It can be fatal, and, anecdotally, it is known as 'dying of a broken heart' (Wells and Browning 2002). This research illustrates that the risk of death is higher in the 3 months immediately following spousal death and, eventually, settles after 1 year into widowhood (Elwert and Christakis 2006). Likewise, rates of depression also stabilise after 1 year of widowhood (Zisook and Shuchter 1991).

International Comparisons

A global report approximates that of the total widows sampled, 14.8% are deprived of basic necessities and live in extremely poor conditions (The Loomba Foundation 2015). This is especially the case in developing countries where 16% of widows encounter severe hostile treatment, such as physical violence; 27% experience certain forms of mistreatment, such as psychological abuse; and 20% of them have undergone some disadvantages, such as losing financial means (The Loomba Foundation 2015; Aderibigbe et al. 2017). A comparison of the quality of life between widows in China, Ghana, India, Russian Federation and South Africa revealed that these disadvantages can vary between country (Lloyd-Sherlock et al. 2015). In China, 0.8% of widows experienced food insecurity compared to 44.1% in Ghana, while in India 42.1% of widows reported moderate/severe conflict compared to 23.9% of married women in the country. These variations can be explained by the acceptability of certain practices by widows. In the Russian Federation, 54.3% of widows live alone compared to 14.6% in South Africa and 7.5% in India, where living alone is associated with low economic status or with pensioners. Thus, these findings indicate the need to support widows, especially, in low- and middle-income countries, where they are seen as more vulnerable (Lloyd-Sherlock et al. 2015).

Widows are placed at a disadvantage in some low-income countries because of rituals following spousal death (see Box 1 for alternative terminology used to describe a widow). Some traditions, such as death and burial rites, sometimes called the cleansing ritual, are extensively performed in sub-Saharan African regions, and underpinned by rigid cultures that often do not allow grieving spouses to opt out (The Loomba Foundation 2015). While performing the widowhood rites, widows often suffer malnutrition and unhygienic conditions, mobility difficulties, hypertension and various bodily diseases, such as typhoid and malaria (Aderibigbe et al. 2017). Those unable to access proper healthcare and those who are vulnerable to such inhumane treatment, unsurprisingly experience physical ailments and psychological distress. Since disclosing these rites is considered taboo, help-seeking is limited. Moreover, inadequate information is available to minimise the harmful behaviours perpetrated against widows. With the considerable understanding of the factors associated with the malpractices of widowhood, the development of community programmes to address this issue are imperative.

In Pakistan, for example, many widows are shunned from society, and many are disadvantaged through the removal of their rights to remarry and inherit property. This is due to a largely patriarchal, conservative situation in which women are under the care of men and do not have the opportunity to gain authority—something that ownership of property would provide. In all religions or ethnicities, people are instructed to adapt, implement and advocate women rights with fairness and equity. Despite all religions favouring the fair treatment of widows, it is evident that traditions and superstition supersede religious instructions in Pakistan (Mirza 2012).

Box 1 Alternative Terms for Widow

Alternative terms: Kulowa kufa, Rundi, husbandless wife, surviving wife, wife, sod widow, dead man's wife.

The Customary Rituals for Widowhood

In many countries, the rites for widowhood are performed as instructed and imposed by the widow's in-laws and are considered to be imperative in the continuation of tradition (Lloyd-Sherlock et al. 2015). For women in particular, widowhood rituals are denoted as a sign of 'cleansing' a widow from the curses that come with defiance, while testing the woman's loyalty towards their late husband. However, Sossou (2002) argues that such traditions have an underlying motive to mistreat women and contribute to women's inequality at a time when they require the most empathy and support. In many widowhood ceremonies, women's rights are neglected significantly. In addition, inappropriate widowhood rites prevail in many rural and population-dense areas such as southern and eastern parts of Nigeria (Aderibigbe et al. 2017). In these areas, women tend to marry as per customary rather than statutory law, which is considered inappropriate as per the widowhood rituals (Durojaye 2013). Box 2 described various abusive practices that widows endure in various cultures.

Box 2 Abusive Practices Experienced by Widows

Sexual cleansing: It is practiced in various countries including Kenya, Zambia, Malawi, Uganda, Tanzania, Mozambique, Angola, Ivory Coast and Congo. The practice is often forced by the deceased husband's family. Those refusing to engage in practice may be subjected to abuse and beating. Cleansing (forced sexual intercourse) can be done by the deceased husband's brother, other relative or, otherwise, by a paid sex worker. Typically, after sex, the widow burns her clothes, and the man shaves the widow's hair. In public the cleansing can be witnessed by whole neighbourhoods. This practice was outlawed in Kenya in 2015.

Widow burning: Also known as sati or suttee is a Hindu practice, now mostly historical, in which a widow sacrifices herself by sitting atop her deceased husband's funeral pyre. These practices were outlawed in 1827 in British India and again in 1987 in independent India by the Sati Prevention Act, which made it illegal to support, glorify or attempt to commit sati.

A similar practice called widow-strangling was practiced in Fiji where a widow was strangled by their brother. The practice was abandoned when Fijian Fijians adopted Christianity.

Widows killed in witch hunts: Witch hunting is still practiced in many parts of the world. And those likely to be accused and killed as witches are often widows. The practice is prevalent in India, Papua New Guinea, Amazonia and sub-Saharan Africa.

Widow inheritance: It is a cultural and social practice, whereby a widow is required to marry a male relative of her late husband, often his brother. It can also take the form of a return to the widow's parents' home, or a more exploitive inheritance to professional traveling widow inheritors who travel to different communities to inherit widows for financial gain, and often coerce widows to comply with sexual rituals in exchange for providing support.

Banned remarriage: In many cultures remarriage of widows is frowned upon, and widows are required to stay married.

The following section discusses rituals followed in Indian, Nigerian, African and Pakistani traditions to demonstrate societal acceptance and behaviours towards widows.

Customs in India

Women who become widows are often subject to live a life of 'social stigma' and anguish, as some traditions require widows to give up everyday pleasures (Perry et al. 2014). An Indian widow said with tears glistening in her eyes 'I lost my husband when I was 40 and there were times that people, especially married women refused to even eat with me. I remember not being invited to events, people looking at me suspiciously if I smiled or laughed or at times even refusing to sit with me. It was almost like I was the reason why my husband died and I was left to live with the guilt. I still remember my mother telling me that I should have died with him. I was treated worse than an untouchable' (Perry et al. 2014). See Box 3 which details a famous case in India.

Box 3 Case Study: Roopkuvarba Kanwar

In 1987 Roop Kanwar, an 18-year-old young woman, took the decision to jump into the funeral pyre of her husband in an act of self-immolation that came to establish a legacy that would live on for years to come. The mass audience who were spectators to this act described it as a voluntary action.

Roop Kanwar had been married to her husband Maal Singh for 8 months prior to his death from gastroenteritis. During the time of their marriage, she lived primarily with her parents in Jaipur, reportedly spending a total of 20 days with Singh as his wife. On 4 September 1987, in the village of Deorala in Rajasthan, the 18-year-old Kanwar mounted Singh's funeral pyre and burned to death in its flames. Thirteen days later, at the traditional chunari ceremony, a crowd of at least 250,000 gathered at the site of her death to worship her as a goddess. 'Sati mata ki jai' was the oft-repeated cry; it is an invocation of the goddess, or 'devi', that Kanwar was said to have become. Despite official warnings against such a ceremony, the small village was crowded with devotees bent on witnessing the miraculous disappearance of the chunari, or bridal finery, into heaven, and the spontaneous reignition of the funeral pyre. Some wished simply to pray to the blessed 'sati'.

https://www.encyclopedia.com/women/encyclopedias-almanacs-transcripts-and-maps/kanwar-roop-c-1969-1987

Nigerian Customs

In Nigeria, a common practice is whereby a widow drinks the water used to clean her husband's corpse. This practice is rooted in the notion that if the widow drinks this water, it proves that she is not responsible for her husband's death. Refusal to drink the water, as interpreted by others, is thought to be proof that she is responsible for her husband's death. According to historians, a widow's refusal to drink the bathwater of her deceased husband would, 'of course', be taken as an admission that she had killed her husband (Mezieobi et al. 2011; UN HR Committee 1989).

Responsibility for the widow is believed to belong to the family of the deceased husband. This involves the inheritance and its transfer. The widow is not allowed to leave the family home, and the younger brother of the deceased spouse ties the knot with the surviving widow of the deceased brother and looks after her. In some cases, the widowed woman nominates someone in her in-law's family to take her charge and protect her and all the belongings associated with her. The decision as to whether she will be cared for depends upon her behaviour during the life of the deceased spouse or if the deceased was influential and in good standing in the community (Olaore et al. 2012). 'If the woman stays in the family, she can either marry the younger brother of the man or remain single in the house. However, as a rule, a widow must not get pregnant from another man outside the husband's family', explained the interview participant of Olaore et al.'s study (2012).

The widow is also expected to perform some burial rituals for the deceased that includes head shaving and staying indoors. Although men are subjected to some of these rituals, such as shaving the head, women are given longer periods of mourning and are often seen as more vulnerable in these situations. This vulnerability can stigmatise a woman because she is seen as a burden to the community, in which she must perform more rituals to 'cleanse' herself from the deceased. A participant in Olaore et al.'s (2012) also depicted controlling regimes for younger widows: 'If she is young, she is to stay indoors for 5 months to see if she is pregnant so that she bears the child for the deceased. Her husband's people give her money to take care of herself and her children after fulfilling the death rite such as scraping her hair, staying indoors for 4 market days'.

African Widowhood Rites in the Phokwane Area

Phokwane is an administrative area in the Frances Baard District of the Northern Cape in South Africa. In this area, widowhood rites, outlined in research conducted by Pauw (1990), are aimed at purifying the widow, following the death of a husband. According to Pauw (1990), there are several other ceremonies for widows in Phokwane including the following:

1. Hands and feet sprinkled with water treated with leilane and the head is shaved.

   The widowed wife and other family members of the deceased are expected to participate in some cleansing rituals which includes washing of the hands and the feet after burial and the sprinkling of water on the grave with leilane. Leilane is a plant found in Phokwane primarily used to nullify the effect of ritual danger to ascertain that the widow or other family members of the dead do not contaminate the community with death impurities. In some communities, the widow is expected to shave her head (Pauw 1990). The ritual of head shaving is also performed by other Africans such as the Igbo of Nigeria, the Zulus of South Africa, Bapedi of Phokwane and in the village of Bakenberg in Mokopane (Pauw 1990; Rosenblatt and Nkosi 2007).
2. Blackening of the widow's body and attire.

   The widow is provided with a black dress and headcloth, accompanying a unique python-skinned headband for mostate women, or cow-skinned for common women. These clothes are considered the clothes of darkness (sefifi or senyama) (Pauw 1990). Furthermore, a widow must offer a path to passers-by when walking down the road and must sit at the back of the bus/taxi to prevent herself from being regarded as bad luck (Kotzé et al. 2012).

Customs Followed in Pakistan

The rituals and traditions associated with widowhood are widely practiced in different areas of Pakistan. In particular, there are several habits and commitments inflicted on a widow to mourn her husband. The grieving process is thought to represent the relationship of husband and wife as being intact. While there are multiple methods to show respect to the dead husband, the widow experiences many diverse practices, including cleansing the widow. Practices including marrying the surviving brother of the deceased, head shaving and forbidding the widow to remarry someone outside the family (Khan 2017). During widowhood rites, widows experience malnutrition and unhygienic conditions and are vulnerable to bodily diseases, such as typhoid and malaria, yet are unable to access proper healthcare. ‘Widows are the symbol of sorrow; we lose all our liberties after the death of our husband and our life is not different from a prisoner locked in a jail’, narrated 26-year-old Rabia, who lost her husband in a blast in Quetta, Pakistan (Khan 2017).

Preventing Remarrying

In Pakistan, many Pakistani widows do not remarry, especially in the underdeveloped areas of Pakistan, where most people think that if a widow is remarried, then this would indicate that she was not a loyal partner. This way, a widowed woman is ridiculed, insulted and has less value as an individual human. The continuation of these practices prolongs gender inequality and the violation of a woman’s basic rights and privileges.

Grieving Periods and Probation from Leaving Home

Widows are expected to stay home during the grieving period, which might be challenging for working women. It is expected that the widow shows a reverential attitude and deep sorrow for her deceased husband, while complying with the mourning rites. Such actions and emotional tendencies are expected of a bereaved widow as a symbol of sorrow. She is expected to appear as if in agony and is often encouraged to publicly mourn the death of her husband, so that those around her can see the pain she must be suffering.

The Islamic law Shari’ah instructs the widow to observe mourning and express sorrow during the period of ‘iddah’. This serves as a mark of respect for the deceased husband and a sense of devotion and loyalty to the relationship. Thus, it is not permissible for a woman who is in iddah to adorn herself with coloured clothing; wear jewellery; use perfumes; apply henna (mehndi), surma (kohl application in eyes) or other make-up; or beautify herself in any way. However, she is certainly allowed to keep herself clean and presentable. If she is used to applying oil to her hair and she fears that not applying hair oil will result in headaches, then she is allowed to use non-scented hair oil, provided the result does not enhance her beauty. Any practice that could mildly provoke another man, or attract someone, is considered immoral and looked down upon by those around. In Christian countries, Muslim women must abstain from wearing black clothes during 'iddah' because this is the Christian way of mourning their dead. Hence all these customs are religiously followed by the women in Pakistan as they are 'entitled' to do so (Das 2016).

Struggles Over Land Ownership

In Pakistan, especially in the interior areas of Sindh and Punjab, a great deal of significance is connected to land titles and ownership. There are implications for woman when their husband dies and there is a son with a hefty entitlement of property and assets. The widowed woman is then no longer considered to have any association with property and assets, often refused the right to her late husband's property (see Chap. 22).

The Concept of Widowhood in Islam

In Islam, there is no specific social or religious ritual or practice that one is compelled to undertake in the case of widowhood. Islam advocates considerable flexibility and understanding of an individual's situation, experiences and emotions, while encouraging them to do whatever they consider to be best and whatever they are most comfortable with. This is within the context of honouring the memory of their departed partner while taking the path that will help them cope best with grief. Islam is the religion that promoted the concept of women's rights to the world about 1400 years ago. The last prophet Muhammad commented on how men should treat their women: 'The best of you is he who is best to his family and I am the best among you to my family' (*Ibn-Hanbal, No. 7396*) (Badawi 1971).

Policy and Practice Recommendations

Protection of Women's Rights

The Universal Declaration of Human Rights states that all humans are born free and equal in terms of rights and dignity and everyone should be treated fairly, and no one should be subjected to any unfair treatment. According to the Committee for the Convention on the Elimination of All Forms of Discrimination against Women (CEDAW), their main objective of the Convention is to eradicate gender-based discrimination (Nwogu 2015). The Convention states that non-discrimination and equality contribute to the right of protection of human rights and that denial of full and equal enjoyment of all rights for all people is a violation of principle of equality. The committee thereby stresses the equal enjoyment of rights are essential whatever a person's gender. It also considers that practices associated with widowhood, such as those described earlier in this chapter, significantly hinders the freedom of women (Durojaye 2013; Cusack and Pusey

2013). Thus, discussion on the discrimination widows face is required to influence and transform their experiences and eradicate discriminatory rituals. To uphold the rights of widows, the establishment and implementation of national laws for the protection of widows' rights to inheritance, as well as protection from harmful practices, would strengthen the judicial framework.

Eradicating Harmful Traditions

The development and implementation of awareness-raising programmes to address the issue are necessary in order to reframe and promote the rights of widows to increase their safety and security. Inclusion of women in these programmes would further facilitate an environment where widows could report safety- and security-related issues and seek help (United Nations Population Fund 2011). There is a particular need to educate traditional elders regarding the consequences of widowhood rituals being followed and their devastating impact on widows and those children who are growing up as part of that society. This is dependent on the ability to address patriarchy in order to accomplish the gender equality needed for widows and women in general (Nwogu 2015).

Public Enlightenment Campaign

According to Nwogu (2015), there is a need for the development of insight among men and women on the devastating impacts of rituals associated with widowhood. To achieve this a public awareness campaign needs to be targeted at places such as mosques and churches to promote activism to eradicate harmful practices associated with widowhood.

Writing of Wills and Family Inheritance

Family and community cultures should change in an endeavour to address gender equality. This can be achieved through policy and practice. It is important that spouses make valid wills during their lifetime that is explicit about the inheritance and protection of their (future) widow. To avoid any harmful and detrimental circumstances, a husband should prepare a valid will bequeathing his immovable assets, such as property, to his wife, as these assets are often acquired through the partnership of both spouses (Nwogu 2015).

On the principal of equality and non-discrimination, daughters should receive shares in their father's property, and wives should inherit a share of husband's belongings. These cultural and policy changes hold the potential to negate those customs that deprive a woman of her inheritance (Nwogu 2015).

Summary

- Widowhood still persists as a stigma in the society that brings immense hardships for women.
- There is a lack of understanding and attention seen on family, societal, cultural and political level to uphold the rights of women and their empowerment. Marking international days will not triumph in making any change in the lives of women unless we educate our coming generations and ourselves.
- Women of our nation, including widows, should have the opportunity to exhibit their powerful qualities and acquire the same status based on their attributes and services as anyone else within the society.

References

Aderibigbe SA, Lawal MO, Olatona FA et al (2017) Knowledge and perception of widowhood rites among adults in Ilorin, Kwara State. Tropic J Health Sci 24:1–7

Badawi JA (1971) Status of woman in Islam

Cusack S, Pusey L (2013) CEDAW and the rights to non-discrimination and equality. Melbourne J Int Law 14(54):1

Das PR (2016) There is a 'village of widows' in Punjab. It's tragic but there's a serious problem here. Scoopwoop

Durojaye E (2013) 'Woman, but not human': widowhood practices and human rights violations in Nigeria. Int J Law Policy Fam 27:176–196. https://doi.org/10.1093/lawfam/ebt001

Elwert F, Christakis N (2006) Widowhood and race. Am Sociol Rev 71:16–41

Elwert F, Christakis N (2008) The effect of widowhood on mortality by the causes of death of both spouses. Am J Public Health 98:2092–2098. https://doi.org/10.2105/ajph.2007.114348

The Loomba Foundation (2015) The Loomba Foundation

Hashim Y, Ezeh P, Lawal S (2018) Does social enterprises empower widows in north-west Nigeria? J Bus Manag 20:1–7. https://doi.org/10.9790/487X-2006030107

Houston K, Shrestha A, Kafle H, Singh S, Mullany L, Thapa L, Surkan P (2016) Social isolation and health in widowhood: a qualitative study of Nepali widows' experiences. Health Care Women Int 37:1277–1288. https://doi.org/10.1080/07399332.2016.1142546

Khan H (2017) Quetta's war widows. The Express Tribune

Koren C, Lowenstein A (2008) Late-life widowhood and meaning in life. Ageing Int 32:140–155. https://doi.org/10.1007/s12126-008-9008-1

Kotzé E, Els L, Rajuili-Masilo N (2012) "women … mourn and men carry on": African women storying mourning practices: a South African example. Death Stud 36:742–766. https://doi.org/10.1080/07481187.2011.604463

Lillard L, Waite L (1995) 'Til death do us part: marital disruption and mortality. Am J Sociol 100:1131–1156. https://doi.org/10.1086/230634

Lloyd-Sherlock P, Corso B, Minicuci N (2015) Widowhood, socio-economic status, health and wellbeing in low and middle-income countries. J Dev Stud 51:1374–1388. https://doi.org/10.1080/00220388.2015.1066497

Martikainen P, Valkonen T (1996) Mortality after the death of a spouse: rates and causes of death in a large Finnish cohort. Am J Public Health 86:1087–1093. https://doi.org/10.2105/ajph.86.8_pt_1.1087

Mezieobi D, Mezieobi S, Iyamu E (2011) Widowhood practices among Igbos of South Eastern Nigeria as a betrayal of the fundamental human rights of women. J Contemp Res 8:72–83

Mirza F (2012) Widowhood: a life interrupted. https://www.dawn.com/news/763493/widowhood-a-life-interrupted

Moon J, Kondo N, Glymour M, Subramanian S (2011) Widowhood and mortality: a meta-analysis. PLoS One 6:e23465. https://doi.org/10.1371/journal.pone.0023465
Nwadinobi E (2014) Conflict intervention on behalf of widows: notes from Enugu State in Nigeria. In: Fritz J (ed) Moving toward a just peace: the mediation continuum. Springer, New York, NY, pp 167–188
Nwogu MIO (2015) THE legal anatomy of cultural widowhood practices in south eastern Nigeria: the need for a panacea. Global J Polit Law Res 3:79–90
Olaore AY, Drolet J, Olaore IB (2012) Nigerian marital cultural practices and implications for human rights. In: Drolet J (ed) The tensions between culture and human rights. University of Calgary Press, Calgary, AB, p 47
Pauw BA (1990) Widows and ritual danger in Sotho and Tswana communities. Afr Stud 49:75–99. https://doi.org/10.1080/00020189008707728
Perry B, Oluoch L, Agot K et al (2014) Widow cleansing and inheritance among the Luo in Kenya: the need for additional women-centred HIV prevention options. J Int AIDS Soc 17:19010. https://doi.org/10.7448/ias.17.1.19010
Rosenblatt PC, Nkosi BC (2007) South African zulu widows in a time of poverty and Social Change. Death Stud 31:67–85. https://doi.org/10.1080/07481180600995214
Sossou MA (2002) Widowhood practices in West Africa: the silent victims. Int J Soc Welf 11:201–209. https://doi.org/10.1111/1468-2397.00217
Streeter J (2020) Gender differences in widowhood in the short-run and long-run: financial, emotional, and mental wellbeing. J Econ Age 17:100258. https://doi.org/10.1016/j.jeoa.2020.100258
UN Human Rights Committee (1989) CCPR General Comment No. 18: non-discrimination upholding the rights of widows. United Nations Population Fund, New York, NY. https://www.unfpa.org/press/upholding-rights-widows
Wells Y, Browning C (2002) Widowhood. Macmillan Publishers, New York, NY
Zisook S, Shuchter SR (1991) Early psychological reaction to the stress of Widowhood. Psychiatry 54:320–333. https://doi.org/10.1080/00332747.1991.11024562

Tazeen Saeed Ali, PhD and Post Doctorate, is a Professor in the School of Nursing and Midwifery and in the Department of Community Health Sciences, Aga Khan University. Her research and expertise are in conducting research in the area of gender-based violence, inequalities in health, sexual and reproductive health, and in academia in teaching healthcare professionals to screen and manage the clients around the same area.

Anum S. Hussaini, BSN, is a Research Coordinator in the Clinical Trials Unit at the Aga Khan University. Her research examines challenges in maternal and child health as well as issues concerning clinical research and the need for exploring innovative regimes and plans through outsourcing.

Parveen Ali, PhD Professor of Gender Based Violence and Professor of Nursing in the Health Sciences School, the University of Sheffield and Doncaster and Bassetlaw Teaching Hospitals. Her research examines gender-based violence, inequalities in health related to gender and ethnicity, and nursing as a profession.

Michaela M. Rogers, PhD, is a Senior Lecturer in Social Work in the Department of Sociological Studies at the University of Sheffield. Her research examines interpersonal violence with a focus on marginalised groups, impacts, help-seeking, service access and service responses.

Part IV

Non-Partner Sexual Violence

Exploring Rape as a Gender-Based Crime

Madhumita Pandey

Learning Objectives
Having read this chapter, you should be able to do the following:

- Critically examine the legal definitions of rape and analyze the nature and prevalence of this gender-based crime
- Use a feminist lens to explain the perpetration of rape, understand the stereotypes, and responses
- Apply the knowledge on rape through different real-world cases and contexts.

Introduction

The feminist movement of the 1960s and 1970s not only highlighted the problem of sexual violence against women but brought forward the issue of rape into the mainstream conversation. However, the fear of rape and level of sexual offences continue to have a profound and damaging effect on individuals and communities all around the world. The World Health Organization (2013) defines sexual violence as any sexual act or any attempt for the purpose of obtaining a sexual act through violence or coercion, which can encompass a variety of situations, such as rape (including marital rape), rape by strangers, sexual abuse, sexual or physical abuse of those with disabilities, sexual abuse of children, forced marriage, and child marriage (Krug et al. 2002). About 36% of women around the world have experienced sexual

M. Pandey (✉)
Helena Kennedy Centre for International Justice, Department of Law and Criminology, Sheffield Hallam University, Sheffield, UK
e-mail: M.Pandey@shu.ac.uk

P. Ali, M. M. Rogers (eds.), *Gender-Based Violence: A Comprehensive Guide*,
https://doi.org/10.1007/978-3-031-05640-6_14

violence, with widely varying prevalence estimates (García-Moreno et al. 2013). Almost all forms of sexual violence are also forms of gender-based violence, but not all gender-based violence (GBV) is sexual in nature.

Defining Rape

What is rape? A simple question yet one possessing such complex depth and existing at the intersection of society, ethics, legality, and morality. It is perhaps the easiest to define rape through the legal framework of society. Most rape definitions around the world use three key components: *penetration*, *force*, and *lack of consent* (Decker and Baroni 2011; Remick 1992). In England and Wales, rape is a statutory offence defined under the Criminal Offences Act (2003) as follows:

> *(1) A person (A) commits an offence if*
> *(a) He intentionally penetrates the vagina, anus, or mouth of another person (B) with his penis.*
> *(b) B does not consent to the penetration.*
> *(c) A does not reasonably believe that B consents.*
> *(2) Whether a belief is reasonable is to be determined having regard to all the circumstances, including any steps A has taken to ascertain whether B consents.*
> *(3) Sections 75 and 76 apply to an offence under this section.*
> *(4) A person guilty of an offence under this section is liable, on conviction on indictment, to imprisonment for life.*

Something that instantly stands out in this definition is how it privileges the 'penis'. It is not unusual for rape and sexual assault definitions to be gendered in nature, and the use of language such as, '*his penis*', leads to females getting statutorily excluded from being able to commit rape. However, while we can see a clear gender bias in terms of who can perpetrate rape, i.e., a person of male sex, the law is not gender-specific in relation to who can be a victim of rape. Other narrower definitions of forms of assault and sexual activity without consent are also included within the Sexual Offences Act (2003), chapter 'Reflections and Way Forward', and have been listed in Table 1.

Definitions of rape pose challenges even in other parts of the world. For instance, according to the Indian Penal Code (IPC) 375 (2015), a man is said to commit 'rape' if he (a) penetrates his penis, to any extent, into the vagina, mouth, urethra, or anus of a woman or makes her to do so with him or any other person or (b) inserts, to any extent, any object or a part of the body, not being the penis, into the vagina, the urethra, or anus of a woman or makes her to do so with him or any other person or (c) manipulates any part of the body of a woman so as to cause penetration into the vagina, urethra, anus, or any part of body of such woman or makes her to do so with him or any other person or (d) applies his mouth to the vagina, anus, and urethra of a woman or makes her to do so with him or any other person, under the circumstances falling under any of the following seven descriptions:

Table 1 Definitions of assault and sexual activity without consent under the Sexual Offences Act (2003) of England and Wales

Assault
Assault by penetration
1. A person (A) commits an offence if
(a) He intentionally penetrates the vagina or anus of another person (B) with a part of his body or anything else.
(b) The penetration is sexual.
(c) B does not consent to the penetration.
(d) A does not reasonably believe that B consents.
2. Whether a belief is reasonable is to be determined having regard to all the circumstances, including any steps A has taken to ascertain whether B consents.
3. Sections 75 and 76 apply to an offence under this section.
4. A person guilty of an offence under this section is liable, on conviction on indictment, to imprisonment for life.
Sexual assault
1. A person (A) commits an offence if
(a) He intentionally touches another person (B)
(b) The touching is sexual
(c) B does not consent to the touching
(d) A does not reasonably believe that B consents
2. Whether a belief is reasonable is to be determined having regard to all the circumstances, including any steps A has taken to ascertain whether B consents
3. Sections 75 and 76 apply to an offence under this section
4. A person guilty of an offence under this section is liable on the following:
(a) On summary conviction, to imprisonment for a term not exceeding 6 months or a fine not exceeding the statutory maximum or both
(b) On conviction on indictment, to imprisonment for a term not exceeding 10 years
Causing sexual activity without consent
Causing a person to engage in sexual activity without consent
1. A person (A) commits an offence if
(a) He intentionally causes another person (B) to engage in an activity
(b) The activity is sexual
(c) B does not consent to engaging in the activity
(d) A does not reasonably believe that B consents
2. Whether a belief is reasonable is to be determined having regard to all the circumstances, including any steps A has taken to ascertain whether B consents
3. Sections 75 and 76 apply to an offence under this section
4. A person guilty of an offence under this section, if the activity caused involved the following:
(a) Penetration of B's anus or vagina
(b) Penetration of B's mouth with a person's penis
(c) Penetration of a person's anus or vagina with a part of B's body or by B with anything else
(d) Penetration of a person's mouth with B's penis is liable, on conviction on indictment, to imprisonment for life
5. Unless subsection (4) applies, a person guilty of an offence under this section is liable on the following:
(a) On summary conviction, to imprisonment for a term not exceeding 6 months or to a fine not exceeding the statutory maximum or both
(b) On conviction on indictment, to imprisonment for a term not exceeding 10 years

Firstly, against her will.

Secondly, without her consent.

Thirdly, with her consent, when her consent has been obtained by putting her or any person in whom she is interested, in fear of death or of hurt.

Fourthly, with her consent, when the man knows that he is not her husband and that her consent is given because she believes that he is another man to whom she is or believes herself to be lawfully married.

Fifthly, with her consent when, at the time of giving such consent, by reason of unsoundness of mind or intoxication or the administration by him personally or through another of any stupefying or unwholesome substance, she is unable to understand the nature and consequences of that to which she gives consent.

Sixthly, with or without her consent, when she is under eighteen years of age.

Seventhly, when she is unable to communicate consent.

Explanation 1. For the purposes of this section, 'vagina' shall also include labia majora.

Explanation 2. Consent means an unequivocal voluntary agreement when the woman by words, gestures or any form of verbal or nonverbal communication, communicates willingness to participate in the specific sexual act, provided that a woman who does not physically resist to the act of penetration shall not by the reason only of that fact, be regarded as consenting to the sexual activity.

Exceptions. (1) A medical procedure or intervention shall not constitute rape; (2) sexual intercourse or sexual acts by a man with his own wife, the wife not being under 15 years of age, is not rape.

Once again, we see a highly gendered and heteronormative definition of rape and one that does not recognize marital rape as a criminal offence. Rape of a woman or girl by her husband is still not criminalized in many jurisdictions around the world. Along with India, these include Ghana, Indonesia, Jordan, Lesotho, Nigeria, Oman, Singapore, Sri Lanka and Tanzania. In four of these, marital rape is expressly legal even where the 'wife' being raped is a child bride and the 'marriage' is in violation of minimum age of marriage laws (Equality Now Report 2017).

Marital Rape

Victorian ideals of womanhood made way for a long-standing history of women being lauded for keeping families together and withstanding any adversity in their martial life. In fact, martial rape was criminalized in the United Kingdom only in 1991 wherein, in R v R, a court judgment delivered in the House of Lords, determined that under the English Criminal Law it is possible for a husband to rape his wife. Until then, there were numerous instances where leading criminal justice professionals had claimed that a husband can never rape his wife. For instance, Sir Mathew Hale, a former Chief Justice of the Court of King's Bench in England famously wrote, 'The husband cannot be guilty of a rape committed by himself upon his lawful wife, for by their mutual consent and contract the wife hath given up herself in this kind unto her husband, which she cannot retract' (History of the Pleas of the Crown 1847).

Consent: 'No Means No' or 'Yes Means Yes'?

Consent poses a major challenge in cases of sexual violence all around the world. According to Coy et al. (2013), it is frequently assumed that nonconsensual sex is the result of miscommunication. In their report for the Office of the Children's Commissioner's Inquiry into Child Sexual Exploitation in Gangs and Groups in the United Kingdom, the authors argue that such ideas create expectations that for sex to be refused, there should be a clear verbal 'no', unlike other forms of human interaction where declining can typically be much less direct. Another key point emerging from this report was that while young people understand what it is meant to give consent for sex, they have very limited sense of what getting consent might involve (Coy et al. 2013). Some researchers have noted that the label of 'miscommunication' as applied to rape is also problematic in that it implies a level of victim responsibility, perpetuating a notion that the problem lies with the victim's sexual communication (Henley and Kramarae 1991).

The rape trial of Welsh international footballer Ched Evans also highlighted this predicament. Evans claimed that he had indulged in consensual sex; however, the prosecutors alleged that the victim, a 19-year-old, was too drunk to consent to sexual intercourse. This case witnessed major public outcry as the court allowed the victim's previous sexual history to be used as evidence. While Evans took responsibility for having sex with a drunk girl, he argued that his actions did not constitute as 'rape'. Similarly, another trial of the two Irish professional rugby players and two of their friends also highlighted the toxic male culture in elite sports industry and the contrasting views on sexual consent. During the trial the victim had to answer grueling questions of the defendant's lawyers, while her underwear was passed around the court for the jury to examine. The defense lawyers claimed that the victim did not physically resist or scream for help from anyone at the party. A common misbelief about sexual violence is that victims 'must' fight back to make it clear that they are resisting the act; however, several researchers have found that fighting back is not the most common response of sexual assault (Kozlowska et al. 2015; Gbahabo and Duma 2021). Furthermore, this case highlighted the harmful notion of sexual conquest and masculinity as the alleged players posted messages on a social messenger application saying 'We are all top shaggers' among several other boastful abusive and misogynistic messages after the party (New York Times 2018).

Case Study: Hollywood Horror

The recent #Metoo movement put heavy spotlight on Hollywood with several allegations on both leading actors and top entertainment executives. One key figure that was accused by 87 women was Harvey Weinstein. Weinstein was found guilty in New York and has been sentenced to 23 years in prison for rape and sexual assault.

Similarly, the man behind overseeing the hit show 'The Big Bang Theory' and many more, Leslie Moonves, was a prominent voice in the #metoo movement and also helped in creating the Commission on Eliminating Sexual Harassment and Advancing Equality in the Workplace which was chaired by Anita Hill. However, the public statements made by one of the most powerful media executives in America and the CEO of CBS Corporation weren't exactly in sync with his private actions as six women came forward with sexual harassment complaints against him. One can't help but notice his statement, 'But I always understood and respected—and abided by the principle—that "no" means "no", and I have never misused my position to harm or hinder anyone's career.' This language dates back to the anti-rape movement of the late 1960s and early 1970s. There's a reason why feminists have gradually moved away from the 'no means no' to focus instead on affirmative, active, and enthusiastic consent—'yes means yes'.

Consent is key in sexual violence. Sex without consent is rape even if the victim is under the influence of drugs or alcohol or as most argue is wearing revealing clothes. Yet only 12 European countries out of the 31 have laws that define rape as sex without consent: Belgium, Croatia, Cyprus, Denmark, Germany, Greece, Iceland, Ireland, Luxembourg, Malta, Sweden, and the United Kingdom (Amnesty International 2020).

Prevalence

People of all genders and ages experience rape; however, there continues to be a disproportionate number of women and girls who are sexually victimized around the world. According to the UN Women (2020), 15 million adolescent girls worldwide, aged 15–19 years, have experienced forced sex. Borumandnia et al.'s (2020) study shows that sexual violence against women in China, North Korea, and Taiwan has increased the most among countries in the world (average rate of 196.68 per 100,000 persons). This is followed by Lithuania and Namibia (average rate of 81.62 per 100,000 persons). In the USA, there are 463,634 victims (age 12 or older) of rape and sexual assault each year (National Crime Victimization Survey 2019).

The Crime Survey for England and Wales (CSEW) year ending March 2020 reported that there were 773,000 adults aged 16–74 years who were victims of sexual assault (including attempts) in the previous year, with 618,000 female victims, almost 4 times as many male victims (155,000). Over the past 15 years, the prevalence of rape or assault by penetration over this time has remained around 0.5% (CSEW 2020). While the volume of sexual offences recorded by the police has almost tripled in recent years, the latest figures for the year ending March 2020 show a decrease of 0.7% to 162,936 offences compared with the previous year. In the year ending March 2021, rape offences recorded by the police fell by 6% (55,696 offences). Rape accounts for 38% of all sexual offences recorded by the police. This is the second year-on-year decrease; prior to the year ending March 2019, the number of rape offences had been increasing annually. This trend is likely to reflect the diminishing impact of recording improvements as well as the effects of national lockdown restrictions. The fall in rape this year was driven by large decreases in April to June 2020, with offences 21% lower than in the respective period in 2019.

Latest estimates from the CSEW showed that fewer than one in six female victims aged 16–59 years of sexual assault by rape or penetration (16%) reported it to the police. Changes in police recording practices and victims' willingness to report are likely to result in annual variations in the number of offences recorded by the police; however, police recorded crimes remain well below the number of victims estimated by the survey.

Issues with Underreporting

Rape and sexual assault are very serious crimes but often go unreported. Back in 2018, when Dr. Christine Blasey Ford came forward with sexual assault allegations against Judge Brett Kavanaugh, a supreme court nominee under the Trump era, one of the first questions asked was, 'You were sexually assaulted 36 years ago, why didn't you report it then?' According to the US Department of Justice's (2020) analysis of violent crime, 80% of rapes and sexual assault go unreported. It is common for many sexual assault and rape survivors, who are mostly women, to not report the offense to authorities and the Rape, Abuse and Incest National Network (RAINN, 2020), largest non-profit anti-sexual assault organization in the USA, outlines various reasons behind this including the following:

- Fear of retaliation
- Belief that the police would not/could not do anything to help
- Belief that it was a personal matter
- Reported to a different official
- Belief that it was not important enough to report
- The victim did not want to get the perpetrator in trouble

In England and Wales, for the majority of female victims of rape or assault by penetration (including attempts), the offender is a partner or ex-partner or someone known to them other than as a partner or family member (CSEW 2017). This makes it even more difficult to report the crime.

Legal Loopholes

It is legally possible for a perpetrator of rape or sexual assault to escape punishment if he marries the victim in at least nine jurisdictions. These are Bahrain, Iraq, Jordan, Kuwait, Lebanon, Palestine, the Philippines, Tajikistan, and Tunisia. It is also possible in Greece and Russia, Serbia, and Thailand, in circumstances where the couple are in a sexual relationship and under the law the girl is otherwise deemed too young to consent to sexual intercourse (Equality Now Report 2017).

False Allegations

Since 1989, when the USA's courts began allowing DNA evidence, 873 cases of wrongful convictions have been documented (Gross and Shaffer 2012), and a substantial number of these have involved men convicted of sexual offenses (Ross et al. 2014). The prevalence of false allegations of rape remains a highly controversial issue. On the one hand, mainstream socio-legal rape research and commentary claims that allegations of rape are rare, or at least no more than false allegations for other crimes. On the other hand, many criminal justice professionals report that false allegations of rape are a common occurrence (Saunders 2012). This disparity has been well documented by researchers (Lees 2002; Kelly et al. 2005; Rumney 2006). Despite several research findings indicating the low prevalence of false rape allegations, many criminal justice professionals stand their ground. In one study from the United Kingdom, while researchers estimated that only 3% of a sample of police rape cases contained 'probable or possible' false allegations, police officers claimed that 'a good half, a lot and even most rape cases are false' (Kelly et al. 2005, p. 50). Such skepticism and stereotypical attitudes in the justice system and society at large adversely affect the treatment of rape victims and the investigation and prosecution of their complaints (Lees 2002; Temkin and Krahé 2008).

Motives for Rape

One of the most common ways to understand how convicted rapists view themselves, their actions, their victims, and to what extent do they take responsibility for their crimes is by studying their motivational accounts (Bryden and Grier 2011). Theories of sexual offending began in early 1950s, with psychiatry dominating the field (e.g., Karpman 1954). With the rise of the feminist movement in the 1970s, feminist scholars stressed on the motivational theories of rape that were governed by sociology and culture (e.g., Brownmiller 1975), and this was later challenged by the evolutionary psychologists who argued that men do not rape as a result of their gender-biased socialization, but rather their chief and most influential motivation is indeed sexual

Table 2 Adult male rape classification by (Blasko 2016)

Classification	Behavioral description
Compensatory	Expression of sexual fantasies with minimal aggression evident
Sadistic	Expression of aggressive sexual fantasies
Anger	Expression of rage
Power/control	Desire to achieve power and dominance
Opportunistic/antisocial	Spur of the moment, impulsive, and situational

(e.g., Thornhill and Palmer 2000). Blasko's (2016) synthesized classification of adult male rapists' sexual and nonsexual motivation have been presented in Table 2.

Risk and Protective Factors for Rape and Sexual Assault

There is no single factor that causes sexual violence, nor is there a single pathway to the perpetration of rape. Heise's (1998) integrated ecological framework, highlighted varying how violence against women is normalized at different levels of social ecology. These levels of layers span from the individual person, to the larger societal actions, and how varying factors affect this. For example, at the individual level, this can be seeen in how victims feel (or are made to feel) responsible for their attack, and the indoctrination of rape victims to blame themselves. This leads to the maintenance of 'rape myths', a term coined by Burt (1980) that refers to 'prejudicial, stereotyped, or false beliefs about rape, rape victims, and rapists'. At the social level, interaction of children with other peers or access to holistic sex education.

Rape Myths

Rape myths are dangerous and cause serious harm. They evoke feelings of shame and blame in the victims which prevents them to come forward to report the crime. It also prevents victims from getting support and affects how services respond to such crimes. Some common rape myths are as follows:

- Women who drink or take drugs deserve to get raped.
- Women who wear revealing clothing or flirt are asking for it.
- If women didn't scream, fight back, or run away, then it wasn't rape.
- Women often play hard to get or they often say no when they mean yes.

Risk factors are generally linked to a greater likelihood of perpetration of sexual violence. They are contributing factors and might not be direct causes, but it is important to note that everyone who is identified as 'at risk' becomes a perpetrator of violence. Protective factors on the other hand can lessen the likelihood of sexual violence victimization or perpetration. The risk and protective factors for the perpetration of sexual violence as outlined by the Center for Disease Control and Prevention (CDC 2022) are presented in Table 3.

Table 3 Risk and protective factors for the perpetration of sexual violence

Risk factors	
Individual risk factors	• Alcohol and drug use
	• Delinquency
	• Lack of concern for others
	• Aggressive behaviors and acceptance of violent behaviors
	• Early sexual initiation
	• Coercive sexual fantasies
	• Preference for impersonal sex and sexual-risk taking
	• Exposure to sexually explicit media
	• Hostility toward women
	• Adherence to traditional gender role norms
	• Hyper-masculinity
	• Suicidal behavior
Relationship factors	• Prior sexual victimization or perpetration family history of conflict and violence
	• Childhood history of physical, sexual, or emotional abuse
	• Emotionally unsupportive family environment
	• Poor parent-child relationships, particularly with fathers
	• Association with sexually aggressive, hypermasculine, and delinquent peers
	• Involvement in a violent or abusive intimate relationship
Anger	• Family history of conflict and violence
	• Childhood history of physical, sexual, or emotional abuse
	• Emotionally unsupportive family environment
	• Poor parent-child relationships, particularly with fathers
	• Association with sexually aggressive, hypermasculine, and delinquent peers
	• Involvement in a violent or abusive intimate relationship
Community factors	• Poverty
	• Lack of employment opportunities
	• Lack of institutional support from police and judicial system
	• General tolerance of sexual violence within the community
	• Weak community sanctions against sexual violence perpetrators
Societal factors	• Societal norms that support sexual violence
	• Societal norms that support male superiority and sexual entitlement
	• Societal norms that maintain women's inferiority and sexual submissiveness
	• Weak laws and policies related to sexual violence and gender equity
	• High levels of crime and other forms of violence
Protective factors for perpetration	
These factors can also exist at individual, relational, community, and societal levels	• Families where caregivers work through conflicts peacefully
	• Emotional health and connectedness
	• Academic achievement
	• Empathy and concern for how one's actions affect others

Responding to Rape and Sexual Assault

As noted by many researchers, various acts of sexual violence against women are actually connected to commonly occurring aspects of everyday male behavior in the society (Scully and Marolla 1985; Kelly 1988; Stout 1991; McMahon and Baker 2011). Kelly (1988) was one of the first researchers to stress the relevance and use of a 'continuum' to understand the perpetration of sexual violence against women. She argued that 'The concept of a continuum can enable women to make sense of their own experiences by showing how typical and aberrant male behaviour shade into one another' (Kelly 1988, p. 75). At one end of the continuum are behaviors that are generally considered sexually violent in our society, such as rape. These acts are recognized as serious crimes in most cultures and societies and are judged more harshly and carry legal ramifications and punishments (Stout 1991).

At the other end of the continuum are behaviors that are more commonly accepted, traditional gender norms, sexually degrading language against women, molestation, and harassment (McMahon and Baker 2011). The behaviors at this end of the continuum are often normalized as a part of our culture, and their connection to sexual violence is not widely recognized nor judged as harmful (Stout 1991). The behaviors on the less severe side of the continuum are important because they contribute to a culture of violence that supports and tolerates the more severe forms of violence against women (Brownmiller 1975; Sanday 2007; Schwartz and DeKeseredy 1997). Kelly's (1988) continuum included women's experiences ranging from flashing, sexual harassment, obscene phone calls, pressure to have sex, domestic violence, sexual abuse, coercive sex, sexual assault, incest, and rape. Guy (2006, p. 6) presented an integrated continuum of sexual violence in which she stressed the importance of including all forms of oppression as 'by providing a visual conception of the continuum that is more inclusive, of class, race, disability status, sexual orientation and anti-Semitism in addition to gender that it will remind and inspire us to develop a vision of comprehensive sexual violence prevention work which routinely encompasses all forms of oppression'.

Several researchers have adopted and modified this continuum to fit the scope of their work, for instance, the Racist Violence Continuum (e.g., Sanders-Phillips and Kliewer 2020), Disability and Hate Crime Continuum (e.g., Hollomotz 2013), and the Homophobic Violence Continuum (e.g., Faulkner 2006). Feminist theory articulates sexual violence in the context of a rape culture, which is a complex system of beliefs that encourages male sexual aggression and supports violence against women (O'Sullivan et al. 1993). Thus, viewing rape as a cultural phenomenon can have a deep impact on the development of sexual violence prevention strategies.

Education is key, and efforts are being made to educate, inform, and challenge young people about healthy relationships, abuse, and consent. The UK Government (2020) has been involved in collaborating with teachers, academics, and other practitioners. The national campaign, 'This is Abuse', made a strong impact, and there is a further investment of £3.85 million in a new campaign to continue to build young people's awareness around issues of consent, 'sexting', and relationship abuse. Involving men as agents of change can be a powerful tool in prevention. The CPS #ConsentIs campaign, focused on creating a public discussion about consent, and the White Ribbon Campaign are good examples of this practice.

It is important to note that the Covid-19 pandemic further exasperated the issues around sexual violence as many women and girls were forced to live with their perpetrators with limited mobility, increased insecurity over health, jobs, and money. As societies try to find a way out of the global devastation caused by the pandemic, stronger financing, better policies, and better service delivery need to be at the core of driving change. Intersectional feminist discourses have continually highlighted how norms that support gender inequities, promote hyper-masculinity, and uphold cultural adherence to traditional gender roles do not only perpetuate sexual violence but also breed homophobia and transphobia. By making these connections explicit and intentionally working toward inclusive advocacy, we can create equitable and safe communities for all marginalized groups who are at the risk of experiencing sexual harm.

Summary

Rape and sexual violence continue to plague our societies. Rape culture is pervasive and embedded in various aspects of our social functioning. This chapter highlighted the following:

- Critical examination of rape and sexual assault definitions within different legal contexts
- Role of consent within rape and issues around how to communicate it
- Prevalence of rape around the world with a focus on perpetration and victimization in the United Kingdom
- Understanding of rape myths, victim blaming, under-reporting, and false rape allegations
- Motivations for rape and classification of rapists
- The risk and protective factors for the perpetration of sexual violence
- Recent cases studies, Harvey Weinstein and Ched Evans, to elucidate the complexity of rape and sexual assault
- And finally, responding to rape and sexual assault

References

Amnesty International (2020) Criminalization and prosecution of rape in Europe. Amnesty International, London. https://www.amnesty.org/en/latest/campaigns/2020/12/consent-based-rape-laws-in-europe/

Blasko BL (2016) Overview of sexual offender typologies, recidivism, and treatment. In: Sexual violence. Springer, New York, NY, pp 11–29

Borumandnia N, Khadembashi N, Tabatabaei M, Alavi Majd H (2020) The prevalence rate of sexual violence worldwide: a trend analysis. BMC Public Health 20(1):1–7

Brownmiller S (1975) Against our will: men. Women and rape. Simon and Schuster, New York, NY

Bryden DP, Grier MM (2011) The search for rapists real motives. J Crim Law Criminol 101:171

Buchwald E, Fletcher PR, Roth M (eds) (1993) Transforming a rape culture. Milkweed Editions, Minneapolis, MN, p 9

Burt MR (1980) Cultural myths and supports for rape. J Pers Soc Psychol 38(2):217

Centers for Disease Control and Prevention (2022) Risk and protective factors. CDC, Atlanta, GA. https://www.cdc.gov/violenceprevention/sexualviolence/riskprotectivefactors.html

Coy M, Kelly L, Elvines F, Garner M, Kanyeredzi A (2013) "Sex without consent, I suppose that is rape": how young people in England understand sexual consent. Office of the Children's Commissioner, London

Crime Survey for England and Wales (2017) Figures on sexual offences from the year ending March 2017 Crime Survey for England and Wales and crimes recorded by police. Crime Survey for England and Wales, London. https://www.ons.gov.uk/peoplepopulationandcommunity/crimeandjustice/articles/sexualoffencesinenglandandwales/yearendingmarch2017

Crime Survey for England and Wales (2020) Figures on sexual offences from the year ending March 2020 Crime Survey for England and Wales and crimes recorded by police. Crime Survey for England and Wales, London. https://www.ons.gov.uk/peoplepopulationandcommunity/crimeandjustice/bulletins/sexualoffencesinenglandandwalesoverview/march2020

Decker JF, Baroni PG (2011) No still means yes: the failure of the non-consent reform movement in American rape and sexual assault law. J Crim Law Criminol 101:1081

Equality Now (2017) Impact report. https://d3n8a8pro7vhmx.cloudfront.net/equalitynow/pages/334/attachments/original/1527683249/Impact_Report_2017.pdf?1527683249

Faulkner E (2006) Homophobic sexist violence in Canada: trends in the experiences of lesbian and bisexual women in Canada. Can Woman Stud 25:154

García-Moreno C, Pallitto C, Devries K, Stöckl H, Watts C, Abrahams N (2013) Global and regional estimates of violence against women: prevalence and health effects of intimate partner violence and non-partner sexual violence. World Health Organization, Geneva

Gbahabo DD, Duma SE (2021) "I just became like a log of wood … I was paralyzed all over my body": women's lived experiences of tonic immobility following rape. Heliyon 7(7):e07471

Gross SR, Shaffer M (2012) Exonerations in the United States, 1989 Through 2012: report by the national registry of exonerations. University of Michigan Law School, Ann Arbor, MI

Guy L (2006) Re-visioning the sexual violence continuum. Partn Soc Change

Hale M (1847) Historia placitorum coronae: the history of the pleas of the crown (No. 61325-61341). RH Small

Heise LL (1998) Violence against women: an integrated, ecological framework. Viol Against Women 4(3):262–290

Henley N, Kramarae C (1991) Miscommunication, gender and power. In: Miscommunication and problematic talk. Sage, Philadelphia, PA, pp 18–43

Hollomotz A (2013) Disability and the continuum of violence. In: Disability, hate crime and violence. Routledge, London, pp 52–63

Indian Penal Code (2015). Section 375. Rape. https://www.indiacode.nic.in/show-data?actid=AC_CEN_5_23_00037_186045_1523266765688&orderno=425

Karpman B (1954) The sexual offender and his offenses. Julian Press, New York, NY

Kelly L (1988) Surviving sexual violence. Polity Press, New York, NY

Kelly L, Lovett J, Regan L (2005) A gap or a chasm. Attrition in reported rape cases. Home Office Research Study

Kozlowska K, Walker P, McLean L, Carrive P (2015) Fear and the defense cascade: clinical implications and management. Harvard Rev Psychiatry 23:263

Krug EG, Mercy JA, Dahlberg LL, Zwi AB (2002) The world report on violence and health. Lancet 360(9339):1083–1088

Lees S (2002) Carnal knowledge: rape on trial. Women's Press Ltd., London

McMahon S, Baker K (2011) Changing perceptions of sexual violence over time. National Online Resource Centre on Violence Against Women, Harrisburg

O'Loughlin E (2018) Acquittal in Irish Rugby rape case deepens debate on sexual consent. The New York Times. https://www.nytimes.com/2018/04/15/world/europe/ireland-rugby-paddy-jackson-stuart-olding.html

O'Sullivan, C. (Ed.). (1993). Transforming a rape culture. Minneapolis: Milkweed Editions.
RAINN (2020) Sexual assault statistics. https://rainn.org/get-information/statistics/sexual-assault-victims?_ga=2.89592798.413442361.1649423343-1707902002.1649161158
Rape, Abuse and Incest National Network (2020) Reasons victims choose to report—or not. https://www.rainn.org/statistics/criminal-justice-system
Remick LA (1992) Read her lips: an argument for a verbal consent standard in rape. Univ Pa Law Rev 141:1103
Rumney PN (2006) False allegations of rape. Camb Law J 65(1):128–158
Sanday PR (2007) Introduction to the second edition. In: Fraternity Gang Rape. New York University Press, New York, NY, pp 1–22
Sanders-Phillips K, Kliewer W (2020) Violence and racial discrimination in South African youth: profiles of a continuum of exposure. J Child Fam Stud 29(5):1336–1349
Saunders CL (2012) The truth, the half-truth, and nothing like the truth: reconceptualizing false allegations of rape. Br J Criminol 52(6):1152–1171
Schwartz MD, DeKeseredy W (1997) Sexual assault on the college campus: the role of male peer support. Sage Publications, Philadelphia, PA
Scully D, Marolla J (1985) "Riding the bull at Gilley's": convicted rapists describe the rewards of rape. Soc Probl 32(3):251–263
Sexual Offences Act (2003) Chapter 42. Rape. https://www.legislation.gov.uk/ukpga/2003/42/part/1/crossheading/rape
Stout KD (1991) A continuum of male controls and violence against women: a teaching model. J Soc Work Educ 27(3):305–319
Temkin J, Krahé B (2008) Sexual assault and the justice gap: A question of attitude (Vol. 5). Bloomsbury Publishing
Thornhill R, Palmer CT (2000) A natural history of rape. MIT Press, Cambridge, MA
UK Government (2020) Ending violence against women and girls. Strategy 2016 – 202. https://assets.publishing.service.gov.uk/government/uploads/system/uploads/attachment_data/file/337608/What-know-need-prevent-E.pdf
US Department of Justice (2020) National crime victimization survey, 2019. Office of Justice Programs, Bureau of Justice Statistics, Washington, DC
World Health Organization (2013) Responding to intimate partner violence and sexual violence against women: WHO clinical and policy guidelines. World Health Organization, Geneva

Madhumita Pandey, PhD is a Senior Lecturer in Criminology at the Helena Kennedy Centre for International Justice situated within the Department of Law and Criminology at Sheffield Hallam University. She works in the area of sexual offending, sex offenders and violence against women, particularly focusing on rape, in the Global South. She utilises a feminist framework to work with victims and perpetrators of gender-based violence to not only highlight women's vulnerability but also men's responsibility. More recently, she has expanded the scope of her research to include women's rights and menstrual health and hygiene in India.

Sexual Harassment: Breastfeeding, Design and the City

Sally Sutherland

Learning Objectives
Having read this chapter, you should be able to understand the following:

- Sexual harassment is pervasive and experienced by people of all genders in the UK public realm.
- Many people are forced to adopt strategies to avoid sexual harassment in public spaces and to breastfeed their infants in public.
- Creative practices can instigate change by promoting new ways of thinking and generating conversation that, in turn, leads to action.

Introduction

Sexual harassment is experienced extensively in the UK public realm by people of all genders (see Box 1), but disproportionately by women and girls. These experiences often lead to fear and a constant need to negotiate the public realm in customary ways. Sexual harassment is a violent and often misogynistic practice that violates people's rights, liberties and dignity. Due to sexual and street harassment and the environment this creates, the public realm can be particularly challenging to traverse for women, girls and people with intersecting marginalised identities (Plan International UK 2021). Most women, mothers and pregnant women will likely have experienced street and/or public sexual harassment at some point in their lives.

S. Sutherland (✉)
Radical Methodologies Research Group, University of Brighton, Brighton, UK
e-mail: S.C.Sutherland@brighton.ac.uk

P. Ali, M. M. Rogers (eds.), *Gender-Based Violence: A Comprehensive Guide*,
https://doi.org/10.1007/978-3-031-05640-6_15

These experiences shape how people experience and negotiate the public realm. Fear of public sexual harassment restricts access for girls and young women to education (getting to and from educational settings) and health-related practices such as exercise and leisure (Plan International UK 2021). This chapter uses an example of breastfeeding and argues that this is one of the many, but perhaps one of the most consequential practices negatively impacted by an often-violent public realm.

Box 1 Terminology

A Note About Language, Breastfeeding and Gender

This chapter recognises the limits of biologically based binary definitions of sex and gender. Due to these binary understandings, literature about breastfeeding and street harassment focuses on the experiences of cisgender women and cisgender mothers (cisgender refers to people whose gender identity is the same as that which was ascribed at birth). Breastfeeding is commonly associated with the gendered practices of being a woman, a mother and motherhood. However, many women and mothers may not have the opportunity or desire to breastfeed. Also, people of different gender identities may breastfeed. Some parents are more comfortable using the term ‘chestfeeding’ to describe feeding their infant from their body. For this chapter, the term ‘breastfeeding’ is inclusive of chestfeeding.

The term gestational parent means the parent who carried the child through pregnancy. Breastfeeding can be practised by people who were not the gestational parent of the child. Feeding in this instance could be due to adoption, fostering or various ‘rainbow family’ relationships. This chapter celebrates breastfeeding and intimate caring practices and the different relations and genders that carry them out. Within this chapter, ideally, the terms would be inclusive of all gender identities and peoples. However, the gaps in knowledge and research make this problematic. There is an urgent need for more gender-inclusive research into breastfeeding and street harassment—specifically, research acknowledging and including experiences of those who do not fit into exclusionary gender categories.

Defining Public

‘Public’ is a highly subjective term. Many different publics exist. For this chapter, the term ‘public’ is used to describe the public realm, away from absolute privacy, in the presence or view of strangers. Physical, offline, and public spaces are the primary focus of this chapter.

Alternative Terminology

Public, public realm, in public, public sphere, public space.

It is widely recognised that breastfeeding is beneficial to mothers, gestational parents and infants throughout their lives (Victora et al. 2016). Despite the known benefits, breastfeeding rates within Western culture remain very low, and many people stop breastfeeding before they are ready (Brown 2017). Multiple contributing barriers to breastfeeding exist at social, cultural and political layers of society (Brown 2017). A factor of particular concern is exposure to violence. Several studies have shown links between impaired breastfeeding rates and experiences of intimate partner violence (Normann et al. 2020). However, very few studies have examined the long-term impacts of violent experiences on breastfeeding rates (Holland et al. 2018). An area that needs further exploration is how neighbourhood violence, including sexual and street harassment, might affect mothers' and parents' ability or willingness to breastfeed their children in the public realm (see Box 2).

This chapter argues that reimagining and redesigning within the context of the public realm presents opportunities and possibilities for change. However, in doing so, it is necessary to acknowledge that the discipline of design is both directly and indirectly complicit in harassment and violence. In the context of breastfeeding, the public domain is a set of systems and structures that host parents and children. Although complex, it embodies the interrelated consequences of design decisions, cultures and actions. Nevertheless, there are opportunities and possibilities that come through creative practice to reimagine and reinvent more safe and equitable environments for care.

Box 2 Personal Reflections

'Sally is overdeveloped' is an odd statement to graffiti. I must have been about 13. I still don't know why someone would write this about my breasts on a street sign. My dad painted over it with white paint. I don't know who wrote it, but the sign is still there, more than 25 years later.

Growing up, my life was governed by almost daily public threats of violence and rape on the streets around my home. At the time, I didn't know any different, and accepted this as a part of my daily life. As I transitioned from girlhood to young womanhood, these threats formatively shaped who I am, how I perceive myself and the world around me. During my adult everyday walking in the urban public realm, I am acutely aware of how my experiences are shaped by my changing (ageing) identity and the neighbourhoods that I traverse. There are cultural, spatial and temporal variables, but me and my thoughts remain constant.

My 28 years of urban life before I birthed my first child taught me that the public realm was as exciting as it was hostile. I do not trust the public realm, its spaces or the people within it. It is a place I love and frequent out of choice and necessity, but this has never been a place of safety. Twelve years ago, I crossed the border into the 'Republic of Motherhood' (Berry 2018). For 12 years, these experiences have also been shaped and restricted by my practices of mothering and my maternal body as 'object'. The most contentious of these public mothering or parenting practices was breastfeeding my children.

Breastfeeding, for me, was a deviant act in any place. In the public realm, my leaky body was both revered and resented. During my first 4 years of motherhood, my children would be nourished, comforted and eat from my body in all kinds of places. I fed them, and they ate from my body in cafes, on busy buses, in filthy public toilets, in a redundancy work meeting, in windowless nursing/changing rooms that smelt so bad it would make me gag, on wet benches, in pubs, on the floor, the grass or beach. How I felt about these experiences was entirely contextual, but I felt—indeed—I felt so many feelings. I still 'feel' about it.

These feelings have activated my wonderings about how to activate changes to create safer and more equitable experiences for others. Indeed, how to reconceive and give form to intersectional feminist futures is a growing area of interest in my field of design. Design, however, is never neutral (Papanek 1974), and how it plays direct and indirect roles in structural violence needs acknowledging. Nevertheless, design and creative practices can shift, unmake and remake these public spatial, temporal and discourse variables. I am drawn to design and creative practices as they can connect culture, everyday lives and work actively to make and introduce change and action.

Breastfeeding and the UK Public Realm

Increasing breastfeeding rates would profoundly impact human and planetary health and wellbeing from individual to global scales. Individual and societal benefits of breastfeeding manifest in many ways. Benefits of breastfeeding include nutrition and immuno-support for the child and through the mother or gestational parent's protection against breast and ovarian cancers, Type 2 diabetes and obesity (Victora et al. 2016). Breastfeeding reduces infant illness rates (Brown 2016) and consequently decreases the need for health services and subsequent health care costs (Renfrew et al. 2012; Brown 2017). An increase in breastfeeding rates would also reduce environmental and ecological damage by reducing the demand for breastmilk substitutes (Karlsson et al. 2019) and minimise the need for teats, bottles and sterilisers to practice bottle feeding (Brown 2016). However, breastfeeding is a divisive and complex subject in the UK, partly due to its promotion as the best way to feed an infant combined with the systematic lack of support to do so.

A recurring theme of UK breastfeeding research is the challenges faced when breastfeeding in 'public' (Hauck et al. 2021). Despite the continued efforts of medical and health services to increase UK breastfeeding initiation and continuation, rates in the UK remain among the lowest in the world (Renfrew et al. 2012). The recorded breastfeeding rates in the UK vary significantly (McAndrew et al. 2012), as breastfeeding is culturally contextual (Cassidy and El Tom 2015). All public breastfeeding experiences will vary significantly, but there are also broader trends across socioeconomic groups and within intersectional variations of race, class and ethnicity (Isherwood et al. 2019).

Paying attention to frightening and gender-related experiences of the public realm is fundamental to supporting breastfeeding practices. Breastfeeding is physiologically, physically, practically and emotionally experienced by an infant feeding dyad—it is an embodied 'intercorporeal' interaction. However, many parents find breastfeeding in public to be a stressful and embarrassing experience (NCT 2009; Sheehan et al. 2019). Stress hormones can interfere with levels of prolactin and oxytocin—the chemicals within the body needed to produce breast milk—these changes can potentially impede milk production (Brown 2016). Current literature rarely discusses the impacts of stress or emotional discomfort on breastfeeding practices.

Breastfed infants need to be fed regularly and 'on demand', meaning that negotiating the public realm is essential if parents wish to participate in public life and engage in the public sphere. How people feel about breastfeeding and behave in the public realm plays a crucial role in breastfeeding duration and whether parents and children have access to spaces and activities with others. Scott et al. (2015) emphasise that people who do not breastfeed in public are more likely to discontinue breastfeeding sooner. The most recent Infant Feeding Survey (2010) showed that more than half of mothers felt uncomfortable feeding in front of others and that 40% of breastfeeding mothers had never breastfed in public (McAndrew et al. 2012). Mothers from socially disadvantaged backgrounds and young mothers are less likely to breastfeed, and those who do are less likely to breastfeed in the public realm (McAndrew et al. 2012)—this is likely due to feeling uncomfortable, potentially unsafe and perceptions of public judgement.

At present, breastfeeding in the public realm is protected by UK law. Yet, in practice, breastfeeding can feel unwelcome, alien and 'out of place, and taking up space in ways that make other people feel uncomfortable' (Kern 2020: p. 28). Many people report receiving negative comments or being asked to stop (NCT 2009; Boyer 2012). Unease with breastfeeding in the public realm is cited as a common reason for stopping (Brown 2016; Boyer 2018).

Social attitudes to breastfeeding have a notable impact on how people feel about breastfeeding in the public realm and in front of others (Brown 2016). These feelings also impact overall infant feeding decisions (Brown 2016). Breastfeeding in public has been associated with negative judgement from strangers (Grant 2016), and disapproval of public breastfeeding is widespread in UK society (Brown 2016). Significantly, infant feeding is not the same for everyone and is particularly challenging for mothers from marginalised contexts to negotiate (Jamie et al. 2020).

Unaccepting attitudes of public breastfeeding relate to ambivalent sexism (Acker 2009) and misogyny. In addition, hypersexual perceptions of women's bodies and breasts are held by some who find public breastfeeding an uncomfortable concept (Acker 2009; Grant 2016). Breasts frequently perceived as *sexual* rather than *nurturing* lead to some breastfeeding women fearing potential predatory attention in the public realm (Sheehan et al. 2019). The uncertainty of potentially revealing a part of a breast or nipple in public can trigger fears of physical and moral danger. Societal misconstruction of bodily identities and functions creates a problematic tension between nurture and eroticism when breastfeeding in the public realm (Sheehan et al. 2019).

Behaviour modifications are often adopted to negotiate people and places when breastfeeding in the public realm (Sheehan et al. 2019; Hauck et al. 2021). Parents adopt strategies such as limiting their time away from home to avoid breastfeeding in public altogether. Other tactics include using breastfeeding covers, avoiding eye contact, not being alone, sitting in specific ways or in discrete corners or moving to private locations. While experiences are spatial and material, they can also be described as constantly changing *assemblages of matters and meanings* that different people experience in different ways.

Nursing, feeding or mother and baby rooms are increasingly common in shopping centres and public spaces. These facilities are immensely beneficial for some (Boyer 2012), especially for very young children or those with complex feeding needs. However, these spaces are usually small white, windowless rooms positioned next to a toilet and integrated with nappy changing facilities (Grant 2016). While the quality of the spaces varies, they can be tricky spaces to breastfeed within (Boyer 2012) as they are often dirty and potentially isolating (Boyer 2012; Grant 2016). Public toilets also become places frequently used to breastfeed and pump milk. They are not dissimilar in design, layout, location and cleanliness to the 'feeding rooms'. Without the simultaneous engagement with broader systemic infant feeding challenges, the provision of nursing rooms can 'other' breastfeeding parents. This othering can be counterproductive when seeking to include parents and infants in the public realm. Instead, there is a need to transition to safe and visible infant feeding in all public and private realms.

Nursing rooms are an example of public health support for breastfeeding in the UK, focusing solely on the individual's responsibility. Yet, in Western culture, complex and varied determinants compromise breastfeeding practices. Many determining factors have been identified at a societal rather than an individual level, therefore beyond the control of breastfeeding mothers or parents (Brown 2017). It is argued that the environment is the principal determining factor of breastfeeding in the UK over and above individual background (Peregrino et al. 2018), and perceived social norms might exert breastfeeding practices over a mother's breastfeeding attitudes and knowledge (Scott et al. 2015). These more complex and culturally embedded challenges that face breastfeeding practices are impossible to address using individualist interventions or simple solutions. How mothers, parents and infants negotiate intimate caring practices in the public realm is one of many opportunities for attention and action.

While the public realm has been recognised as a site of street and sexual harassment for many years, there is very little research or information about how these experiences impact other practices, such as intimate acts of caring. As the average age of women having a child in England and Wales is 30 (ONS 2020), it is likely that these people will have reported or experienced sexual harassment in a public space. The sexual nature of public harassment mirrors the hypersexualisation of the maternal and breastfeeding body. Even though the term MILF (mum I'd like to fuck) is a common slang term in the UK, maternal and parental experiences of harassment are not explicitly mentioned in reports about UK harassment.

Supporting breastfeeding in the public realm sustains the significant benefits of breastfeeding and being breastfed. Conversely, not supporting breastfeeding in the public realm results in real and perceived physical, emotional and moral danger. This contradiction is one of the many ways new mothers and parents are set up to fail in the UK. Without action and change, stress, shame, guilt and grief will continue to be felt by new mothers and parents, regardless of how they feed their infants.

> … understanding the problem of infant feeding in terms of violence originating at multiple levels beyond the individual gets us away from the 'educating the mother' interventions so often used. Shifting the focus can stimulate interventions designed at multiple levels to change policies, institutions, and cultural attitudes. (Chin and Dozier 2012: p. 65)

So far, this chapter has been discussing the issue of breastfeeding in the public realm. It will now examine the public realm as a site of sexual and street harassment for girls, women, mothers and parents, as an external but related violence.

Street Harassment and the UK Public Realm

> Regardless of the level of severity, catcalls, sexual comments, ogling, wolf-whistling and groping in public spaces by strangers debilitate the survivor's liberty to freely enter public spaces without fear. (Baptist and Coburn 2019: p. 115)

Relentless public sexual harassment is the daily norm for many young women and girls in city neighbourhoods worldwide (see Box 3 for alternative terminology). Recent surveys and reports document and draw attention to experiences of harassment in the UK public realm. For example, the House of Commons Women and Equalities Committee (2018) has recently reported that sexual harassment in the UK is widespread and the most common type of violence encountered by UK women and girls. The APPG for UN Women report (2021) has established the high prevalence of sexual harassment experienced by women and girls in UK public spaces and the urgency for this to be addressed. Crucially the report reveals that almost all women in the UK have experienced sexual harassment in a public space. Typical forms of harassment in the UK include catcalls or wolf whistles, being stared at and unwelcome touching or groping (APPG for UN Women 2021). Unwelcome sexual advances or calls for sexual 'favours' are common (APPG for UN Women 2021). Experiences of harassment are contextual and situated in radically different neighbourhoods; factors that impact street harassment include location and time of day or night (APPG for UN Women 2021).

Box 3 Alternative Terminology: Sexual Harassment
Public sexual harassment, street harassment, public harassment, sexual harassment, stranger harassment.

Girls and women of varying ages in the UK experience street and public sexual harassment, and young women are most at risk. The APPG for UN Women (2021) report that 86% of UK women aged 18–24 have experienced sexual harassment in a public space. Reports of harassment when wearing a school uniform are not uncommon (Plan International UK 2021). Harassment often starts when people are very young, with girls aged 7–10 experiencing unwanted attention and feeling unsafe in public (Girl Guiding 2020).

It is, however, unhelpful and impossible to consider girls and women as a homogenous group. Simultaneous, intersecting inequalities and oppressions affect experiences of public sexual harassment, providing unique experiences of violence (Imkaan 2019). Girls and young women who identify as lesbian, gay, bisexual, trans or queer are more likely to record being stared at and receiving unwanted attention (Girl Guiding 2020). These figures correlate with research into adults' experiences that demonstrate that people who hold multiple marginalised identities are more likely to experience online (Plan International UK 2020) and street harassment (Baptist and Coburn 2019).

This harassment shapes urban lives in countless conscious and unconscious ways (Kern 2020). Work by Plan International illustrates how normalised sexual harassment is in different parts of the world and how common consequences of sexual harassment include fear and anger. The *Our Streets Now* campaign documents the prevalence and impact of UK sexual harassment, demonstrating it as broad-ranging and far-reaching. The consequences of this harassment of girls and children are that many feel worried and unsafe in public from a young age (Girl Guiding 2020). While physical public spaces are the focus of this chapter, it is important to acknowledge that online harassment is just as frightening and dangerous. Both are sites where problematic social and cultural behaviours can be deeply harmful, and as part of everyday lives, these online and physical public realms interconnect.

To avoid sexual harassment in the public realm, women and girls consciously and unconsciously modify behaviours and practices due to both real and perceived threats. These behaviour modifications include not walking alone, not smiling, wearing modest clothing (Sen 2019) and not going out (Girl Guiding 2020). Feminist Geographer Leslie Kern argues that a woman alone in a city learns a set of primarily unconscious embodied habits moulded by the navigation of our urban environment (Kern 2020). Kern argues that these bodily responses stay with us, shaping all kinds of things, such as how we walk, our posture and if and how we make eye contact (Kern 2020).

The strategies that breastfeeding mothers and parents employ are not dissimilar to those by women avoiding unwanted sexual attention or harassment. Significant effort is used in negotiating the public realm, which is often unnoticed and becomes second nature. Spatial decision-makers, including policymakers, developers, designers and architects, have responded similarly to sexual and street harassment and public breastfeeding practices. However, common responses are to 'solve' these 'problems' by offering site-specific solutions for the autonomous individual, to keep women safe and out of sight of offenders or the problematic public realm. These approaches often frame the issue as a problem for the individual rather than engaging with the multiple levels of violence that underpin the situation.

These universalist solutions also typically focus solely on supporting an anonymous homogenised interpretation of an individual without acknowledging the broader contexts of gendered, mothering or parenting, experiences in the public realm. White windowless rooms to breastfeed a child, single-sex spaces to avoid unwanted attention or phone numbers to call when people fear their safety act like sticking plasters for vastly more urgent, significant cultural and societal challenges. On their own, these solutions feel short term. At best, they provide spaces for some people to feel safe and private in the public realms. At worst, they reinforce structural and systemic violence. In creating spaces for women's safety, or private places for breastfeeding practices—presented under the guise of neoliberal ideals of 'choice'—these interventions reinforce gender stereotypes and cultural attitudes that breastfeeding is unwelcome in public and should be practised in private and out of sight (Boyer 2012). Oversimplified interventionistic strategies, such as those outlined above, can reinforce narrow ideas that women's or breastfeeding bodies are problems for cities. As Kern describes, these bodies are 'too fat, too fertile, too sexual, too messy, too vulnerable' (Kern 2020: p. 166).

Cheer Up Luv as Form-Giving Action

> Cities are made up of invisible boundaries, intangible customs gates that demarcate who goes where … We claim our right to disturb the peace, to observe (or not observe), to occupy (or not occupy) and to organise (or disorganise) space on our own terms. (Elkin 2017: p. 288)

This chapter introduces and showcases the work *Cheer Up Luv*, an ongoing campaign by UK-based photographer and activist Eliza Hatch. This example presents a counter conventional approach demonstrating how creative practice can provide site of care, and opportunity for form-giving action. This action sits in direct contrast to the more common solutionist approaches outlined above. This work is complex and tangential and provides genuine insight from lived experiences—providing a more authentic representation of the nature of the challenges faced. The Cheer Up Luv project sensitively and actively pervades the violent territory of street harassment, manifesting as an international photojournalism-online platform-community-podcast-exhibitions-talks-workshops-campaign that spans digital and physical realms. *Cheer Up Luv* retells accounts of sexual harassment, with Hatch photographing survivors in the location or a similar location to where the harassment occurred. The location becomes a stage for the narrative and acts to reclaim the space and body within the public realm. The photos and stories are posted on the Cheer Up Luv Instagram account and website. These stories are also exhibited in pop up exhibitions in urban community settings, often associated with talks and workshops such as bystander intervention or self-defence classes.

The project gives form to individual experiences and moves beyond raising awareness to enable understanding, generate empowerment and provoke online and offline action. Cheer Up Luv demonstrates how creative practice as an act of form giving can provide new insights into public sexual and street harassment that, in turn, enable alternative futures.

The voices and images in the Cheer Up Luv campaign provide examples, including maternal and post-natal experiences of harassment, misogyny, intimidation and the overt hypersexualisation of bodies, breasts and nipples in the everyday public realm. The following texts and images are three examples of the many stories within the Cheer Up Luv project.

Korantema, Asiyah, and Kelsey

Korantema, Asiyah, and Kelsey's stories shown in Figs. 1, 2, and 3 are powerful, and their situated and embodied experiences of harassment are crucially platformed. Through the Cheer Up Luv platform, streets, bodies, sexuality and problematic encounters are taken seriously and reclaimed through the action of collective storytelling that recognises and gives form to these experiences. Hatch's creative practice outputs are 'agentic objects'—they can shift narratives about the present by reclaiming bodies, agency and voice within the public realm.

Cheer Up Luv does not tell anyone what to do or claim to solve anything; instead, it invites thinking, conversation and action. The stories and conversations shift narratives and expose violent normative practices. They challenge myths and misrepresentations. Spanning the digital and physical realms, the act of taking and

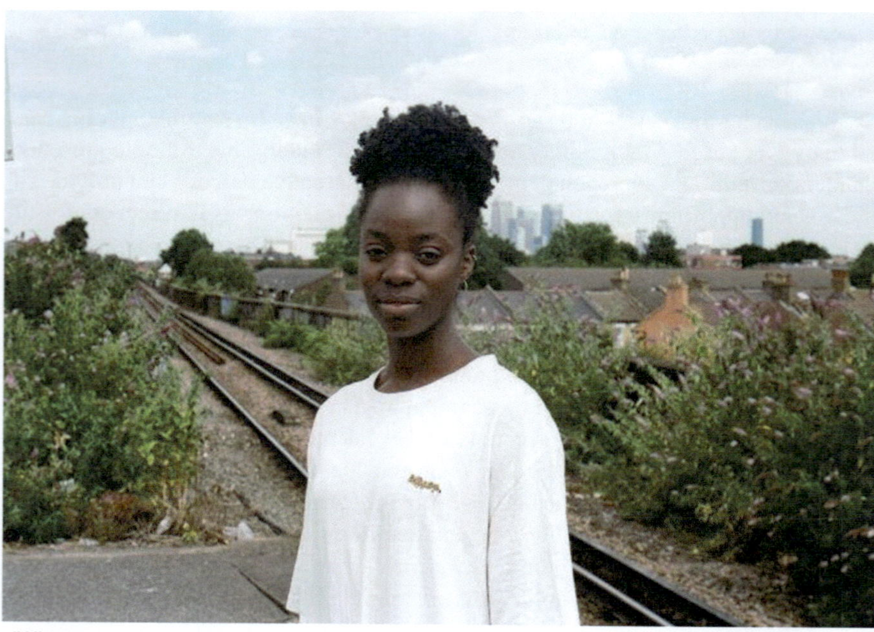

'When I was in year 7, I was walking home in east London and a man stopped me and asked for directions. After I told him, he asked me, "Are your nipples big or small?" I thought I misheard so I said, "What?" He stepped closer and asked me again . - I ran all the way home.' Korantema

Fig. 1 Korantema, 2017, by Eliza Hatch. (© Cheer Up Luv)

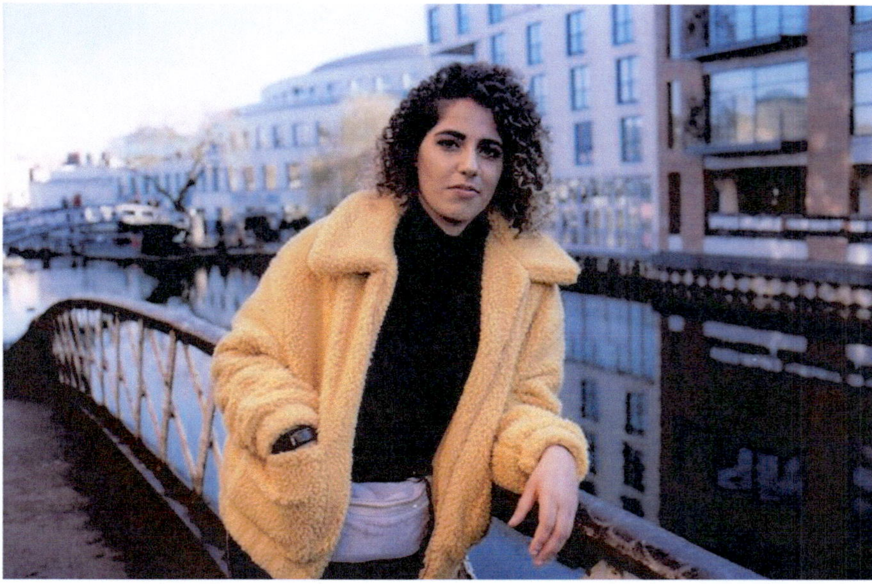

'I was walking my children to school early one morning, when a group of men in a building site started whistling and making sexual noises. One of them shouted, "Come on turn around love, don't be shy we don't bite." I was horrified that certain men think that this behaviour is acceptable. My children had to witness the filth that was said to me. These individuals choose a time when they know a woman is vulnerable and won't be able to fight back. To make matters worse, when I explained to a friend, she replied saying, "Oh don't worry babe, it's because your pretty, don't take no notice of it."' Asiyah

Fig. 2 Asiyah, 2019, by Eliza Hatch. (© Cheer Up Luv)

exhibiting photography serves to reclaim the public realm for participants and observers—it takes up space. Cheer Up Luv provokes alternatives by reclaiming narratives and by promoting social and political change.

The Cheer Up Luv project provides snapshots of unique experiences of violence. These stories reveal the often-violent public landscapes that women, girls and parents negotiate daily. This chapter argues that designers and creative practitioners have the skills, insight and visionary capabilities to facilitate alternative futures. More specifically, creative practice can challenge dominant narratives to shift power, dismantle myths and disrupt invisible but problematic social and cultural norms. Significantly, this work argues for practices that move beyond raising awareness or individualistic 'solutions' to instead move towards more radical and long-term change. These critical change-making actions present opportunities to resist violence originating beyond the individual. Collective action must be taken to activate more equitable and just everyday experiences for girls, women, mothers and parents. This chapter argues that this is especially relevant where they impact infant feeding practices, not least due to the significant impacts on individual and global health.

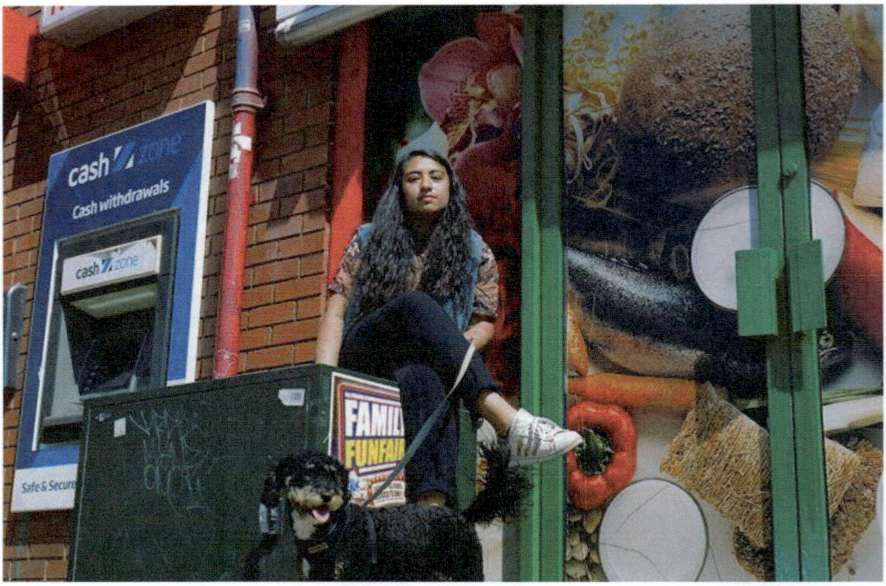

'An old man came up to me and my friend at a bus stop and said we were beautiful. We explained that we didn't care what he thought of our appearance, but he cut us off and said, "I'm going to walk over there now, and when I do, I'm going to turn around and look at your bottoms!" As we turned to glare at him, laughing he said, "See, you're scared now." And carried on laughing.' Kelsey

Fig. 3 Kelsey, 2017, by Eliza Hatch. (© Cheer Up Luv)

Summary

- The UK public realm is a site of frequent violent harassment for many girls, women, mothers, people and parents in the UK.
- Action and change are needed to reflect this situation in the UK's physical, cultural, social and moral public realms.
- An intersectional approach is necessary for understanding unique experiences of violence (Imkaan 2019) and their consequences on infant feeding practices.
- There are similarities between the behaviours adopted when negotiating the public realm wanting to avoid sexual harassment and wanting or needing to breastfeed.
- Action and change within the gendered and hypersexualised public realm could lead to gender-related health-promoting and equalising practices.
- Cheer Up Luv is an example of a project that actively spans the digital and the physical, bringing conversation and change.
- Cheer Up Luv is an example of creative practice as activism and action, joining up experiences and action and crucially giving form to alternative futures.

- Challenges of public sexual harassment and public breastfeeding originate with levels of violence beyond the individual, meaning that individualistic solutions to these problems often act as sticking plasters for broader and deeper societal and cultural issues.
- Creative practice can engage in challenging narratives to shift power, dismantle myths and disrupt invisible norms.

Special Thanks Enormous gratitude goes to Eliza Hatch for allowing the use of the photos in this chapter and to Korantema, Asiyah, and Kelsey for permitting their pictures and stories to be shared in this context.

References

Acker M (2009) Breast is best … but not everywhere: ambivalent sexism and attitudes toward private and public breastfeeding. Sex Roles 61(7–8):476–490

APPG for UN Women (2021) Prevalence and reporting of sexual harassment in UK public spaces. https://www.unwomenuk.org/site/wp-content/uploads/2021/03/APPG-UN-Women-Sexual-Harassment-Report_Updated.pdf. Accessed 17 Oct 2021

Baptist J, Coburn K (2019) Harassment in public spaces: the intrusion on personal space. J Fem Fam Ther 31(2–3):114–128

Berry L (2018) The republic of motherhood. Chatto & Windus, London

Boyer K (2012) Affect, corporeality and the limits of belonging: breastfeeding in public in the contemporary UK. Health Place 18(3):552–560

Boyer K (2018) The emotional resonances of breastfeeding in public: the role of strangers in breastfeeding practice. Emot Space Soc 26:33–40

Brown A (2016) Breastfeeding Uncovered: who really decides how we feed our babies? Pinter & Martin, London

Brown A (2017) Breastfeeding as a public health responsibility: a review of the evidence. J Hum Nutr Diet 30(6):759–770

Cassidy T, El Tom A (eds) (2015) Ethnographies of breastfeeding: cultural contexts and confrontations. Bloomsbury Academic, London

Chin N, Dozier A (2012) The dangers of baring the breast: structural violence and formula feeding among low-income women. In: Smith P, Hausman B, Labbok M (eds) Beyond health, beyond choice: breastfeeding constraints and realities. Rutgers University Press, New Brunswick, NJ, pp 64–73

Elkin L (2017) Flâneuse: women walk the city in Paris, New York, Tokyo, Venice and London. Vintage, London

Girl Guiding (2020) Girls Attitudes Survey 2020: a snapshot of girls' and young womens' lives. https://www.girlguiding.org.uk/globalassets/docs-and-resources/research-and-campaigns/girls-attitudes-survey-2020.pdf. Accessed 25 Oct 2021

Grant A (2016) "I … don't want to see you flashing your bits around": exhibitionism, othering and good motherhood in perceptions of public breastfeeding. Geoforum 71:52–61

Hauck Y, Bradfield Z, Kuliukas L (2021) Women's experiences with breastfeeding in public: an integrative review. Women Birth J Austr Coll Midwiv 34(3):217–227

Holland M, Thevenent-Morrison K, Mittal M et al (2018) Breastfeeding and Exposure to Past, Current, and Neighborhood Violence. Matern Child Health J 22(1):82–91

House of Commons Women and Equalities Committee (2018) Sexual harassment of women and girls in public places https://publications.parliament.uk/pa/cm201719/cmselect/cmwomeq/701/701.pdf. Accessed 25 Oct 2021

Imkaan (2019) The value of intersectionality in understanding violence against women and girls (VAWG). https://eca.unwomen.org/en/digital-library/publications/2019/10/the-value-of-intersectionality-in-understanding-violence-against-women-and-girls. Accessed 25 Oct 2021

Isherwood J, Boyer K, Dowling S (2019) Local landscapes of breastfeeding: a comparison of breastfeeding amongst mothers in low- and high-income neighbourhoods in Bristol, UK. Health Place 59:102125

Jamie K, McGeagh L, Bows H et al (2020) 'I just don't think it's that natural': adolescent mothers' constructions of breastfeeding as deviant. Soc Health Illn 42(7):1689–1708

Karlsson J, Garnett T, Rollins N et al (2019) The carbon footprint of breastmilk substitutes in comparison with breastfeeding. J Clean Prod 222:436–445

Kern L (2020) Feminist city: claiming space in a man-made world. Verso, London

McAndrew F, Thompson J, Fellows L et al (2012) Infant feeding survey - UK, 2010. https://digital.nhs.uk/data-and-information/publications/statistical/infant-feeding-survey/infant-feeding-survey-uk-2010. Accessed 25 Oct 2021

NCT (2009) Mother and baby survey reveals mothers worries about breastfeeding in public. https://nctwatch.wordpress.com/2009/07/24/mother-and-baby-survey-reveals-mothers-worries-about-breastfeeding-in-public/#_msocom_1. Accessed 25 Oct 2021

Normann A, Bakiewicz A, Kjerulff M et al (2020) Intimate partner violence and breastfeeding: a systematic review. BMJ Open 10(10):1–9

ONS, Office of National Statistics (2020). Birth characteristics in England and Wales: 2019. https://www.ons.gov.uk/peoplepopulationandcommunity/birthsdeathsandmarriages/livebirths/bulletins/birthcharacteristicsinenglandandwales/2019. Accessed 25 Oct 2021

Papanek V (1974) Design for the real world: human ecology and social change. Paladin, St Albans

Peregrino AB, Watt RG, Heilmann A et al (2018) Breastfeeding practices in the United Kingdom: is the neighbourhood context important? Matern Child Nutr 14(4):1–15

Plan International (2020) Free to be online? Girls' and young women's experiences of online harassment. https://www.planinternational.nl/uploaded/2020/09/SOTWGR2020-CommsReport-EN.pdf?x10967. Accessed 25 Oct 2021

Plan International UK (2021) What works for ending public sexual harassment, September 2021. https://plan-uk.org/file/what-works-for-ending-public-sexual-harassment-full-report/download?token=wtUTx1DM. Accessed 25 Oct 2021

Renfrew MJ, Pokhrel S, Quigley M et al (2012) Preventing disease and saving resources: the potential contribution of increasing breastfeeding rates in the UK. UNICEF, London

Scott JA, Kwok Y, Synnott K et al (2015) A comparison of maternal attitudes to breastfeeding in public and the association with breastfeeding duration in four European Countries: results of a cohort study. Birth 42(1):78–85

Sen P (2019) What will it take? Promoting cultural change to end sexual harassment. UN Women, New York, NY. https://www.unwomen.org/en/digital-library/publications/2019/09/discussion-paper-what-will-it-take-promoting-cultural-change-to-end-sexual-harassment. Accessed 17 Oct 2021

Sheehan A, Gribble K, Schmied V (2019) It's okay to breastfeed in public but .... Int Breastfeed J 14(1):1–11

Victora C, Bahl R, Barros A et al (2016) Breastfeeding in the 21st century: epidemiology, mechanisms, and lifelong effect. Lancet 387(10017):475–490

Sally Sutherland is an AHRC Design Star-funded doctoral candidate at the University of Brighton. Her creative, exploratory, practice-based design research focuses on design, culture and gender and aims to support more inclusive breastfeeding and infant feeding practices.

Part V

Harmful Practices

Acid Attacks

Lucy Neville, Matt Hopkins, and Teela Sanders

Learning Objectives
Having read this chapter, you should be able to understand the following:

- The definition and characteristics of acid attacks and the historic use of corrosives in acts of violence
- The difficulties involved in ascertaining the global prevalence of acid attacks
- International differences in who is more commonly victimised by acid-based violence
- Productive ways forward in reducing the volume and severity of acid attacks

Introduction

This chapter presents an exploration of violence involving corrosive substances, widely referred to as 'acid attacks'. While by no means common, acid attacks occur around the globe and lead to significant physical and emotional harms to survivors and their families. However, while acid attacks have attracted significant media and policy attention, they remain an under-researched and poorly understood phenomenon. The majority of academic work that has focussed on acid attacks has been epidemiological, examining the type and extent of injuries sustained by survivors;

L. Neville (✉) M. Hopkins T. Sanders
School of Criminology, University of Leicester, Leicester, England, UK
e-mail: lucy.neville@leicester.ac.uk; matt.hopkins@leicester.ac.uk; teela.sanders@leicester.ac.uk

P. Ali, M. M. Rogers (eds.), *Gender-Based Violence: A Comprehensive Guide*, https://doi.org/10.1007/978-3-031-05640-6_16

far less attention has been paid to understanding offender motivations for using corrosive substances as weapons or to identifying potential preventative strategies. Much of the work attempting to draw attention to the harm caused by acid attacks has thus far been carried out by nongovernmental organisations (NGOs) such as the Acid Survivors' Trust International (ASTI) and the Acid Survivors' Foundation (ASF). Charities such as these work to support survivors, pressure governments into taking action on corrosive crime and to monitor the numbers of attacks. In this chapter, acid attacks are defined and described, with a brief history of their occurrence and prevalence offered for context. Some of the difficulties in obtaining prevalence rates are explained, with some discussion about how acid attacks follow very different patterns in different countries. The impact acid attacks can have on survivors, families and communities are described. Finally, an overview of some useful explanatory theories for acid attacks is provided, before outlining some suggestions for future policy, practice and research.

Definition and Types

A range of labels have been used to describe the phenomenon known as 'acid attacks' (see Box 1). The term 'vitriolic' attack, referring to vitriol—a sulphuric acid-based substance used in the treatment of precious metals—was used throughout the nineteenth and early twentieth centuries (Watson 2017), but more recently the term 'acid attack' has been widely adopted.

While acid is often used in such attacks, other corrosive substances are also common, particularly strong and easily accessible alkalis, such as caustic soda or lye (often contained in household cleaning products). In the UK, alkali-based household products (such as bleach) are the most frequently used corrosives in violent assaults (Hopkins et al. 2021). The broad range of substances used in 'acid' attacks is recognised in the wording of acid laws in countries such as India and Pakistan, as well as in the UK, where the National Police Chiefs Council defines substances used in acid attacks as 'those that cause visible destruction and/or permanent change in human skin tissue at the site of contact' (Hopkins et al. 2021: 5). Damage to skin tissue is caused by a substance with a particularly high or low pH value. The acidity or alkalinity of a substance is determined using the power of hydrogen (pH) scale (which ranges from 0 to 14), with 7 indicating a neutral substance, low pH values indicating acids and high pH values indicating alkalis. While the exact chemical composition of a corrosive substance used in an attack may make little difference to the suffering experienced by the victim (or mean much to the media or public), it is nevertheless important in terms of potential criminal justice sanctions and crime prevention.

Acid attacks have therefore been defined as 'intentional acts of violence in which perpetrators throw, spray, or pour (corrosives) onto victims' faces or bodies' (Kalantry and Kestenbaum 2011: 1)—often leading to long-lasting physical damage and scarring. Many scholars have argued that a unique factor of acid attacks is that often the primary intent is not to kill the victim (or even simply to physically hurt them per se), but to permanently disfigure them (Mannon et al. 2007; Tan et al. 2015).

In their review of the global literature on acid attacks, Mannon et al. (2007: 149) identify two broad motives for acid attacks: enforcement of a violent/acquisitive crime or as part of a 'crime of passion' between current or former romantic partners. A more recent review suggests four general motives for the use of corrosives in violent assaults (Hopkins et al. 2021):

- Relationship breakdown/refusal of marriage/rejection of romantic advances
- Robbery and street fights
- Racially motivated assaults and other types of hate crime
- Business competition, violence against officials and political rivalry

Box 1 Alternative Terminology
Acid violence, acid throwing, corrosive crime, noxious substance attacks, vitriol attacks, vitriolage, burns violence, chemical attacks, chemical assault.

Historical Context

The coverage of acid attacks in the global media would suggest that this form of violence is a relatively new phenomenon. However, acid attacks have a long history worldwide, with accounts of 'vitriolage' stretching back to at least the sixteenth century, and an upsurge of accounts in the nineteenth century when highly concentrated acids started to be regularly used in industry (Tan et al. 2015).

Historically, such crimes were often reported as 'crimes of passion' with a particular focus on women who used this form of violence to exact revenge upon erstwhile male lovers (Tan et al. 2015). Indeed, writing in the early twentieth century, Blackham (1936: 146) notes that acid attacks constitute 'a particularly cruel crime which is almost exclusively confined to females'. Acid was also often used as a weapon of choice in street-based violence, with a Judge at The Old Bailey commenting in 1889 that 'it is the crime of the Apache of Paris (a Parisian street gang), who is said to go about with a dagger in one pocket and a bottle of vitriol in the other' (in The Daily Mail, 10th September 1924: 10).

Similar cases of acid used in street-based violence were reported throughout the eighteenth, nineteenth and twentieth centuries in the UK and the USA, where sulphuric acid was mass manufactured, easily available and unregulated (Yousaf and Purkayastha 2016). In addition, there are numerous accounts of vitriol throwing being used as a form of industrial protest, with trade unionists targeting masters and business owners (see Hopkins et al. 2021). Certainly, acid attacks were firmly established in the public consciousness by the nineteenth century, with Arthur Conan Doyle incorporating vitriol throwing into the plot of an 1890s Sherlock Holmes novel.

Acid attacks also have a long history in South Asia, with burning being historically viewed as a 'semi-legitimate' form of punishment against women, who were regarded as the property of their male relations (Chowdhury 2005). Faga et al. (2000) describe husbands burning disobedient wives, traditionally with lit kerosene, but in some cases with the use of acids. Discussing the prevalence of domestic violence in Pakistan, Yousaf and Purkayastha (2016) state that acid violence is viewed as a normative form of domestic 'punishment' within some rural communities.

Prevalence

There have long been concerns over high rates of acid violence in countries such as India, Pakistan, Bangladesh, Nepal, Uganda and Cambodia (ASTI 2015), for example, in India the case of Reshma Qureshi, who was just 17 when her former brother-in-law poured acid over her face in an attack (The Guardian 2019) gathered significant attention, as did that of Laxmi Agarwal, who was attacked at the age of 16 by a family 'friend' after she had rejected his romantic advances (The Times of India 2005). However, while acid attacks are viewed as a social problem in many countries around the globe, accurate measurement of the extent of acid attacks remains a challenge (Haque and Ahsan 2014). While some international literature provides estimates of the extent of acid attacks, particularly in South Asian countries (e.g. Kalantry and Kestenbaum 2011; ASTI 2015), the likely under-reporting of crimes involving corrosives is a significant barrier to assessing the true prevalence of this type of violence. Some countries keep no record of acid attacks at all, having no requirement to record an attack as a separate category from any other weapon-based violent crime; or, when attacks are recorded, the type of corrosive used and/or the most basic details about the attack are not noted (ASTI 2015).

The best estimates as to the prevalence of acid attacks come from the UK and India. In the UK it is estimated that around 800 corrosive attacks occur nationally per year (Hopkins et al. 2021). In India, data from the National Crime Records Bureau (2018) shows that there are generally around 200 cases per year. Across other countries, the number of attacks tends to be lower than the UK and India, though such figures tend to come from estimates made by organisations such as the ASTI, and are therefore perhaps less accurate. ASTI warns that the true global rates of such crimes are likely to be much higher, noting that their work suggests that acid violence is also common in Iran (which does not record the offence) and Afghanistan. ASTI has also expressed concern about the lack of any attempt to systematically collect data on the number of corrosive attacks in Europe, though they estimate as many as 3000 attacks occur annually across the continent.

Even in countries which do keep records of acid attacks, officers on the scene often do not have access to testing kits, and gathering samples to send for testing and analysis is difficult and costly. Police reports therefore tend to rely on victim/witness accounts to identify acid attacks, and victims often (and understandably) initially panic when they experience a tingling or burning sensation when a substance is thrown at them and assume they have been sprayed with something extremely corrosive—only for it later to be identified as something less noxious, such as lemon juice or washing-up liquid (Hopkins et al. 2021). Typically, the exact substance used in a violent attack will remain unknown (Beare 1990).

In December 2017, the British media claimed that the UK had one of the highest rates of acid attacks in the world (The Independent 2017), with Rachel Kearton, the National Police Chiefs Council lead on corrosive attacks stating, 'The UK now has one of the highest rates of recorded acid and corrosive substance attacks per capita in the world and this number appears to be rising ... It appears that ... we will again exceed previous records for the number of attacks [but] I strongly feel that this is an under-reported crime at this time' (Kearton cited in Gayle 2017).

Prevalence and Gender: An International Comparison

Traditionally, acid attacks have been viewed as a particular problem with the 'developing' world or within low- and middle-income countries (LMIC), and as such they have been linked to wider global issues with gender inequality and violence against women (Chowdhury 2011). However, to conclude that acid violence only happens towards women in LMICs or that all acid violence is domestic is misleading. In many high-income countries, as well as in LMIC like Jamaica and Uganda, the victims of acid attacks are more likely to be male, and the attack often happens during the course of another crime event, such as a robbery or burglary.

While some studies have found that women are more likely to be victims of acid attacks than men (e.g. Kalantry and Kestenbaum 2011; ASTI 2015), most studies have observed that, with the exception of Bangladesh and Taiwan, men generally comprise the majority of victims (Mannon et al. 2007; Nagarajan et al. 2020). In Bangladesh, which can be viewed as an anomaly with its proportionally high number of female victims, acid attacks have been described as a 'gender crime' (Faga et al. 2000), with women often being targeted because of proposal rejections and/or the spurning of romantic/sexual advances. It has been theorised that in low- and middle-income countries (LMIC) like Bangladesh, acid attacks are often perpetrated with the 'intent to disfigure' rather than the intent to kill, in order to spoil the life chances and marriage opportunities for women victims (ActionAid 2017). However, Mannon et al. (2007) note that this trend is reversed in both Jamaica and the USA, where, in the context of domestic or romantic disputes, the victims are more often men.

The highest male-to-female ratio of victims has been observed in the UK (see Hossain et al. 2019; Nagarajan et al. 2020). Data gathered from a number of UK police forces suggests that both the victims and offenders involved in acid attacks are much more likely to be male, with men constituting 72% of the victims of corrosive-based crimes and 88% of the offenders (Hopkins et al. 2021). This is not surprising if we consider a corrosive to be yet another potential weapon in a criminal's arsenal: an abundance of cross-cultural evidence suggests that men are more likely to carry and use weapons than women (see, e.g. Pickett et al. 2005) and are correspondingly more likely to be the victims of violent crime. Feminist commentators have argued that the growing awareness in the UK that victims of acid attacks are often male and White has led to the increasing political and media attention paid to the issue. ‘When we thought they mostly affected Asian women with jealous exes, acid attacks weren’t on anyone’s radar’, Rabina Khan (2017, emphasis added) wrote in *The Independent*, ‘It’s only because we’re *all* vulnerable that we’re starting to address the issue’.

In the UK, the majority of attacks occur in public settings against young, male victims (Tan et al. 2015; Hopkins et al. 2021). Offenders are often younger (Home Office 2017), and attacks are more concentrated in economically deprived urban areas (Hopkins et al. 2021). The demographic profile of offenders and victims, and the geographic clustering of attacks, has led to perceptions that acid attacks in the UK are carried out by ‘urban street gangs’ (Twoon et al. 2016). An usually high number of attacks in the UK involve more than one offender. The Office for National Statistics suggests that 75% of all violent crime in recent years involved an offender acting alone (ONS 2019). However, in the case of acid attacks, police data suggests that around 42% of attacks involve two or more offenders (Hopkins et al. 2021). It seems there is a particular appeal of corrosives as a weapon to those engaged in gang activity and other kinds of joint enterprise. In Hopkins et al.’s (2021) police dataset, 30% of cases involved the throwing of corrosives during the committing of another crime (generally robbery or burglary), 17% were unprovoked attacks, and 10% were related to gang activity (generally, disputes over territory or access to drug markets).

Explanatory Theories

Explanatory theories for acid attacks are divided along similar lines to prevalence, with different theoretical models attempting to explain acid violence towards women in LMIC, and men in high-income counties. In LMIC where acid attacks are generally targeted at women, Baruah and Siddika (2017) describe acid violence as a symptom of ‘toxic masculinity’, where the goal of male offenders is to permanently disfigure their female victims under ‘the patriarchal reasoning that a woman’s appearance is her only asset’.

In high-income countries such as the UK, there seems to be a clear distinction between seemingly unplanned assaults that happen between cohabiting individuals in a domestic setting—where corrosives are used because they are convenient and ‘to hand’ and premeditated acquisitive and violent crime that happens between strangers or associates on the streets (Hopkins et al. 2021). Much like other forms of weapon carrying and use, many explanations for the second ‘type’ of acid attack ground themselves in social learning theory and differential association, as well as rational choice theory. As such, theories to explain why acid attacks occur can be derived from Brennan’s (2019) work on the use of weapons more generally. Brennan notes that explanatory factors for weapon-based violence can be divided into individual-level, interpersonal (e.g. the influence of peers), community (e.g.

neighbourhood deprivation and exposure to violence) and societal (e.g. availability of weapons). Brennan (2019) also observes how teasing out the differences between predictors of offending and victimisation are very difficult, as many offenders will also have been victims of the same types of crime they perpetuate (and, indeed, may be carrying weapons to protect themselves from further victimisation).

Hopkins et al. (2021) outline the key reasons why offenders choose acid over other types of weapons:

- Acid and other corrosives are easy to obtain.
- Corrosives are easy to carry and conceal—in particular, the ease with which household or industrial bleach can be decanted into sports drinks bottles means that, as a weapon, acid is very straightforward to disguise and does not arouse suspicion (even when searched by police).
- Acid is accurate (e.g. compared to guns or knives). Furthermore, interviews with offenders suggest that many of them do not view acid as a 'proper' weapon and believe they can control the damage incurred (by diluting the corrosive to reduce the pH level). There is frequently therefore a denial of the seriousness of the weapon, a denial of its potential harms and a denial of the intent to injure, in line with Sykes and Matza's (1957) techniques of neutralisation, where offenders develop a rationale to justify their behaviour.
- Corrosives can bring about instant visual incapacitation, which makes committing an offence like robbery or burglary easier, as well as reducing the likelihood of the victim being able to identify the offender.
- Corrosives allow a physical distance to be kept between the offender and a (possibly physically stronger) victim.
- Corrosives are silent.
- The use of corrosives ends crime events quickly.

Risk Factors

A key risk factor for acid attacks is the wide and easy availability of corrosives (Haque and Ahsan 2014; ASTI 2015; Kalantry and Kestenbaum 2011). Generally corrosive substances, even those with very high or low pH values, are not illegal or well regulated. They are easy to acquire through links to tradespeople in businesses such as building or industrial cleaning, and the market rarely runs dry as corrosives are continuously needed by industry (Kalantry and Kestenbaum 2011). Corrosives are also often far cheaper than other dangerous weapons, such as guns. For example, campaigners in India have noted that not only is acid easily available but sells for as little as the cost of a soft drink in many stores (Deswal 2020). Bond et al. (1998) found that as the possession of firearms became more regulated at state and federal levels in the USA, acid attacks rose.

Recent work has also looked at the meanings and rewards of carrying and using corrosives for offenders—such as self-protection and reputation—and why this is important in the context of their lives. Offenders in Hopkins et al.'s (2021) study talked about a cycle of risk—where fear of victimisation and of other people carrying weapons, particularly acid, both normalised acid carrying and meant offenders felt it was necessary to carry for their own protection. The higher volume of acid carriers inevitably led to more acid use in violent attacks, meaning that offenders felt further vindicated in their decision to carry a corrosive substance when going about their day-to-day business (Fig. 1).

In turn, this may lead to the issue of acid attack 'amplification', whereby the intense media focus on acid attacks suggests that they are very common and that many people regularly carry acid. This leads to the perception that the risk of an attack is high and that there is therefore a need to arm oneself to prevent future victimisation.

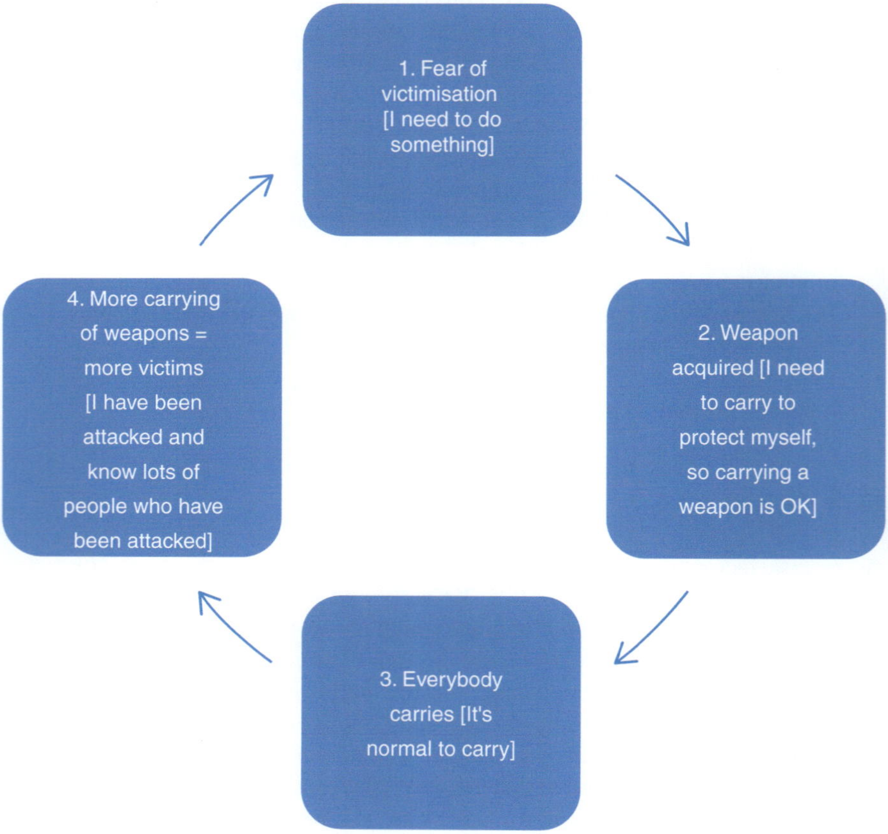

Fig. 1 The cycle of protection and the carrying of acid. (In Hopkins et al. 2021: 94)

Case Study

Laxmi Agarwal was 15 and still in school in New Delhi, India, when she was approached by a much older family 'friend', Naeem Khan, who proposed to her. Agarwal rejected him and ignored his subsequent attempts to contact her. Almost a year later, Agarwal was attacked while waiting at a local bus stop by Khan and his brother's girlfriend, who threw acid in her face as they drove past her on a motorbike. Unfortunately, before she was admitted to hospital, concerned onlookers doused Agarwal's face in water, which caused the acid to run down her body and burn her neck as well as her face. Once in hospital, Agarwal underwent multiple operations for the extensive damage done to her face and neck, including eye surgery. Khan was initially released on bail, but following widespread public protests, he was eventually sentenced to 10 years in prison. Since her recovery, Agarwal has become a passionate campaigner for acid attack awareness, both in India and globally, and has called for a ban on the sale of acid. She works with the Chhanv Foundation, which assists acid attack survivors with rehabilitation, legal and medical aid, counselling and job opportunities. She also set up a café, Sheroes Hangout, which employs acid attack survivors and works towards making survivors feel confident about interacting in public, without hiding their faces. The award-winning 2020 film *Chhapaak* is based on Agarwal's life story.

Impact

Strong acids and alkalis can cause severe permanent physical damage, such as blindness, hearing loss, loss of hair, facial disfigurement (including loss of facial features), scarring, organ damage, breathing impairment, loss of mobility, paralysis and death (Faga et al. 2000; Kalantry and Kestenbaum 2011). The effects of disfigurement are thought to be more severe within developing countries and LMICs (Chowdhury 2005, 2011; Shah 2009), due to the associated social stigma and limited burn-treatment facilities. Acid burns also leave a victim particularly vulnerable to infection such as septicaemia (Behera et al. 2014). One example of this is the case of Joanne Rand in the UK. Rand was covered in sulphuric acid when she happened to witness an assault in progress and she died from sepsis following her release from hospital.

An acid burn can also have serious, long-lasting psychological and social impacts on not only the victim but their family and friends (Griffiths et al. 2017), with some survivors stating that having to live with physical and psychological impacts is 'worse' than a fatal attack. Many survivors of acid attacks suffer from anxiety and depression. ASF (2015) estimates that this affects as many as 80% of victims. PTSD, phobias, insomnia, nightmares, social avoidance and isolation, low self-esteem and fear of further attacks are also commonly reported impacts (Mannon et al. 2006). All of this can have a substantial effect on survivors' quality of life, and sometimes the long-term psychological effects coupled with the physical damage experienced by survivors is so extreme that the victims take their own lives (Burd and Ahmed 2010) or report the desire to do so (e.g. Piper 2017). In 2017, Mark Van Dongen, who had had acid poured over his face and body by his ex-partner while he slept, was allowed to end his life via euthanasia in Belgium. Van Dongen had spent 14 months in a UK hospital after the attack and had suffered widespread scarring, the loss of sight in one eye, had had his lower left leg amputated and was paralysed from the neck down (see Storey 2018).

Because of the profound impact they can have on victims and their loved ones, acid attacks have been the focus of a number of autobiographical books and films, for example, the best-selling memoir of Katie Piper (2011) who was attacked with sulphuric acid by an ex-boyfriend (and his accomplice), sustaining injuries so serious that she spent 12 days in an induced coma. These stories allow the realities of the physical and emotional pain experienced by survivors to be better understood by the general public and have also demonstrated the ways survivors have been able to rebuild their lives after being attacked. In addition, such media has helped to raise awareness about the need for policy and regulatory reform when it comes to the production and purchase of corrosives. The release of the film *Chhappaak* in 2019, which told the story of Laxmi Agarwal, provoked a national debate on the regulation of acid sales in India. *Chhappaak* (the Hindi word for 'splash') was described by the director, Meghna Gulzar, as a film about not just trauma but triumph and a way of bringing attention to the issue of acid violence to a wider audience (The Daily Excelsior 2019).

Policy and Practice

NGOs such as ASTI and ASF have long campaigned for a global tightening of the regulation surrounding the purchase and carrying of acid and other corrosive substances. By framing acid attacks as a form of gender-based violence, ASTI has reminded governments of their obligations to protect women and girls from discriminatory forms of violence according to the 1992 United Nations Committee on the Elimination of Discrimination against Women and Children. This has led to greater control over the sale of corrosives in countries such as Bangladesh, India and Cambodia.

However, many countries do not have specific laws or policies regulating the sale and use of corrosives and do not treat acid attacks as different from any other kind of violent assault. Those that do have specific legislation regarding the control of corrosives have attempted to put systems in place based on similar principles:

- Regulating the sale of corrosives
- Licencing and recording who is manufacturing and purchasing corrosives
- Restricting sales to those over 18 years of age

For example, in India, the government revised the Poison Act (1919) to include the 'Model Rules to Regulate the Sale of Acid and Other Corrosive Substances' (2013). These rules developed licensing for the sales of acid ensured that buyers need proof of identity to purchase acid and that sellers keep a list of purchasers and restricted sales to adults. Punishments range from imprisonment for 1 month on the first occasion of breaking one of these rules to 6 months for subsequent offences. Similar laws have been brought in in Bangladesh and Cambodia, including laws which limit and regulate the importation, production and transportation of corrosives.

Up until 2019, the UK did not have tight controls on the sale of acid or have legislation specific to acid attacks. Growing concerns over this lack of regulation led to the development of the 2017 Acid Attacks Action Plan (Lipscombe and Hutton 2017). Acid attacks were specifically covered in the 2018 Serious Violence Strategy, and new possession offences were created in the 2019 Offensive Weapons Act (Home Office 2017, 2018). Prior to this, the onus was on the police to prove *intent* to use the acid as a weapon (as well as to identify a substance carried as a corrosive in the first place). Many sellers also subscribe to a voluntary government scheme setup to encourage the responsible sales of corrosives, including not selling them to those under 18.

Implications for Policy, Practice and Research

Current research suggests that the best way to reduce acid attacks is to focus on tighter regulation of acids and other corrosive substances and to borrow from the 'what works' literature with regard to violent crime more generally. Hopkins et al. (2021) suggest potential opportunities for prevention that fall into four broad categories:

- **Control of corrosive/acid availability**—interventions that make it more difficult for potential offenders to access or use corrosives. By making it more difficult to acquire corrosives, their situational availability is reduced, and they become a less attractive weapon to prospective offenders. However, while controlling the availability of corrosives may be an important strategy, there has also been a suggestion that some action should be taken to reduce the ease with which corrosive substances can be decanted into sports drinks bottles that allow for 'ease of disguise' and 'easy firing' (Hopkins et al. 2021). It is likely that making it more difficult for potential offenders to place corrosives into drinks bottles (e.g. by changing the design of the bottle or making it change colour on contact with substances with low or high pH values) would be a simple but effective way to design out many acid attacks.
- **Deterring potential throwers through corrosive/acid law**—interventions that deter potential offenders from carrying and using corrosives through the use and threat of criminal justice sanctions. Such laws make the throwing of acid an aggravating feature in a crime, resulting in heavier sentences. This is presumed to act as a deterrent, meaning that offenders will refrain from carrying/using cor-

rosives as they are concerned that they will be severely punished (Hopkins Burke 2014). Bangladesh, Uganda, Cambodia and Colombia have all recently imposed laws which create lengthy sentences (up to and including life) for violence involving acid. In the UK, the media attention surrounding acid attacks has led to increasing pressure for judges to use the highest available tariff when sentencing acid offenders. For example, Arthur Collins, who was convicted after throwing acid in a crowded nightclub, was sentenced to 20 years and 5 months in November 2017. As Tilley (2009) suggests, widespread publicity about lengthy criminal sanctions can act as a general deterrent mechanism to would-be offenders.
- **Focusing on individual carriers/throwers**—interventions that make individuals less receptive to the idea of carrying and using corrosives. Much of the recent literature on weapon crime prevention has recommended treating violence as a public health problem rather than a crime and justice problem. Doubtless acid attacks could be reduced by taking such an approach, which involves early interventions in cases where multiple risk factors (be they individual, relational, community or societal) are present (Grimshaw and Ford 2018). No interventions in the UK currently engage with individuals directly in relation to acid crime. However, it is likely that approaches aimed at violent crime more generally, such as the 'pulling levers' approach which targets individuals involved in gang violence or drug dealing, could be effective. In this approach youth workers, probation officers and social services directly communicate the risks and consequences of actions to gang members; as such this method aims to reduce violence through the threat of strict law enforcement and the encouragement of community engagement and social service provision. In a global sense, such a transformation requires that various forms of disadvantage—such as poverty and gender inequality—are confronted and that long-term macro solutions are developed.
- **Focusing on communities**—interventions aimed at communities where the prevalence of carrying and violent use of acid is high. The importance of developing campaigns aimed at highlighting the damage done by acid attacks on victims, their loved ones and the wider society is well-recognised (ASTI 2020). Evidence from the global literature suggests that efforts to change perceptions about corrosives, along with the receptiveness of individuals to carry acid, is a fruitful avenue for prevention. The evidence from many LMIC countries where acid violence is high has revealed that attitudes towards women and forms of toxic masculinity are key factors in decisions to use acid (Baruah and Siddika 2017), and campaigns targeting these issues have been successful (ASTI 2020). Schemes involving talking to school children about the harms of acid attacks and detailing the potential damage that corrosives can cause to people on the packaging they are sold in, similar to the contemporary health warnings on cigarette packets in the UK, could be effective (Hopkins et al. 2021).

However, little work has been conducted to date on 'what works' with acid attack prevention in a specific sense, nor on whether schemes aimed at restricting access to acid (such as stricter regulations and laws) simply displace corrosive crimes by encouraging the use of alternative weapons, or if, instead, they have a diffusion effect by discouraging the use of *any* form of violence.

Future research needs to focus on furthering our understanding of the extent and nature of corrosive substance crime, identifying preventative strategies and establishing 'what works' in relation to preventing acid attacks.

Summary

- Acid attacks are a global problem, but obtaining accurate prevalence rates is difficult.
- While acid attacks in some low- and middle-income countries predominantly affect women and can be viewed as a form of gender-based violence, in many high-income countries, the majority of victims are men, and attacks often take place during the commission of other offences, such as robberies or burglaries.
- The wide availability of acid and the ease and low cost of purchasing it contributes towards making it an attractive weapon for offenders.
- Further work needs to be done, especially with offenders, to identify preventative strategies and ascertain 'what works' in relation to reducing acid-based violence.

References

Acid Survivors Trust International (ASTI) (2015) Justice? What justice? Tackling acid violence and ensuring justice for survivors. https://www.trust.org/contentAsset/raw-data/4d72e4f4-4ea7-445d-b636-d8023944a859/file. Accessed 18 Mar 2020

ActionAid (2017) 'My scar in no way is my stigma': acid attacks against women and girls; motives, means and survivors reclaiming power. Action Aid, London

ASF Pakistan (2015) Acid violence in Pakistan: a situational analysis. http://www.asfpakistan.org/wp-content/uploads/2017/02/SAAV-report-2015.pdf. Accessed 30 Jul 2020

ASTI (2020) Acid survivors trust international homepage. http://www.acidviolence.org/. Accessed 24 Mar 2020

Baruah B, Siddika A (2017) Acid attacks are on the rise and toxic masculinity is the cause. Conversation. https://theconversation.com/acid-attacks-are-on-the-rise-and-toxic-masculinity-is-the-cause-82115. Accessed 13 Mar 2020

Beare JDL (1990) Eye injuries from assault with chemicals. Br J Ophthalmol 74:514–518

Behera C, Rani A, Pradhan M, Dikshit PC (2014) Fatal corrosive attack: a study of 13 cases from central Delhi, India. Am J Foren Med Pathol 35(2):9–112

Blackham RJ (1936) Women in honour and dishonour. Sampson Low, Marston & Co., London

Bond SJ, Schnier GC, Sundine MJ, Maniscalco SP, Groff DB (1998) Cutaneous burns caused by sulphuric acid drain cleaner. J Trauma 44:523–526

Brennan IR (2019) Weapon-carrying and the reduction of violent harm. Br J Criminol 59(3):571–593

Burd A, Ahmed K (2010) The acute management of acid assault burns: a pragmatic approach. Ind J Plast Surg 43(1):29–33

Chowdhury EH (2005) Feminist negotiations: contesting narratives of the campaign against acid violence in Bangladesh. Meridians 6(1):163–192

Chowdhury EH (2011) Transnationalism reversed: women organizing against gendered violence in Bangladesh. State University of New York Press, New York, NY

Daily Excelsior (2019) "Chhappaak" is about trauma and triumph, says Meghna Gulzar. https://www.dailyexcelsior.com/chhappaak-is-about-trauma-and-triumph-says-meghna-gulzar/. Accessed 11 Feb 2020

Daily Mail (1924) Judge of vitriol throwing. Daily Mail (8862):733–739

Dearden L (2017) UK has one of highest rates of acid attacks in the world, police reveal. Independent. https://www.independent.co.uk/news/uk/crime/acid-attacks-uk-highest-world-figures-police-revealed-a8098236.html. Accessed 10 Feb 2020

Deswal V (2020) Acid attacks – need to regulate acid sales. Times of India. https://timesofindia.indiatimes.com/blogs/legally-speaking/acid-attacks-need-to-regulate-acid-sales/. Accessed 4 Mar 2020

Faga A, Scevola D, Mezzetti MG, Scevola S (2000) Sulphuric acid burned women in Bangladesh: a social and medical problem. Burns 26:701–709

Gayle D (2017) Acid attacks: 2017 likely to set new record in UK. The Guardian. https://www.theguardian.com/world/2017/dec/07/uk-acid-attacks-2017-likely-new-record. Accessed 20 Sep 2021

Griffiths C, Guest E, White P, Gaskin E, Rumsey N, Pleat J, Harcourt D (2017) A systematic review of patient-reported outcome measures used in adult burn research. J Burn Care Res 38(2):e521–e545

Grimshaw, R, Ford, M (2018) Young people, violence and knives – revisiting the evidence and policy discussions. https://www.crimeandjustice.org.uk/publications/young-people-violence-and-knives-revisiting-evidence-and-policy-discussions. Accessed 24 May 2020

Guardian (2019) "He thought he'd ruin me": Indian acid attack survivor and model speaks out. The Guardian. https://www.theguardian.com/global-development/2019/apr/02/indian-acid-attack-survivor-and-model-speaks-out-reshma-qureshi. Accessed 12 Feb 2020

Haque AE, Ahsan H (2014) Human rights violations against women: acid violence in Bangladesh. Am J Prev Med 46(2):216–217

Home Office (2017) Acid attack action plan. https://www.gov.uk/government/news/home-secretary-announces-action-plan-to-tackle-acid-attacks. Accessed 23 Jan 2020

Home Office (2018) Serious violence strategy. https://www.gov.uk/government/publications/serious-violence-strategy. Accessed 23 Jan 2020

Hopkins Burke R (2014) An introduction to criminological theory, 4th edn. Routledge, London

Hopkins M, Neville L, Sanders S (2021) Acid attacks: theory, motivation, and context. Palgrave, London

Hossain RR, Papamichael E, Coombes A (2019) East London deliberate corrosive fluid injuries. Eye 34:733–739

Kalantry, S, Kestenbaum JG (2011) Combating acid violence in Bangladesh, India, and Cambodia. Avon Global Center for Women and Justice and Dorothea S. Clarke Program in Feminist Jurisprudence, Paper 1. http://scholarship.law.cornell.edu/avon_clarke/1. Accessed 28 Jul 2020

Khan R (2017) Acid attacks have been happening in the UK for 200 years, so why are we only talking about them now? The Independent. https://www.independent.co.uk/voices/acid-attacks-victims-uk-impact-women-disproportionately-muslim-niqab-media-only-just-reporting-a7877531.html. Accessed 20 Sep 2021

Lipscombe S, Hutton G (2017) Acid attacks: briefing paper number CBP 8041. House of Commons Library, London

Mannon A, Ghani S, Clarke A, White P, Salmanta S, Butler PEM (2006) Psychosocial outcomes derived from an acid burned population in Bangladesh, and comparison with Western norms. Burns 32:235–241

Mannon A, Ghani S, Clarke A, Butler PEM (2007) Cases of chemical assault worldwide: a literature review. Burns 33:149–154

Nagarajan N, Mohamed S, Asmar O, Stubbington Y, George S, Shokrollahi K (2020) Data from national media reports of 'acid attacks' in England: a new piece in the Jigsaw'. Burns 46:949–958

National Crime Records Bureau (2018) Crime in India: statistics vol 1. Ministry of Home Affairs, New Delhi. http://ncrb.gov.in/StatPublications/CII/CII2018/cii2018.html. Accessed 12 Feb 2020

Office for National Statistics (ONS) (2019) The nature of violent crime in England and Wales: year ending March 2018. https://www.ons.gov.uk/peoplepopulationandcommunity/crimeandjustice/articles/thenatureofviolentcrimeinenglandandwales/yearendingmarch2018#how-is-violent-crime-defined-and-measured. Accessed 20 Sep 2021

Pickett W, Craig W, Harel Y, Cunningham J, Simpson K, Molcho M, Mazur J, Dostaler S, Overpeck M, Currie CE (2005) Cross-national study of fighting and weapon carrying as determinants of adolescent injury. Pediatrics 116:e855–e863

Piper K (2011) Beautiful: a beautiful girl. An evil man. One inspiring true story of courage. Ebury Press, Reading

Piper K (2017) A survivor's perspective of acid attacks in the UK: an open letter from Katie Piper. Scars Burns Heal 3:1–2

Shah H (2009) Brutality by acid: utilizing Bangladesh as a model to fight acid violence in Pakistan. Wisconsin Int Law J 26:1172–1199

Storey T (2018) Court of appeal: voluntary acts and the chain of causation in homicide cases: the need for "free and unfettered volition" R v Wallace [2018] EWCA Crim 69. J Crim Law 82(4):292–295

Sykes GM, Matza D (1957) Techniques of neutralization: a theory of delinquency. Am Sociol Rev 22:664–670

Tan A, Kaur Bharj A, Nizamoglu M, Barnes D, Dziewulski P (2015) Assaults from corrosive substances and medico legal considerations in a large regional burn centre in the United Kingdom: calls for increased vigilance and enforced legislation. Scars Burns Heal 1:1–10

Tilley N (2009) Crime prevention. Willan, Collumpton

Times of India (2005) Hate, obsession trapped acid attack victim. Times of India. https://timesofindia.indiatimes.com/city/delhi/Hate-obsession-trapped-acidattackvictim/articleshow/1091028.cms. Accessed 12 May 2020

Twoon M, Tan A, Dziewulski P (2016) Letter to the editor: acid attacks: a growing problem in the UK. Burns 42:1141–1159

Watson KD (2017) Love, vengeance and vitriol: an Edwardian true-crime drama. In: Kilday A, Nash D (eds) Law, crime and deviance since 1700. Bloomsbury, London, p 111

Yousaf FN, Purkayastha B (2016) Beyond saving faces: survivors of acid attacks in Pakistan. Women's Stud Int Forum 54:11–19

Lucy Neville is a Lecturer in Criminology at the University of Leicester. Her research explores sex and sexuality in different forms, and she has worked with a variety of marginalised groups. She has a strong commitment to radical pedagogy, working with scholars from across disciplinary boundaries (#IAF), and to moving research findings into the public arena.

Matt Hopkins is Associate Professor in Criminology at the University of Leicester. He has researched extensively on violent crime and public space violence. His work has included studies of violence against employees in retail outlets, disorder at sports events, and the use of weapons in violent crime. He is co-author of *Acid Crime: Context and Motivation* (with Teela Sanders and Lucy Neville).

Teela Sanders is Professor of Criminology and Dean of Research and Enterprise in the College of Social Sciences, Arts and Humanities at the University of Leicester. She is a specialist in gender, violence, and policing.

Bride Abduction

Lisa Wiebesiek

Learning Objectives
Having read this chapter, you should be able to understand the following:

- The distinction between consensual and nonconsensual bride abduction
- How the practice is shaped by the social, historical, economic and political context in which bride abduction takes place
- The important role that ideas and beliefs about culture and tradition play in the practice
- How the tension between cultural and human rights discourse can undermine efforts to address nonconsensual bride abduction

Introduction

This chapter provides an overview of bride abduction and illuminates the centrality of consent. It sets the discussion against a backdrop of varying social, historical, economic and political contexts and draws sharply into focus the ways in which cultural discourse and human rights discourse compete and how such tensions operate to undermine efforts to address the problem of nonconsensual bride abduction.

L. Wiebesiek (✉)
Centre for Visual Methodologies for Social Change, University of KwaZulu-Natal, UKZN, Durban, KwaZulu-Natal, South Africa
e-mail: WiebesiekL@ukzn.ac.za

P. Ali, M. M. Rogers (eds.), *Gender-Based Violence: A Comprehensive Guide*,
https://doi.org/10.1007/978-3-031-05640-6_17

Broadly defined, bride abduction is the abduction of a girl or woman for the purposes of marriage. Various forms of bride abduction have been practised throughout history and are still practised by several social, religious and ethnic groups in diverse contexts across the globe (see Box 1).

Box 1 Where Is Bride Abduction Practised?

- *Africa*: Egypt, Ethiopia, Kenya, Rwanda, South Africa, Ghana
- *Central Asia*: Kyrgyzstan, Kazakhstan, Turkmenistan, Uzbekistan
- *The Caucasus*: Dagestan, Chechnya, Ingushetia, Azerbaijan, Georgia
- *East and South Asia*: Pakistan, Indonesia, China
- *The Americas*: the USA (among, e.g. the Hmong ethic group), Mexico, Chile
- *Europe and United Kingdom* (among, e.g. certain Romani (Roma) and Traveller communities)

It is difficult to estimate the global prevalence of bride abduction partly because of variation in the practice. Rates vary across and within country contexts or regions, and underreporting and a lack of (good-quality) data further complicates attempts to establish the number of girls and women affected by bride abduction worldwide (Becker et al. 2017). The variation in the practice is reflected in the range of names or terms for the practice (see Box 2) which both frame and reflect how bride abduction is understood and perceived by those who experience it, the communities in which it is practised, researchers, practitioners and policy-makers. For example, Werner (2009) observes that the word 'kidnapping' implies that the bride is a child or is childlike, feeding into the infantilization of women and implying that bride abduction specifically involves underage girls. Following Werner (2009), the term bride abduction is used in this chapter because it is less problematic than the other available terms.

There are a number of practices similar or related to bride abduction and with which the practice is sometimes conflated (see Box 2). For example, bride abduction is sometimes defined as a type of forced marriage, that is, a marriage concluded without the consent of one or both of the individuals involved. However, because the marriage that is the motive for the abduction is not *always* the outcome, some scholars argue that the abduction and the marriage are two separate but linked events (see, e.g. Mwambene and Sloth-Nelson 2011).

Box 2 Alternative and Related Terminology

Alternative Terminology

Wife capture, marriage by capture, marriage by abduction, abduction marriage, kidnapping for marriage, bride kidnapping, bridenapping and bride theft.

Related Terms

Forced marriage, early and forced marriage, child marriage, arranged marriage, and groom abduction.

Types of Bride Abduction

There are a number of factors that distinguish one form of bride abduction from another, including whether or not the intended bride and the intended groom knew each other prior to the abduction, who is involved in the abduction, the manner in which the abduction itself occurs and what takes place after the abduction. A crucial distinction across all forms is that between consensual and nonconsensual bride abduction.

Consensual Bride Abduction

As the name suggests, in consensual abductions (Werner 2009; Kim and Karioris 2020), also known as mock or staged abductions (Handrahan 2004), the girl or woman who is the target has agreed to the abduction. Such abductions may be motivated by the bride and/or groom's family (sometimes both) objecting to the proposed marriage, the desire of the bride and/or groom to avoid an arranged marriage and marry the person of their choice or to avoid the expense associated with the celebrations accompanying marriage rites or ceremony(ies). In communities where bride price is still expected, a couple might stage an abduction to relieve the financial pressure on the groom and his family (Kleinbach and Salimjanova 2007).

Although consensual abductions take place with the agreement of the girl or woman, the process may, nevertheless, at least appear to involve a degree of resistance from the target and violence from the abductor(s). The display of resistance and force may be entirely staged for the benefit of on-lookers or witnesses as a demonstration of the girl or woman's virtue, innocence and honour (see, e.g. Borbieva 2012).

Nonconsensual Abductions

In nonconsensual (Kim and Karioris 2020; Kleinbach and Salimjanova 2007) or forced (Handrahan 2004) abductions, the girl or woman who is the target has not agreed to be abducted. Although there are cases where she has consented to the marriage but not the abduction, more often than not, nonconsensual abductions are undertaken with the intention of forcing the girl or woman into a marriage. In nonconsensual abduction, the intended bride and the intended groom may not know each other at all, may be acquainted to some degree or may even be in a relationship with each other. Nonconsensual bride abduction tends to involve more genuine resistance and violence than consensual abductions. In certain contexts, the abductor may rape his victim as part of the abduction or as part of attempts to persuade the abducted girl or woman to proceed with the marriage.

There is a lack of consensus between scholars, activists and policy-makers on the one hand, and the local communities in which bride abduction is practised, on the other, about whether it is a legitimate and harmless cultural practice or a form of gender-based violence (GBV). This lack of consensus can undermine efforts to address bride abduction by local and international NGOs, policy-makers, researchers and practitioners. From a human rights perspective, nonconsensual bride abduction is considered to be a violation of the rights of girls and women and a form of GBV.

Examples of Bride Abduction

In this section of the chapter, two examples of bride abduction are presented in order to anchor the discussion of the practice that follows.

Ala Kachuu

Ala kachuu is a form of bride abduction practised among the Kyrgyz people in the Kyrgyz Republic (also known as Kyrgyzstan) in Central Asia. Once a constituent republic of the Soviet Union, Kyrgyzstan declared independence in 1991, becoming a democratic state. Although there are historical accounts of *ala kachuu* in pre-Soviet Kyrgyzstan, it was rare. It went against both customary law (*adat*) and Sharia law, was not socially accepted (causing serious conflict between families and tribes) and was punished (Kleinbach and Salimjanova 2007; Kleinbach et al. 2005; Werner 2009).

Although key details of the abduction vary from case to case (Werner 2009), described in broad strokes, *ala kachuu* involves the abduction of a girl or woman by a man, often with the help of a group of his friends. The girl or woman resists her abductors, this resistance being real or feigned depending on whether the abduction is consensual or nonconsensual. The girl or woman is then taken to the home of a member of her abductor's family, usually that of his parents. She is given into the care of female members of her abductor's family who attempt to place on her head the scarf traditionally worn by married Kyrgyz women which would indicate that she will proceed with the marriage. Again, the abducted girl or woman resists either genuinely or as part of the performance of the staged abduction. She is pressured to write to her family to inform them of her abduction and her intention to marry her abductor.

In theory, a girl or woman can refuse to proceed with the marriage, and if her parents support her, she can return to her natal home. However, more often than not, even if she does not want to, the girl or woman proceeds with the marriage motivated by the shame associated with being considered stubborn and disobedient and therefore undesirable as a wife, whose virtue may well be considered comprised as a result of the possibility that she may no longer be a virgin, and with returning home to a family that can now only ask for a smaller amount in bride price. The abducted girl or woman may also agree to proceed with the marriage as a result of coercion in the form of threats or experiences of violence, even rape, at the hands of her would-be husband. As part of concluding the marriage, the groom's family presents the bride's family with bride wealth in the form of gifts.

In post-Soviet Kyrgyzstan, there has been a dramatic increase in, particularly nonconsensual, *ala kachuu*. Many Kyrgyz have come to believe that both consensual and nonconsensual *ala kachuu* are an authentic and legitimate cultural practice that was common among the Kyrgyz prior to the Soviet period in spite of the fact that research has consistently shown that this is not the case.

The increase in *ala kachuu* in post-Soviet Kyrgyzstan has been attributed to the desire to develop and solidify a Kyrgyz national, cultural and ethnic identity as a reaction to the policies, laws and ideologies imposed by the Soviet state which served to undermine the Kyrgyz way of life (Werner 2009; Werner et al. 2018). Part of this process involves reclaiming customs and traditions such as *ala kachuu* that are believed to have been central to ancient Kyrgyz culture. During the Soviet period, state laws banned what were referred to as 'crimes of custom' (Werner 2009: 320), including practices like bride wealth, polygamy, arranged marriage, forced marriage and bride abduction. These laws formed part of Soviet efforts to increase gender equity and emancipate women across the Union. As a result of these laws and other measures, during the Soviet period, young people, including women, had far more independence in the selection of their marriage partners than they had in pre-Soviet times when parents had significant if not total control over who their children married and when.

Ukuthwala

In pre-colonial South Africa, a form of bride abduction called *ukuthwala* was practised among the amaZulu and amaXhosa peoples. Described as a legitimate though unconventional route to marriage, the historical practice of *ukuthwala* involved the consensual (staged) abduction of a woman by her suitor (Nkosi 2011; Van der Watt and Ovens 2012). The practice was undertaken by couples whose families, for whatever reason, would not consent to their marriage. Similar to *ala kachuu*, *ukuthwala* usually involved a woman being abducted, by prior arrangement, by her suitor aided by a small group of his male friends and younger family members. The woman would pretend to resist and would appear to onlookers to be forcefully carried away to the would-be groom's family homestead where she would be given into the care of his female family members. A messenger would then be sent to the woman's family to inform them about the abduction after which the senior male members of both families would enter into a process of negotiating *lobolo* (often translated into English as bride wealth). If an agreement was reached between the two families, the marriage proceedings would commence (Koyana and Bekker 2007). *Ukuthwala* continued to be practised throughout the colonial and apartheid eras in South Africa although more and more rarely.

Similar to Kyrgyzstan under Soviet rule, during the colonial and apartheid (a white supremacist ideology, system of legislation and institutionalised racial segregation that served to disenfranchise and oppress especially Black South Africans) eras, concerted efforts were made to systematically undermine, damage and destroy the ways of life of the Indigenous people of South Africa. This history has shaped ideas about culture and tradition in post-apartheid South Africa in important ways (Hunter 2010; Moletsane 2011, 2013) such that in recent decades, there has been a strong desire to retrieve, reclaim, restore, preserve and protect indigenous culture, tradition and practices, *ukuthwala* among them (Moletsane 2011, 2013).

Unfortunately, in contemporary South Africa under the guise of *ukuthwala*, girls and women are being abducted without their consent, held against their will, subjected to various forms of violence including sexual violence and forced into marriage. Like Kyrgyz girls and women who are abducted, enormous pressure is exerted on girls and women who are abducted against their will under the guise of *ukuthwala* to proceed with the marriage to their abductor.

By claiming these actions to be *ukuthwala*, perpetrators lend an air of legitimacy to what is otherwise seen as a violation of the rights of the victim(s)/survivor(s). Although historians and experts in customary law in South Africa contend that this form of abduction is a distortion of the consensual historical practice, many individuals and communities insist that nonconsensual abduction of a girl or woman for the purposes of marriage is a legitimate cultural practice (Mwambene and Kruuse 2017; Nkosi and Wasserman 2014; Koyana and Bekker 2007).

The Impacts of Bride Abduction

The impacts of nonconsensual bride abduction include the immediate and long-term trauma of the abduction and the associated violence including sexual violence. Girls and women in marriages concluded as a result of nonconsensual abduction experience higher rates of psychological stress, depression and other mental health issues including suicide (Becker et al. 2017). Rates of domestic violence are higher in forced marriages that are the outcome of nonconsensual abduction (Werner et al. 2018). Poor maternal and child health outcomes including low birth weight are associated with forced marriages as a result of bride abduction, particularly in cases of early and unwanted pregnancy (Nkosi 2009). An additional issue in a context like South Africa is the increased risk of contracting HIV and other sexually transmitted infections among girls and women married through nonconsensual bride abduction.

Just the threat of bride abduction can compromise girls' education as they are frightened to leave home to walk to and from school for fear of abduction. Once they have been abducted and married, girls are rarely able to finish their education which contributes to the perpetuation of the cycle of poverty in the communities in which bride abduction is practised (see, e.g. Nkosi 2014). Higher rates of divorce among couples married as a result of nonconsensual bride abduction often leave the women in extremely vulnerable positions as they are unable to find work to support themselves and their children (Becker et al. 2017). The impacts of bride abduction extend to those girls and women who refuse to proceed with the marriage through shame, loss of reputation and diminished prospects for marriage in the future associated with refusal (Borbieva 2012; Werner 2009).

Understanding Bride Abduction

As the examples discussed above demonstrate there are important similarities between them which make it possible to identify common themes across different forms of bride abduction that contribute in important ways to understandings of these practices. There are a number of theories that can be used (sometimes in combination) to understand bride abduction in a nuanced and holistic way, including feminist theory more broadly, intersectionality, social constructionist theories of gender, feminist post-colonial theories and cross-cultural frameworks.

Bride Abduction as a Gendered Practice

Bride abduction is clearly a gendered practice. It is, after all, girls and women who are the targets of abduction, and it is they who are often, but not always, forced into marriage following abduction. Even in consensual abductions, the groom takes on the active role of the abductor, while the girl or woman is the passive target. These roles reflect traditional gender roles that a husband and wife will be expected to assume in a traditional or customary marriage.

From a social constructionist perspective,[1] the abduction process can be seen as a performance or enactment of idealised constructions of gender. Highly valued feminine traits that signal successful femininity in contexts where bride abduction is practised include innocence, passivity, obedience and virtue. These are precisely the traits that are demonstrated through a girl or woman's display of resistance to consensual bride abduction, for example. These are also traits that make a girl or woman desirable as a potential wife. The forceful, even violent, act of exerting control and dominance over a woman by abducting her and potentially forcing her into marriage can similarly be understood as a demonstration of traits associated with constructions of successful masculinity within a patriarchal gender order (Connell and Messerschmidt 2005).

The extremely high value placed on a girl or woman's virginity and the careful surveillance and policing of female sexuality that surround and play a central role in bride abduction is further evidence of the gendered nature of this practice. Shepherd's (2008: 50) understanding of violence as both gendered and gendering, as 'one of the sites where culturally and historically specific understandings of gender as a power relationship are reproduced' is useful for understanding bride abduction as a gendered practice and specifically nonconsensual bride abduction as a form of GBV.

[1] Social constructionism is the theory that people develop knowledge of the world in a social context. Social constructs are created through language and social interactions, and, as such, much of what we perceive as reality relies on shared assumptions and understandings.

Context

Drawing on feminist post-colonial[2] scholars, Chandra Talpade Mohanty (1988) and Uma Narayan (1998), Werner et al. (2018: 584) point out that 'like other issues related to gender equality and GBV, bride kidnapping can too easily be told as a "single story", divorced from local contexts (social, political, cultural, economic, religious, historical, etc.) and mobilized in ways that perpetuate stereotypes and unequal power relations'. It is important to be mindful of and try to avoid cultural and gender essentialism in efforts to understand, theorise about and address nonconsensual bride abduction.

A careful study of bride abduction in its social, historical, political and economic context reveals that it is not simply a manifestation of gender inequality, but rather that it takes place at the intersection of multiple mutually reinforcing dimensions of inequality and oppression. For example, poverty and ideas about culture influenced by the historical context as they intersect with gender inequality play an important role in the current practice of bride abduction. In impoverished rural communities in South Africa, for example, *lobolo* (bride wealth) is often thought of as a powerful motivator for nonconsensual abduction perpetrated under the guise of the historical traditional practice of *ukuthwala*. For many families *lobolo* can not only do much to relieve the, often dire, financial circumstances but also reduce the number of mouths to feed in the household, provide *lobolo* to enable a son to marry and (hopefully) secure a more prosperous future for a daughter. Kim and Karioris (2020: 50) argue that the conditions in which *ala kachuu* occur are shaped by 'interconnected insecurities related to the rise of [an] ethno-nationalist state, stagnating pastoral livelihoods, environmental degradation, [and] rural poverty'. It is crucial to understand these conditions in order to effectively address nonconsensual bride abduction.

The Tradition/Rights Binary

In the lack of consensus about whether bride abduction is a legitimate and harmless cultural practice or a violation of the rights of girls and women, two competing discourses are at work. The first is a discourse of the sacred and unassailable culture and the second a discourse of human rights. Through these discourses the tradition/rights binary (Hunter 2010) is established and perpetuated. Tradition and human rights are presented as mutually exclusive positions 'with the result that efforts to change these [traditional] practices become framed as a struggle between culture and the law' (Werner 2009: 329).

[2]Postcolonialism is the theory that people develop a postcolonial identity resulting from interactions between different identities (cultural, national, and ethnic as well as gender- and class-based) which are assigned varying degrees of social power by the colonial society.

Love and Marriage

That nonconsensual bride abduction is still practised points to the abiding importance of marriage as a (gendered) social institution. For women in particular, marriage is often central to constructions of successful femininities (Shai 2018). A failure to get married, then, implies a failure to achieve successful femininity. In addition to this, for women, marriage is often a strategy to achieve financial and social security in contexts where poverty and changing social and political norms and circumstances make life precarious. Certainly, men and boys are also under pressure to get married in many contexts, but it is often a less urgent need for men than it is for women. Men are able to achieve successful masculinity via other means (see, e.g. Connell and Messerschmidt 2005), and in contexts where paid employment is scarce, are more likely than women to secure a job (Hunter 2010).

A study of bride abduction in context also exposes changing ideas about love and marriage. The idea that marriage should be based on romantic love is a relatively new one in human history. It became established in so-called Western contexts in the late eighteenth and early nineteenth centuries with the influence of enlightenment thinking, urbanisation and the growth of the wage labour economy (Coontz 2005). Prior to this, marriage was seen as a practical arrangement to secure alliances, wealth, labour or influence. With migration and globalisation, the romantic idea of the love-based marriage has spread at the same time as ideas about individualism and the right to personal happiness (Coontz 2005). As a result, growing numbers of young people across the globe have begun to long for and feel that it is their right to choose who and when they marry based on romantic love. This independent approach to marriage is at odds with practices like bride abduction in which the bride in particular has little or no choice and which are concluded for far more pragmatic reasons. Marriage becomes the site of struggle between modernity and culture and tradition, age and gender hierarchies (Borbieva 2012).

Consent and Coercion

Consent is central to understanding and addressing bride abduction and other forms of GBV, particularly sexual violence. Although, on the surface, consent may appear to be fairly straightforward, a matter of whether someone said 'yes' or 'no', in real-world conditions, it is a complex and contested concept. From a legal perspective, how can consent or the absence thereof can be proven? An unambiguous definition of coercion is also elusive. A particular complication associated with bride abduction is the fact that the girl or woman is expected to resist her abductor (and the marriage) even when the process is undertaken with her full and unreserved consent. If a girl or young woman initially refuses to proceed with the marriage, but then later agrees following intense and sometimes prolonged efforts to convince her to change her mind, can this be considered consent? At what point does convincing become coercion?

The use of violence, including sexual violence, to force a woman to proceed with the marriage is much less ambiguous than verbal threats of violence and ruin, for example. Gill and Anitha (2011) contend that conceptualising consent and coercion as a binary does not account for women's lived experiences of bride abduction and other forms of forced marriage. Consent and coercion can instead, more usefully be understood as 'two ends of a continuum between which lie degrees of sociocultural expectation, control, persuasion, pressure, threat, and force' (Anitha and Gill 2009: 165).

Legal Framework

There are several international legal instruments, conventions and agreements that are applicable to the practice of nonconsensual bride abduction, including the Universal Declaration of Human Rights (1948); the Convention on the Elimination of all forms of Discrimination against Women (CEDAW) (1981) and the Convention on Consent to Marriage, Minimum Age for Marriage and Registration of Marriages (1962) (see Handrahan 2004). There are also relevant regional instruments such as the African Charter on the Rights and Welfare of the Child (ACRWC) (1990) (Mwambene and Sloth-Nelson 2011) and the European Convention on Human Rights (1950). According to these international and regional conventions and agreements, nonconsensual bride abduction is a violation of the human rights of girls and women and should be treated as such by all signatories to them.

At country-level there are laws to specifically address nonconsensual bride abduction or that are applicable to the practice as a violation of the rights of girls and women. In Kyrgyzstan, for example, the Kyrgyz criminal code states that nonconsensual bride abduction is prohibited and punishable by a fine or imprisonment (Kleinbach and Salimjanova 2007). In South Africa, *ukuthwala* itself is not considered a crime. However, nonconsensual bride abduction committed under the guise of *ukuthwala* is prosecuted in South Africa under kidnapping, human trafficking and sexual offences laws. In South Africa, the right of all South Africans to practise their culture is enshrined in the Constitution. In cases where nonconsensual bride abduction is perpetrated under the guise of *ukuthwala*, the exercising of this right infringes on girls' and women's right to, among other things, live free from all forms of violence. This precedent was established in the landmark case of The State v Jezile (see Mwambene and Sloth-Nelson 2011; Mwambene and Kruuse 2017), when the defence attempted to use culture as a defence in the trial of a man charged with abducting, raping and trafficking a girl of 14.

Implications for Research, Policy and Practice

In spite of the international, regional and national legal and policy frameworks to address nonconsensual bride abduction that are in place, the practice continues in local communities. This suggests that, while important, a legal and policy framework implemented using a top-down approach is not sufficient to effectively address nonconsensual bride abduction. As discussed above, these practices are often highly valued by local communities as an integral part of their culture and traditions and calling them into question can be perceived as an attack on culture. Further, criminalising nonconsensual bride abduction does more to treat a symptom than it does the cause.

Efforts to address nonconsensual bride abduction may benefit from including a focus on working with communities to better understand, challenge and change the patriarchal attitudes and beliefs and unequal gendered power relations underlying bride abduction as a form of GBV. Further, engaging with communities in critical dialogue about the dynamic, constantly evolving nature of culture and both the value and limitations of remembered histories may defuse the often highly charged debates about attacks on and threats to culture. To this end, community-based participatory research (Coughlin et al. 2017) might be a useful approach to working with communities towards social and policy change to end nonconsensual bride abduction.

Summary

- Bride abduction is practised by different social and ethnic groups in various parts of the world.
- There is a lack of consensus between researchers, activists, practitioners and policy-makers and local communities in which bride abduction is practised as to whether it is a form of GBV or a legitimate cultural practice.
- From a human rights perspective (and the position taken in this chapter), when it is not consensual, when it involves coercion or force and when it is experienced by girls and young women as violence, bride abduction is a form of GBV.
- The distinction between consensual and nonconsensual abduction is central to understanding and addressing bride abduction.
- Criminalising the practice is not a sufficient response to nonconsensual bride abduction because of the support the practice still receives in communities where it is practised.
- Efforts to address nonconsensual bride abduction may benefit from including a focus on working with communities to change attitudes and beliefs about gender equality and the nature of culture and tradition.

References

Anitha S, Gill A (2009) Coercion, consent and the forced marriage debate in the UK. Fem Leg Stud 17:165–184

Becker CM, Mirkasimov B, Steiner S (2017) Forced marriage and birth outcomes. Demography 54(4):1401–1423

Borbieva NO (2012) Kidnapping women: discourses of emotion and social change in the Kyrgyz Republic. Anthropol Q 85(1):141–169

Connell RW, Messerschmidt JW (2005) Hegemonic masculinity: rethinking the concept. Gend Soc 19(6):829–8599

Coontz S (2005) Marriage, a history: from obedience to intimacy, or how love conquered marriage. Viking, New York, NY

Coughlin SS, Smith SA, Fernandez ME (2017) Handbook of community-based participatory research. Oxford University Press, Oxford

Gill AK, Anitha S (eds) (2011) Forced marriage: introducing a social justice and human rights perspective. Zed Books, London; New York, NY

Handrahan L (2004) Hunting for Women. Int Fem J Polit 6(2):207–233

Hunter M (2010) Love in the time of AIDS: inequality, gender, and rights in South Africa. Indiana University Press, Bloomington, IN

Kim E, Karioris FG (2020) Bound to be grooms: the imbrication of economy, ecology, and bride kidnapping in Kyrgyzstan. Gend Place Cult 28:1627. https://doi.org/10.1080/0966369X.2020.1829561

Kleinbach R, Salimjanova L (2007) *Kyz ala kachuu* and *adat*: nonconsensual bride kidnapping and tradition in Kyrgyzstan. Cent Asian Surv 26(2):217–233

Kleinbach R, Ablezova M, Aitieva M (2005) Kidnapping for marriage (*ala kachuu*) in a Kyrgyz village. Cent Asian Surv 24(2):191–202

Koyana DS, Bekker JC (2007) The indomitable Ukuthwala custom. De Jure 40(1):139–144

Mohanty C (1988) Under Western Eyes: feminist scholarship and colonial discourses. Fem Rev 30(1):61–88

Moletsane R (2011) Culture, nostalgia, and sexuality education in the age of AIDS in South Africa. In: Mitchell C, Strong-Wilson T, Pithouse K, Allnutt S (eds) Memory and pedagogy. Routledge, Oxfordshire

Moletsane R (2013) Nostalgia. AIDS review 2013. University of Pretoria, Pretoria, SA

Mwambene L, Kruuse H (2017) The thin edge of the wedge: ukuthwala, alienation and consent. S Afr J Hum Rights 33(1):25–45

Mwambene L, Sloth-Nelson J (2011) Benign accommodation? *Ukuthwala*, 'forced marriage' and the South African Children's Act. J Fam Law Pract 2(1):5

Narayan U (1998) Essence of culture and a sense of history: a feminist critique of cultural essentialism. Hypatia 13(2):86–106

Nkosi M (2009) Bride abduction in KwaZulu-Natal schools and its effects on education. Agenda 23(80):109–114

Nkosi S (2011) *Lobola*: black students' perceptions of its role on gender power dynamics. Masters Thesis, University of the Witwatersrand, Johannesburg, South Africa. http://wiredspace.wits.ac.za/handle/10539/10376. Accessed 6 Nov 2021

Nkosi M (2014) Ukuthwala "bride abduction" and education: critical challenges and opportunities faced by school principals in rural Kwazulu-Natal. J Soc Sci 41(3):441–454

Nkosi M, Wasserman J (2014) A history of the practice of *ukuthwala* in the Natal/KwaZulu-Natal region up to 1994. New Contree 70:131–146

Shai PN (2018) Constructions of Femininity in the Context of Sexual Relationships among Women living in the rural Eastern Cape Province, South Africa. [Doctoral Thesis, University of the Witwatersrand]. http://wiredspace.wits.ac.za/handle/10539/26910

Shepherd LJ (2008) Gender, violence and security. Zed Books, London

Van der Watt M, Ovens M (2012) Contextualizing the practice of Ukuthwala within South Africa. Child Abuse Res South Afr J 13(1):11–26

Werner C (2009) Bride abduction in post-Soviet Central Asia: marking a shift towards patriarchy through local discourses of shame and tradition. J R Anthropol Inst 15:314–331

Werner C, Edling C, Becker C, Kim E, Kleinbach R et al (2018) Bride kidnapping in post-Soviet Eurasia: a roundtable discussion. Cent Asian Surv 37(4):582–601

Lisa Wiebesiek, PhD is the research manager of the Centre for Visual Methodologies for Social Change at the University of KwaZulu-Natal. Her research interests include community-based participatory research, participatory visual methodology, gender-based violence, adolescent sexual and reproductive health and rights, and rural education.

Colourism

Monica Majumdar

Learning Objectives
Having read this chapter, you should be able to

- Understand the definition of colourism and its associated practices/terminology within different cultural groups
- Understand how colourism and skin tone bias evokes psychological, emotional and physical pressure on women of colour
- Recognise indicators of colourism and help prevent and support victims.

Introduction

Colourism is a form of discrimination against individuals with 'dark' complexions, usually within the same ethnic group. Thus, a racial hierarchy is formed, placing 'light' and 'fair' skin tones as highly coveted and 'dark' as undesirable. Colourism can occur in many forms, including discrimination towards body parts or 'ethnic' features such as hair texture and facial features.

A key response to colourism is to engage in skin lightening. Skin lightening or bleaching includes the application of creams, lotions or soaps over the face and body, in addition to other practices including vaginal bleaching, chemical peels, laser treatments, glutathione whitening tablets, injections or drips, avoiding sunlight or outdoor environments and Ayurvedic/home remedies such as consumption of almond milk (Badaam Doodh) or application of Haldi (turmeric paste) to lighten the complexion.

M. Majumdar (✉)
Queen Mary University of London, London, UK

P. Ali, M. M. Rogers (eds.), *Gender-Based Violence: A Comprehensive Guide*,
https://doi.org/10.1007/978-3-031-05640-6_18

Colourist values and practices can impact both men and women. However, women, in particular, are succumbing to the pressures of colourism and to a 'white is right' ideology, thus, placing the value of dark skin tones as undesirable and light skin as a way of developing their socioeconomical position (Hargrove 2019). Hall (2006) advocates that colourism impacts women more than men, as a women's status and social mobility is assigned to their visual representation and 'beauty'.

Skin-lightening products and the mass messaging around Eurocentric looks are heavily marketed towards women. Consumption patterns also indicate a gendered connotation. For instance, Pollock et al.'s (2020) report indicates 75% of women use skin-lightening products vs. 25% of men, one in two Filipino women use skin-lightening products as part of their daily skin care routine, and over 60% of Jordanian women use skin-lightening products for cosmetic reasons. Furthermore, a study by Owusu-Agyei et al. (2020) found women in Ghana are four times more likely to use skin-lightening products in comparison to men. The demographic characteristics may vary; however, the rationale for women remains the same—to conform to community and societal pressures, to avoid abuse and shame and to appear 'beautiful'.

To further explore the link between gender and colourism, this chapter will cover the historical context and the role of the female body. An outline of the current skin-lightening market and its prevalence internationally. A look at the risk factors associated with colourist practices and the subsequent impact on women. The chapter finishes with a discussion on culturally sensitive approaches to changing the narrative around colourism.

Historical Context

Contextualising the origin and history behind colourism requires an understanding of colonialism. Sommer (2011: 190) describes colonialism as 'domination of people from another culture'. Colonisation involved establishing foreign control and settlement amongst people and land traditionally by the West, for the purpose of cultivation and 'civilisation'.

During colonisation, people of 'darker' tones were positioned as slaves, loafers, convicts, prostitutes and other groups deemed of lower status: visuality of darkness being associated with labour work and poverty. Consequently, the virtue of 'Whiteness' or 'lighter' skin tone represented the economic, social, legislative and cultural leadership over the less privileged.

The formation of colourist ways and ideologies cannot be pinpointed to one moment or movement, yet the division between races, the civilisation of 'non-Whites' by the British and the establishment of racial hierarchies can be implicated. In British history, light skin provided access to privileges, wealth, status and dominance. As Phoenix (2014) contends, the colonial mentality operates a political beauty, symbols of power and an inherent preference for light skin, placing historical baggage on people today to conform to a 'cosmopolitan Whiteness' and yearn for lighter complexions. What has been brought on by previous colonial rule has created an avenue for skin tone modification, heavily driven by the skin-lightening industry and its products.

The marketing of soap demonstrates how the skin colour continuum and ideology of 'Whiteness' have transpired through the eighteenth and nineteenth century and the colonial discourse of today. Interpretations from several scholars, including Mehaffy (1997), White (1999) and McClintock (1995), corroborate the view that race and skin tones were moulded as fetishes within the imperial world. Light and fair complexions held symbolic salience and were central to modernity, ethnic hybridity, civilisation and the iconography of empire. The colonial disdain perpetuated a negative connotation of filth, dirt, ugly and odour towards people of colour; consequently, soap as a commodity offered the solution of physical cleanliness and tool for civilisation.

For colonised women, specifically, those of dark complexions dealt with a constant restructuring of identity to indicate femininity and strategy for survival. As Kyeremateng (2020) contends, the dehumanisation of dark skin often made women question the normality of their own complexion as well as that of their offspring; exemplified in N.K. Fairbank's advert, 'Why doesn't your mamma wash you with Fairy soap?'. As a result, misogynistic messages within skin-lightening adverts were normalised, as they offered women a route into Western modernity, universal feminism and a tool for navigation for their children.

Gill's (2006) insight to honour supports this, as she recalls the terms 'Mother Russia', 'Mother India' and 'Mother Ireland'. Signposting how women are assigned to a symbol of nationalism and how women are held accountable on how their children are identified and positioned within society. Women are situated as either a hindrance or aid for the native man's civilising movement. The advert articulates how integrating the white and cleansed ideal is a mother's (woman's) job, even if this comes as the loss of her own ethnic identity.

Risk Factors

Despite the physical modification to a lighter complexion, skin-lightening products have a detrimental impact on users. First and foremost, there are health implications. The most harmful chemicals found in these products are hydroquinone, mequinol and retinoid. The long-term use of which interrupts melanin production and creates irreversible damage to melanocytes, causing skin irritation, which paradoxically will darken the skin (Pollock et al. 2020). Other reported health implications from the prolonged use of skin-lightening creams include hypertension, nephrotic syndrome, dermatitis, mercury poisoning, diabetes, ochronosis, kidney failure and cancer within the skin and liver (Cobb 2019).

Second is the assimilation experience and the emotional/psychological repercussions of having an 'undesirable' complexion. Hill (2002: 80) explains that the bearing of skin colours weighs more on women, in comparison to men, noting that 'Black women seeking to be perceived by others as feminine and attractive feel compelled to emulate Whiteness; often painfully through the use of skin bleaches, hair dyes and straightening combs'. Social media imagery and adverts advocate messaging around 'pure' and 'innocent' skin, often positioned with light-skinned complexions.

On the other hand, skin tanning, another body modification process, is glorified to a certain extent, consumed by men and women of fair complexion, exoticising brown skin. Tanning carries little social stigma; rather, it is considered to be a mainstream beauty regime. Martin et al. (2009) highlights the attitudes towards tanning. Women are said to be liberated and making a fashion statement; on some social media platforms, tanning is described as the 'orange is the new black' effect. The perception of tanning offering glowy, healthy and desirable skin is often linked to power dynamics, as people of White heritage or complexions drive the movement. Moreover, social media has created a space for body dysmorphia, in particular for women of colour.

Figure 1 is an adaptation of skin-lightening adverts showcasing lexicon, symbols and vocabulary used by brands such as Fair & Lovely, Garnier and L'Oréal. Terminology such as 'younger', 'radiant' and 'perfect skin' exemplifies how focusing on Whiteness/lightness is a manipulative indoctrinating method to encourage consumers that fairness is better and is the only way to be beautiful. Furthermore, it heightens the 'lack' of beauty in darkness by eliminating dark marks, hyperpigmentation and even melanin.

Charles (2003) suggests that the pressure of colourism and the resulting act of skin lightening is not an indication of self-loathing, but is promoted and sustained through the mainstream presence of a Eurocentric western look. In the twenty-first century, women translate their perception of beauty from online trends and the digital look. Instagram and Snapchat are highly influential. The current trend is 'Instagram Face', a look that combines lip fillers, pore-free skin, high cheekbones, large eyes and light complexion as a single, cyborgian look (Tolentino 2019). Consequently, creating a representation of desire, the images hold meaning; the beholder rebounds and realigns their looks to fit in. Subhasini and Angel (2020: 3760) extend this by suggesting there is an investment in white bodies. Elements such as whitewashing within Hollywood and Bollywood, even the representation of Caucasian or 'lightened' complexions of dark-skinned models, emphasises Whiteness 'variably as a norm and a mode of superiority'. Tiffany & Co's recent 'About Love' campaign with Beyonce mirrors this ideology. Observers have claimed that Beyonce's skin tone appears 'artificially lightened'. Sources such as the Independent (2021) and Lipstick Alley (2021) describe her appearance as white European and camouflage of her natural skin. One particular snippet highlights the challenges for the BAME community:

> It's a really trendy advert; however, you can't disguise the truth that Beyonce's skin seems considerably lighter than it often does. You solely must flick again via her Instagram and see she's so much darker than in that advert. She's sporting plenty of make-up, there's plenty of filters happening—she seems a totally different shade.

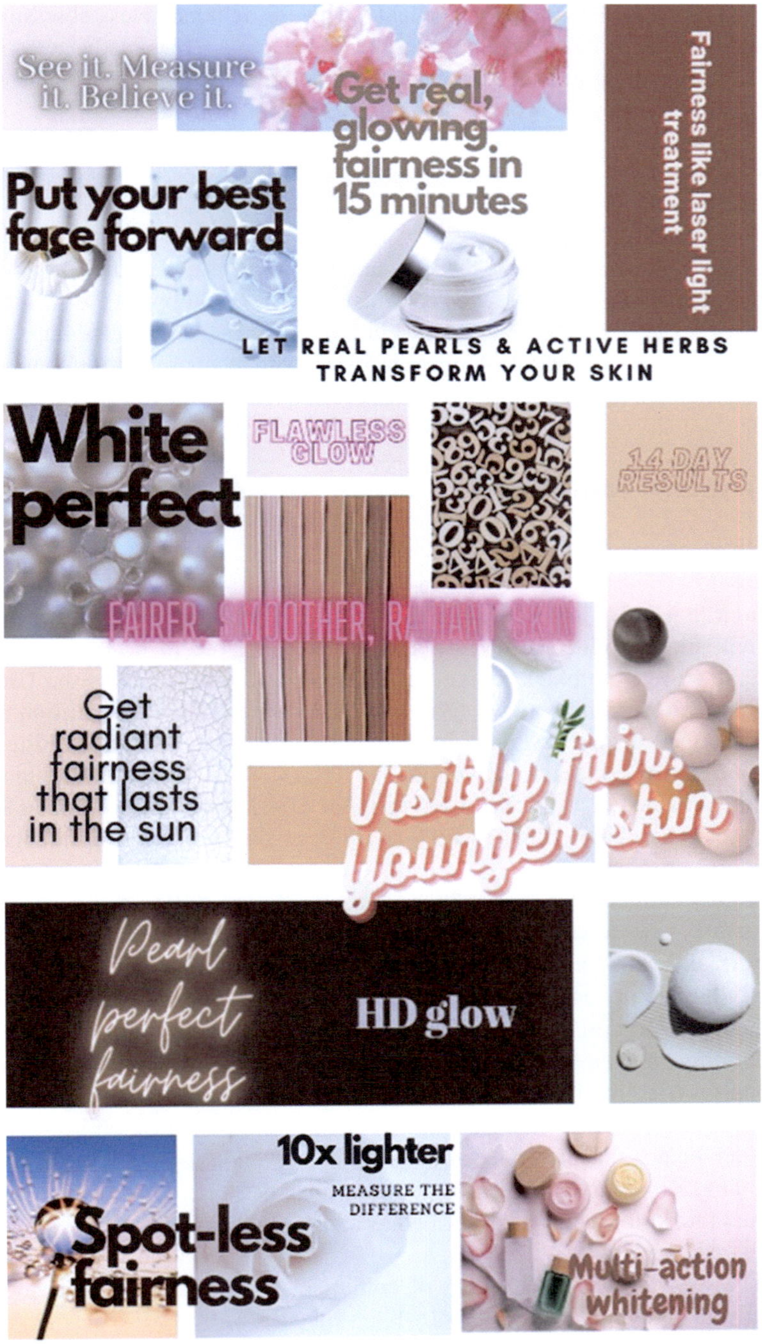

Fig. 1 Mood board showcasing vocabulary and symbols found in skin-lightening adverts

There must be steadiness. On the one hand, why are we nonetheless obsessing over what folks appear to be? On the opposite, for Beyonce, as a black lady, her skin tone sends out a worrying message to her younger and older followers. It sends out the message that lighter skin is best. (Samuels 2021: para 16).

Prevalence

Despite the contentious nature of skin-lightening products and criticism by activists and social movements, the practice continues to grow and impose the 'white gaze' upon users (Yancy 2008). The global skin-lightening market is valued at £3.7 billion and forecasted to reach £6.8 billion by 2027, with most users from Bangladeshi, Chinese, Indian, Nigerian, Pakistani and Thai ethnicities (Shahbandeh 2018).

International Comparison

The UK

Although legislation is attempting to control the availability of the most toxic skin-lightening products, they are still easily available in beauty complexes, ayurvedic stores, the black market, pharmacies and online across the UK. In a simple Google search using the term 'skin bleaching', over eight million results are available, with the first page including options to buy skin-lightening products via eBay or 20 treatment options via Treatwell. Though skin lightening is not widely discussed, the demand exists in the UK. Most users are from a British African or Asian background, who heavily draw on 'homeland' influences and community pressures.

A survey conducted by the British Skin Foundation (2019) established that a third of users perceived light skin as more attractive, thus opting to use skin bleachers and skin-lightening treatments. In addition, 11% cited pressure as a key driving factor, usually exerted by family and friends, and another 11% referred to cultural pressure. Furthermore, despite sustaining side effects such as skin thinning, uneven skin tone and rashes, 21% carried on using the products as the long-term solution of lighter-skinned 'outweighed' the short-term issues. Finally, 5% admitted to using a skin-lightening product on a child. Phoenix's (2021) advocates that 'Colourism in general is a taboo topic and until recently people haven't wanted to talk about it in the UK' (2021: para 4). Her research indicated that colourism was described as a barrier when entering the job market or for career development.

Conversely, the knock-on effect of colourism for the white female body can result in isolation and fetishisation of white skin (Box 1).

Box 1 Exploring the Role of Colourism on the White Female Body

The Knock-On Effect of Colourism on the White Body

Research from Grant (2020) suggests that as the 'white/light' skin is glorified, this creates a fetishisation. Women are labelled with terms such as 'Gori (*white skinned girl*), Barbie doll and blonde bimbo'—all due to her looks and appearance. Colourist values has created a desirability for light skin tones, but women who naturally possess this can be segregated in interracial relationships as they are perceived as an outsider. As Zambelli (2021) describes, women in this scenario may ultimately become the object of disapproving gazes and commentaries by strangers. There is an expectation within some communities, to marry within the same culture, to preserve traditions and caste systems. There may be a desire for light-skinned brides, but this is usually with the caveat of them being from the same culture/religious group.

Africa

At present, Africa has the highest number of users and consumers of skin-lightening products. Countries such as Ghana, Rwanda, South Africa and Uganda have either full or partial bans on skin-lightening products. However, the technicalities around which products impose a health risk or are deemed illegal due to the active ingredients have made the ban difficult to monitor and enforce. Statistics from the World Health Organization suggest that over 40% of African women bleach their skin through soaps, creams, tablets and drips. These products are prominent in some areas, with 77% of women in Nigeria, 59% in Togo (*described as Akonti*), 35% in South Africa, 27% in Senegal and 25% in Mali (*referred to as xessal, caco/tcha-tcho*). Across South Africa, tribes place different values on the practice as reflected in the name, such as ukutsheyisa/isiXhosa (*to chase beauty*) and isiZulu equivalent to 'applying creams on the skin' (Thomas 2020). Across south-central Africa, the acronym FBI (formerly Black individuals) is widely used about skin bleachers. However, regardless of tribe/nation differences, the motivations are similar, the potential of increased privileges, superior social standing, increased marital and employment prospects.

Observed for over four decades, skin bleaching in Africa is largely attributed to colonialism, Westernisation and allowing movement across a racial hierarchy. As Lewis et al. (2011: 30) suggest, 'Colonialism ultimately left behind a social psychology and an African consciousness of submission and imitation—a psychological colonisation'. Historically, skin bleaching was observed by rural and poor African women; however, the practice has become a norm for mobile working/educated professional Black women, increasing the demand for skin-bleaching products and the number of users in Africa.

The materiality of skin bleaching in some parts of Africa, such as Nigeria, resides in enforcing constructions that reflect femininity, aesthetics and beauty. To characterise the practice, alternative terminology such as 'skin toning', 'body decoration', 'body art', 'blemish removal' or 'body modification', thus positioning the act of bleaching as a source of self-expression (Mangezvo 2018). Despite recent social movements such as Black Lives Matter creating dialogue around colourism, and the need to regulate skin lightening products, there is an advocation around freedom of choice. Insight from sellers and users in Uganda offers an alternative perspective. Many describe skin bleaching as a form of liberation and a process of reverting to their natural state:

> Whiteness has been elevated and presented as a universal standard of progress. When people say it's about Whiteness, it's not necessary to physically be white; it's about wanting to access things white people have easy access to—privileges, economic and social status.
>
> Light skin is what men want; it makes sense for women to assimilate to the standard that men want to increase the chances of getting married. And marriage serves as a form of social capital—being someone's wife, a child bearer and esteemed member of society. So, it will elevate a woman. (Rao 2019: para 22)

South Asia

Whether it is perceived as a fixation on Whiteness or an anti-blackness problem, the presence of skin lightening across Bangladesh, India and Pakistan is very much at the forefront. The influence of colonialism on beauty standards has become the midst of Asian culture, with 'white/fair' skin being the pinnacle of beauty and prosperity. India's fascination with fair skin stems from a combination of colonialism, colourism and patriarchy. Therefore, it is imperative to explore British colonisation to understand skin lightening in India and the trickle effect on Bangladesh and Pakistan.

While establishing their position, the British defined themselves as the superior race, placing them within a higher social class than the native communities—Bangladeshi, Indian and Pakistani people. In doing so, dark skin was associated with discriminatory and stereotypical connotations such as evil, ugly, lazy and corrupt. Consequently, being 'white' in Bangladesh, India and Pakistan represented an imperial race; this Western reign of colonialism has revolved from intergroup racism into today's generation perception of colourism.

Today, some of the biggest brands in the skin-lightening industry have a strong foundation in India. It is reported that the likes of Hindustan Unilever—Fair & Lovely, Procter & Gamble, Nivea, Garnier and Emami—saturate the skincare market. The World Health Organization (2018) shows that 61% of skin products available in India are intended for skin lightening. Products include creams, face washes, deodorants, vaginal whiteners and creams targeted towards children aged 6 months+. It is estimated that 60% of Indian women and 10% of Indian men use at least one skin-lightening product as part of their skincare regime (Dixit 2019). The push and dominance reside on various factors but undoubtedly across South Asia; specifically, India is prominent because of Bollywood and caste systems.

Emmanuel (cited in Abraham 2017: para 8) explores this in further detail, explaining:

> In India, codified with caste systems, ancient Hindu classification determined occupation and social stratum. At the top, Brahmins were priests and intellectuals. Bottom, outcastes were confined to the least-desired job: the darker you looked, the lower your place in the social hierarchy. This preference for fair skin was perpetuated and strongly reinforced by colonialism. It was a fact that the rich could stay indoors versus the poor who worked outside and were dark-skinned. The driving force in modern-day globalisation is the rampant dark stigma where western beauty ideals predominate worldwide; with these ideals come products to service them and rigid cultural perceptions across South Asia.

The Bollywood industry has notably used white filters and whitewashing, while household names such as Shah Rukh Khan, Deepika Padukone, and Sonam Kapoor become the face of skin lightening and the epitome of beauty.

There is a cynical pattern, dark skin is masked as the dangerous, unattractive side of beauty and the state that needs to be improved, and as ethnic minorities are underrepresented, it perpetuates ethnic and racial stereotypes. Even when native members of the South Asian community are used as public figures or in advertising, they are shown in a considerably lighter skin tone. For instance, L'Oréal's 'White Perfect' skin-lightening campaigns present actresses Sonam Kapoor and Aishwarya Rai with lighter and brighter skin tones. Tools such as Photoshop and Facetune aid the construction of fictitious imagery and unattainable beauty ideals. As demonstrated below (Fig. 2), body- and face-sculpting options within Photoshop means skin tone and facial features can be easily changed. However, in doing so, it promotes body image disturbance and fosters a culture of colourism.

Though such depictions can be easily aligned to other modelling/marketing campaigns, the constant messaging around light skin, especially towards women, becomes problematic.

Colourism and the bias towards skin tones can have detrimental impacts on women, including dowry abuse, physical abuse, emotional abuse and in some cases, death. It is apparent, the idealisation of light skin starts for women at a young age, as demonstrated in the case of M Lavanya (Box 2).

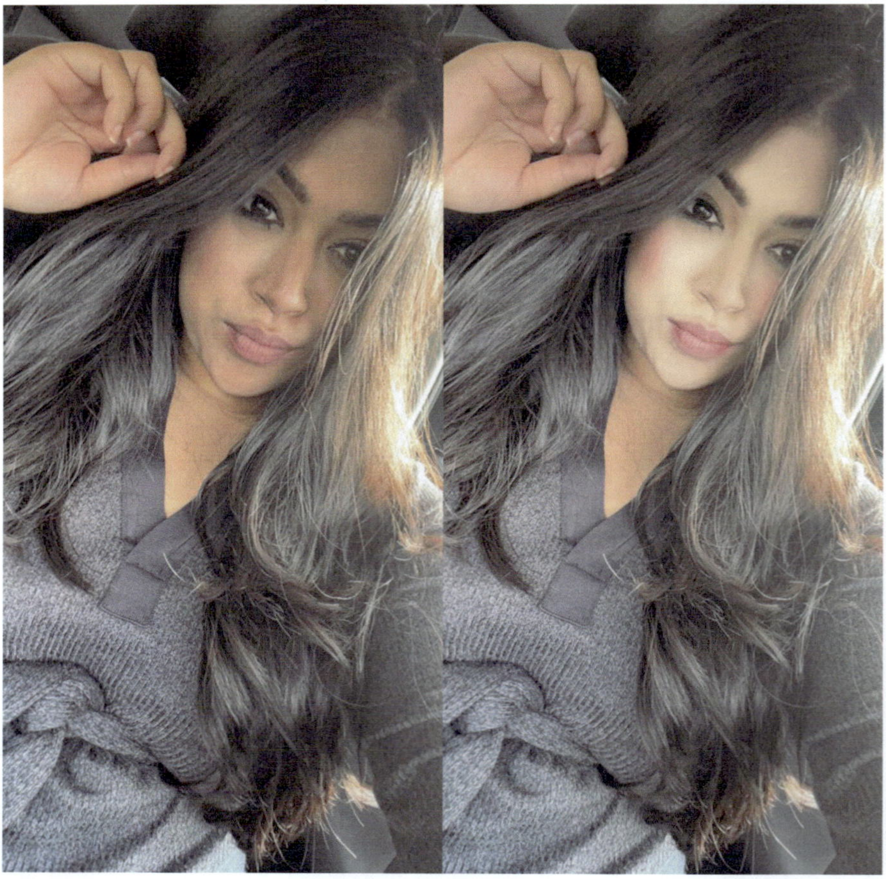

Fig. 2 Before and after photos showcasing the difference in skin tones after using Photoshop and Facetune

Box 2 Case Study: M Lavanya

In 2018, 14-year-old M Lavanya from Hyderabad, India, set her body on fire after months of verbal and physical abuse over her dark complexion. Alongside taunts about her skin tone and appearance, she was subjected to character assassination, whereby her peers would assign derogatory labels and blackmail her into silence. Lavanya attempted suicide once at her home and this was reported to the school. According to Samaa News (2018: para 6), 'The principal decided to shame her and put the onus on her, instead of taking action against her classmates'. Unfortunately, her second attempt resulted in her death; after setting her body on fire with kerosene, she suffered 45% burn injuries.

In addition, India's Ayurvedic system encourages pregnant women to improve/lighten their foetus's complexion by consuming saffron milk, oranges, coconut and fennel seeds. The onus remains on women throughout childhood as they are encouraged to stay out of the sun and integrate potentially harmful skin-lightening solutions into their skincare routine. By the age of marriage, women are conforming to familial and societal pressures and the male gaze.

Wang (2019) discusses how first-generation mothers recognise skin-lightening practices as a measure of survival for daughters and secure their place in society. On the other hand, fathers are deemed not to mirror the same concerns with their sons. As a result, their sons and the male autonomy can compensate for their looks, unlike daughters that may get caught up in a vicious cycle of misogyny and sexism, where their value is defined on aesthetics and desirability. Wives are subjected to a patriarchal system as the male gaze hones in on beauty being submissive. Womanhood becomes fixed to pleasing the male expectation, and women are subjected to unattainable ideals.

Insight from Hashmi (2018) highlights how Whiteness is deeply embedded within Pakistani culture and ways of being. For example, the lack of representation across mainstream media and social media. The idea of fair skin is perceived to bring success and acceptance, and this carries the ideology of behavioural qualities, moral values and the ideal woman for generation after generation. Jago Pakistan, a morning chat show, is notorious for showcasing an array of skin-lightening products on the show and during breaks and depicting black faces in several 'comedy skits'. One notable episode held a segment where makeup artists were challenged to make dark skin look beautiful, described as 'near enough impossible'. Other references include using natural home remedies, including applying lemon or sandalwood on the face to lighten the skin and spectrum of foundation shades. Most makeup courses are designed and catered towards light and fair women. Heavily used within mainstream media, lyrics and generally in the South Asian community, the terminology 'Gori' refers to light-skinned women, thus narrowing the notions of beauty and removing femininity and attractiveness of darker women.

Within Pakistani media and soap operas, there is a clear distinction between light-skinned and dark-skinned models. Light-skinned models are highly sought after, whereas dark-skinned models are rarely seen. Light skin is portrayed as a representation of beauty and success. The skin-lightening market is waiting to cash in on people's hidden aspirations. In principle, through the constant visual portrayal of lighter skin tones and Caucasian models, there is a notion of normalising Whiteness by making it visible. Iqbal (2015: 3) extends this:

> These dramas are meant to be reflective of Pakistani lifestyles and the characters portrayed are envisioned to represent the everyday Pakistani, yet instead, they represent the vision of a fair-complexioned society with only the minor and villainous characters being those with darker skin. In western culture, the media and television are associated with playing a huge role in the concept of our self-image and Pakistan's media is no different, portraying fair skin as the epitome of beauty. Thus, programmes meant to represent the Pakistani culture portray an image that is not of the general population, but instead of an ideal that society envisions.

In Bangladeshi culture, the translation of the word 'dark' can often align to descriptions of dirt, burnt, burden and dirt, whereas the interpretation of 'white' symbolises purity, wellbeing and cleanliness. When exploring Bengali vocabulary, these distinctions are made evident, for instance, *forsha* (*fair or light-skinned*), *ujjal shamla* (*medium yet bright*), *shamla* (*not too dark or light*) *and kalo* (*black or dark*). These distinctions between skin tones and proverbs highlight the discursive formation of 'fair' or 'white' skin; thus, Bangladeshi women are bound by a lifestyle instilled with racial meaning. In the case of Aklima (Box 3), her eligibility for marriage and the success of it was determined by her complexion.

Box 3 Case Study: Aklima

Aklima's story focuses on dowry abuse. From a young age, her parents perceived her dark skin as a huge burden in finding a suitable candidate. The majority of her suitors would complain about her shyamla (dark)/moyla (dirty) complexion. One that stuck in Aklima's mind is 'I cannot marry a shyamla girl without five lakhs and a job, none of which you can offer. So, you've disrespected me by showing your daughter; you've wasted my time' (Rob 2019: para 2).

Not being able to compensate and meet these requests took a toll on Aklima's father, in regard to health—in the upkeep of three jobs. Aklima was eventually successful in finding a suitor, based in Dubai. The Nikkah (Islamic marriage) was conducted, and Aklima was advised by the groom and his family to wait in Bangladesh until her visa application was complete. After a month of no contact, Aklima received a phone call from her husband. Within this phone call, Aklima received the news that her husband had remarried to someone of a lighter complexion, and he would not return the dowry, as it was deemed as compensation. Aklima was not only subjected to dowry abuse but is a victim of bride abandonment.

Bride abandonment is when husbands deliberately 'dispose' of unwanted brides in their countries of origin. Where they are often at risk of violence, exploitation, poverty, destitution and social stigma. Sometimes women are separated from their children; others are abandoned with their children in situations of near destitution (Southall Black Sisters 2014).

As Rozario (2002) observes, in Bangladesh, the colour hierarchy is ongoing, dictating the value of a woman's body, their value and worth, an expression of power relations which women must naturally conform to and play 'survival of the skin tone' when competing for resources available for men. Thus, South Asian women do not have the essence of being but are interpreted via multiple social systems.

Impacts of Colourism

Women, particularly women of colour, accept a negative connotation about their skin tones and react to the bleached ideals manifested in social environments. There is a discourse of 'Whiteness' representing intelligence, honesty, happiness, chastity, moral virtue, motherhood and beauty, whereas 'dark' corresponds to laziness, immorality, criminality and ignorance. A study conducted by Rondilla and Spickard (2007) identified four key themes when discussing colourism and the notion of 'Whiteness': 'beauty is light', 'stay out of the sun', 'avoid being romantically linked with or married to dark people' and 'white equals upper class'. Rondilla and Spickard (2007) advocate that individuals' perceptual filtering induces 'Whiteness' as a relatable ideal and a power dynamic.

Focusing on economic and social movements, aesthetic preferences and the physical appearance of white skin socially constructed the notion of beauty and the chances of finding a suitable partner. As Utley and Darity (2016: 130) depict, 'Colourism adds a colour component to the social capital women might seek to possess to present themselves as marriageable'. Notably, within India, colourism affects marriage choices and the institution of marriage, as dowries (a traditional marriage custom in India) dictate the 'marketability' of a bride, usually attributed to appearance, domestic skill set, education and virginity. Women are treated as products in these circumstances, and their best features are highlighted—predominately their 'light' skin. Dowry can be used to overcome the so-called disadvantages such as dark skin, subsequently increasing dignity and status. Being dark categorises brides as one of the 'unmarriables' due to the association of lower caste, wealth and unattractiveness. For fathers and brothers arranging suitors, women of the house with dark complexions are often deemed a burden.

Financial incentives through dowries ensure desire from grooms as well as guaranteeing a 'happy' marriage life. The dowry amount is argued to be substantially higher in comparison to a 'fair' bride, who offers the asset of an 'appealing light' complexion that would be socially accepted by 'higher castes'. In the case of Pooja Prakash (Box 4), dowry abuse was used to compensate for her 'dark' skin.

Box 4 Case Study: Pooja Prakash

In 2014, Pooja Prakash (29) from India committed suicide due to dowry abuse and verbal abuse after marriage from her husband and in-laws about her skin tone. According to India Today (2014: para 6), Pooja's husband Virendra from the start of their marriage (2010) would taunt her daily saying 'you are black, so you will have to bring money from your parents'. Her parents reportedly offered 8 Lakh (£7000) to 'compensate' for her complexion but due to financial constraints could not keep up with the demands from Virendra and his family.

Pooja found it difficult to remove herself from the situation due to community pressures and perceived shame. Pooja has left behind a young infant daughter. Virendra and his parents were arrested and booked under various sections of the Indian Penal Code.

Sahay and Piran (1997: 167) argue that 'Within South Asian culture, the words beautiful and fair are used synonymously, and there is often a preference for a female with a light complexion in marriage if other considerations are equal'. The thought of beauty is used to allocate women into a 'beauty queue' where one's complexion determines how socially and physically desirable it is regarding marriage (Hunter 1999).

By default, dark skin is associated with menial labour, whereas fairness is aspirational; a woman with light skin is perceived as not needing education or well-paid jobs to prove her worth. A bride with a dark complexion can result in emotional, physical and financial abuse from her husband and in-laws. A notable case is the one of Somera Bibi. Her in-laws demanded 100,000 rupees (£1000) and farmland to compensate for her dark skin. After the marriage, Somera's family were victimised and forced to give up a further 250,000 rupees. Eventually, Somera's family were unable to keep up with the demands, and Somera became a victim of physical abuse, subjected to taunts that 'she's too dark and not wanted in the family'. Eventually, this led to bride burning by her mother-in-law and husband, which resulted in her death (Marszal 2016).

To the preference of their mothers, men are expected to bring home a daughter in law that conforms to society's ideal of beauty, elevate or maintain their social standing, ensure future offspring carry this social capital and not blacken the family's face and legacy.

'Dark' skin can even be grounds for divorce, whereas being light indicates stability or, as Hunter (2002: 177) suggests, 'Women who possess this form of capital (beauty) can convert it into economic capital, educational capital, or another form of social capital'. So, there is a 'woman's place, a hierarchy of beauty, and being at the bottom could threaten both your future as well as your family's. As Rondilla and Spickard (2007: 13) suggest, 'women's bodies are manipulable commodities objectified for male consumption, the entire beauty industry is built on the foundational principle that women will alter their bodies through makeup, coloured contact lenses, plastic surgery and many more to increase their amount of beauty, or capital'. The perspective is that you will stand out from the crowd only when you have a 'white face'. There is also the desire to mimic the west, to appear modern and advanced.

Violence inflicted on women because of their complexions often goes unreported, primarily due to the normalisation of the light skin ideal; anything outside of this would be perceived to go against the norm, but 'honour' plays a role whether women are placed as the keepers of honour through their skin and body, or protecting the honour and the perception of others within the community. Unfortunately, a few case studies have highlighted the disposition of women due to their gender, standing in the community, and complexion. What has been made apparent in both reported and unreported cases is that women of darker skin tones are treated differently compared to men.

Previous research conducted, specifically on skin-lightening users from the Bangladeshi community, provides insight. For example, one participant describes the pressure of gender and power dynamics concerning skin tones:

> Lighter skinned girls are desirable for marriage—a wealthy and handsome man comes by and takes you away. It's a 'twisted fairy tale', I guess. Having darker skin just makes it harder for her parents to send her off for marriage. You're also pitied; I hate being pitied; everyone just says things like 'oh poor girl, how will you marry her? It will be hard to find a good lad for her'. My brother is darker than me; however, there is no need for him to use it—there shouldn't be an issue of marriage for him, and I don't think anyone would expect it of him; he's a boy at the end of the day, and I'm a girl. (Majumdar 2015)

In the spectrum of colourist views and values, men, regardless of skin tone, are placed in the mindset of accepting society's traditional outlook of being a man while embracing their ethnic heritage without ridicule. Discourses of the superiority of Whiteness linked to power (colonial or patriarchal) present in the British Bangladeshi community and perpetuated by women (mothers, aunties) and men alike prescribe the importance of bringing home a fair bride. The women in the study were drawn to men with different brown shades; however, they feel that men do not have this attitude towards them. There was a sense of intimidation, insecurity and colour consciousness in a discussion about brothers, fathers and spouses. Although various driving factors for attaining a lighter skin tone were discussed, one participant described light skin to give her 'superpowers', which helped combat the criticism from men and show their degree of privilege.

Implications for Education and Awareness Raising

As signposted throughout this chapter, government and social movements have encouraged society and brands to realign their thoughts and messages around skin lightening. Several authors such as Layla Saad, Ijeoma Oluo, Reni Eddo-Lodge and Lynn Thomas are leading conversations around antiracism education and how to tackle different forms of structural racism, including colourism. However, it is evident that skin lightening is a habitual practice, and it requires culturally sensitive interventions to evoke a behavioural change. One example includes adapting terminology. For instance, commentary such as 'I'm almost as tanned as you' or 'you're pretty for a dark-skinned girl'—though this may be said in admiration of someone's skin tone, this can often be demeaning and heighten preferential treatment of light skin over dark skin.

Second is tackling colourist thoughts and views. Many of the practices above and those that exist within cultural groups are often passed through generations. Challenging these mindsets and practices requires a scope of self-acknowledgement. For example, it recognises how your body language, response to the imagery and 'White privilege' could impact a member of the BAME community. In the words of Monk Kidd (2001), 'We can't think of changing our skin. Change the world, that's how we got to think'. Being part of the South Asian community, I can reflect on the so-called norms I have challenged, such as interrogating family members who think it is acceptable to label and describe women by their appearances, often using words like that 'kali (black) girl'. Showcasing how being sunburnt is acceptable, often within the South Asian community, young children are encouraged to stay out of the sun, all in all, to avoid looking dark.

Applying interventions and offering support can be difficult. However, dialogue, education and representation provide a solid structure, as not only does this combat any labels assigned to dark skin but normalising how there is more than one look and way of being; each carries its own merits and beauty. Several community pages and forums are available online to help aid the conversation around colourism, including UK-based initiatives such as the Sapphire Community Group, Mind UK (charity), Raang.uk (Instagram), Show Racism the Red Card (charity), Race On The Agenda: ROTA, Stand Up To Racism UK and Race Equality First.

Summary

- Colourism is a prevalent problem, affecting people from different ethnicities, in particular women from the BAME community.
- A common practice to offset the pressures of colourism is skin lightening.
- Skin lightening can entail the application of creams, soaps, drips and home remedies. Skin-lightening solutions can potentially lead to physical/mental health issues, body dysmorphia and a loss of ethnic identity.
- Exploration of case studies, risks factors and impacts has shown that much of a woman's self-worth is determined by her appearance. As a result, women engage in skin lightening to gain acceptance in many domains, i.e. community, societal positioning and marriage. Colourist values and practices have often meant women are victims of domestic abuse, bride abandonment, financial abuse, rape and bullying.
- Challenging colourism not only requires an antiracist approach, but dialogue and culturally sensitive practices. These need to address the mindset of different generations but also men and women, to help dismantle racist systems and reflect on personal accountability.

References

Abraham M (2017) Emmanuel K: Skin lightening: India's obsession that is becoming a medical problem. https://scroll.in/pulse/850030/skin-lightening-indias-obsession-that-is-becoming-a-medical-problem. Accessed 26 Jul 2021

British Skin Foundation (2019) Skin Lightening. https://www.britishskinfoundation.org.uk/skin-lightening. Accessed 18 Feb 2021

Charles ADC (2003) Skin bleaching, self-hate and black identity in Jamaica. J Black Stud 33(6):711–728

Cobb C (2019) Side Effects and Precautions of Skin Bleaching. https://www.healthline.com/health/skin-bleaching. Accessed 17 Feb 2021

Dixit N (2019) Fair, but not so lovely: India's obsession with skin whitening. https://brightthemag.com/fair-but-not-so-lovely-indias-obsession-with-skin-whitening-beauty-body-image-bleaching-4d6ba9c9743d. Accessed 27 Mar 2021

Gill A (2006) Patriarchal violence in the name of 'honour'. Int J Crim Justice Sci 1(1):1–12

Grant C (2020) What is Colourism? https://www.verywellmind.com/what-is-colorism-5077380. Accessed 18 Sep 2021

Hall ER (2006) The bleaching syndrome among people of color. J Hum Behav Soc Environ 13(3):19

Hargrove TW (2019) Light privilege? Skin tone stratification in health among African Americans. Soc Race Ethnicity 5(3):370–387

Hashmi M (2018) Pakistan's problem with colourism. https://shadesofnoir.org.uk/pakistans-problem-with-colourism/. Accessed 19 Jun 2021

Hill ME (2002) Skin color and the perception of attractiveness among African Americans: does gender make a difference? Soc Psychol Q 65(1):77–91

Hunter M (1999) Colorstruck: skin colour stratification in the lives of African American women. Sociol Inq 68(1):517–535

Hunter M (2002) If you're light, you're alright: light skin as social capital for women for colour. J Gend Soc 16(2):175–193

Independent (2021) What is the controversy around Beyonce's Tiffany Campaign. Independent. https://www.independent.co.uk/life-style/fashion/beyonce-tiffany-campaign-diamond-controversy-b1909722.html. Accessed 30 Sep 2021

India Today (2014) Gurgaon woman commits suicide as husband taunts her for black complexion. India Today. https://www.indiatoday.in/india/north/story/gurgaon-woman-kills-herself-after-husbands-taunt-on-skin-colour-195893-2014-06-06. Accessed 27 Apr 2021

Iqbal A (2015) Ab Gora Hoga Pakistan (now Pakistan will be white): a study into the phenomenon of skin lightening in Pakistan. In: CERS Working Paper 2015. https://www.leeds.ac.uk/. Accessed 15 May 2021

Kyeremateng T (2020) How colourism and misogynoir affected a generation of dark-skinned black women on and off the timeline. https://gal-dem.com/how-colourism-and-misogynoir-affected-a-generation-of-dark-skinned-black-women-twitter/. Accessed 12 Nov 2021

Lewis KM, Robkin N, Gaska K, Njoki LC (2011) Investigating Motivations for Women's Skin Bleaching in Tanzania. Psychol Women Q 35(1):29–37

Lipstick Alley (2021) Beyoncé looking a little white in New Tiffany Ad. Lipstick Alley. https://www.lipstickalley.com/threads/beyonc%C3%A9-looking-a-little-white-in-new-tiffany-ad.4694588/. Accessed 23 Oct 2021

Majumdar M (2015) The twisted fairy-tale behind how light skinned girls are 'trending': perceptions of skin lightening products among British Bangladeshi women. Dissertation, Oxford Brookes University

Mangezvo PL (2018) The (re)making of bodies and enforcement of masculinities: aesthetics and aspiration at Zimbabwean. Afr Dev 43(1):113–126

Marszal A (2016) Indian bride 'burnt alive by husband's family because her skin was too dark'. https://www.telegraph.co.uk/news/2016/06/09/indian-bride-burnt-alive-by-husbands-family-because-her-skin-was/. Accessed 22 Apr 2021

Martin JM, Ghaferi JM, Cummins DL, Mamelak AJ, Schmults CD, Parikh M, Speyer LA, Chuang A, Richardson HV, Stein D, Liégeois NJ (2009) Changes in skin tanning attitudes: fashion articles and advertisements in the early 20th century. Am J Public Health 99(12):2140–2146

McClintock A (1995) Imperial leather: race, gender, and sexuality in colonial context. Routledge, New York, NY

Mehaffy MM (1997) Advertising race/racing advertising: the feminine consumer nation 1876-1900 signs. J Women Cult Soc 23(1):131–174

Mohdin A (2021) Phoenix A: Meghan's claims about Archie highlight colourism problem in UK. https://www.theguardian.com/uk-news/2021/mar/08/meghan-claims-archie-highlight-colourism-problem-uk. Accessed 22 Aug 2021

Monk Kidd S (2001) The secret life of bees. London: Tinder Press.

Owusu-Agyei M, Agyei M, Ogunleye AT (2020) Skin-lightening practices among shoppers in select markets in Kumasi, Ghana: a cross-sectional survey. JAAD Int 1(2):104–110

Phoenix A (2014) Colourism and the Politics of Beauty. Fem Rev 108(1):97–105

Pollock S, Taylor S, Oyerinde O, Nurmohamed S, Dlova N, Sarkar R, Galadari H, Manela-Azulay M, Chung SH, Handog E, Kourosh S (2020) The dark side of skin lightening: an international collaboration and review of a public health issue affecting dermatology. Int J Women's Dermatol 7(2):158–164

Rao P (2019) Paying a high price for skin bleaching. https://www.un.org/africarenewal/magazine/april-2019-july-2019/paying-high-price-skin-bleaching. Accessed 28 Feb 2021

Rob R (2019) The dark dowry: white supremacy in communities of colour. https://www.thedailystar.net/star-weekend/perspective/news/the-dark-dowry-1762825. Accessed 14 Jan 2021

Rondilla LJ, Spickard P (2007) Is lighter better? - Skin-tone discrimination among Asian Americans. Rowman and Littlefield publications, Lanham, MD

Rozario S (2002) Poor and 'dark,' What is my future: identity construction and adolescent women in Bangladesh. In: Manderson L, Rice LP (eds) Coming of age in south and southeast Asia: youth, courtship and sexuality, 1st edn. Routledge, London, pp 16–32

Sahay S, Piran N (1997) Skin colour preferences and body satisfaction among South Asian-Canadian and European-Canadian female university students. J Soc Psychol 1(2):167–171

Samaa News (2018) Indian teen sets herself on fire over dark skin taunts. https://www.samaa.tv/global/2018/01/indian-teen-fire-dark-skin-taunts/. Accessed 16 Jan 2021

Samuels D (2021) Critics claim Beyonce's skin tone 'artificially lightened' in new Tiffany & Co ad with Jay-Z. https://travelguides.buzz/topstories/critics-claim-beyonces-skin-tone-artifically-lightened-in-new-tiffany-co-ad-with-jay-z/. Accessed 27 Oct 2021

Shahbandeh M (2018) Forecasted market value skin lightening products worldwide from 2017 to 2027. https://www.statista.com/statistics/863876/globalforecasted-market-value-of-skin-lightening-products/. Accessed 5 May 2021

Sommer M (2011) Colonies - colonisation - colonialism: a typological reappraisal. J Ancient West East 10(1):183–193

Southall Black Sisters (2014) Transnational Marriage Abandonment. https://southallblacksisters.org.uk/campaigns/transnational-marriage-abandonment/. Accessed 12 Feb 2021

Subhasini G, Angel S (2020) Undoing whiteness: post-colonial identity and the unfinished. J Matematik 1(2):3760–3762

Thomas LM (2020) Beneath the surface: a transnational history of skin lighteners. Duke University Press, Durham

Tolentino J (2019) The age of the Instagram face. The New Yorker. https://www.newyorker.com/culture/decade-in-review/the-age-of-instagram-face. Accessed 27 Feb 2021

Utley TJ, Darity W (2016) India's colour complex: one day's worth of matrimonial. Rev Black Polit Econ 43(2):129–138

Wang S (2019) The role of gender role attitudes and immigrant generation in ethnic minority women's labor force participation in Britain. J Res Sex Rol 80(3):234–245

White L (1999) Sex, soap, and colonial studies. J Br Stud 38(4):478–486

World Health Organisation (2018) Mercury in skin lightening products. WHO, Geneva. https://www.who.int/ipcs/assessment/public_health/mercury_flyer.pdf. Accessed 15 Feb 2021

Yancy G (2008) Black bodies, white gazes: the continuing significance of race. Rowman & Littlefield Publishers, Inc, Lanham, MD

Zambelli E (2021) Interracial couples and the phenomenology of race, place, and space in contemporary England, Identities. Global Stud Cult Power 28(6):1–12

Monica Majumdar is a PhD student at Queen Mary University of London. Her research examines colourism, colonialism, the skin lightening phenomenon and identity construction. She is also a Facilitator for Oxford Against Cutting, with expertise in Colourism, Honour Based Abuse, Body Image and Social Media.

Dowry-Related Abuse and Dowry Death

Tazeen Saeed Ali, Zohra Jetha, Shagufta Parveen, Parveen Ali, and Michaela M. Rogers

Learning Objectives

Having read this chapter, you should be able to understand the following:

- The concept and custom of dowry in different countries
- The concept of dowry-related abuse and dowry death
- The prevalence and impacts of dowry-related abuse
- The trend of dowry deaths in India
- The types of interventions to address dowry-related abuse

T. S. Ali (✉)
School of Nursing and Midwifery, The Aga Khan University, Karachi, Pakistan

Department of Community Health Sciences, The Aga Khan University, Karachi, Pakistan
e-mail: tazeen.ali@aku.edu

Z. Jetha
School of Nursing and Midwifery, Aga Khan University, Nairobi, Kenya
e-mail: zohra.jetha@aku.edu

S. Parveen
Health Sciences School, University of Sheffield, Sheffield, UK
e-mail: perveen.shagufta@aku.edu

P. Ali
The Health Sciences School, University of Sheffield, Sheffield, UK
e-mail: parveen.ali@sheffield.ac.uk

M. M. Rogers
Department of Sociological Studies, University of Sheffield, Sheffield, UK
e-mail: m.rogers@sheffield.ac.uk

P. Ali, M. M. Rogers (eds.), *Gender-Based Violence: A Comprehensive Guide*,
https://doi.org/10.1007/978-3-031-05640-6_19

Introduction

Transfers of wealth and resources at the time of marriage have existed historically in many parts of the world, from the Babylonian civilization to Renaissance Europe. Such exchanges still take place in many parts of the world, and especially in the developing world. There are two types of exchanges: bride price (transfer from the groom's side to the bride's) and dowry (transfer of wealth from the bride's family to the groom or his family). The practice of bride price is widespread in parts of East Asia and some African countries, whereas the practice of dowry is most common in South Asian and Middle Eastern countries, including Afghanistan, Bangladesh, India, Iran, Nepal, Pakistan, Sri-Lanka, Turkey, Azerbaijan, Tajikistan, Egypt, Morocco, Bosnia and Serbia. In most of these countries, and others, the custom of dowry is practised very religiously with the exchange of sizable dowries amounting to several times more than a household's annual income (Ali et al. 2013; Anderson 2007). In the past, dowry was considered a compensation for taking the bride from her birth family and therefore depriving them of her. As time evolved, the proportion of dowry to income has increased to the extent that it has led to families to live in poverty conditions and accruing debt through multiple loans. It has also become a compulsion for the families of girls to spend beyond their means on wedding expenses, and a family may be forced to sell significant assets solely to cover the cost of a wedding. Over time, people have started expecting this exchange, and when expectations are not met, it results in negative consequences. The practice, therefore, has been associated with gender-based violence (GBV), particularly, intimate partner violence (IPV) and family violence in developing countries where there is a lack of social and legal support for women. This chapter aims to explore the concept of dowry-related abuse. We start by defining dowry and dowry-related abuse before providing information on prevalence, impacts and causes. We use Pakistan and India as case studies to explore dowry-related abuse and dowry deaths; however, as discussed in the chapter, such practices are not limited to these two countries. We end by highlighting interventions that can be effective in addressing dowry-related abuse.

Defining Dowry, Dowry-Related Abuse and Dowry Death

Dowry is considered to be a payment in exchange for accepting the bride into the family, or as a compensation for wedding costs incurred by the groom's family. It takes the form of cash or material goods including jewellery, electrical appliances, furniture, bedding, crockery or even motorcycles or cars (Suran et al. 2004). Another interpretation of dowry is that it is given to brides and grooms to help them start their new life effectively. It may also be seen as the bride's rightful share in her parents' property as often girls and women do not inherit any property from their natal family in many countries. The practice itself is not abusive and was meant to support the new family; however, it can result in abuse. The practice is known by different names in various parts of the world, and Box 1 provides definitions, alternative terminology and related concepts.

Box 1 Definitions, Alternative Terminology and Related Concepts

Definition: A payment, such as property or money, paid by the bride's family to the groom or his family at the time of marriage.

Alternative Terminology

Bride price, kanyadhan, stridhan, trousseau, jahez, dahez, dāj, daaj, daijo, çeyiz, joutuk, jiazhuang, varadhachanai, streedhanam, miraz, serotwana, idana, saduquat, mugtaf.

Related concepts: bride price and dower

Bride price or bride service is a payment by the groom, or his family, to the bride, or her family.

Dower is the property settled on the bride herself, by the groom at the time of marriage, and which remains under her ownership and control.

As noted, giving or receiving or dowry is not abusive in itself; however, when the groom or his family demands more money or commodities, and the bride's family is unable or unwilling to pay, dowry-related violence can occur. The UN Division for the Advancement of Women defines dowry-related violence or harassment as 'any act of violence or harassment associated with the giving or receiving of dowry at any time before, during or after the marriage' (UN Women 2009). Physical violence, marital rape, acid attacks and burning alive (where a woman is covered in kerosene or some other accelerant and deliberately set on fire) are the most common forms of dowry-related violence (Ramakrishnan 2013). Forms of coercion may be used, such as the denial of clothing, evictions and fake imprisonment as a kind of extortion. The most severe impact of this violence is termed dowry death, referring to the death of any married woman who was murdered by her in-laws or husband, whereas suicide-related dowry is a crime where dowry is the principal cause for the death of a married woman (Babu and Babu 2011).

The practice of dowry is not new and is widely found in many cultures and traditions. Available evidence suggests it used to be practised in Rome, Greece, China, India, Europe, England, Russia, Romina, Mexico, the United States and Brazil. Over time, the practice prevalence has reduced—though not fully eliminated—in many of the countries. In the following, we provide some examples of how it is practised in different countries is shown in Box 2.

Box 2 Examples of Dowry Practices in Different Countries

Afghanistan: Dowry is a common practice in Afghanistan. The items included in a dowry are determined by the resources of the bride's family and the desires of the groom's family and can be sizeable. The dowry is transported from the bride's house to the groom's house in a ritual ceremony with a band and huge crowd 1 day before the wedding day, with the bride's family taking the longest route in the residential area, so the community can see the dowry being offered by the bride's family. When a bride arrives at her husband's home, the type of dowry she provides typically has an impact on how she is treated.

India: Dowry has been an integral part of India for centuries. During British rule, women were prohibited from buying or owning any property, land or assets, meaning that the men in a family owned all the gifts given to the bride by her parents. This rule led to significant cultural shifts in culture with the emergence of female infanticide, foeticide and sex selective abortions, for example. In 1961, India passed the Dowry Prohibition Act to make mandatory dowry illegal. Even though anti-dowry laws have been in place for decades, they have been widely criticised as ineffective (Manchandia 2005) with the continued and widespread practice of dowry. In modern India, it is reported that in cases of dowry, it is not uncommon that a groom's family will be dissatisfied with the dowries brought by the bride, resulting in physical and psychological abuse, and extreme acts including homicide or forced suicide of women (Kumar 2003; Rocca et al. 2009).

The Middle East: In Morocco, dowry is usually agreed upon before a marriage for the groom to the bride. Depending on the woman's martial state, she may receive a higher or lower payment. Virgin females, for example, receive a much higher Mahr than dowry compared to widows or divorcees. The marriage is usually postponed or cancelled if the elders of the two households cannot agree on the dowry sum. The dowry's value and composition are determined by social class, family wealth and regional customs (Shaheed 1994). In Turkey, dowry is referred to as çeyiz, and weddings can be called off if the groom's family is not satisfied with the dowry at the displaying ceremony. The wedding is marked complete once the entire dowry is sent to the groom's place in a ceremonial ritual (Sandikci and Ilhan 2004).

For women, marriage is an essential ritual to maintain their social status in society. Once married, a woman is expected to take the responsibility for her husband, in-laws and the entire household. Thus, women are often restricted to the duties of the household and are treated as submissive by the in-law's family (Tichy et al. 2009). However, the amount of dowry plays an important role in disputes between the families, with the dowry being demanded more than the bride's family can offer, resulting in various crimes including harassment of brides to dowry-related deaths (Reshma and Ramegowda 2013). There are various reasons for dowry-related abuse, and these include attitudes towards women, women's position and status in society, lack of participation of women in political spheres due to socioeconomic constraints and lack of appropriate legal sanctions against such practices. As the abuse is against a newlywed bride who has moved in with in-laws and has less contact with her natal family and other friends, it is often difficult for the victim to disclose their experiences and for others to spot abuse. The culturally accepted practice of abuse means that the victim and her birth family stay silent about the issue and do not seek help or even talk about it. The way to improve the condition of women is by increasing women's education, enhancing their participation in political decision-making and improving the status of women in the community and society (Reshma and Ramegowda 2013).

Prevalence

As mentioned earlier, dowry is common in many countries and so is dowry-related violence as over time, families have started expecting dowries from the bride's families and when dowry is not provided or provided as less than expected, it becomes a reason for intimate partner violence (IPV) and/or family violence. Women who are unable to pay dowry are at risk of being killed, especially if the groom and family are inflexible and insistent (Rudd 2001). Determining the actual prevalence of dowry-related abuse is very difficult as the issue is often under-reported; however, there is ample evidence to demonstrate its existence. For instance, in Bangladesh, between 2014 and 2017, the total number of dowry deaths was 750 women, with the average number of 187 dowry deaths per year (Rehman 2018).

Pakistan has the greatest documented number of dowry-related fatalities per 100,000 women in the world, with over 2000 dowry-related deaths per year with yearly rates exceeding 2.45 deaths per 100,000 women from dowry-related violence (Home Office 2011). In Pakistan, following other South Asian countries, the amount of dowry to be paid has risen in recent years. Yet, compared to other parts of the country, rural Pakistan's dowry prices have managed to stay low with only about 12% of the household's yearly expenses (nondurable goods) going towards each dowry. Rural brides seem to have more control over their dowry than their in-laws. The prevalence of dowry practices range from 87% to 97% in both rural and urban areas of Pakistan; however, there is little to understand the association between dowry practices and IPV (Ali et al. 2021).

Pakistan became the first Muslim country to make receiving dowry illegal as per the tenets of Islam in October 2020 (Tribune 2020). The only dowry allowed under the new law will be clothes (for the bride only) and bedsheets. In the event of a divorce, the groom's family is responsible for returning all gifts and dowry to the girl. Pakistan has enacted several pieces of legislation to combat the issue of excessive dowry demands, including Dowry and Bridal Gifts (Restriction) Act, 1976, and West Pakistan Dowry (Prohibition of Display) Act, 1967. Other, more religion-oriented legislations, such as the Muslim Personal Law of Shariat of 1948 and the

Muslim Family Laws Ordinance of 1961, specifically note protections for women and their inheritance rights, even outside of the dowry.

In India, although the practice of dowry has been prohibited by the Dowry Prohibition Act of 1961, it is still widespread owing to social and cultural expectations. If a person gives or takes dowry, then such a person is liable to be punished for a period of 6 months and pay a fine of INR 5000. Despite this act, India has recorded the highest number of deaths related to dowry worldwide, with an approximate of 8000 deaths in the year 2011 (Jeyaseelan et al. 2015). In 2020, nearly 7000 dowry death cases were reported in India. This was a gradual decrease from 2014, in which this number was approximately 8500 (Kanwal 2021). This figure is likely to be a gross underestimate due to under-reporting on the account of social stigma (Hitchcock 2001). Unfortunately, even with dowry, nearly 44% of married adolescent girls report experiencing some form of physical, emotional or sexual violence (Srivastava et al. 2021). The likelihood of violence is substantially higher among girls who said their husbands requested money (54% for emotional abuse, 42% for physical and 40% for sexual abuse (Srivastava et al. 2021).

Dowry is associated with suicide and homicide (Khalid et al. 2017; Mohanty et al. 2013). Babu and Babu (2011) undertook an analysis of data collected by India's National Crime Records Bureau (NCRB) finding that the total of dowry-related deaths was 8093 and for suicide the figure was 3148. There was a 74% increase in dowry-related murders from 1995 to 2007 and 31% increase for suicides by victims (Babu and Babu 2011). Other research has found similarly high rates. For example, 140 cases of dowry deaths were reported in a 2-year period from 2007 to 2009 (Mohanty et al. 2013). One hundred twenty-seven cases of dowry deaths were reported during the period of 2010–2014 (Belur et al. 2014). The total number of deaths as reported were 8391 in 2010; 8331 in 2011; 8233 in 2012; 8083 in 2013 and 8455 in 2014 (Khalid et al. 2017). Across this body of research, the unnatural deaths of victims were recorded as resulting from accidents, murders, sudden deaths and suicides. Burning, poisoning and hanging were also major causes of deaths (Mohanty et al. 2013; Belur et al. 2014).

The most concerning outcomes of the practice of dowry are dowry deaths, murders and suicides (Babu and Babu 2011). Research has been conducted to explore the factors associated with dowry deaths, IPV and family violence among married women, and these include the level of education, economic status, age at marriage, alcoholism, duration of married life, type of family, employment status, religion and caste (Shrivastava and Shrivastava 2013; Khalid et al. 2017; Jeyaseelan et al. 2015; Nongrum et al. 2014; Chhabra 2018; Bhattacharya and Singh 2017; Mohanty et al. 2013; Babu and Babu 2011; Pallikadavath and Bradley 2019). Victims are often young women aged between 18 and 26 years (Mohanty et al. 2013). Women's literacy plays a major role in the relationship with dowry deaths (Babu and Babu 2011). The higher the educational qualification of women, the less likelihood is the occurrence of violence (Babu and Babu 2011; Bhattacharya and Singh 2017). Those women who married between 20 and 25 years faced less violence than women who married before 20 years (Bhattacharya and Singh 2017). More dowry deaths were reported in nuclear families and among lower socioeconomic strata of society (Khalid et al. 2017). The economic status of the husband's family is also another factor explaining violence faced by married women (Pallikadavath and Bradley 2019). A study reveals that the majority of the cases of dowry deaths occurred between the first 4 years of marriage (Mohanty et al. 2013; Bhattacharya and Singh 2017).

The practice of dowry has spread to other countries as well, especially due to immigration of individuals from one country to another (Ghafournia and Easteal 2018). In Australia, for example, a Queensland-based social worker reported dealing with over 30 domestic violence cases in the Indian community across Queensland, New South Wales and South Australia (O'Connor and Lee 2022). A clinical audit of 56 South Asian victims of family violence presenting to one psychiatric outpatient setting revealed dowry abuse in 50% of cases (O'Connor and Ibrahim 2018).

It may be impossible to estimate the actual number of victims of dowry-related violence as the victims are hesitant to report the violence to authorities due to fear of revenge. Furthermore, for fear of being involved in the violence, families may often fail to report a dowry-related fatality. Overconcern for the perpetrator, shame or stigma associated with being a victim, belief in the futility of the complaint procedure or fear of being blamed for the violence all contribute to low reporting rates. Existing laws in some countries may prevent women from reporting acts of assault. In countries where dowry is illegal, such as India, seeking police assistance could result in the woman's family being criminally punished or imprisoned for paying a dowry. When dowry-related deaths or injuries are disguised as just cooking mishaps or suicides, the problem of underreporting becomes much more problematic (Dhillon 2018).

Impacts

Dowry-related abuse is perpetrated not only by the husband, but family members and the manifestations may include subjecting the victim to silent treatment, ignoring and isolating her within the family. It can take the form of physical, psychological or sexual abuse. Various studies have been conducted to explore the impact of dowry-related abuse on victims (Pandey et al. 2009; Bhattacharya and Singh 2017; Nongrum et al. 2014; Chhabra 2018). It can result in physical and psychological impacts for the victim. Physical symptoms include muscle strain, head injury and physical injuries, during pregnancy leading to abortions, placental abruption, rupture of the uterus, death of an unborn child (Chhabra 2018), chronic pain and gastrointestinal infections (Pandey et al. 2009; Bhattacharya and Singh 2017).

The girl/bride may be sent to her birth family for some time to pressurise, humiliate and embarrass them. The abuse can be in the form of publicly taunting and humiliating the bride and/or her family, controlling her movements and access to other people or facilities that she has, including food. Effects on mental health include depression, anxiety (Chhabra 2018), psychosomatic symptoms and post-traumatic stress disorder (Pandey et al. 2009). The effects of emotional/

psychological abuses include the phobias, anxiety and suicidality (Chhabra 2018), maternal depression (Nongrum et al. 2014), pregnancy complications due to gestational pre-eclampsia and problems in giving birth (Bhattacharya and Singh 2017). The effects of sexual abuse include HIV, unwanted pregnancies and complications during pregnancy (Chhabra 2018), sexually transmitted diseases, pre-term delivery and low-birth-weight babies (Nongrum et al. 2014). Box 3 provides two examples of extreme impacts of dowry-related violence, one from India and another one from Nepal. Both examples demonstrate that dowry related violence impacts women from all social stratas.

Box 3

Case 1: The State of Bihar vs. Mirityunje Kumar

Charu Lata, a resident of Patna, Bihar was married to Mirityunje Kumar in 2012. At the time of marriage, 20 Lacs were provided as dowry, but Charu's family, soon after the wedding, demanded another 15 Lacs. The in-laws pressurized Charu by harassing, torturing and beating her daily. In the meantime, Charu started working in a bank, creating another issue. Despite having a degree in hotel management from Australia, Mirityunje was unemployed and was jealous of his wife's success.

While Charu was working in the bank, all of her salary was being deposited in her father-in-law's account. An additional 2 Lacs were also provided by the bride's family. However, this was not enough.

Mirityunje continued to be jealous and abusive, and one day when Charu Lata refused to give any more money to her husband and in-laws, he tied her up with ropes and tortured her firstly and then killed her through strangulation in front of his family. On 24 July 2016, the family ran away with Charu Lata's 30-month-old son, locking the body in the house. The body was recovered a few days later, and cases were filed against the husband and family.

The husband was arrested 3 days later on 28 July and confessed his crime in front of the police.

Mobeen, L (2021). Dowry Deaths in India: A Harrowing Reality. https://www.paradigmshift.com.pk/dowry-deaths/.

Read the original post at ParadigmShift.com.pk: https://www.paradigmshift.com.pk/dowry-deaths/.

Case 2: Sunita Yadav: Dowry Death in Nepal

Sunita Yadav was beaten and burnt by her husband Sachitananda Yadav, a medical doctor. Sunita was taken to Kathmandu for treatment at the Tribhuvan University Teaching Hospital but died due to her injuries.

Sunita was in an abusive marriage for 16 years ago. At the time of marriage, Sachitananda Yadav's family demanded a huge amount of dowry. Sunita's family tried to give as much as possible. Yet, Sachitananda kept

demanding more and warned not to take her to his home until her family relented. The cruelty did not stop here. Sunita was tormented for not bringing enough dowry to her husband's house, and on 4 June 2015, Sachitananda's family tried to kill Sunita by burning her alive. The case was filed at the District Administration Office, Parsa, but it was settled through a meeting by village elders. To ensure that Sunita was safe, her family spent over 2 million rupees to pay dowry to her in-laws. Yet, Sachitananda demanded even more: new Maruti car and additional money. When her family could not meet this demand, he beat her to death.

Rage against dowry death: https://myrepublica.nagariknetwork.com/news/rage-against-dowry-death/.

In the extreme case, violence leads to death in the form of bride burning, homicide and forced suicide. Anecdotal evidence indicates common practices are to gaslight the person or put so much intense pressure that they see no option other than taking their own life. The abuse is intended to force the woman to pressure her family to pay more dowry. Even when demands are met, the abuse can continue to escalate to ensure further demands are met without resistance.

Interventions for the Protection of Girls and Women from Dowry-Related Abuse

To deal with the practice of dowry and its negative impact, a multidimensional approach is needed. It needs an attitudinal change across society which can be brought through various interventions at various levels.

Role of Education

To eliminate the harmful and the ruthless tradition of dowry and dowry-related violence, measures such as education can play a significant role in today's world. Girls and women should be well-educated, well-versed and well-aware of the laws and rights of women that promise safety and security. They need to understand the significance of education and pursue a viable career that will enable them to be independent in male-dominated, patriarchal societies. At the same time, males in the same society and their families should benefit from the same education so that they an be aware of the consequences they may have to face in the case they demand or accept dowry in any form. The act of giving women an equal right and eliminating social discrimination due to gender is amongst the significant measures that can minimize and potentially eliminate dowry customs and eventually dowry-related violence.

Role of Media

Nowadays, social media is available to every community, regardless of status and geographical region and social media platforms, and can play a vital role in breaking the customary practice of dowry. Television has a significant role as the effects of dowry-related issues can be portrayed through television soaps and movies. People are highly influenced by what they watch on television and are most likely to see the actors and actresses as their role models. Moreover, television shows can play an essential role in creating awareness about the culture of dowry and its negative impact. Young people see celebrities as their role models, and it is increasingly common that young people participate in writing blogs and platforms such as Twitter, Instagram and Facebook can be used to convey clear and concise messages to younger populations.

Role of Matchmaker

There are many cultures that do not favour love marriages; therefore, families consult with matchmakers to select partners for marriage. These matchmakers scrutinise marriage proposals according to the family's expectations and in relation to the proposal of money and asset provision. Sometimes they fix the amount of dowry with the consent of both parties. As such, matchmakers still have a considerable role to play in many communities. Therefore, matchmakers should be educated on dowry and dowry-related abuse in order to discourage giving and accepting dowry, and, as such, they have a pivotal role to play in eradicating this practice.

A Whole System Approach

Where dowry is still practised, governments should adopt a whole system approach to include screening for dowry-related abuse, assessment and referral pathways to support. All healthcare professionals in medical facilities should be made aware of dowry-related abuse and be able to offer therapeutic counselling along with medical care. Furthermore, specialized public health professionals should be introduced in community health centres to ensure that dowry-related awareness, and screening is carried out in the community. Moreover, there is a need for systems to develop for referring women and/or family to pursue redress through the judicial system and to receive social support from the community or social workers. Finally, there is a need for pathways and protocols to enable different professionals and agencies to work together to respond to the individual, family and community needs resulting from dowry-related abuse.

Summary

- Dowry-related abuse and dowry deaths are commonplace where the practice of dowry continues.
- Dowry deaths and suicides remain constantly high in some countries, including Pakistan and India.
- There are various interventions that can address dowry-related abuse and countries where dowry continues should adopt strategies and action plans to embed such interventions and adopt a whole system approach.

References

Ali TS, Árnadóttir G, Kulane A (2013) Dowry practices and their negative consequences from a female perspective in Karachi, Pakistan—a qualitative study. Health 5(7D):84

Ali TS, Hussain N, Zeb S, Kulane A (2021) Association of dowry practices with perceived marital life and intimate partner violence. J Pak Med Assoc 71(10):2298–2303

Anderson S (2007) The economics of dowry and brideprice. J Econ Perspect 21(4):151–174

Babu GR, Babu BV (2011) Dowry deaths: a neglected public health issue in India. Int Health 3(1):35–43

Belur J, Tilley N, Daruwalla N, Kumar M, Tiwari V, Osrin D (2014) The social construction of 'dowry deaths'. Soc Sci Med 119:1–9

Bhattacharya S, Singh A (2017) 'The more we change, the more we remain the same': female feticide continues unabated in India. BMJ Case Rep 2017:bcr2017220456

Chhabra S (2018) Effects of societal/domestic violence on health of women. J Women's Health Reprod Med 2(1):6

Dhillon A (2018) Death by dowry' claimed by bereaved family in India. Guardian. https://www.theguardian.com/global-development/2018/jul/18/death-by-dowry-claim-by-bereaved-family-in-india

Ghafournia N, Easteal P (2018) Are immigrant women visible in Australian domestic violence reports that potentially influence policy? Laws 7(4):32

Hitchcock A (2001) Rising number of dowry deaths in India. World Soc. http://www.wsws.org/en/articles/2001/07/ind-j04.html

Home Office (2011) Operational guidance note: Pakistan, August 2011. Pakistan OGN 11. https://www.refworld.org/docid/4e4213da2.html

Jeyaseelan V, Kumar S, Jeyaseelan L, Shankar V, Yadav BK, Bangdiwala SI (2015) Dowry demand and harassment: prevalence and risk factors in India. J Biosoc Sci 47(6):727–745

Kanwal S (2021) Total number of reported dowry death cases in India from 2005 to 2020. https://www.statista.com/statistics/632553/reported-dowry-death-cases-india/. Accessed 31 May 2022

Khalid MA, Venkatesulu B, Prasad KJ (2017) Socio-etiological aspects of dowry deaths: an autopsy based study. Ind J Foren Med Toxicol 11(1):84

Kumar V (2003) Burnt wives—a study of suicides. Burns 29(1):31–35

Manchandia P (2005) Practical steps towards eliminating dowry and bride-burning in India. Tulane J Int Compar Law 13:305

Mohanty S, Sen M, Sahu G (2013) Analysis of risk factors of dowry death–a south Indian study. J Forensic Legal Med 20(4):316–320

Nongrum R, Thomas E, Lionel J, Jacob KS (2014) Domestic violence as a risk factor for maternal depression and neonatal outcomes: a hospital-based cohort study. Indian J Psychol Med 36(2):179–181

O'Connor M, Ibrahim S (2018) Suicidality and family violence in Australian immigrant women presenting to out-patient mental health settings. Austr Psychiatry 26(2):224–225

O'Connor M, Lee A (2022) The health impacts of dowry abuse on South Asian communities in Australia. Med J Aust 216:11

Pallikadavath S, Bradley T (2019) Dowry, 'dowry autonomy' and domestic violence among young married women in India. J Biosoc Sci 51(3):353–373

Pandey GK, Dutt D, Banerjee B (2009) Partner and relationship factors in domestic violence: perspectives of women from a slum in Calcutta, India. J Interpers Viol 24(7):1175–1191

Ramakrishnan V (2013) A broken promise: dowry violence in India. Pulitzer Center, Washington, DC. Crisis reporting

Rehman V (2018) Revisiting the fairness paradigm in India: synthesis of literature and application of the self-concept theory. Soc Bus Rev

Reshma MA, Ramegowda A (2013) Dowry – The Cancer of Society, Journal of Humanities And Social Science 17(4):35–45

Rocca CH, Rathod S, Falle T, Pande RP, Krishnan S (2009) Challenging assumptions about women's empowerment: social and economic resources and domestic violence among young married women in urban South India. Int J Epidemiol 38(2):577–585

Rudd J (2001) Dowry-murder: an example of violence against women. Women's Stud Int Forum 24(5):513–522

Sandikci O, Ilhan E (2004) Dowry: a cherished possession or an old-fashioned tradition in a modernizing society? Contemp Consump Rit Res Anthol 20:149–178

Shaheed F (1994) Controlled or autonomous: identity and the experience of the network, women living under Muslim laws. Signs J Women Cult Soc 19(4):997–1019

Shrivastava PS, Shrivastava SR (2013) A study of spousal domestic violence in an urban slum of Mumbai. Int J Prev Med 4(1):27

Srivastava S, Kumar P, Govindu M, Muhammad T Dowry demand and other risk factors for intimate partner violence against adolescent girls: a cross-sectional study in India. 2021. https://www.researchsquare.com/article/rs-139794/v1

Suran L, Amin S, Huq L, Chowdury K (2004) Does dowry improve life for brides? A test of the bequest theory of dowry in rural Bangladesh. Population Council, New York, NY

Tichy LL, Becker JV, Sisco MM (2009) The downside of patriarchal benevolence: ambivalence in addressing domestic violence and socio-economic considerations for women of Tamil Nadu, India. J Fam Violence 4(8):547–558

Women UN (2009) Good practices in legislation on "harmful practices" against women. UN, New York, NY

Tazeen Saeed Ali, PhD and Post Doctorate, is a Professor in the School of Nursing and Midwifery and in the Department of Community Health Sciences, Aga Khan University. Her research and expertise are in conducting research in the area of gender-based violence, inequalities in health, sexual and reproductive health, and in academia in teaching healthcare professionals to screen and manage the clients around the same area.

Zohra Jetha, MSCN and senior instructor at the School of Nursing and Midwifery, Aga Khan University. Her research interests include breast oncology screening and rehabilitation and in academia.

Shaugfta Perveen is a PhD student at the Aga Khan university School of Nursing and Midwifery. Her research examines the nutritional status of the school-going early adolescents in both genders at school level in Pakistan and also to see the efficacy of school-based nutrition education strategies as well.

Parveen Ali PhD Professor of Gender Based Violence and Professor of Nursing in the Health Sciences School, the University of Sheffield and Doncaster and Bassetlaw Teaching Hospitals. Her research examines gender-based violence, inequalities in health related to gender and ethnicity, and nursing as a profession.

Michaela M. Rogers PhD is a Senior Lecturer in Social Work in the Department of Sociological Studies at the University of Sheffield. Her research examines interpersonal violence with a focus on marginalised groups, impacts, help-seeking, service access and service responses.

Female Genital Mutilation

Peggy Mulongo, Andrew Rowland, and Sue McAndrew

Learning Objectives

Having read this chapter, you should be able to understand the following:

- The historical and cultural contexts in which FGM
- The different types of female genital mutilation (FGM) and its effects
- The legislation surrounding the protection of women and girls from FGM in England and Wales, as an example of protective legislation
- Implications for practice, policy and research regarding FGM

P. Mulongo (✉)
Mental Health Nursing & Practice, University of Central Lancashire (UCLan), Preston, Lancashire, UK

Equality, Diversity and Inclusion, School of Nursing, University of Central Lancashire (UCLan), Preston, Lancashire, UK

School of Nursing, Faculty of Health & Wellbeing, University of Central Lancashire (UCLan), Preston, Lancashire, UK
e-mail: PMulongo@uclan.ac.uk

A. Rowland
Manchester, England, UK

Children's Rights, Law, and Advocacy, University of Salford, Salford, UK

M'Lop Tapang, Sihanoukville, Cambodia

SicKids Charity, London, UK
e-mail: A.Rowland@salford.ac.uk

S. McAndrew
Mental Health and Young People at the University of Salford, Salford, England, UK
e-mail: s.mcandrew@salford.ac.uk

P. Ali, M. M. Rogers (eds.), *Gender-Based Violence: A Comprehensive Guide*,
https://doi.org/10.1007/978-3-031-05640-6_20

Introduction

Female genital mutilation (FGM) is a global issue (BBC 2019), with estimates suggesting over 200 million females are affected by it (Wood et al. 2021). While it could be considered a mainly sub-Saharan problem, trends in migration have played a major role in transferring cultural and traditional beliefs attached to the practice to Western society (Mathews 2011). For those originating from practicing countries, such cultural and traditional beliefs are strongly rooted, and moving to live in the West has not simply change their beliefs and cultural practices, but rather FGM has become a reality in Europe, Northern America and Australia (Mathews 2011). For this reason, gaining knowledge about and understanding FGM is important for all those involved in health and social care.

Definition, Common Terminology and Types of FGM

FGM refers to procedures involving partial or total removal of the external female genitalia or other injury to female genital organs for nonmedical reasons (World Health Organization (WHO) 2020). 'Female genital cutting', 'female circumcision' and 'female genital mutilation/cutting' are all common terms used synonymously with FGM. Within this chapter, all the above terms will be referred to as FGM.

FGM has four classifications:

- *Type 1—Clitoridectomy*: referring to partial or total removal of the clitoris
- *Type 2—Excision*: referring to partial or total removal of the clitoris and the labia minora, with or without excision of the labia majora
- *Type 3—Infibulation*: requiring the narrowing of the vaginal opening through the construction of a covering seal
- *Type 4*: involves all other harmful procedures to the female genitalia for non-medical purposes, for example pricking, piercing, incision or scraping and cauterization (WHO 2018)

As FGM is culturally bound and often deemed a rite of passage to womanhood in countries where it is practised (WHO 2018), the procedure is often named by the more neutral expression of female genital surgery (FGS) (Hastings Center Report 2012). However, the term 'surgery' is misleading as an assortment of 'instruments' are used to perform the procedure, including knives, glass, razor blades and scissors (Mulongo et al. 2014a).

The Global Prevalence of FGM

The total number of women worldwide who have undergone FGM is unknown; however, it is estimated that 200 million women and girls around the world have had FGM performed (Wood et al. 2021). While over the last three decades, there has been an overall decline in the prevalence of the practice, not all countries have made progress in eradicating FGM, and the pace of decline has been uneven (United Nations Children's Fund (UNICEF) 2016).

Although FGM is declining in many of the countries where it is prevalent, most of these are also experiencing a high rate of population growth, meaning that the number of girls who have had FGM performed will continue to grow if the practice continues at current levels (United Nations Population Fund (UNFPA) 2020). For example, most girls and women in Guinea (76%), Mali (73%), Sierra Leone (69%), Somalia (65%) and Egypt (54%) still support the tradition of FGM (Llamas 2017). It is estimated that 68 million girls are at risk of having FGM performed by 2030 (UNFPA 2020), unless efforts to end the practice are intensified. Furthermore, due to the COVID-19 pandemic, UNFPA estimates there may be a further two million cases of FGM by 2030 that would have otherwise been prevented. Whereas the higher prevalence of FGM is recorded in the African continent, it is reported to be present in 92 countries worldwide (UNICEF 2016), making this an undeniably global issue.

FGM is reported in some Asian countries, the Middle East, among some ethnic groups in Central and South America and in Eastern Europe (WHO 2016). Furthermore, international migration has increased the number of women and girls who have had FGM performed (UNFPA 2020), making it a reality in the UK, Europe, Scandinavia, Canada, Northern America, Australia and New Zealand (Jacobson et al. 2018), with significant variations in the type of FGM performed.

A study by the European Institute for Gender Equality (EIGE 2015) estimated that as many as 1600 girls in Ireland, 1300 girls in Portugal and 11,000 girls in Sweden may have had FGM performed in 2011. In the UK, estimates suggested that approximately 60,000 girls aged 0–14 were at risk of having FGM performed, 103,000 women aged 15–49 and 24,000 women aged 50 plus, all residing in England and Wales, live with the consequences of this 'hidden crime' (HM Government 2016). Between April 2015 and March 2020, the NHS Digital Report (2020) recorded, via the FGM Enhanced Dataset, 24,420 individual women and girls, having had a total of 52,050 attendances, were identified as having been subjected to FGM.

In the UK, there have been increased efforts to eradicate FGM since 2012. A surveillance report found low numbers of children presenting with FGM over a 2-year period (Hodes et al. 2020). In this epidemiological surveillance study, a low number of children having had FGM were identified in the UK, the numbers being consistent with other sources of data. Most children in the study had FGM performed prior to arrival in the UK. These results appear to be consistent with very little FGM happening in the UK, but do not exclude the possibility that it may be continuing as a hidden practice (Hodes et al. 2020). This is, therefore, a good time to discuss new approaches to help ensure its eradication within the UK and further afield (Rowland et al. 2021).

Sociocultural Contexts

While the origin of FGM is uncertain due to the absence of tangible evidence determining when and where this practice started, some researchers suggest it predates Christianity, Judaism and Islam, FGM being performed within these different faith communities (Ahmady 2015). The literature further suggests, from a review of mummies, that FGM was performed in ancient Egypt (Gharib 2019). A Greek papyrus dated 163 BC in the British museum refers to the operations performed on girls in Memphis at the age when they received dowries (Gharib 2019). Nile Nubians circumcised 9- and 10-year-old girls with either type 1 FGM or with type 3 FGM also known as Pharaonic circumcision (Colon and Colon 2001, cited in Gharib 2019). In ancient Rome, the practice was performed on women slaves, whose labia minora were sealed with metal rings to prevent procreation (Gharib 2019). Further evidence demonstrates the practice of FGM in Western cultures in the eighteenth century to regulate masturbation, lesbianism, clitoral enlargement, hysteria and other psychiatric conditions (Andro and Lesclingand 2016).

FGM encompasses several sociocultural factors thought to be crucial for a girl's 'best interest', in becoming a 'proper' woman, ready for marriage (HM Government 2016). A number of sociocultural factors impacting on the practice of FGM include improving fertility, enhancing sexual pleasure for men, suppressing female sexuality, better hygiene, preventing infidelity or to comply with the demands of religious institutions (WHO 2020; Kandala et al. 2019). However, there is no description of the practice in the Quran or the Bible (HM Government 2016). FGM is a patriarchal practice usually performed by older women but embedded in a system that sustains men's power (Sakeah et al. 2019). For the Masai of Tanzania, for example, a woman who has children can only be called 'mother' if she has had FGM performed (Mulongo et al. 2014b). For women and girls brought up in Western society, and possibly still at risk of FGM, the effects of acculturation may impact on their wellbeing given the mix of prevailing cultural norms (Ali et al. 2020). The stigma inherent in the above is likely to further compromise a woman's mental wellbeing, particularly those who are opposed to FGM, yet reside in communities where it is part of their culture.

The motivations for performing FGM vary according to the specific family or community. Some of the sociocultural factors within families and communities that are commonly cited in favour of FGM include: it is a social convention, with many fearing rejection if they refuse to perform it, to prepare a girl for adulthood and marriage and to ensure premarital virginity and fidelity due to the pain of sexual intercourse experienced by some who have had FGM. Some communities argue it has religious origins which is highly contested, but community leaders and medical personnel still contribute to upholding FGM (WHO 2020).

Legislation and Policy

Across the world, the migrant population is represented by vulnerable groups of refugee and asylum seeker families, many of them having experienced various forms of gender oppression. FGM is a serious breach of human rights of women and girls, requiring the granting of refugee status to female asylum seekers escaping this practice from their home country, under the United Nations High Commissioner for Refugees (UNHCR) (WHO 2018). The United Nation General Assembly's Human

Rights Committee (2012) placed FGM in a human rights framework, highlighting the need for a holistic approach including recognising the importance of empowering women, promotion and protection of sexual and reproductive health and breaking the cycle of discrimination and violence (Díaz 2012).

Article 3 of the European Convention on Human Rights (1984) defends the right to be free from torture and inhumane or degrading treatment. These protections are also expressed in the UK Human Rights Act (HRA) 1998. However, evidence in the UK for successful asylum applications on the basis of FGM remains scarce. The UK has been criticised for rejecting women seeking asylum based on FGM, due to an unfounded belief that it could open the 'floodgates' and lead to unmanageable numbers of female asylum seekers arriving at the UK borders (Burrage 2014). Paradoxically this appears to jeopardise the human rights of women and encourages women's health inequality.

FGM Law in England and Wales

It is estimated that at least 59 countries around the world have introduced anti-FGM legislation. A review of such extensive legislation is beyond the scope of this chapter, and therefore FGM law in England and Wales will be used as one example. All forms of FGM have been prohibited in England and Wales since 1985, first by the Prohibition of Female Circumcision Act (1985) and latterly by the Female Genital Mutilation Act (2003). An FGM mandatory reporting duty now applies to teachers and health and social care professionals.

The FGM Act (2003) makes it an offence for UK national or permanent residents to carry out FGM, or to aid, abet, counsel or procure the carrying out of FGM abroad, even in countries where the practice may be legal (Cook 2016). Preventative measures, including the introduction of FGM Protection Orders (FGMPOs) aimed at protecting those at risk of FGM, were introduced by the Serious Crime Act (2015).

FGMPOs

An FGMPO can be made to protect either a girl or woman at risk of FGM without immediate criminal sanctions for parents (Re 2015). The terms of such an order can be broad and flexible, enabling the court to include whatever terms it considers necessary and appropriate to protect the girl. For example, provisions requiring a person to surrender his or her passport. Breach of the order is a criminal offence (Home et al. 2020).

An application for a FGMPO can be made by the girl who is to be protected by the order, or a relevant third party such as a Local Authority, or any other person with permission of the Court (Female Genital Mutilation Act 2003). Once granted, FGMPOs can be extended, added to or revoked. The court has set out what were referred to as *contextual considerations* as relevant factors to consider in making an FGMPO (Suffolk CC v RD and others 2020; Home et al. 2020) (Table 1).

Table 1 Factors for the Court to consider when considering an FGMPO application

Macro factors	Micro factors
The prevalence to FGM in the country and, if known, the relevant region, to which it is proposed to take the child	Any history of FGM within the family
The societal expectations of FGM in that country	The attitudes of the wider family towards FGM
Is FGM illegal in that country and, if so, how effective is the prohibition?	The safeguards that the family can put in place to protect the person from FGM
Is there an extradition treaty if FGM were to be carried out on a child taken abroad to allow a prosecution in the UK?	Whether, and if so how and to what extent, the family have cooperated

Duty to Notify the Police of FGM

In addition to voluntary reporting child abuse and neglect in accordance with professional codes of conduct required by regulators of healthcare professionals, the FGM Act (2003) places a duty on persons who work in a regulated profession in England and Wales (health and social care workers and teachers), to notify the police when, in the course of their work, they discover that an act of FGM appears to have been carried out on a girl who is under 18 years of age (Home et al. 2020). An example of such a code of conduct includes ‘Good Medical Practice’ (GMC 2013).

Child protection procedures would also be engaged should a regulated professional (such as a social worker) believe that a child has suffered from, or is at risk of, FGM (because FGM involves physical harm). Therefore, in addition to making a report to the police where a regulated professional discovers an act of FGM appears to have been carried out on a girl who is under 18 years of age, local child protection procedures should be followed for both suspected cases of FGM and for those children at risk of FGM (Home et al. 2020).

Alongside the legal duty of regulated healthcare professionals, social care professionals and teachers in England and Wales to report cases of FGM to the police, there is existing professional guidance on their obligations to protect people who are vulnerable or at risk from harm, abuse or neglect (Home et al. 2020). Health professionals should be aware that it has been suggested that patients do not always know the law on FGM, even after a clinical consultation (Larsson et al. 2018). However, concern has also been raised about a lack of awareness and training within the health and social care profession on the issue of FGM (B and G (Children) (No 2) 2015).

The Impact of FGM on Physical and Emotional Wellbeing

Overall, there is no doubt that women suffer significant physical, psychological, obstetric and sexual health issues as a result of FGM (Pastor-Bravo et al. 2018).

Physical Health

The use of unsterile instruments during FGM can cause infections after the procedure, particularly due to the wound's close proximity to urine and faeces. Long-term health complications can arise from any type of FGM (WHO 2001). Types 1, 2 and 3 can account for mild to serious physical health consequences, such as keloid scarring, chronic pain, dysuria, infection, pelvic inflammatory disease, haemorrhage, infertility, birth complications and sexual dysfunction (Young et al. 2020; Reisel and Creighton 2014). In contrast, others (Abdel-Azim 2013; Esho 2010) espouse many positive outcomes for women who have experienced FGM, which include enhanced sexual desire, arousal, orgasm, satisfaction and more frequent sexual activity. Nonetheless, the physical consequences associated with FGM often impact on a woman's sexual health and as such can compromise her enjoyment of the relationship.

It is often at the onset of pregnancy and/or during childbirth that the effects of FGM become heightened, with midwives often being the first healthcare professional to recognise that the woman has subjected to it. Although midwives do not have long-term involvement with their clients, offering support and empathy for complications of FGM at an early stage may prompt women to seek out further help (Costello 2015).

Emotional Health

In the last decade, several studies acknowledge that FGM is associated with mental health problems, citing mainly post-traumatic stress disorder (PTSD), anxiety and depression (Smith and Stein 2017). Furthermore, the importance of addressing, assessing and managing mental health issues experienced by those affected by FGM has been constantly recommended (WHO 2018). Factors thought to impact on the severity of the distress include severe forms of FGM, immediate post-FGM complications, chronic health problems and/or loss of fertility secondary to FGM, nonconsensual circumcision in adolescence or adulthood and FGM as being used as punishment (Mulongo et al. 2014b). In the UK, young women receiving counselling for FGM have reported feelings of betrayal by parents, incompleteness, regret and anger (Mulongo et al. 2014b). The literature (Bendiksen et al. 2021; Abdalla and Galea 2019) indicates a high probability of women and girls who have had FGM performed, being at greater risk of psychiatric diagnosis. While there are only a relatively small number of empirical research studies on the psychological consequences of FGM, what is evident is that the mental health of women who have undergone, or who are at risk of FGM, will be compromised (Abdalla and Galea 2019; Knipscheer et al. 2015; Mulongo et al. 2014b). Common mental health problems, such as affective disorder, anxiety and somatization, are evident for women who have undergone FGM and have implications for health and social care professionals working with them. In addition, it would appear that women exposed to FGM are more likely to report symptoms commensurate with post-traumatic stress (PTS), and in particular recurrent flashbacks, the latter being more common among women exposed to more severe forms of FGM (Knipscheer et al. 2015).

Impacts, Coping and Resilience

The practice of FGM is culturally embedded, and consideration is now given to available evidence related to not being circumcised and its effect on wellbeing (Abdalla and Galea 2019). While FGM is condemned within Western society, the psychosocial implications of not having FGM performed could adversely impact on females living in practicing communities. Not undergoing FGM could lead to loss of cultural identity or anomie, resulting in mental distress, and the fear of becoming socially excluded from their community. Some studies report that women who have been subjected to FGM have minimal psychological morbidity, often feeling proud and believing they are a better person (Omigbodun et al. 2020; Mulongo et al. 2014b). Such beliefs may have a protective role against the emergence of psychological distress following FGM, as these women may develop resilience as a way of coping and minimising emotional distress. However, Behrendt and Moritz's (2005) study refutes the idea that cultural embedment may have a protective aspect against the development of PTS and other mental illnesses.

For migrant women and girls brought up in Western society, and possibly still at risk of FGM, the mix of prevailing cultural norms is likely to impact on their wellbeing. The stigma inherent in moving away from sociocultural norms is likely to compromise a woman's mental wellbeing, particularly those who are opposed to FGM, yet reside in communities where it is part of the cultural practice. The strong belief that a woman needs to have FGM performed to be seen as *good* and *acceptable* is often inherent within the culture and passed from one generation to another without question (Mulongo et al. 2014b).

This presents a challenge for those in Western society who consider FGM in the context of human rights and wellbeing and wish to eradicate this harmful practice. While Western society encourages the above approach, this simultaneously highlights the underlying issue of mental health implications surrounding the practice at different levels. Indeed, FGM campaigners may also be vulnerable and experience re-traumatisation of previous emotional struggles, while delivering the message. Equally, it is important to acknowledge the mental wellbeing of women who listen to the messages, as it could adversely impact on their mental health, given the perceived and accepted cultural belief attached to FGM.

To prevent mental distress and reinforce the need to address mental health problems related to FGM, utilising effective coping mechanisms will work towards a successful shift in mentality. Coping strategies are also important to consider when developing services for those exposed to FGM. Vloeberghs et al.'s (2011) study identified four categories of women (the adaptive, religious, disempowered and traumatised woman), providing insight regarding the different ways women coped in each category, in terms of whether or not they seek support.

Implications for Practice, Policy and Research

Health and Social Care Interventions

There is minimal research and/or evaluation of the effectiveness of interventions that have been developed to meet the emotional needs of those who have experienced FGM. Many women who have been exposed to FGM, and living away from their country of origin, will be from an asylum seeker or refugee background. Potentially these women and girls need appropriate therapeutic interventions to address their special needs. While the physical health consequences of FGM are well documented (WHO 2018; Reisel and Creighton 2014), knowledge regarding the impact it has on emotional wellbeing has been slow to develop, with an evident dearth of studies exploring therapeutic interventions that are culturally sensitive and could benefit those affected by the practice of FGM (Smith and Stein 2017; Mulongo et al. 2014a).

Therapeutic Interventions and Guidelines for Healthcare Professionals

Radical acceptance, and in the case of FGM cultural connections, needs to be considered and acknowledged during the healing process. This approach was initially proposed by Linehan (1993), in her bio-social theory and the interaction between these two factors. For example, Linehan's 'invalidating environment' theory could equate to the family's rejection of the uncircumcised woman, and her consequential fear of expressing emotions related to the FGM. Incorporating a bio-social approach may assist in acknowledging reasons for the practice of FGM and the contexts within which it occurs, as well as offering opportunity to validate and respect the woman's experience rather than dismissing it as a cultural issue. When developing therapeutic interventions for women exposed to FGM, account needs to be taken of the deep-rooted beliefs in the practice of FGM, as well as the cultural and social pressures women from practising communities are likely to experience.

A number of countries, such as the UK, Germany, Belgium and Sweden, have established guidelines on FGM for medical providers (WHO 2018), but little attention is paid to effective interventions addressing psychological needs associated with FGM. The WHO (2018) lately provided a comprehensive guideline focusing on FGM and mental health, where cognitive behavioural therapy (CBT) was recommended as intervention for women and girls subjected to FGM who are experiencing symptoms consistent with anxiety disorders, depression or PTSD. Smith and Stein (2017) discussed the importance of psychological interventions for girls and women before and after surgery related to health complications of FGM. Coho et al. (2019) recently developed guidelines for psychological therapists and counsellors working with survivors of FGM, opening doors for further investigations around effective delivery of therapeutic interventions to address FGM.

Sociocultural Factors

Holistic approaches taking account of sociocultural factors could contribute to a better understanding of the psychological traits of women exposed to FGM, whether they remain living in practicing countries or have migrated to Western countries. It is important for health and social care professionals to acquire appropriate knowledge and cultural competence to ensure the use of sensitive therapeutic approaches that address the needs of women and girls who have experienced FGM. Research around blended approaches using cultural and religious values with mental health/psychological therapies increased in the last decade (Koç and Kafa 2019), recognising the roles culture and spirituality play in a person's life, as well as their contributions in therapeutic healing processes (Abu-Raiya et al. 2015). To promote healing, cognisance needs to be taken of the emotional and physical consequences of FGM and the cultural issues surrounding it (Mulongo et al. 2014a). Many women and girls affected by FGM may have to deal with specific, complex health beliefs related to their culture and traditions, often requiring specialist knowledge. Cultural behaviours or attitudes relating to FGM would often have short- and long-term impacts on the mental health of women and girls who have had, or are at risk of having, FGM, hence the continuous necessity to address their complex mental health needs.

Public Health

Public Health Approaches to the Prevention and Identification of Women and Children Who Have Undergone FGM

Previous research has considered the need for an anti-FGM Commissioner (Rowland et al. 2021; Home et al. 2020). In doing so it was suggested that the role of an anti-FGM Commissioner would encompass increased oversight of data collection. In addition, the role would involve coordinated legal, health and educational approaches to the prevention and identification of FGM, avoiding the risk of each sector working in silos and thus coordinating approaches towards the eradication of FGM. Public health research priorities to address FGM have also been set out (Atkinson et al. 2019).

Mulongo and McAndrew (2020) supported the proposed introduction of an anti-FGM Commissioner, emphasising the need for standard coordination. They highlighted mainly challenges surrounding legal demands attached to medical examinations amongst other issues, which are sometimes in conflict with the Nursing and Midwifery Council's (NMC) requirements of protecting and caring for vulnerable people, and not always prioritising the client's emotional wellbeing (NMC 2018). For example, when producing an FGM expert medical/therapeutic report required by the Family Court of Justice, time constraints might be a negative factor when emotionally supporting the individual affected by FGM and her relatives, ahead of the medical examination. Such pressure may often lead to conflict between the different actors involved, each party considering their respective targeted outcomes as a priority (Mulongo and McAndrew 2020), while breaches of Human and Women's Rights may be overlooked, undermining their rights for equality in health.

While tradition and culture play a central role in the practice of FGM, it is never the less a breach of women's human rights that impacts on their mental and physical wellbeing. Globally, transcultural health and social care is an important facet of the twenty-first century, and while the sociocultural aspects of FGM bring complexity in addressing the needs of this group of women, healthcare and social care professionals are best placed to explore how service provision can be improved to better support the estimated 200 million girls and women worldwide who have undergone FGM.

Summary

- Preventing FGM involves professionals often confronted with different challenges when trying to address related physical, mental health, sociocultural and FGM legal issues affecting their clients/patients.
- Women and girls affected by FGM require support for their bio-psychosocial and environmental needs. However, evidence suggests there are limited intervention approaches that could contribute to enhancing their health and wellbeing.
- While global progress is occurring in advancing awareness on FGM, current prevalence demonstrates that the problem persists, and this may intensify over time if existing practice, policies and research are not sustained and developed further.
- FGM legislation has been introduced in many countries; however, it may be crucial to focus on a global public health approach to prevent FGM in the future.
- In the UK, there is strong evidence supporting the need to introduce FGM Commissioners to monitor and evaluate the progress of current legislation protecting women and girls from FGM in England and Wales. Such structure could also play an advocacy role for relevant stakeholders involved in developing strategies to eradicate FGM and promote good practice.

References

Abdalla SM, Galea S (2019) Is female genital mutilation/cutting associated with adverse mental health consequences? A systematic review of the evidence. BMJ Glob Health 4(4):e001553. https://gh.bmj.com/content/4/4/e001553. Accessed 2 Jun 2021

Abdel-Azim S (2013) Psychosocial and sexual aspects of female circumcision. Afr J Urol 19(3):141–142

Abu-Raiya H, Pargament KI, Krause N et al (2015) Robust links between religious/spiritual struggles, psychological distress, and well-being in a national sample of American adults. Am J Orthop 85(6):565

Ahmady KA (2015) Comprehensive research study on female genital mutilation/cutting (FGM/C) in Iran

Ali S, de Viggiani N, Abzhaparova A et al (2020) Exploring young people's interpretations of female genital mutilation in the UK using a community-based participatory research approach. BMC Public Health 20:1132. https://doi.org/10.1186/s12889-020-09183-6

Andro A, Lesclingand M (2016) Female genital mutilation. Overv Curr Knowl Popul 71(2):215–296

Atkinson HG, Ottenheimer D, Mishori R (2019) Public health research priorities to address female genital mutilation or cutting in the United States. Am J Public Health 109(11):1523–1527

B and G (Children) (No 2) (2015) EWFC https://www.bailii.org/cgibin/format.cgi?doc=/ew/cases/EWFC/HCJ/2015/3.html&query=(LJ13C00295). Accessed 2 Jun 2021

BBC (2019) What is FGM, where does it happen and why? https://www.bbc.co.uk/news/world-47131052. Accessed 5 Nov 2021

Behrendt A, Moritz S (2005) Post-traumatic stress disorder and memory problems after female genital mutilation. Am J Psychiatry 162:1000–1002

Bendiksen B, Heir T, Minteh MM et al (2021) The association between physical complications following female genital cutting and the mental health of 12-year-old Gambian girls: a community-based cross-sectional study. PLoS One 16(1):e024723

Burrage H (2014) The UK Home Office (says it) has no data on FGM asylum claims. http://hilary-burrage.com/2014/05/19/uk-home-office-has-no-data-on-fgm-asylum-claims/

Coho C, Parra SR, Hussein L et al (2019) Female genital trauma: guidelines for working therapeutically with survivors of female genital mutilation. Dahlia Project, London. www.dahliaproject.org/resources. Accessed 21 Jun 2021

Colon AR, Colon PA (2001) A history of children: a socio-cultural survey across millennia. Greenwood Press, Westport, CT

Cook K (2016) Female genital mutilation in the UK population: a serious crime. J Crim Law 80(2):88–96

Costello S (2015) Female genital mutilation/cutting: risk management and strategies for social workers and health care professionals. Risk Manag Healthc Pol 8:225–233

Council of Europe (1984) European convention on human rights. https://www.echr.coe.int/documents/convention_eng.pdf

Díaz JL (2012) Fight against Female Genital Mutilation wins UN backing. Amnesty International

Esho T (2010) Female genital cutting and sexual function: in search of an alternate theoretical model. Afr Ident 8(3):221–235

European Institute for Gender Equality (EIGE) (2015) Estimation of girls at risk of female genital mutilation in the European Union. EIGE, Vilnius. https://eige.europa.eu/news/estimating-number-girls-risk-female-genital-mutilation-eu. Accessed 10 May 2021

Female Genital Mutilation Act (2003) An Act to restate and amend the law relating to female genital mutilation and for connected purposes. https://www.legislation.gov.uk/ukpga/2003/31/contents. Accessed 31 Mar 2021

General Medical Council (22 April 2013 amended on 29 April 2019). Good medical practice. Manchester: General Medical Council. https://www.gmc-uk.org/-/media/documents/good-medical-practice%2D%2D-english-20200128_pdf-51527435.pdf. Accessed 15 Mar 2021

Gharib EL (2019) The challenge of female genital mutilation. Sci J Res Rev 1(3):2019

Hastings Center Report (2012) The public policy advisory network on female genital surgeries in Africa: seven things to know about female genital surgeries in Africa. Hastings Cent Rep 42(6):19–27

HM Government (1988) Human Rights Act. https://www.legislation.gov.uk/ukpga/1998/42/contents

HM Government (2016) Multi-agency statutory guidance on female genital mutilation. www.official-documents.gov.uk. Accessed 10 Mar 2021

HM Government (1985) Probition of Female Circumcision Act. https://www.legislation.gov.uk/ukpga/1985/38/contents

HM Government (2015) Serious Crime Act. https://www.legislation.gov.uk/ukpga/2015/9/contents/enacted

Hodes D, O'Donnell NA, Pall K et al (2020) Epidemiological surveillance study of female genital mutilation in the UK. Arch Dis Child 106:372. https://doi.org/10.1136/archdischild-2020-319569

Home J, Rowland AG, Gerry F et al (2020) A review of the law surrounding female genital mutilation protection orders. Br J Midwifery 28(7):418–429

Jacobson D, Glazer E, Mason R et al (2018) The lived experience of female genital cutting (FGC) in Somali-Canadian women's daily lives. PLoS One 13(11):e0206886. https://doi.org/10.1371/journal.pone.0206886

Kandala NB, Nnanatu CC, Atilola G et al (2019) A spatial analysis of the prevalence of female genital mutilation/cutting among 0-14-year-old girls in Kenya. Int J Environ Res Public Health 16(21):4155

Knipscheer J, Vloeberghs E, van der Kwaak A et al (2015) Mental health problems associated with female genital mutilation. BJPsych Bull 39(6):273–277

Koç V, Kafa G (2019) Cross-cultural research on psychotherapy: the need for a change. J Cross-Cult Psychol 50(1):100–115

Larsson M, Cohen P, Hann G et al (2018) An exploration of attitudes towards female genital mutilation (FGM) in men and women accessing FGM clinical services in London: a pilot study. J Obstet Gynaecol 38(7):1005–1009

Linehan MM (1993) Skills training manual for treating borderline personality disorder. Guilford Press, New York, NY

Llamas J. (2017) Female circumcision: the history, the current prevalence and the approach to a patient. https://med.virginia.edu/family-medicine/wp-content/uploads/sites/285/2017/01/Llamas-Paper.pdf. Accessed 21 Jun 2021

Mathews B (2011) Female genital mutilation: Australian law, policy and practical challenges for doctors. Med J Aust 194(3):139–141

Mulongo P, McAndrew S (2020) Female genital mutilation protection orders. Br J Midwifery 29(1):1. https://doi.org/10.12968/bjom.2021.29.1.48. Letter to the Editor

Mulongo P, Hollins-Martin C, McAndrew S (2014a) The Psychological impact of Female Genital Mutilation/Cutting (FGM/C) on girls/women's mental health: a narrative literature review. J Reprod Infant Psychol 32(5):469–485

Mulongo P, McAndrew S, Hollins-Martin C (2014b) Crossing borders: discussing the evidence relating to the mental health needs of women exposed to female genital mutilation. Int J Ment Health Nurs 23(4):296–305

NHS Digital (2020) Clinical Audit and Registries Management Service. Female Genital Mutilation (FGM) enhanced dataset: England, April 2019 to March 2020, experimental statistics. Annual report. Health and Social Care Information Centre, Leeds. https://files.digital.nhs.uk/0B/7A41CB/Female%20Genital%20Mutilation%20%28FGM%29%20-%20April%20 2019%20to%20March%202020%20-%20Report.pdf. Accessed 1 Mar 2021

Nursing & Midwifery Council (2018) The code: professional standards of practice and behaviour for nurses, midwives and nursing associates. NMC, London. http://www.nmc.org.uk/globalassets/sitedocuments/nmc-publications/revised-new-nmc-code.pdf. Accessed 10 May 2021

Omigbodun O, Bella-Awusah T, Groleau D et al (2020) Perceptions of the psychological experiences surrounding female genital mutilation/cutting (FGM/C) among the Izzi in Southeast Nigeria. Transcult Psychiatry 57(1):212–227

Pastor-Bravo MDM, Almansa-Martínez P, Jiménez-Ruiz I (2018) Living with mutilation: a qualitative study on the consequences of female genital mutilation in women's health and the healthcare system in Spain. Midwifery 66:119–126

Re E (Children) (Female Genital Mutilation Protection Orders) (2015) EWHC 2275 (Fam). https://www.bailii.org/cgi-bin/format.cgi?doc=/ew/cases/EWHC/Fam/2015/2275.html&query=(FD15FO7001). Accessed 2 Jun 2021

Reisel D, Creighton S (2014) Long term health consequences of Female Genital Mutilation (FGM). Maturitas 80(1):48–51

Rowland AG, Gerry F, Proudman C et al (2021) The time is right for the UK government to introduce an independent anti-FGM Commissioner. Br J Midwifery 29(1):50–51

Sakeah E, Debpuur C, Aborigo RA et al (2019) Persistent female genital mutilation despite its illegality: narratives from women and men in northern Ghana. PLoS One 14(4):e0214923

Smith H, Stein K (2017) Psychological and counselling interventions for female genital mutilation. Int J Gynecol Obstet 136:60–64

Suffolk CC v RD and others (2020) EWHC 323 (Fam) https://www.bailii.org/cgi-bin/format.cgi?doc=/ew/cases/EWHC/Fam/2020/323.html&query=(NR18F05001). Accessed 2 Jun 2021

United Nations (2012) General assembly strongly condemns widespread, systematic human rights violations in Syria, as it adopts 56 resolutions recommended by third committee. https://press.un.org/en/2012/ga11331.doc.htm

United Nations Children's Fund (2016) Female genital mutilation/cutting: a global concern. UNICEF, New York, NY

United Nations Population Fund (2020) Defying the practices that harm women and girls and undermine equality. State of World Population 2020. UNFPA, New York, NY

Vloeberghs E, Knipscheer J, van der Kwaak A et al (2011) Veiled pain. A study in the Netherlands on the psychological, social and relational consequences of female genital mutilation. Pharos-Dutch National Knowledge and Advisory Centre on Refugee and Migrant's Health, Utrecht

Wood R, Richens Y, Lavender T (2021) The experiences and psychological outcomes for pregnant women who have had FGM: a systematic review. Sex Reprod Healthc 29:100639. https://doi.org/10.1016/j.srhc.2021.100639

World Health Organization (2001) Female genital mutilation. WHO, Geneva. https://www.who.int/gender/other_health/Studentsmanual.pdf. Accessed 2 Jun 2021

World Health Organization (2016) WHO guidelines on the management of health complications from female genital mutilation. WHO, Geneva. http://www.who.int/reproductivehealth/topics/fgm/management-health-complications-fgm/en/. Accessed 15 Mar 2021

World Health Organization (2018) Care of girls and women living with female genital mutilation: a clinical handbook. WHO, Geneva. Accessed 21 Feb 2021

World Health Organization (2020) Female genital mutilation. Key facts. WHO, Geneva. https://www.who.int/news-room/fact-sheets/detail/female-genital-mutilation. Accessed 28 Mar 2021

Young J, Nour NM, Macauley RC, Narang SK et al (2020) Diagnosis, management, and treatment of female genital mutilation or cutting in girls. Section on global health, committee on medical liability and risk management, committee on bioethics. Paediatrics 146(2):e20201012. https://doi.org/10.1542/peds.2020-1012

Andrew Rowland, BMedSci (Hons), BMBS (Hons), PhD, SFFMLM, FAcadMEd, FRCEM, FRCPCH, FRSA, CF is a Consultant Paediatrician in Manchester, UK; Honorary Professor (Children's Rights, Law, and Advocacy) at the University of Salford, UK; a Fellow of the Churchill Fellowship; Non-Executive Director of M'Lop Tapang, Cambodia; and Chair of the Board of Trustees of SicKids charity (1164131). Professor Rowland's research particularly focuses on protecting and promoting the rights of children, humanitarian healthcare for children in difficult circumstances and safeguarding vulnerable people.

Sue McAndrew is Honorary Professor of Mental Health and Young People at the University of Salford. Sue's research explored gay men and suicidality, young carers and service users, childhood sexual abuse and its implications for adulthood, self-harm and suicide and therapeutic engagement.

Honour Crimes

Sadiq Bhanbhro

Learning Objectives
Having read this chapter, you should be able to understand the following:

- The definition and features of honour that underlies abuse, violence and killings
- The scale of honour crimes, including honour killings
- The characteristics of social and cultural structures that shape, justify and maintain violence and killings in the name of honour
- Possible solutions to prevent honour crimes

Introduction

This chapter introduces the notions of honour and honour crimes, including honour-based violence (also known as honour-based abuse; see Box 2) and honour killing. The notion of honour has been a central concept across cultures throughout history. At *prima facie*, honour has positive connotations and characteristics such as high respect, great esteem and prestige. However, it becomes contentious when honour is combined with violence, abuse or killings, creating a new category of violent crime mainly associated with certain cultures and communities. Therefore, I have adopted the term honour crimes in this chapter to avoid unnecessary cultural specifications.

S. Bhanbhro (✉)
Health Research Institute, Sheffield Hallam University, Sheffield, UK
e-mail: S.Bhanbhro@shu.ac.uk

P. Ali, M. M. Rogers (eds.), *Gender-Based Violence: A Comprehensive Guide*,
https://doi.org/10.1007/978-3-031-05640-6_21

Honour crime involves violence and abuse, including murder, committed by people who want to defend or restore the honour of an individual or a social group, which can be a family, clan, class, caste, community, kinship or tribe. This crime may affect men, boys, lesbians, gays, bisexuals and transgender people, but honour-based violence is more prevalent against women and girls. In some cases, both men and women are killed together in honour killings. However, when a woman is murdered in an honour killing, she is killed by her family. In contrast, male victims are killed by the family or relatives of the woman with whom he was accused of inflicting dishonour to the family, for example, by having a pre- or extramarital affair or eloping with the woman for marriage.

In this chapter, I describe the key concepts relating to notions of honour, honour crimes and honour killings. The chapter also provides a historical background of the phenomenon of honour crimes and the prevalence of honour-based violence and killings. I also introduce the sociocultural, political and economic structures that shape, justify and maintain honour crimes.

Definition of the Concepts

Honour, Dishonour and Shame

The notions of honour, dishonour and shame are universal. Still, their understanding, meaning, value and applications vary from culture to culture, region to region and class to class. Thus, there is not a single definition of these concepts. Nevertheless, the most widely used definition of the notion of honour in the literature is 'a person's value in his own and others' eyes'. This explanation of honour has three key aspects: (a) honour as sentiment means it is a matter of feelings; (b) manifestation of the feelings in conduct refers to tangible behaviours as the expression of the feelings; and (c) the appraisal of the conduct by others refers to the reception and evaluation of the conduct by others (Pitt-Rivers 1968, p. 503). The key roles of honour include maintaining and assessing the social position of an individual, family or a social group in the social structure that is subjected to damage through their social and moral behaviours, specifically, the sexual conduct of women and girls (Campbell 1964; Abou-Zeid 1965; Pitt-Rivers 1968).

The above conceptualisation shows honour as a personal attribute of an individual and a collective feature of the social group: family, lineage, clan, kinship, caste group and nation. A man's honour (and in the discussion of honour crimes, it is almost always a man) is reflected in the family, group or lineage to which he belongs. Honour provides or manifests social status since a person receives one's identity from affiliation to a social group. Thus, validation of claims of honour from the group members becomes important. Though honour is a personal quality, the value of a person in their own eyes ultimately depends upon recognition from the group members or people who matter to the person in the social group—the 'significant others' (Moxnes 1993, p. 168). This suggests honour operates within a close social group that can be an extended family, clan, community, caste or kinship group. In honour crimes, including honour killing, honour is considered 'a highly valued and fiercely protected currency in many social groups and communities across cultures that consider women and girls the objects of the currency' (Bhanbhro 2021). In the discussion of honour abuse, the English term 'honour' is widely used; however, there are local terms for honour in different cultures and regions.

Dishonour and shame are secondary concepts to honour and play a vital role in the implication of honour through violence. They are brought about by women's and girls' actions or alleged actions in a social group. By contrast, a male family member's same action or type of action is not viewed as a source of dishonour for the family, although it may be considered his personal dishonour.

In honour-related violence and killings, the sources of dishonour refer to a woman's sexuality, including body, behaviours, clothes, communication and virginity. These are mainly related to men exercising power and control over women and girls, restricting them from crossing three borders. These are sexual, bodily and social and are fundamental for preserving an individual or social group's honour (Bhanbhro 2021). Various behaviours and actions of women and girls are interpreted as sources of dishonour and shame for an individual man or a social group (see Box 1).

Box 1 Sexual, Bodily and Social Borders

Sexual	**Bodily**
• Premarital sex	• Wearing revealing/tight clothes
• Extramarital sex	• No proper purdah
• A woman or girl being raped	• Adopting a Western lifestyle by migrant women and girls living in the Western countries
• Getting pregnant from the sexual relationship	
• Having a boyfriend	
Social	**Social predominantly related to marriage**
• Asking for a share in the inheritance	• Marriage
• Disobedience to parents and/or family men	– Without consent of family
• Working outside of the home	– Outside one's social group (concerned norm circles)
• Moving away from their family house before marriage	– By eloping with a man of her own or another social group
• Going out without the permission of parents or other male members of a family	– With a man from a lower caste
• Talking to an unrelated man	– With a non-Muslim man
• Using a mobile phone	• Asking for a divorce
• Using social media	• Saying no to cousin marriage
	• Complaint to relevant authorities against parents who tried to arrange a forced marriage

The notions of honour, dishonour and shame have different meanings and functions but do not operate separately. The concepts are interconnected and underpin an organised set of social structures called the honour system. The system is informal and customary, but it gets support from state and government institutions such as the police, judiciary and district administration. For instance, in many countries, courts give lenient punishment to perpetrators of honour killings. Also, in some countries, honour killing disputes are settled through the village, tribal or elderly councils. These councils not only condone honour crimes and honour killings but provide infrastructure to the honour system to manifest its power through violence and killings. So, violence against a female relative by a man in the name of family honour is not an individual act; it is a collective social practice that comes from the honour system. Above all, this system considers women as the property of the males in their family, irrespective of their class, ethnicity or religious identity. The owner of the property has the right to decide its fate. The concept of ownership has turned women into a commodity that can be exchanged, bought, sold (Khan 2006) and killed when a woman or girl loses her honour. And the system is deep-rooted to the extent that, in many cases, even family women take part in other women's honour killings, sometimes as instigators, collaborators or abettors (Bates 2018).

Honour Crimes and Honour Killing

Honour crimes is an umbrella term which includes a range of harmful practices shaped by notions of honour, such as domestic abuse; death threats; sexual and psychological abuse; economic abuse and acid attacks; forced marriage; forced suicide; forced abortion; female genital mutilation; assault; blackmail and being held against one's will (see Box 2) (Hester et al. 2015; Nesheiwat 2005). An incidence of honour crime is explained in Fig. 1.

In most cases, killing or the attempted killing of a woman, or a girl to save or restore the honour of an individual man or a social group (commonly known as honour killing) is an extreme form of honour crime.

> in order to save or restore honour, the perpetrators (predominantly male family members) killed a woman or a girl perceived as having brought or tried to bring dishonour or shame (as a result of any action or behaviour described in Box 1) for the social group. (Bhanbhro 2021)

The most widely used definition of honour killing in the literature is the murder of a woman or girl by male family members who have been accused of having engaged in 'sexually immoral' actions such as having premarital or extramarital sex—consequently, becoming a source of dishonour and shame for the family. However, I argue that this definition is narrow because women and girls can be killed for various reasons (e.g. even when they are victims of rape) that are believed to be a source of dishonour and shame for the social group, which can be a family, lineage, caste, clan or tribe. Hence, the above definition of honour killing encompasses the murders of women and girls that occur for many reasons and involve perpetrators outside a family.

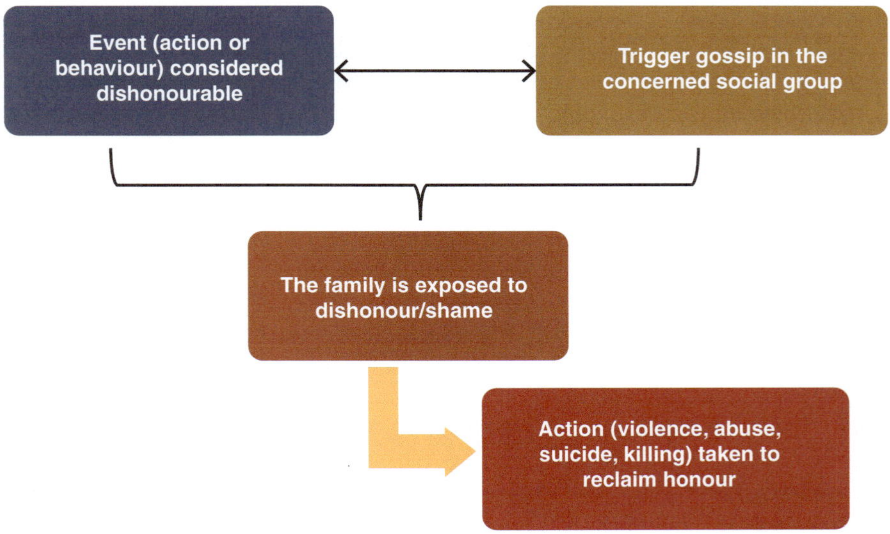

Fig. 1 A model to show how honour is implicated through violence and killings

Box 2 Definition and Terminology of Honour Crimes

Definition

Honour crime involves violence and abuse, including murder, committed by people who want to defend or restore the honour of an individual or a social group, such as a family, clan, class, caste, community, kinship or tribe.

Alternative Terminology

Honour crimes, honour-based violence, honour-based abuse, honour-related violence, patriarchal violence, honour killing, murder in the name of honour.

The Historical Context

Throughout history, women have been held responsible for upholding the honour of their families—often with deadly consequences. Similarly, violence, abuse and murders of women and girls in defending one's family honour have a long history. However, after condemnation from the United Nations in a resolution in 2000, honour crimes in general and honour killings, in particular, have received considerable academic and public attention from the media, human rights organisations, public health professionals, politicians and wider society. It was the first time the UN officially acknowledged crimes against women and girls in the name of honour and included them in the previous resolution 'elimination of all forms of violence against women, including crimes identified in the outcome document of Beijing Plus Five'.

Goldstein (2002), in his historical accounts of honour crimes and honour killings in the Roman Empire, explains that the concept of honour was the desire of men to ensure the children their wives bore were their own. By placing the responsibility for this 'honour' on the shoulders of women, those women could be more easily controlled, and, therefore, men could be more certain of their children's offspring. Fathers were in control of the life and death of their daughters. Once a woman married, her father's authority over her was transferred to her husband. Also, honour was attributed as an underlying reason for horrible violent practices, including duelling in England, foot binding in China, wife immolation in India and the honour-based system of retribution in the Southern States of the USA.

It is important to acknowledge that despite the universality of the notion of honour and its enforcement through violence when it comes to honour crimes and honour killings in Western countries, it has been associated with Muslims, Asians, South Asians, immigrants and Black and ethnic minorities.

Explanatory Theories

Whilst progress has been made towards understanding the nature, causes and extent of violence against women and girls, little is known about honour-related violence and killings beyond its two popular explanations. First, it is condoned by a specific culture type known as 'honour culture'. This authorises its members, mainly males, to resort to violence and murders to save family honour (Lowe et al. 2018; Khan et al. 2018; Kurkiala 2003). The second dominant explanation suggests that violence against women and girls is committed by men using any available excuse; honour is merely one such excuse that serves as a reason where the real cause is down to the socioeconomic and political structures of society that are essentially patriarchal in nature and universally oppressive for women (Begikhani 2005; Pimentel et al. 2005; Sev'er and Yurdakul 2001).

Both explanations are likely to have some truth within them. However, neither is supported by sufficient empirical data. In addition, the first explanation, probably the most prevalent, is reactionary. It appears to close the door to the potential for change; culture is treated as essential and beyond criticism. In the 'cultural explanation' of honour crimes, the culture, traditions and religion of particular communities are taken as causes of violent crime for the sake of honour.

Conversely, some scholars have criticised the cultural explanation. For example, Montoya and Agustín (2013) argue that the 'culturalised forms of violence' largely ignore the gendered nature of violence, and the cultural framing of violence creates a dichotomy between non-violent Europeans and violent others. Similarly, Meetoo and Mirza (2007) argue that in 'domestic violence' discourses, including honour killings, the victim women have been highly 'ethnicised'. In turn, the cultural/racial classification not only stigmatises particular acts of violence but entire communities (Montoya and Agustín 2013; Abu-Lughod 2011; Bhanbhro et al. 2016).

Thus, when honour-related violence is dismissed as a cultural issue, the communities in which it prevails are stigmatised, and those who suffer violence also face their suffering being brushed off as a cultural problem (Montoya and Agustín 2013; Ewing 2008). In addition, some scholars argue that cultural understating and representation of violence conceals more pressing and central structures of violence affecting women and political processes that shape it, in those parts of the world where culture is usually blamed for such violence. It is necessary to be mindful of this when analysing and understanding violence in cultural terms per se (Abu-Lughod 2011; Ewing 2008; Shah 2007).

Prevalence

Honour-based violence and killings occur worldwide in various cultures, some regions being hotspots, such as South Asia and the Middle East. The United Nations has identified honour crimes, including honour killings, that occur in more than 30 countries (see Box 3). There are no reliable statistics on the prevalence of violence and killings for the honour. In 2000, the UN Population Fund estimated that at least 5000 women and girls worldwide are murdered yearly in the name of the so-called honour—although these figures are contested. Some researchers and activists believe that the rates are much higher. For example, the annual reports published by the Human Rights Commission of Pakistan (HRCP) show that over 15,222 honour killings have been recorded in the country between 2004 and 2016. This figure excludes attempted honour killings and other forms of honour-related violence. This means an average of 1170 honour killings annually and 22 per week (HRCP 2019). More recent statistics show that the problem persists. In 2021, 128 women were killed in Sindh province in the name of honour (Soomro 2022), and in Punjab province, between July and December 2021, 90 women were killed, 2439 were raped, and 9529 women were kidnapped for honour (The News 2022).

Similarly, more than 11,000 honour-related violence incidents, including 29 honour killings and attempted killings of women, were recorded by the UK police forces from 2010 to 2014 (Talwar and Ahmad 2015). More recent figures show that the number of honour-based abuse offences recorded by police forces in England has soared over the past 5 years. The data collected through freedom of requests suggests that honour abuse, including rape, death threats and assault, have increased from 884 in 2016 to 1599 in 2021 (Siddique 2021). Overall, no national data exist on the scale of honour crimes in any country because it is not a recorded crime category. Consequently, the actual numbers of the crime are inaccurate.

The stories and reports related to honour crimes, particularly honour killings from the Middle East and South Asia or immigrant communities living in Europe and North America, are almost always linked with Islam (Abu-Lughod 2011). In contrast, in their analysis of various Western legal systems, Giordano (2016) and Fournier et al. (2012) argue that honour and its related practices have origin in

Western legal systems and are not associated with any particular religion. Additionally, the analysis of the newspaper coverage and policy documents on honour-related violence and killings in the Netherlands, Germany, Sweden and the UK found that the issue of honour-related violence in general and honour killings, in particular, is routinely associated with Islam and represented in the media as being ingrained in the values of Islam (Hong 2014; Korteweg and Yurdakul 2010). By contrast, it should be noted that honour crimes and honour killings are also reported among Hindus, Sikhs (see Box 4, Case Study 1) and Christians (Gill 2008; Shafak 2012).

Box 3 Countries Where Honour Crimes Are Reported

Afghanistan, Albania, Australia, Bangladesh, Brazil, Canada, Chechnya, Egypt, Greece, Germany, India, Iran, Iraq, Israel, Italy, Jordan, Lebanon, Netherland, Mexico, Morocco, Norway, Palestine, Sweden, Syria, Turkey, Uganda, United Arab Emirates, United Kingdom, the USA, Yemen.

Box 4 Case Study 1: Forced Marriage Leading to Honour Killing

Surjit Kaur Athwal, 27, a British Indian woman, was killed in December 1998. At 16, she was forced to marry a man 10 years older than her. She barely knew the man she had married as she had only met him once before the wedding. Surjit tried, by all means, to adjust as a new family member but struggled with some of the rules. She described them as harsh and unreasonable compared to where she came from. Reportedly domestic and emotional abuse was involved. She voiced her desire to end the abusive marriage. Surjit was forced to rebel with no other choice in changing things. This didn't go well with her husband, who felt she was forcefully challenging his authority as the man of the house—a taboo in their Sikh tradition—and her mother-in-law was also outraged by her actions. So, Surjit's husband and mother-in-law conspired to murder her to save family honour by duping her when she was attending a wedding with her mother-in-law in India, where she disappeared.

In 2007, the victim's sister Sarbjit was the first person in the history of British honour crimes to stand and testify against her own family. Eventually, the mother and son were found guilty. The victim's mother-in-law was given a minimum life sentence of 20 years, and her husband was sentenced to life.

This case study demonstrated how a crime shaped by the notion of honour starts with abuse and ends with it. Surjit's ordeal started with forced and early marriage; she survived domestic and emotional abuse, and she was killed for the sake of the so-called family honour. This case also shows the involvement of family women in the honour killing of another woman.

Impact

Violence against women and girls committed in the name of honour is a form of gender-based violence. It can negatively affect women and girls' emotional and mental wellbeing if they are directly victimised or witnessed it. As they may live in constant fear for their safety within households, it can impact their day-to-day life, for example, their ability to access social and healthcare services. The Her Majesty's Inspectorate of Constabulary (HMIC) inspection study (2015) in the UK found that 2 of the 36 victims and survivors of honour-based violence, including forced marriage, had attempted self-harm, including suicide, and 11 reported taking medication for anxiety or depression (Hester et al. 2015). Similarly, the negative impact of honour-based abuse, including anxiety, depression, desperation, hopelessness, mental abuse, reduced self-esteem and suicide, was highlighted in research studies (Sedem and Ferrer-Wreder 2015; Dickson 2014; Sabbe et al. 2013).

Implications for Policy, Practice and Research

Common approaches have been suggested to address violence against women and girls in the name of honour and otherwise: introducing strict laws, training police, cultural competency building of prosecutors, more shelter homes for victims, etc. For example, despite Pakistan's landmarking Anti-Honour Killings Laws (Criminal Laws Amendment) Bill 2016, honour-related violence and honour killings continue in the country. This legislation on honour killings includes strict punishment for the perpetrators, making it more challenging than ordinary murder cases. It was passed after the honour killing of Pakistan's social media celebrity Qandeel Baloch (see Box 5, Case Study 2). Despite this law, Qandeel's brother, who killed her, was set free by the court.

Introducing tougher laws and other efforts are necessary but not sufficient to stop honour crimes, including honour killings. Therefore, there is a need to bring the change from within to alter the social structures and narratives that create a viable environment and enable men to harm or kill women and girls for honour.

Public and policy discourses on honour killings often arise from journalism and demotic discourse rather than empirical research, scholarship and theory. Moreover, the perspectives of communities where honour killings are prevalent have been afforded less attention. Therefore, further empirical research is needed to investigate and understand underlying narratives and assumptions behind honour-related violence.

There is a need to keep an official record of honour crimes, including honour killings, both nationally and globally. In Western countries, cultural and religious sensitivity attached to honour crimes may be reduced by focusing on specific social groups with specific social forces that support honour crime instead of certain cultures and communities. This could be achieved by encouraging conscious efforts, including the following:

- By engaging targeted social groups to bring change from within
- Ensuring a change in attitudes, perceptions and behaviours of community members, particularly young people, about the notions of honour
- Bringing a clear understanding of young people concerning family honour, and their communication skills are developed to discuss these sensitive issues in a family

Box 5 Case Study 2: Flawed Trials Concerning Honour Killing

Fouzia Azeem, famous by her stage name Qandeel Baloch, was a model, actress, activist and Pakistan's first social media celebrity. Qandeel rose to prominence due to her videos on social networks covering her daily routine, her rights as a Pakistani woman, and various controversial issues. Qandeel Baloch was murdered by her brother, Waseem Khan, in July 2016, for the sake of family honour. Baloch was drugged and strangled to death at her family home in Multan.

Her younger brother Waseem Khan publicly confessed to the murder, citing the videos and photographs she had posted on social media to bring dishonour to their family. She was subsequently sentenced to life imprisonment. After Qandeel's honour killing, a landmark piece of legislation passed the 2016 Criminal Law (Amendment) (Offences in the name or pretext of Honour) Act. This amendment mandates life imprisonment for those who kill women in the name of 'honour'. It states that even if the victim's parents pardon the killer, the murderer has to go to prison for 12 years. As Khan's case demonstrates, however, some loopholes can be exploited. Waseem's lawyers used what is known as the Qisas and Diyat law to circumvent the new legislation. This legal mechanism allows victims' families to voluntarily pardon or accept financial compensation from the perpetrators, which translates into a judicial acquittal.

In February 2022, 3 years after Waseem Khan was convicted, the high court of Pakistan ordered his acquittal. This shocked the activists and public figures who had campaigned for justice for Baloch and marked a significant step backwards in working to end violence against women and girls, including murders, in the name of honour. The new 2016 law appears to have had little effect: ineffective implementation of that legislation and the resulting flawed trials have created a culture of impunity for honour killings of women and girls.

Summary

- The notion of honour and its corollary concepts are universal, but their meaning, value and applications vary from culture to culture, region to region and class to class.
- Not a single community, culture or class has the monopoly on defending one's honour through violence. It has been a historical and cross-cultural phenomenon.
- Honour crimes, including honour-based violence and killings, occur worldwide. Some regions are hotspots, such as South Asia and the Middle East and migrant groups living in Europe and the USA.
- Further empirical research is required to investigate and understand the sociocultural, political and economic structures that shape, justify and maintain honour crimes.

References

Abou-Zeid A (1965) Honour and shame among the Bedouins of Egypt. In: Peristiany JG (ed) Honour and shame: the values of Mediterranean society. Weidenfeld and Nicolson, London

Abu-Lughod L (2011) Seductions of the "honour crime". Differences 22(1):17–63

Bates L (2018) Females perpetrating honour-based abuse: controllers, collaborators or coerced? J Aggress Confl Peace Res 10(4):293–303. https://doi.org/10.1108/JACPR-01-2018-0341

Begikhani N (2005) Honour-based violence among the Kurds: the case of Iraqi Kurdistan. In: Welchman L, Hossain S (eds) 'Honour': crimes, paradigms, and violence against women. Zed Books, London, pp 209–230

Bhanbhro S (2021) Uncovering Community notions of honour and their relation to honour killings. Doctoral Thesis

Bhanbhro S, Chavez A, Lusambili A (2016) Honour based violence as a global public health problem: a critical review of literature. Int J Hum Rights Healthc 9(3):98–215. https://doi.org/10.1108/IJHRH-10-2015-0032

Campbell JK (1964) Honour, family, and patronage: a study of institutions and moral values in a Greek mountain community. Oxford University Press, Oxford

Dickson P (2014) Understanding victims of honour-based violence. Commun Pract 87(7):30–33

Ewing KP (2008) Stolen honour: stigmatising Muslim men in Berlin. Stanford University Press, Stanford, CA

Fournier P, Mcdougall P, Dekker A (2012) Dishonour, provocation, and culture: through the beholder's eye? Can Crim Law Rev 16(2):161–193

Gill A (2008) Crimes of honour' and violence against women in the UK. Int J Comp Appl Crim Just 32(2):243–263

Giordano C (2016) Honour between different cultures and legal systems: social status, reputation, struggles for recognition. Eur Rev 24(3):417

Goldstein MA (2002) The biological roots of heat-of-passion crimes and honour killings. Polit Life Sci 21:28–37

Hester M, Gangoli G, Gill AK, Mulvihill N, Bates L, Matolcsi A et al (2015) Victim/survivor voices–a participatory research project. A report for Her Majesty's Inspectorate of Constabulary Honour-based violence inspection. HMIC, London

Hong T (2014) Discourses on honour-related violence in Finnish policy documents. Nord J Fem Gend Res 22(4):1–16

Human Rights Commission Pakistan (2019) 2004 and 2016 honour killings in Pakistan. HRCP, Lahore

Khan TS (2006) Beyond honour: a historical materialist explanation of honour-related violence. Oxford University Press, Oxford

Khan R, Saleem S, Lowe M (2018) "Honour"-based violence in a British South Asian community. Saf Commun 17(1):11–21. https://doi.org/10.1108/SC-02-2017-0007

Korteweg AC, Yurdakul G (2010) Religion, culture and the politicisation of honour-related violence. A critical analysis of media and policy debates in Western Europe and North America. United Nations Research Institute for Social Development, Geneva

Kurkiala M (2003) Interpreting honour killings: the story of Fadime Sahindal (1975-2002) in the Swedish press. Anthropol Today 19(1):6–7

Lowe M, Khan R, Thanzami V, Barzy M, Karmaliani R (2018) Attitudes toward intimate partner "honour"-based violence in India, Iran, Malaysia, and Pakistan. J Aggress Confl Peace Res 10(4):283–292. https://doi.org/10.1108/JACPR-09-2017-0324

Meetoo V, Mirza HS (2007) "There is nothing 'honourable' about honour killings": gender, violence and the limits of multiculturalism. Women's Stud Int Forum 30(3):187–200

Montoya C, Agustín RL (2013) The othering of domestic violence: the EU and cultural framings of violence against women. Soc Polit 20(4):534–557

Moxnes H (1993) Honour and shame. Biblic Theol Bull 23(4):167–176

Nesheiwat F (2005) Honour crimes in Jordan: their treatment under Islamic and Jordanian Criminal Laws. Penn State Int Law Rev 23(2):251–281. http://elibrary.law.psu.edu/psilr/vol23/iss2/2

Pimentel S, Pandjiarjian V, Belloque J (2005) The "legitimate defence of honour," or murder with impunity? A critical study of legislation and case law in Latin America. In: Welchman L, Hossain S (eds) 'Honour': crimes, paradigms, and violence against women. Zed Books, London, pp 245–262

Pitt-Rivers J (1968) Honour. Int Encycl Soc Sci 6:503–511

Sabbe A, Oulami H, Zekraouni W, Hikmat H, Temmerman M, Leye E (2013) Determinants of child and forced marriage in Morocco: stakeholder perspectives on health, policies and human rights. BMC Int Health Hum Rights 13(43):1–12

Sedem M, Ferrer-Wreder L (2015) Fear of the loss of honour: implications of honour- based violence for the development of youth and their families. Child Youth Care Forum 44(2):225–237

Sev'er A, Yurdakul G (2001) Culture of honour, culture of change: a feminist analysis of honour killings in rural Turkey. Viol Against Women 7(9):964–998

Shafak E (2012) 'Honour killing': murder by any other name. The Guardian. https://www.theguardian.com/uk/2012/apr/30/honour-killings-spreading-alarming-rate

Shah N (2007) Making of crime, customs and culture: the case of karo kari killings of upper Sindh. In: Bennet J (ed) Scratching the surface: democracy, traditions, gender. Heinrich Boll Foundation, Lahore, pp 135–155

Siddique H (2021) 'Honour-based' offences soared by 81% in last five years. The Guardian. https://www.theguardian.com/society/2021/oct/31/honour-based-offences-soared-by-81-in-last-five-years
Soomro I (2022) Karo-Kari claimed 176 lives in Sindh in 2021: study. The News International. https://www.thenews.com.pk/print/930710-karo-kari-claimed-176-lives-in-Sindh-in-2021-study
Talwar D, Ahmad A (2015) Honour crime: 11,000 UK cases recorded in five years. British Broadcasting Corporation, London. http://www.bbc.co.uk/news/uk-33424644
The News International (2022) In the name of honour in six months: '2,439 women raped, 9,529 kidnapped, 90 killed in Punjab'. The New International. https://www.thenews.com.pk/print/931530-in-the-name-of-honour-in-six-months-2-439-women-raped-9-529-kidnapped-90-killed-in-Punjab
United Nations Population Fund (2000) The state of the world's population (Research Report). UNFPA, New York, NY. http://web.unfpa.org/swp/2000

Sadiq Bhanbhro, PhD is a Senior Research Fellow at Health Research Institute, Sheffield Hallam University. He researches global public health, women's health and well-being, gender, sexuality, violence (particularly honour crimes and honour killings) and racism.

Violence, Land and Gender: Exploring Connections

Susie Jacobs

> **Learning Objectives**
> After reading this paper, you should be able to understand the following:
>
> - Women's disadvantaged access to and control over agricultural land in many tenure systems
> - Broad issues concerning women's land rights and gender-based violence
> - Complexities of land titling initiatives
> - Potential benefits of women's land rights and underlying reasons for backlashes against these

Introduction

This chapter links two traditions of scholarship and activism: discussion of gendered violence and women's land rights within an agrarian political economy frame—that is, a perspective linking wider political and socioeconomic trends with social policies and practices. It asks: What roles do household and community-level violence play in depriving rural women of land access and control? And where women gain access to and control over land, does this affect the incidence of gender-based violence (GBV) experienced?

S. Jacobs (✉)
Sociology at Manchester Metropolitan University, Manchester, England, UK
e-mail: S.Jacobs@mmu.ac.uk

P. Ali, M. M. Rogers (eds.), *Gender-Based Violence: A Comprehensive Guide*,
https://doi.org/10.1007/978-3-031-05640-6_22

These questions are lent complexity by the fact that historically and in the present, land claims and property regimes have been tied in almost inextricably with violence, apart from questions of gender. This is true both of land as territory and as a productive resource. Additionally, although causation of conflicts should not be simplified (van Leeuwen and van der Haar 2017), land scarcity or lack of access to land are often a background or precipitating factor in armed conflicts. In Chiapas, Mexico, the EZLN ('Zapatista') uprising was at core an agrarian movement (van Leeuwen and van der Haar 2017). In Rwanda, severe land shortages were a contributory factor to the 1994 genocide (Polavarapu 2011): armed conflicts themselves greatly exacerbate GBV against women and girls (see chapter 'Wartime Violence and Intimate Partner Violence'). Thus, violence may be integral to control over land, including gendered aspects of land access and control.

The chapter is structured as follows: the next section focuses on the backdrop to the question of gender-based violence and women's land rights: women's greatly inferior control over land and agriculture. The third section discusses empirical work exploring land titling and the incidence of gender-based violence (GBV) (see Box 1 on terminology). The fourth examines violence as an impediment to women's claims to land. The fifth section explores some of the reasons for backlashes against women's land rights as well as helpful policy directions.

Box 1 Alternative Terminology
Violence against women (VAW); domestic violence: abuse; gendered land rights; land tenure systems; land security; land titling.

Background

Women across the world play key or predominant roles in agricultural production. The UN's Food and Agriculture Organisation (FAO) writes that in low-income countries, 45% of the measured agricultural workforce is female, rising to 60% in parts of Asia and Africa (FAO 2022). The FAO also notes that figures on women's participation tend to be underestimates (FAO 2018). Women's labour on farms is usually unremunerated and little-acknowledged.

Gender, Land and Land Tenure

Women's control over land is highly unequal to men's across much of the world, as is (now) well-known. This is particularly the case in patrilineal kinship systems, although male control over land can also extend to matrilineal societies. Even where kinship is reckoned bilaterally (on both mother and father's sides), as is the case in most of Europe and the Americas, women usually still have inferior access and rights (e.g. Brandth 2002; Jacobs 2017). Across the world, women have less direct access to land than do men; their access tends to be through male family members, particularly husbands and fathers. Where land is held privately and is owned outright, women's land is usually of lower quality and on smaller plots compared with men (FAO 2018). Where women own or hold land, their rights tend to be less secure. For the 20 countries for which sufficient information is available, the FAO reports that fewer than 15% of agricultural landholders (who may not own land outright) are women—including those who have joint tenure with husbands (FAO 2018). Women also constitute a much smaller proportion of landowners than do men.

In much of sub-Saharan Africa (henceforth, SSA) and among some indigenous peoples elsewhere, land is held communally; thus, no one 'owns' the land—although commodification of land is increasing rapidly. Land is traditionally allocated and administered by a clan/lineage elder, although worked by individual households. Although in SSA, women are (usually) the main agriculturalists, their access to land is mediated through husbands or fathers. However, in most African societies, wives should by right have access to a plot of land on which to cultivate food crops, and often have rights of disposal over such crops. A wife should retain this, and access to the husband's land more generally, so long as a marriage lasts. A woman who is divorced, or who is single with children, is meant to be able to access land from her father's patrilineage. However, in practice such access is often insecure and very difficult to negotiate (Murugani et al. 2014). Access to land for lone women, as elsewhere, is usually dependent on maintaining 'good' relationships with partners and within the extended family. Lack of success in such negotiations can lead to eviction and destitution.

In most of the world, land is held privately rather than communally, but it is often held in informal arrangements. Customary arrangements may also exist alongside formal laws, and farmers commonly lack documentation. Additionally, a parcel of land can be subject to claims by various people or groups.

Where legislation exists to give women land rights (see below), this does not always translate into effective control. Doss and Meinzen-Dick (2020) formulate a framework for analysis of land security for women. They suggest that the following bundles of rights be considered: use rights; management and transformation (*abusus*); economic ownership (for instance, the right to profit); exclusion; transfer and future interests (e.g. inheritance). Rights may or may not overlap (FAO 2018). Thus, in most of SSA, married women *do* have rights of access, and (occasionally) of management. However, it is less likely for them to be able to exercise rights to transfer land or to exclude others from its use.

Relatedly, social impediments to women's land rights often exist, such as the expectation that women not appear overly assertive (see later). Taboos may also apply to women and farming—e.g. the idea in China, that women's menses might pollute crops, or South Asian strictures against women ploughing. These stigmatise women's bodies and affect their ability to farm or to act as farm managers.

Land Titling

Land titling has been a main policy initiative to address women's insecure and unequal land rights. 'Titling' is a type of codification and legalisation of land claims, especially in contexts where land is held communally or in informal systems. The movement to codify or to grant land titles to women has (at least) two motivations. One has been feminist campaigns to empower women through greater economic independence. Land rights and landholding in agrarian contexts are seen to increase women's food security; to reduce poverty; to lead to greater decision-making power and to enhance community standing. The important role of land in livelihoods has also been underlined by a number of Southern women's movements—as one example, the Tanzania Women Lawyers Association (Whitehead and Tsikata 2003).

The other motivation, however, is the wider move to formalise—and potentially, to commodify—land by international institutions. The World Bank and other institutions have for several decades, pushed for titling or formalisation of claims and use-rights; this is seen to stimulate investment, to make it possible to use land as collateral and in theory, to protect land from predation by others. The International Institute for Environment and Development comments with regard to Africa, that for more than two decades, the majority of international actors' support for women's land claims has concentrated on titling—assuming the desirability of individual titles (IIED 2021).

Improving the security of women's land rights is also put forward as a rationale for titling (Manji 2006). The common (although not universal) link of titling with commodification and privatisation means that this is a fraught issue. If land becomes commodified, it can be alienated – for instance, used as collateral to raise loans. Since the majority of rural women are poor, they are unlikely to fare well in a marketised economy (Manji 2006; Jacobs 2017) and may lose their land.

Titling can be individual or can allow more than one name on permits or deeds—typically, of both husband and wife. A number of countries have moved to joint or (less commonly) sole titling as well as to more secure rights, especially for widows. Measures enacted include equality in the right to control property regardless of marriage type (e.g. formal or customary); spousal consent required to alienate property and specific representation for women in land-related institutions. Despite much progress in the legal realm, discrimination in law limits women's land rights in at least 75 countries (Roberts 2021).

Where egalitarian laws exist, it has proved difficult to implement them. Women's land rights often remain 'on paper' rather than 'on the ground' as these may contradict existing gendered social structures and practices.

Landholding and IPV

The various frames that might address GBV and land issues each tend to bypass or to ignore selected issues. Literature on land occupations and corporate land 'grabs' (or acquisitions) has sometimes acknowledged that women land activists are subject to sexualised violence—over and above the violence commonly meted out to land activists (Global Witness 2020). However, less attention is given to intimate partner violence (IPV) within households (Brickell 2015). On the other hand, discussion of GBV in low- and middle-income countries has not tended to engage with agrarian contexts, and research specifically on GBV/IPV in agrarian settings is scarce. The International Fund for Agricultural Development notes that rural and indigenous women may be at higher risk of IPV and are less likely to report (IFAD 2019). Factors that may heighten the risk of IPV and that make reporting difficult or dangerous in rural areas include lack of services; geographical and social isolation; lack of other (e.g. nonagricultural) livelihood options and greater community acceptance of IPV against women and girls (Bellows et al. 2015).

Most studies of the relation between GBV and women's landholding have been linked with moves to land titling. One of the benefits of land titling for women, along with potentially enhanced decision-making powers, is posited to be reduction in violence. Selected studies of this topic are summarised below.

A number of studies of land titling and IPV have come from India; most indicate a decrease in violence associated with property ownership, including with landholding. Constraints of space allow detail here for only one, recent study. (Kelkar et al. 2020) led a quantitative and qualitative study in three Indian states: two—Karnataka and Telengana, 'patriarchal'—and the third in the matrilineal context of Meghalaya. This was a study of 256 women and 106 men across six villages; only women with land in their own (sole) names were included. Kelkar found that women's land ownership was associated with decreased GBV due, among other, to their greater economic empowerment and increased agency, among other.

In other geographical regions, Grabe et al. (2015) built on an earlier Nicaraguan study by Grabe, comparing land ownership by women in Nicaragua and in Tanzania, among Maasai people. This study was of 267 women in Nicaragua and 225 in Tanzania. In both countries, traditional norms prohibit or discourage married women—and most other women—from having title to land. In both settings, landowners reported less psychological and physical violence. In Tanzania, reduction in psychological violence against women approached levels of statistical significance. Maasai women also felt that landholding increased their community status and security. In both sites, structural changes in women's land ownership related to greater power in the marriage relationship.

The studies above report results that appear optimistic for the potential of land rights/ownership to reduce GPV. However, others report ambiguous results.

For instance, in a Zimbabwean national health survey (Wekwete et al. 2014), 4094 married/partnered women were sampled. The study found joint ownership of land to be associated with *increased* physical violence in partnerships as well as with GBV overall. Relatedly, K. Jacobs and Kes' (2015) research on titling and joint tenure in Uganda and South Africa found that spouses, especially in Uganda, held very different views of 'joint ownership'. This could lead to misunderstandings and conflict: in particular, husbands often did not acknowledge the wife's claims to joint land titles.

Peterman et al. (2017) conducted a systematic review of 28 international surveys concerning women's individual asset ownership and experiences of IPV. Results for the impact of land ownership on IPV were found to be highly variable: in five countries on different continents, the association of women's or land ownership with VAW was positive.

In another, Caribbean/Central American review, Gahramanov et al. (2021) found in the four countries studied that *sole* property ownership—unlike joint ownership—did not reduce IPV. However, the study also found that in rural areas, women's property ownership was a factor in reduction of IPV and that joint land ownership was a negative predictor. The authors posit that joint ownership of land may be less of a challenge to male control over women's household and farm labour.

Thus, associations between women's land ownership and GBV vary and are highly context- and culturally-specific (Peterman et al. 2017; IIED 2021). Evidence from three continents supports the finding that women with more secure rights may be less at risk of IPV or violence within communities. But in highly male-dominated contexts in which land is an important resource, challenges to men's traditional land rights are often seen as a threat which can itself exacerbate violence.

GBV as an Impediment to Land Rights

Violence often prevents realisation of women's claims to land, even where customary rights exist. This is even more strongly the case for newer rights—e.g. in cases where state-backed land redistribution allocates land to women as well as men, or in more contemporary situations of legal rights to land or titling. As Bellows et al. (2015) found in their research on GBV as an impediment to women's food security, this is largely a hidden narrative.

Many accounts, however, do exist of violence against widows as well as divorcees when they attempt to retain or to claim land. This increase in visibility is a result of NGO and women's movement campaigning and signals growing acknowledgement that widows should not be disinherited and potentially, left destitute.

Murugani et al. write that in southern Africa, there are numerous instances of female farmers having land taken upon divorce and/or the death of the husband (2014: 205). Widowhood brings insecurity for many women, who can face violent eviction and disinheritance. Izumi (2007) documented this in Zimbabwe, where the husband's patrilineal relatives often appropriated the land on which a widow lived, claiming customary law as justification. Mootz et al. (2017) note that in northeastern Uganda, women lack land rights without the presence of the husband, so widows are frequently evicted unless they are 'inherited' by one of the husband's patrilineage kinsmen.

In Rwanda, the 1994 genocide meant that women—many of whom had suffered rape—became a large majority of the population. Nonetheless they continued to face evictions and conflict with regard to land claims. The post-conflict context was one of breakdown of communal structures (Polavarapu 2011), emphasising the need for codification and of stronger rights for women. Despite Rwanda's egalitarian land laws, abuses had not ceased. Another Rwandan/Liberian study notes that when women try to exercise their legal land rights – for example when objections are made to a husband's sale of land without consent they are often met with violence (Hughes and Richardson 2015).

In Kenya, a grassroots project helped to carry out care for HIV-affected households (Dworkin et al. 2013). Caregivers found that in a number of cases women would suddenly disappear from households, because they had been 'chased away' by in-laws or were denied the use of the husband's land (see also Box 2 on GROOTS-Kenya).

Abuse of widows is not confined to particular world regions. A pilot study in Bangladesh, India and Sri Lanka (Swaminathan et al. 2007) found that even if widows were not evicted immediately, they often were abused until they left the marital home and land. Additionally, appropriation of property by the husband's lineage or kin often takes place during funeral preparations, when the widow is in mourning.

Women may try to minimise conflict through acceptance or negotiation of an existing gender order. The need for many rural sub-Saharan African women to maintain 'good' kinship and marriage relationships to maintain access to land has been noted. But similar norms are widespread in other regions. In much of Asia including China, Vietnam, Cambodia, Myanmar and India, it is a woman's role to maintain family 'harmony'. Park (2019) notes that in Cambodia, the formal code governing expected female behaviour (*Chbab Srey*)—enjoining (among other) respect for husbands, frugality and the need to speak softly, were omitted from the school curriculum only in 2007.

Doss et al. (2014) found that in Orissa state, India, women felt that it was their duty to minimise conflict within the family. Doss et al. note that the threat of violence—or simply a desire to fit into expectations of wives and mothers—can lead women to 'trade away' decision-making authority. In an example with some parallels, in Muslim *shari'a* law, women are entitled to shares of family property amounting to one-half of a man's. However, it not uncommon for women to cede rights in religious law to maintain relationships with brothers (Kabeer 1991; Chaturvedi 2004), as their support may be needed in case of later marital difficulty.

If the above are examples of attempts to maintain the gendered status quo through blocking access to/control over land, there exist examples in which existing social structures have changed dramatically. The Chinese revolution was a rare instance in which wives and daughters gained land rights in the initial land redistribution in the late 1940s and early 1950s. Women—particularly single women who were often destitute—had joined in enthusiastically in land reform campaigns (Jacobs 2010). Redistribution of land and title deeds to women, virtually unknown in Han China, was highly symbolic. Women asserting land rights and taking possession of their new title deeds were, however, often subject to violence, including murder. Hundreds of thousands of women lost their lives attempting to assert land rights (Jacobs 2010, citing Delia Davin).

Some 70 years on, Park (2019) notes that Cambodian studies (see also Brickell 2015) find that women land activists against state and corporate land 'grabs' themselves suffered from impacts on the family, including IPV.

Thus, women asserting land rights—particularly when these are not on behalf of a community or social movement but within households—are often seen as disloyal to their marriages and families (Murugani et al. 2014). This implies that women who do not display 'feminine' attributes of compliance, including ceding land and property rights, may face coercion. This may be indirect, through divorce/desertion or may be enacted through forms of GBV.

The next section turns to discussion of some of the reasons for GBV in the context of women's land claims.

Underlying Factors and Policy Implications

Resistance to land rights for women has been very widespread: perhaps more so than to women's entry into paid work in industry. Women can face violence, as the examples above indicate, not only in asserting desired claims but in cases where they have already won land, either through legislation, state-backed land redistribution or social movement activity. Such violence can be physical and sexual, along with psychological coercion.

This section briefly discusses some underlying explanations of GBV with regard to land rights, before exploring directions for policy. First, the observation with which the chapter began is apposite: land claims are not infrequently backed with violence or its threat. Land is both a material resource and a signifier of social status and power, and social structures around land ownership sustain gendered power relations that themselves put women at risk of violence (Grabe et al. 2015). Peterman et al. (2017) note that women 'tied' to immovable property may be at particular risk.

Women's labour—however little-acknowledged—is crucial to agrarian households and economies (Jacobs 2010), and loss of control over this labour may be perceived as an economic and practical risk. As Gahramanov et al. (2021) note, women's sole ownership/holding of land may be a threat to male control, and this may precipitate IPV.

Beyond the practicalities of the need for household labour, landholding may be linked not only with control over land as economic resource but also with identity and masculinity. In South Africa, for instance, struggles for women's land rights were first initiated by the government (the ANC), NGOs and by local women in the 1990s. Cross and Friedman (1997) found that many rural men—and some women—saw the suppression of women's attempts to hold and dispose of land to be an urgent moral concern. Strengthening of women's rights in this lineage-based context was feared as potentially leading to the destruction of the family and of rural society itself.

Control over land in most smallholding households and communities is thus bound up with the nexus of kinship and gendered, household-based agriculture.

Given the entrenched nature of gendered inequality in landholding and control, and the emotive nature of land rights, policies which would effectively address 'backlashes' and resultant GBV are not straightforward.

Certainly, where land is already privately owned, women should enjoy the same rights to titles as men, regardless of marriage status. As the IIED (2021) argues, where land is held communally, recognition of communal rights would need to be complemented by rendering void any customary arrangements that discriminate against women. There may also exist alternatives and safeguards to land privatisation, such as cooperatives, or enacting strict land ceilings and blocks to alienation of land (Jacobs 2010; Agarwal 2016).

Changes in the legal sphere are key, but as seen, these often prove difficult to enforce. Women's land rights are arguably most secure when there already exists wide gendered equity (see Kelkar et al. 2020; Doss and Meinzen-Dick 2020). This implies an holistic and long-term strategy that includes but also goes beyond land rights.

Where possible, changes in gendered land tenure should attempt to engage the community, including elders and men in affected households. For instance, the carefully structured WOLTS (Women and Land Tenure Security) initiative by the NGO Mokoro (Daley et al. 2021) includes young male champions' of women's land rights in Mongolia and Tanzania. The WOLTS programme has been promising in terms of increasing women's community participation as well as in protecting community land rights.

Relatedly, it is important that women's land rights be publicly acknowledged and made visible (e.g. Jacobs 2010; K. Jacobs and Kes 2015). Increase in social and normative acceptance is a key aspect.

Despite educational and political campaigns, social acceptance of women's land rights is often less than universal. Peterman et al. (2017) suggest that at a minimum, there must be monitoring for GBV in the wake of tenure changes. 'Enforcement' policies are also key, as is institutional backup. Thus, mechanisms to report GBV—ideally to local government or law enforcement officials—or else to other relevant bodies such as Women's Committees or other, are needed (see Box 2). Secure land rights for women—which may take various forms—are likely in the long term to be an important element in reduction of GBV. Landholding—or more secure land rights—may benefit women economically, may lead to greater freedom of mobility and can enhance women's social status (Agarwal 2016; Kelkar et al. 2020). In the shorter term, however, backlashes may occur against rights for women and in defence of existing gender orders within households and communities.

In enactment of more gender-egalitarian land rights, implementation of measures against GBV remain key.

Box 2 Case Study: GROOTS-Kenya Community Watch Dog Model

The GROOTS-Kenya Community Land and Property Watch Dog Model (CWDG) is a structural intervention including programming to support women's land and property rights and to reduce violence against women.

Although Kenyan statutory law now outlaws gender discrimination in inheritance, disputes are mainly regulated through customary law. Some 45% of Kenyan women experience violence and/or sexual abuse during their lifetimes, and in one study cited, 60% of widows/divorcees experienced violent asset-stripping or disinheritance. The CWDGs are comprised of volunteer men and women; of community health workers; paralegals; traditional leaders and government stakeholders. Their functions are to monitor disinheritance at local levels, to mediate land disputes and to refer unresolved cases to formal adjudication mechanisms.

Hillyard et al. (2016) discuss a small, in-depth study carried out in two provinces with especially high rates of GBV. The 30 women interviewed had all experienced property rights violations and also had been assisted by CWDGs. Nearly all reported that violence had ceased when reported to the CWDGs, whether or not the dispute was fully resolved.

Participants offered four rationales for the reduction in GBV:

- Improved awareness of women's land rights and of violence
- Improved community-level reporting
- A comprehensive response to reports of GBV
- Perpetuators' fears of legal or other consequences of their actions

Summary

- GBV/IPV with regard to women's land claims and rights has been a little-studied area.
- Formal land titling has been one of the main policies to address women's lack of control over agricultural land, and some studies indicate benefits. Because this has often been linked with privatisation, however, there are clear risks for poorer women—including loss of their land.
- Research examining links between land titling (on sole or joint bases) and reduction in GBV is so far not definitive. A number of studies do point to reduction in GBV and IPV; but others indicate increases in IPV.
- The latter could indicate a 'backlash', and some men worry about loss of status as well as loss of control over women's household labour.
- It is important to safeguard communal rights while at the same time rescinding gender discriminatory aspects of customary law.
- Policies promoting secure land rights for women should be accompanied by measures to combat GBV as well as promoting gender equity more broadly.

References

Agarwal B (2016) Gender challenges: Vols. 1, 2 and 3. Oxford University Press, Oxford

Bellows A, Lemke S, Jenderedjian A, Scherbaum V (2015) Violence as an under-recognized barrier to women's realization of their right to adequate food and nutrition: case studies from Georgia and South Africa. Viol Against Women 21(10):1194–1217

Brandth B (2002) Gender identity in European family farming: a literature review. Sociol Rural 42(3):181–200

Brickell K (2015) Towards intimate geographies of peace? Trans Inst Br Geogr 40(3):321–333

Chaturvedi A (2004) Muslim women and law. Commonwealth Publishers, New Delhi

Cross C, Friedman M (1997) Women and land: marginality and the left hand power. In: Meer S (ed) Women, land and authority. Oxfam, Oxford, pp 17–34

Daley E, Grabham J, Narangerel Y, Ndakaru J (2021) Women and community land rights: investing in local champions. Mokoro Ltd. With HakiMadini (Tanzania) and PCC (Mongolia), Oxford

Doss C, Meinzen-Dick R (2020) Land tenure security for women: a conceptual framework. Land Use Policy 99:105080

Doss C, Kim S, Njuki J, Hilenbrand E, Miruka M (2014) Women's individual and joint property ownership: effects on household decision-making. Discussion Paper 01347. IFPRI/CGIAR, Washington, DC

Dworkin S, Grabe S, Lu T, Hatcher A, Kwena Z, Bukusi E, Mwaura-Muira D (2013) Property rights violations as a structural driver of women's HIV risks: a qualitative study in Nyanza and Western Provinces, Kenya. Arch Sex Behav 42:703–713

FAO (2018) Briefing: the gender gap in land rights. FAO, Rome. http://www.fao.org/family-farming/detail/en/c/1119178/

Food and Agriculture Association of the United Nations [FAO] (2022) When you think farmer, think female!: the FAO and UNDP are empowering women for a sustainable future. FAO, Rome. https://www.fao.org/in-action/naps/newsevents/detail/en/c/1379336/

Gahramanov E, Gaibulloev K, Younas J (2021) Women's type of property ownership and domestic violence: a theoretical note. Rev Econ Househ 18:223–232

Global Witness (2020) Press release: "Global Witness records the highest number of land and environmental activists murdered in one year – with the link to accelerating climate change of increasing concern". https://www.globalwitness.org/en/press-releases/global-witness-records-the-highest-number-of-land-and-environmental-activists-murdered-in-one-year-with-the-link-to-accelerating-climate-change-of-increasing-concern/

Grabe S, Grose R, Dutt A (2015) Women's land ownership and relationship power: a mixed methods approach to understanding structural inequalities and violence against women. Psychol Women Q 38(1):7–19

Hillyard S, Buusi E, Graebe S, Lu T, Hatcher A, Kwena Z, Mwaura-Muiru E, Dworkin S (2016) Perceived impact of a land and property rights program on violence against women in rural Kenya: a qualitative investigation. Viol Against Women 22(14):1682–1703

Hughes A, Richardson A (2015) Land and gender-based violence: experiences from Rwanda and Liberia. Resource equity report

International Fund for Agricultural Development of the United Nations (IFAD) (2019) Briefing: putting an end to violence against women in rural communities. IFAD, Rome. https://www.ifad.org/zh-TW/web/latest/-/putting-an-end-to-violence-against-women-in-rural-communities

International Institute for Environment and Development (IIED) (2021) Briefing: why simple solutions won't secure African women's land rights. IIED, London. http://pubs.iied.org/20336IIED

Izumi K (2007) Gender-based violence and property grabbing in Africa: a denial of women's liberty and security. Gend Dev 15(1):11–23

Jacobs S (2010) Gender and agrarian reforms. Routledge, New York, NY; London

Jacobs S (2017) Beneficial for women? Global trends in gender, land and titling. In: Bock B, Shortall S (eds) Gender and rural globalization. CABI, Wallingford, Oxon, pp 322–336

Jacobs K, Kes A (2015) The ambiguity of joint asset ownership: cautionary tales from Uganda and South Africa. Fem Econ 21(3):23–55

Kabeer N (1991) Gender dimensions of rural poverty: analysis from Bangladesh. J Peasant Stud 18(2):241

Kelkar G, Gaikwad S, Mandal S (2020) Women's land ownership and its ramifications for gender-based violence, working paper 4. GenDev: Centre for Research and Innovation, Gurgaon, Haryana

van Leeuwen M, van der Haar G (2017) Theorizing the land-violent conflict nexus. World Dev 78:94–104

Manji A (2006) The politics of land reform in Africa. Zed Books, London

Mootz J, Stabb S, Mollen D (2017) Gender-based violence and armed conflict: a community-informed socioecological conceptual model from Northeastern Uganda. Psychol Women Q 41(3):1–21

Murugani V, Thamaga-Chitja J, Koanisi U, Shimelis H (2014) The role of property rights in rural women's land use security and household food security for improved livelihood in Limpopo Province. J Hum Ecol 15(11):1311–1330

Park CMY (2019) 'Our lands are our lives': gendered experiences of resistance to land grabbing in rural Cambodia. Fem Econ 25(4):21–44

Peterman A, Pereira A, Bleck J, Palermo T, Yount K (2017) Women's individual asset ownership and experience of intimate partner violence: evidence from 28 international surveys. Am J Public Health 107(5):747–755

Polavarapu A (2011) Procuring meaningful land rights for women of Rwanda. Yale Hum Rights Dev J 14(1):105–154

Roberts B (2021) Securing women's land rights: challenges and solutions. Feed Fut. https://agrilinks.org/post/securing-womens-land-rights-challenges-and-solutions

Swaminathan H, Bhatla N, Chakraborty S (2007) Women's property rights as an AIDS response: emerging efforts in South Asia. ICRW (International Center for Research on Women), Washington, DC

Wekwete NN, Sanhokwe H, Murenjekwa W, Takavaraha F, Madzingira N (2014) The association between spousal gender-based violence and women's empowerment among currently-married women aged 15-49 in Zimbabwe: evidence from the 2010-11 Zimbabwe demographic and health survey. Afr Popul Stud 28(3):1413–1431

Whitehead A, Tsikata D (2003) Policy discourses on women's land rights in Sub-Saharan Africa: the implications of the return to the customary. J Agrar Stud 3(1–2):67–112

Susie Jacobs, D.Phil is an Hon. Research Fellow and emerita Reader in Comparative Sociology at Manchester Metropolitan University. Her research has focused on gender, agriculture and land issues, particularly agrarian reforms. Other key areas include gendered violence in wars and conflicts; labour organisation and sexual harassment in agribusiness farms; and 'race', racisms and ethnicity in higher education.

Menstruation and Gender-Based Violence

Richard Whitecross

Learning Objectives
Having read this chapter, you should be able to understand the following:

- How cultural, religious and social traditions and practices in relation to menstruation are multifaceted and impact on the wellbeing and safety of women and girls
- The vulnerability of women and girls, mainly living in the Global South, associated with menstruation
- Why it is important to be aware of and support locally lead challenges to cultural, religious and social norms that place restrictions on women during menstruation
- How the practice of social isolation and seclusion, as illustrated by the example of *chhaupadi* in Nepal, makes women and girls vulnerable to gender-based violence

Introduction

This chapter introduces the cultural, religious and social practices around menarche and menstruation that impact on women and girls (see Box 1 for definitions). The anthropologist Chris Knight notes that menstruation attracts 'extraordinary attention … in virtually all cultures' (Knight 1996: 363). Gottlieb (2020: 144) notes that 'despite shared biological roots, individuals and communities perceive and

R. Whitecross (✉)
Law, The Business School, Edinburgh Napier University, Edinburgh, UK
e-mail: R.Whitecross@napier.ac.uk

P. Ali, M. M. Rogers (eds.), *Gender-Based Violence: A Comprehensive Guide*,
https://doi.org/10.1007/978-3-031-05640-6_23

experience in enormously different ways'. Across a range of cultures, menarche represents a symbolic transition from childhood to womanhood linked with sexual maturation (Lee 2009). Acknowledging the universality of menstruation in 2019, human rights experts noted that 'the stigma and shame generated by stereotypes around menstruation have severe impacts on all aspects of women's and girls' human rights' (United Nations 2019).

Social science research reminds us that how women and girls experience menstruation depends on the complex interrelationship between social, cultural, religious and political contexts which shape and inform their experiences. It is important to understand that a practice may reflect social mores, as well as religious or other cultural influences. As a result of the stigma and shame highlighted by the United Nations, women and girls experience inequality in access to health care, housing, water, sanitation, education, freedom of religion or belief, safe and healthy working conditions. Nor are they able to participate in cultural and public life without discrimination. These can be difficult to untangle. However, it is this intertwined nature of customs and practices associated with menstruation that make challenging culturally informed practices difficult. For many women, the cultural, religious and social traditions and practices associated with menarche and menstruation can be highly restrictive and damaging as illustrated in the main case study presented in this chapter.

Buckley and Gottlieb (1988) and Paige and Paige (1981) provide anthropological studies of menstruation that demonstrate the importance of menarche as a sign of physical maturity and fertility. In some cultures, for example, menarche is celebrated with girls receiving gifts (Uskul 2004). Other cross-disciplinary studies highlight cultural and social perspectives that hold menstruation as physically, psychologically and spiritually problematic (Delany et al. 1977). Anthropologists and other social scientists have recorded a range of practices that prohibit menstruating women and girls from engaging in various activities and often being required to seclude themselves.

Whilst sexual relations are possible during menstruation, many cultures treat sexual relations during menstruation as either inappropriate or risk laden. Stubbs (2008: 58) notes that even in the United States until the 1980s, 'this negative characterisation … was supported by psychodynamic theorists who believed that menarche was a traumatic intrapsychic event, provoking anxiety … as well as diminished self-esteem'. In her study of the cultural perceptions and practices of adolescent girls in the United States, Stubbs reflects on the ongoing negative characterisation of the menstrual cycle. She notes the tension between menstruation as a normal physiological process and greater availability of menstrual products with mixed messages in menstrual education that it should be hidden (2008). Significantly, she demonstrates the impact of these mixed messages on adolescent girls' negative perception of menstruation and how this contributes to self-objectification, body shame and their lack of agency in their own sexual decision-making. The enduring cultural tension over menstruation in the Global North is succinctly captured by Stubbs who notes '[a]dvertisements for contraceptives that promote the notion that menstruation is unimportant, unnatural, unhealthy, and a generally negative experience, do the same thing. In a culture that objectifies women, who wouldn't want to avoid such an experience?' (Stubbs 2008: 64).

Therefore, although there are physiological similarities in the experience of menarche and menstruation, it is important to understand that how both are understood and perceived is linked to a range of culturally and religiously informed social practices that impact on women and girls. In fact, there is a 'striking diversity of menstrual experiences, especially in the Global South' (Gottlieb 2020: 144). Indeed, a number of studies illustrate how varying perceptions of menstrual practices may allow women to demonstrate their own agency by deciding whether or not to engage with those practices (Mirvis 2020). This chapter focuses on outlining how restrictive menstrual practices endanger women and girls. The chapter illustrates these practices by drawing on recent social science and health research conducted in South Asia. The role of religion, as well as social and cultural norms such as caste, shapes and informs the experience of menarche and menstruation. In particular, it focuses on a widespread practice, called *chhaupadi*, in Nepal where women and girls are required to seclude and isolate themselves during menstruation.

Definitions and Types

There are three main terms in relation to menstruation that are set out in Box 1. As the definition of menstruation suggests, the focus of this chapter is on the physiological process as experienced by women and girls in a variety of social and cultural settings. The chapter does not discuss menopause, which like menstruation is experienced differently across cultures and societies with its meaning and management highly contested. This chapter does not adopt a biomedical approach to understanding menstruation and gender-based violence. Rather it draws, as illustrated in the introduction, on the complex interrelationship and meaning making of social, cultural and religious factors that define the experience of this universal physiological process.

Historical Context

Box 1 Definition

Menses refers to the time of menstruation (period) and the menstrual discharge.

Menarche refers to the first experience of menstruation and to the age at which this occurs.

Menstruation refers to the physiological process of discharging blood and other material from the lining of the uterus through the vagina, which occurs in sexually mature women (except during pregnancy and for a time after pregnancy) at intervals of about one lunar month until menopause.

Menopause is the final cessation of the menstrual cycle (Shorter Oxford Dictionary 2007).

In South Asia attitudes towards and beliefs about menstruation impact on women and girls through a range of social restrictions and religious/cultural practices. Due to widely held beliefs that view menstruation as impure, women and girls during menses are prohibited from touching certain people, usually men, as well as livestock, crops and drinking water sources. As a result of such beliefs and practices associated with menstruation, women and girls during menstruation have limited access to food, water and other necessities. Significantly, research highlights that because of such beliefs women and girls are unable to practice good menstrual hygiene (House and Mahon 2013). To illustrate the cultural, religious and social practices and stigma around menstruation, one such practice, *chhaupadi* (isolation) in Nepal, is the main focus of this chapter. Although the geographical focus is on Nepal, it is important to understand that similar practices and their negative impact on the lives of women and girls during their menses are not restricted to either Nepal, India or the region of South Asia.

Various authors have explored the taboos and restrictions around menstruation in Hinduism (e.g. Narayanan 2005). It is claimed that Hindus believe that when women menstruate, the menstrual blood is impure; therefore, during menstruation their body is impure. Narayanan (2005) argues that the menstruation taboo is one of the reasons that women are not permitted to be priests. A study conducted in Cuddalore district in Tamil Nadu, in southern India, highlights the belief that menstruation is religiously impure and ceremonially unclean and was responsible for compliance by women especially by women from higher socioeconomic backgrounds where purity is emphasised (Selvi and Ramachandra 2012). Menstruation is not perceived as a natural physiological process, and in those communities in Nepal in which chhaupadi is practised, it is believed that the touch of a menstruating woman or girl is impure, requiring husbands and family members to bathe if touched. In their detailed qualitative study in Nepal, Rothchild and Piya (2020) observed that menstruation was framed by their informants as a concern about men or boys, rather than about the physical process they were experiencing.

The dyad of purity and pollution is one that is recognised across cultures and is not restricted to Hinduism or to South Asia. Guterman et al. (2007) note that all major religions contain, to varying degrees, restrictions on menstruating women, including the requirement to isolate themselves and not engage in various activities. Jun and Jang (2018: 50) argue that religious beliefs are not 'solely responsible for the menstruation taboo'. Rather, they see the menstruation taboos and the practice of chhaupadi in Nepal as reflecting the wider and complex interrelationship between religious beliefs and social norms and values.

Nepal: The Context

Located in the Himalayas, Nepal is a multi-ethnic, multilingual and multicultural country. Approximately 90% of Nepalese are Hindu (Asian Development Bank 1999). In 2020, the United Nations Development Program ranked Nepal 142nd out of 189 countries in terms of its human development index and 110th out of 160 countries in its gender inequality index. The Asian Development Bank (1999) noted women in Nepal are excluded from education and have limited labour market opportunities and decision-making over their property. A republic since 2006 when the monarchy was abolished, Nepal is a predominantly, though not exclusively, Hindu country. This is important for two reasons. The first is that a caste system remains in place in Nepal. Second, as will be discussed below, the practice of *chhaupadi* is rooted in the Hindu belief that menstruating women and girls are impure (Bhandari 2013). As a result of social, cultural and religious beliefs and practices, Nepalese women have limited or no social capital. This lack of power is further exacerbated by the caste system.

Menstruation and Impurity: The Basis of the Practice

The Nepalese Ministry of Health reported in 2012 that about a quarter of women did not know about menstruation before the onset of menarche. Similarly, Rothchild and Piya (2020) in their qualitative study on menstruation in Nepal found that Nepalese women were unprepared for menarche. Rothchild and Piya note that whilst some were able to access advice, many women reported being discouraged by their mothers from discussing what was happening to them or asking questions and advice. This lack of information and support has practical consequences in terms of hygiene. However, one of the main features of Rothchild and Piya's findings is the social requirement for women to isolate and the cultural and taboos and religious rituals associated with menstruation.

Chhaupadi: Isolation and Vulnerability

The practice of *chhaupadi* (alternatives spelling include: *chaupadi*, see Box 2) in Nepal refers to the requirement for women and girls to move to a remote makeshift hut during menses. The term *chhaupadi* is based on two words: *chhau* refers to being 'untouchable' and *padi* meaning 'women' (Dahal et al. 2017: 3). When girls experience their first menstruation, they are required to be sequestered for between 11 and 15 days, with a similar period of sequestration at the second menses, then up to 7 days for their third. Thereafter women and girls are banished to the *chhaupadi goth* or *chhau* shed for on average 4–7 consecutive days (Robinson 2015). At the end of their period, the women and girls bathe and wash their clothes before returning home.

The *chhaupadi goth* are built from stone and mud, typically long and dark with no windows or doors that can be locked. Women using the *chhaupadi goth* report being unable to control the temperature which ranges from freezing in winter to stifling in summer months. Research conducted in 2011 suggests that the number of dedicated *chhaupadi goth* are decreasing (UNRHCO 2011). This is not because the practice is diminishing but that resources are not available to maintain the huts. The areas in which the practice continues are among the poorest in Nepal. As a result, women and girls have stayed in cattle sheds during menstruation (UNRHCO 2011: 4). The use of cattle sheds increases the vulnerability of women and girls to a range of infections as they are required to eat and sleep in the cattle sheds. In one study, a woman described that she felt reduced to being an animal during her period and seclusion (Khadka 2020).

Box 2
Alternative terms used for the practice of *chhaupadi*: *chhue* or *bahirhunu* in Dadeldhura, Baitadi and Darchula, *chaupadi* in Accham and *chaukulla* or *chaukudi* in Bajhang district.

Prevalence of Chhaupadi

The research evidence from Nepal suggests that *chhaupadi*, despite official steps to prohibit the practice, remains widespread. In particular, various studies suggest that it continues to be widely practiced in the hill districts of Far West and Mid-West regions of Nepal. In 2011, it was estimated that more than 95% of women were practicing *chhaupadi* in Achham District (UN Resident and Humanitarian Office 2011). Recent research highlights that as families migrate from the hill districts in search of work, they bring the practice with them. A series of studies between 2014 and 2017 suggested a significant increase in the number of women practicing *chhaupadi* in Tikapur in Kailali District (Khadka 2020). Jun and Jang (2018) in their study of non-compliance with the state prohibition of *chhaupadi* argue that policy or law-making to address the practice is insufficient. Their study demonstrates the importance of engaging with established norms and challenging them, for example, through local level education programmes that highlight the human harm caused by *chhaupadi*.

Research highlights that social pressure remains the primary reason for the continued practice of *chhaupadi* (Jun and Jang 2018). Although there have been high-level moves to prohibit the practice and legislation passed in 2017 criminalising those requiring women and girls to seclude themselves during menstruation, traditional social norms and religious beliefs reinforce and maintain the practice (Thapa and Aro 2021). This is particularly the case in the far western districts of Nepal where up to 60% of women still practice *chhaupadi*. It is important to understand that in many communities, support for the practice remains strong among village elders, husbands, mother-in-law, Hindu priests and traditional healers, as well as older women who believe that it is necessary to maintain purity and not anger the gods.

Jun and Jang's research suggests that both bonding and bridging social capital contribute to ignoring legal prohibitions. This appears to be because those respondents with strong bonding and bridging social capital appear to value and uphold *chhaupadi* because the practice is viewed as socially necessary, and as a caste related social norm that builds solidarity. One Nepalese woman explained that 'I follow it because my family members and ancestors followed it and it will bring bad luck to my family if I do not follow it and something bad will surely happen' (Amayta et al. 2018: 7).

The Experience of Chhaupadi

As the case study of Geeta and Ishu (Box 3) suggests, Nepali women and girls who practice *chhaupadi* experience a range of physical and mental impacts. The banishment to the *chhaupadi goth* or shed means that they are forced to live in unhygienic and exposed conditions. According to the beliefs about menstruation, women and girls are viewed as impure and unclean during menstruation and are not permitted to eat ghee (clarified butter), yoghurt, curd or drink milk. Instead, they are only permitted to eat a restricted range of foods, for example, flatbreads with salt. This deprives women and girls of a balanced diet and important nutrition during menstruation. In addition to prohibitions on foodstuffs, women and girls often are required to engage in physically demanding work during the period that they are effectively banished to the *chhaupadi* shed. For example, they undertake digging, collecting firewood and farm labour.

Although there are no accurate statistics, it is reported that women and girls staying in the *chhaupadi goth* die as the result of snake bites, scorpion stings or animal attacks. In addition, the sheds offer little or no protection from the weather, with some women being reported to have died of exposure. Whilst the women and girls are sent to the *chhaupadi* huts because they are viewed as impure, during their menstruation, they are also vulnerable to sexual assault. Isolated and removed from other houses, the women are unprotected, and research suggests that sexual assaults are not reported due to stigma associated with rape (UN 2011). Research suggests that women and girls are too afraid to sleep in the *chhaupadi goth* due to concerns about sexual assault or being bitten by snakes (Action Aid 2021). A female community health volunteer observed:

> the sheds are not secure and safe. They are small, with no proper ventilation, light, electricity and other necessities. There are many cases in which women have died of cold and suffocation. The things get worse in winter when the women light fires for heat inside the shed with no ventilation. Sanitation and hygiene is another problem. (Amayta et al. 2018: 10)

Women and girls practising *chhaupadi* report a range of physical and psychological problems. The unsanitary conditions of the *chhaupadi goth*, or shed, mean that they experience diarrhoea, dehydration and a range of reproductive and urinary tract infections. Research suggests that reproductive health problems, for example, itching in the genital region, painful and smelly menstruation, abnormal discharge and burning sensation when urinating, were significantly higher among women and girls practising *chhaupadi* than those not required to follow this practice (Ranabhat et al. 2015).

Legislation and Education

Sandbakken (2011) notes that the practice is directly linked to local cultural understandings and local power structures. Recognising the need to challenge these cultural practices, nongovernmental organisations (NGOs) have used drama and other public education approaches to make women and girls aware of their rights and to challenge social pressure to engage in the practice of *chhaupadi*.

Women's rights in Nepal have been slowly recognised. The protracted civil war between 1996 and 2006 impeded progress. However, in May 2005, the Supreme Court of Nepal banned the practice of *chhaupadi*. The Supreme Court issued the Government of Nepal with a directive to introduce laws to eliminate the practice throughout Nepal. The Interim Constitution of Nepal 2007, issued after the overthrow the royal government in 2006, set out the end of discrimination based on gender, and it sought to promote rights of equality and social justice, including caste discrimination. In theory, the Interim Constitution provided the legal basis for further state backed efforts to bring the practice of *chhaupadi* to an end. The Interim Constitution stated the following:

- There shall be no discrimination because of gender.
- Every woman shall have the right to reproductive health and reproduction.
- No physical, mental or other kind of act of violence shall be committed against any woman; and there shall be equal rights to parental property for sons and daughters.

However, *chhaupadi* continued to be practised, especially in far western districts of Nepal. Newspaper articles continued to report stories of women and girls sexually assaulted, bitten by snakes or dying from cold (Bhandaree et al. 2013). Importantly, the practice was identified as responsible for the high rate of uterine prolapse in women, a high rate of neonatal mortality (32 deaths per 1000) and a range of menstruation disorders (Bhandaree et al. 2013). In 2017, following the newspaper reports of three deaths of women and girls practising *chhaupadi* the Nepali Parliament introduced and enacted a new law to criminalise *chhaupadi* (Kathmandu Post 2017). The new law, which came into effect in August 2018, imposes a fine (3000 rupees) and/or a 3-month prison sentence for anybody forcing women or girls to follow the practices of *chhaupadi* (Preiss 2017). However, a local study in 2017 highlighted that up to 60% of people in Karnali, one of the Western districts, were unaware that the practice is illegal (Dahal et al. 2017).

Aligned to the legislation, the Nepal authorities, along with other member states of the South Asian Association of Regional Cooperation (Afghanistan, Bangladesh, Bhutan, India, Pakistan, the Maldives, Sri Lanka), responded to concerns over menstruation hygiene by committing to the Dhaka Declaration in 2016 (Sixth South Asian Conference on Sanitation, 2016). The Dhaka Declaration recognises the need to work to change social norms and behaviours that negatively impact on women and girls during menstruation.

In a recent study, Jun and Jang (2018), conducted in south-eastern Nepal highlighted the social aspects underlying the continued practice of *chhaupadi* despite the legislative measures by the Supreme Court and the Nepali Government. Their research suggests that the practice continues to be carried out based on social capital built and reinforced by tradition and social norms. The findings of their research suggest that 'government interventions should be geared toward reconceptualizing the prevailing norms around *chhaupadi*' (Jun and Jang 2018: 66).

One area that appears to be changing are attitudes around menstruation and attending school. It was believed that the goddess, Sarasvati, would become angry if a menstruating girl reads, writes or touches a book (UN 2011). In a recent study conducted in 2017, it was found that the number of girls attending school during their monthly cycle had significantly increased, possibly reflecting state and non-governmental emphasis on education (Amayta et al. 2018: 12).

Box 3 Case Study: Geeta and Ishu, Western Nepal

Geeta lives with her parents, aunt and nephew in a remote village in western Nepal. Although the practice of chhaupadi has been prohibited, it continues to be practised in her village. When she experienced her first period aged 11, Geeta was sent to a small mud hut, removed from her family home and village for 21 days. Unable to go to school, Geeta spent her days cleaning, sweeping and cutting grass. Since her menarche, she continues to spend 4 days each month on her own in the chhaupadi goth or menstruation hut or animal shed. She is not allowed to sleep in her own bed, to eat certain foods or touch her parents. Geeta does not like being sent to the hut. She is afraid of snakes and of being assaulted.

Her mother, Dhauli, believes in the practice of chhaupadi. She, like many of those living in remote rural communities, believes that if menstruating women and girls do not follow chhaupadi, the 'gods' will become angry and there will be serious consequences, for example, a poor harvest or livestock will become ill and die.

Ishu is 14 years old and is sent away from her home when her period starts. The hut where she stays has no windows and is very warm in summer but freezing in winter. To wash, she must walk 2 hours to wash in the nearest river. Lacking access to sanitary towels, Ishu uses rags which can cause serious infections. Her mother, Durga, is anxious for her safety when she is sent to the hut, particularly her vulnerability to sexual assault.

Source: Action Aid 2021 *Chhaupadi and menstruation taboos*.

Menarche and menstruation are universal features of women and girl's lives. As illustrated above, subtle and not so subtle forms of gender violence are experienced by women and girls following the onset of menarche. Tackling these forms of gender violence, particularly when embedded in social, cultural and religious practices, is challenging. However, the example of female-led initiatives to educate local communities, including other women, shows that such forms of gender violence can be challenged and open up the opportunity for girls and young women to access education and enable them to support their families.

Summary

- Although women, and girls, experience menarche and menstruation in similar physiological ways, how menarche and menstruation are perceived and understood varies across societies and cultures, reflecting a range of cultural and social factors.
- Whilst menstruation is viewed as morally neutral or ambivalent in some societies, menarche and menstruation are often represented as impure.
- As a result of the perceived impurity and pollution brought about by menarche and menstruation women are restricted in what they can do, eat and required to seclude or isolate themselves.
- In the widespread practice of *chhaupadi*, isolation makes Nepalese women and girls vulnerable to illness and to sexual assault.
- Activities to challenge local beliefs and to educate local communities about menstruation are more successful and meaningful than hard to enforce legal prohibitions.

References

Action Aid (2021) Chhaupadi and menstruation taboos. https://www.actionaid.org.uk/our-work/period-poverty/chhaupadi-and-menstruation-taboos Accessed 9 April 2021

Amayta P, Ghimire S, Callahn KE, Baral BK, Poudel KC (2018) Practice and lived experience of menstrual exiles (chhaudpai) among adolescent girls in far-western Nepal. PLoS One 13(2):e0208260. https://doi.org/10.1371/journal.pone.0208260

Asian Development Bank (1999) Country briefing paper: women in Nepal. ADB, Mandaluyong. https://www.adb.org/sites/default/files/instutional-document/32561/women-nepal.pdf. Accessed 6 Nov 2021

Bhandaree R, Pandey B, Rajak M, Pantha P (2013) Chhaupadi: victimizing women of Nepal. Sci Commit Rev:141–143

Bhandari S (2013) Cultural conceptions and silent acceptance of stereotypes: a critical study on Nepalese women's situation. Thesis, Master of Global Studies, Stavanger, Norway

Buckley T, Gottlieb A (1988) Blood magic: the anthropology of menstruation. University of California Press, Berkeley, CA

Dahal BP, Acharya S, Munakarmi R, Sunar T, Parajuli B (2017) Implementing status of national laws, policies, and guidelines – a study on situation of implementation status of national laws, policies and chhaupadi elimination guidelines in Karnali. Action Works Nepal & BEE Group, Nepal

Delany JM, Lupton MJ, Toth E (1977) The curse: a cultural history of menstruation. Mentor, New York, NY

Gottlieb A (2020) Menstrual taboos: moving beyond the curse. In: Bobel C et al (eds) The Palgrave handbook of critical menstruation studies. Palgrave Macmillan, Singapore

Guterman MA, Mehta, P and Gibbs, M (2007) Menstrual Taboos Among Major Religions. The Internet Journal of World Health and Societal Politics. 2007;5(2). https://ispub.com/IJWH/5/2/8213 Accessed 9 April 2021

House, S, Mahon, T and Cavill, S (2013) Menstrual Hygiene Matters: a resource for improving menstrual hygiene around the world. Co-published WaterAid and 17 other organisations, 2012, Reproductive Health Matters, 21(41):257–259.

Jun M, Jang I (2018) The role of social capital in shaping policy non-compliance for chhaupadi practice in Nepal. Asian Women 34(3):47–70.

Kathmandu Post (2017) 60 percent people unaware of Chhaupadi ban. Kathmandu Post 18 August. https://kathmandupost.com/national/2017/07/18/60-percent-people-in-karnali-unaware-of-chhaupadi-ban-report Accessed 10 April 2021

Khadka N (2020) Chhaupadi Pratha: women's experiences and perceptions about social suffering. Molung Educ Fron 10:81–92. (Special Issue)

Knight C (1996) Menstruation. In: Barnard A, Spencer J (eds) Encyclopaedia of social and cultural anthropology. Routledge, London

Lee J (2009) Bodies at Menarche: stories of shame, concealment and sexual maturation. Sex Roles 60(9–10):615–627

Menarche (2007) Shorter Oxford Dictionary. University of Oxford Press, Oxford, 1750

Mirvis TA (2020) Personal narrative: let girls be girls – my journey into forced womanhood. In: Bobel C et al (eds) The Palgrave handbook of critical menstruation studies. Palgrave Macmillan, Singapore

Narayanan V (2005) Gender and Priesthood in the Hindu Traditions. Journal of Hindu-Christian Studies, vol.18, 22–31

Paige JM and Paige, KE (1981) The Politics of Reproductive Ritual. University of California Press, Berkeley.

Preiss D (2017) Law in Nepal sets penalties for forcing a woman into a menstrual shed. National Public Radio. https://www.npr.org/sections/goatsandsoda/2017/08/10542585664/law-in-nepal-sets-penalites-for-forcing-a-woman-into-a-menstrual-shed. Accessed 10 Aug 2021

Ranabhat C, Kim CB, Choi EH, Aryal A, Partk MB (2015) Chhaupadi culture and reproductive health in women in Nepal. Asia Pac J Public Health 27:785–795

Robinson H (2015) Chaupadi: the afflictions of menses in Nepal. Int J Women's Dermatol 1:193–194

Rothchild J, Piya PS (2020) Rituals, taboos, and seclusion: life stories of women navigating culture and pushing for change in Nepal. In: Bobel C et al (eds) The Palgrave Handbook of critical menstruation studies. Palgrave Macmillan, Singapore

Sandbakken LD (2011) The Practice of Chhaupadi: the link between local cultural understanding and women's rights in rural Nepal. Norwegian University of Science and Technology, Norway

Selvi KT, Ramachandra S (2012) Socio-cultural taboos concerning menstruation: a micro level study in the Cuddalore district of Tamil Nadu, India. Int J Sci Res Publ 2(8):1–7

Sixth South Asian Conference on Sanitation (2016) Better sanitation better life. The Dhaka Declaration. http://www.endwaterpoverty.org.sites/default/files/oldfiles/SACOSAN_VI_declaration.pdf. Accessed 6 Nov 2021

Stubbs M (2008) Cultural perceptions and practices around menarche and adolescent menstruation in the United States. Ann N Y Acad Sci 1135:58–66

Thapa S, Aro AR (2021) Menstruation means impurity': multilevel interventions are needed to break the menstrual taboo in Nepal. BMC Womens Health 28(1):84

United Nations (2019) International Women's Day – 8 March 2019 women's menstrual health should no longer be a taboo. UN, New York, NY. http://www.ochr.org/EN/NewsEvents/Pages/DisplayNews.aspx?NewsID=24258&LangID=E. Accessed 7 Oct 2021

United Nations Resident and Humanitarian Coordinator's Office (2011) Field bulletin: chaupadi in the far west. http://www.ohchr.org/Documents/Issues/Water/ContributionsStigma/others/field_bulletin_issue1_april_2011_-_chaupadi_in_far_west.pdf. Accessed 9 Apr 2021

United Nations Resident and Humanitarian Coordinator's Office (2020) The Next Frontier: human development and the anthropocene: briefing note for countries on the 2020. Human Development Report, Nepal. http://hdr.undp.org/sites/default/files/Country-Profiles/NPL.pdf. Accessed 5 Nov 2021

Uskul AK (2004) Women's menarche stories from a multicultural sample. Soc Sci Med 59(4):667–679

Richard Whitecross, MA, LLB, LLM, PhD is Professor of Law at Edinburgh Napier University. His research areas include legal anthropology, specialising in South Asia and the Himalayas, citizenship, inequalities, access to justice and gender-based violence. He is currently conducting funded research on child contact and domestic abuse in the Scottish civil courts.

Spiritual Abuse and Gender-Based Violence

Emma Tomalin

Learning Objectives

Having read this chapter, you should be able to understand the following:

- Different types of spiritual abuse that take place in faith settings, the family and the public sphere
- The links between spiritual abuse and gender-based violence
- The pros and cons of using the term 'spiritual abuse'
- The benefits of promoting spiritual abuse as a recognised category alongside other types of abuse

Introduction

The term 'spiritual abuse' is often used interchangeably with religious abuse (Swindle 2017) and increasingly attracts the interest of scholars, faith actors and organisations with a mandate to protect and support people experiencing gender-based violence (GBV). Swindle suggests that there are three broad types: '(a) abuse perpetrated by religious leadership, typically an individual leader; (b) abuse

E. Tomalin (✉)
School of Philosophy, Religion and History of Science,
University of Leeds, Leeds, UK
e-mail: e.tomalin@leeds.ac.uk

P. Ali, M. M. Rogers (eds.), *Gender-Based Violence: A Comprehensive Guide*,
https://doi.org/10.1007/978-3-031-05640-6_24

perpetrated by a religious group, directed either towards an individual or towards a group of people and (c) abuse in which the abuse itself has a religious component to it' (Swindle 2017: 34). GBV, the topic of this volume, has psychological, physical and sexual dimensions and has been defined by the United Nations as referring to 'harmful acts directed at an individual based on their gender. It is rooted in gender inequality, the abuse of power and harmful norms'.[1]

As with GBV, power relations, including gender relations, play a key role in spiritual abuse where existing dynamics intensify and are intensified by the abuse. Women, children and the elderly are most often the targets. Spiritual abuse is predominantly, but not always, perpetrated by men in positions of authority within faith traditions, the family or the public sphere. As such, spiritual abuse is likely to also be a case of gender-based violence (GBV) where, I argue, all cases of religiously based gender discrimination amount to spiritual abuse, whether or not that label is used. The link between spiritual abuse and GBV is particularly acute since most religious traditions have strongly patriarchal elements justified by recourse to religious texts and teachings that maintain women's subordinate status to men and can therefore make women more vulnerable to spiritual abuse and less likely to challenge it. Moreover, most religious traditions are not only patriarchal but also heteronormative, therefore establishing a basis upon which to marginalise lesbian, gay, bisexual, transgender, queer and intersex (LGBTQI+) people, with the risk of psychological and physical and sexual abuse that is justified with respect to normative teachings upheld by the tradition. This includes gay conversion therapy promoted by some faith groups (Greenough 2018).

The chapter begins with a discussion about researching and defining spiritual abuse. It follows with an examination of the pros and cons of using the label and concerns that the lack of recognition of it as a separate category of abuse makes it difficult for statutory agencies and third sector organisations to address it. Next, literature about and approaches to spiritual abuse is examined in three main areas: within faith settings, within the family and within the public sphere. Finally, the chapter concludes with a discussion of why it is important for spiritual abuse to be more widely recognised as a specific type of GBV.

Researching and Defining Spiritual Abuse

Oakley et al. (2018: 3) mentions that spiritual abuse 'is a relatively new term in literature, policy and discourse' with one of the first texts in this area being Johnson and VanVonderen's 1991 text *The Subtle Power of Spiritual Abuse* (2005). The term originated in the USA and then spread to other areas including Australia and the UK. Earlier material on the topic also exists but does not explicitly use the term

[1] https://www.unhcr.org/uk/gender-based-violence.html#:~:text=Gender%2DBased%20violence%20refers%20to,threatening%20health%20and%20protection%20issue.

spiritual abuse (e.g. Plowman 1975). With respect to religious traditions outside of Christianity and in non-Global North settings, the term is less frequently used, although this does not mean that the practices it points to are absent. Increasingly, the term is used for a wider range of faith traditions and contexts. For instance, the organisation *In Shaykh's Clothing* was founded in North America in 2010 'to help Muslims understand and recover from spiritual abuse', and in 2019, it published *The Code of Conduct of Islamic Leadership* with guidance about how to avoid spiritual abuse.[2]

Before one starts labelling social phenomena as spiritual abuse, it must be remembered that this is a subjective and political act, and one needs to ask who is involved in making the decisions about what is included and what is left out, and when and why the label is used. A large amount of the literature on spiritual abuse is either by or about people who claim to have experienced spiritual abuse at the hands of previously trusted authority figures. However, what is experienced as spiritual abuse by some people, others might understand to be a legitimate and desired part of engaging in a spiritual path where teachings and actions are intended to challenge the individual to transcend their normal state of being and to engage in activities that might be physically and psychologically uncomfortable or painful. Additionally, just as the term 'cult' is widely perceived to be a derogatory label, where Harrison argues 'Labeling a group a cult is a cowardly way of tolerating, condoning, appeasing, or promoting favored religions while simultaneously rejecting and disparaging a minority religion' (2016), there a danger that the term spiritual abuse might be used by those who are hostile to certain spiritual practices and traditions.

Reflecting this complexity, in 2018, the Evangelical Alliance published a report critiquing the term spiritual abuse, rather than the practices it encompasses, 'because of its own inherent ambiguity, and also because attempts by some to embed it within statutory safeguarding discourse and secular law would be unworkable in practice, potentially discriminatory towards religious communities, and damaging to interfaith relations' (Evangelical Alliance 2018: 1; Goodwin 2020). Relatedly, some people might feel uneasy about labelling certain practices as spiritual abuse from not wanting to reinforce supremacist or racist stereotypes or to be seen as interfering in and judging other cultural and religious traditions.

While these considerations are valid, others highlight as problematic that 'spiritual abuse' is not formally recognised by third sector and statutory bodies in the UK or internationally as a category of abuse that has distinctive attributes that may require special knowledge and strategies (Gatiss 2019). Oakley and Kinmond (2014) suggest that although some Christian churches are beginning to take it seriously as part of their safeguarding duties, the attention it receives is sparse and often confined to the ways that it impacts children. Despite the growing interest in spiritual abuse, there is no agreed upon definition nor what should be included in its scope, yet as Oakley et al. write, 'a clear, shared definition is surely required for a

[2] https://inshaykhsclothing.com/about-our-code-of-conduct-of-islamic-spiritual-leaders/.

positive movement forward in research, understanding, awareness, policy and practice' (2018: 4). For instance, Oakley and Kinmond (2013: 25) confine their definition of spiritual abuse to its emotional and psychological dimensions and define it as follows:

> coercion and control of one individual by another in a spiritual context. The target experiences spiritual abuse as a deeply emotional personal attack. This abuse may include: manipulation and exploitation, enforced accountability, censorship of decision making, requirements for secrecy and silence, pressure to conform, misuse of scripture or the pulpit to control behaviour, requirement of obedience to the abuser, the suggestion that the abuser has a 'divine' position, isolation from others, especially those external to the abusive context.

By contrast, Swindle finds this definition too vague and narrow since 'there is no attention given to physical or sexual abuse in a religious setting' (2017: 40). Accounts within the wider literature support both Oakley and Kinmond's exclusive definition and Swindle's more inclusive approach, with survivors reporting experience of the psychological damage they have experienced as well as sexual and physical abuse in religious settings. Gatiss (2019) attempts to provide some clarification in highlighting the specific nature of spiritual abuse as opposed to other types, arguing that 'the "spiritual" aspect … is the context of the abuse'. However, if by spiritual context one means a faith setting such as a place of worship or religious community, then instances where spiritual abuse takes place outside faith settings such as in the family are missed out. Perhaps how one defines it depends on the purpose of one's analysis, with Gatiss writing about the 'Church of England's definitions of "spiritual abuse", and how it can be avoided' (2019) and Oakley and Kinmond (2013) wanting to highlight the need for a specific category of spiritual abuse that can sit alongside other definitions of abuse in policy settings.

Box 1 Types of Spiritual Abuse

Spiritual abuse within a faith setting

- Where scripture or beliefs are used to humiliate or embarrass
- Where there is coercion to give money or other resources
- Where force is used to be intimate or to have sex
- Where there is pressure or obligation to do things against one's will[3]

[3] https://www.webmd.com/mental-health/signs-spiritual-abuse.

Spiritual abuse in the family

- Where religious beliefs or practices are ridiculed
- Where the free practice of religion is prevented
- Where beliefs are to manipulate or bully
- Where it is demanded that children be raised with/without a certain religion
- Where religious texts or beliefs are used justify other kinds of abuse (physical, sexual, financial, etc.)[4]

Spiritual abuse in public settings

- Where the state discriminates against people because of their religion, using threats of or actual violence
- Where public/private institutions (e.g. schools, prisons, workplaces) discriminates against people because of their religion
- Where individual perpetrators use faith to coerce people to engage in activities they would otherwise have not participated in

In the following sections, the literature that focuses on different types of spiritual abuse within faith settings, within the family and within public settings (see Box 1) is discussed, while recognising that these are not clearly demarcated domains.

Spiritual Abuse Within Faith Settings

Many of the first-hand survivor accounts of spiritual abuse relate to faith settings, including places of worship and their associated communities; religious communities where trained religious specialists or those seeking to train or ordain in a religious tradition live; retreat centres or religious classes and religious schools. The trust placed in faith leaders can bring many positive outcomes, but where the power imbalance is abused or where the views and advice of faith leaders are ill informed, the consequences can be disastrous. Several extreme examples of spiritual abuse that have led to mass violence are well known. These include the famous 'Jonestown Massacre' where the Rev Jim Jones ordered over 900 of his followers to commit mass suicide at their temple in Guyana (Barker 1986) and the deadly Sarin attack on Tokyo's subway in 1995 by members of the new Buddhist movement Aum Shinrikyo (Reader 2000).

[4] https://www.thehotline.org/resources/what-is-spiritual-abuse/.

The majority of books written for a general audience originate from the USA and look at spiritual abuse in Christian Churches as well as 'cults'. These include books by and about survivors, self-help books and books written for pastors and church institutions about how to avoid spiritual abuse (Blue 1993; Diederich 2017; Johnson and VanVonderen 2005 [1991]; Langone 1995; Oakley and Humphreys 2019; Orlowski 2010). There is also a body of literature that has grown rapidly, no doubt under the impact of the #MeToo movement, looking at abuse scandals within Tibetan Buddhism, particularly with respect to the Lamas/teachers Chogyam Trungpa (Chandler 2019) and Sogyal Rinpoche (Finnigan and Hogendoorn 2019). Some yoga teachers have also attracted high numbers of Western female devotees, although men are sometimes also affected, who experienced abuse at the hands of trusted gurus and yogis. These include Yogi Bhajan (Dyson 2020; Ellis-Petersen 2018) and Bikram Choudhury, the founder of Bikram or 'hot' yoga (Delaney 2019), also the topic of a 2019 Netflix documentary *Bikram: Yogi, Guru, Predator*.[5]

Another prominent manifestation is the spiritual abuse of LGBTQI+ people in faith settings. This can include psychological and emotional damage inflicted by the message that their sexuality is immoral and should be kept hidden, to damaging conversion therapy and rituals that aim to 'cure' people of their queer identity, carried out by faith groups as well as healthcare professionals (Yates and Snodgrass 2019; Craig et al. 2017). In settings where it has not yet been banned, there are campaigns to make conversion therapy illegal, including in the UK (Parker and Lawrie 2021).

Abuse in faith settings impacts children as well as adults. For instance, cases of abuse within religious institutions was one of the major areas of focus of the *Australian Royal Commission into Institutional Responses to Child Sexual Abuse*, set up in 2012. As McPhillips explains 'religious institutions are treated as "special" institutions in Australian public life' which means that they enjoy 'certain legal, cultural and economic privileges legitimated by the state … embedded in the constitutional right to freedom of religious belief and expression' (2020: 3). This includes the recognition that 'religious organisations have jurisdiction over internal matters, including … responses to allegations of child sexual abuse' (2020: 3–4). Although since the Royal Commission Report was published in 2017, several states have put in laws to prevent this; some faith actors have refused to cooperate arguing that it is a restriction of their religious freedom. This is particularly the case with respect to requirements to report all allegations of child sexual abuse to the authorities, which could break the sacred bond of the Catholic confessional when such crimes are admitted to a priest (2020: 10).

Another area involving religion and child sexual abuse was the satanic ritual abuse scandal of the 1980s/1990s. The first major case that came to public attention was via a book published in the USA called *Michelle Remembers* (1980), which, as Goodwin writes, was 'a first-hand account of Michelle Smith's memories of captivity, torture and molestation by a group of devil worshipping cultists' (2020: 283).

[5] https://www.netflix.com/gb/title/80221584.

There are many books that have been written on the so-called 'satanic panic', particularly from the point of view of survivors and therapists, undergirding a widespread belief that individual cases were part of larger organised networks. Journalist Rosie Waterhouse reports in her PhD thesis on the topic that she was 'tasked to investigate the evidence for the existence of Satanic ritual abuse' by the UK newspaper she worked for at the time, *The Independent* (Waterhouse 2014: 31). Her research revealed 'two polarised camps—with believers who were campaigners, therapists, social workers and "survivors" on one side, and sceptics including criminal investigators and academics on the other' (2014: 40). Waterhouse, with others, concluded that there was no evidence for ritual child abuse and that instead certain 'claims-makers' and a globalised media were spreading myths about this to serve their own ends (2014: 41). There was also evidence that the therapeutic process was instrumental in the phenomenon of false memory syndrome (Waterhouse 2014: 16). Others, however, are critical that the dominance of discourses about ritual satanic child abuse being a fabrication have meant that genuine accounts have not been taken seriously (Scott 2001).

More recently, social services, medical practitioners and the police in the Global North have become aware of a form of child abuse where children are trafficked from their homes in Africa for witchcraft or *juju* rituals, where 'they are exposed to violent and degrading treatments, often involving the forced extraction of their blood to be used for clients demanding blood rituals' (Rogers 2011; Nagle and Owasanoye 2016). While this form of spiritual abuse is often initiated by religious specialists, family members can also be complicit in facilitating it for financial gain or because they have been coerced themselves through spiritual abuse. A report by the UK organisation AFRUCA, which works in 'BME communities to protect and safeguard children from abuse and harm',[6] explores the branding of African immigrant children as witches by 'rogue faith leaders', who resort to this as a means of helping families address a range of stressful issues around 'job loss, unemployment, business failures, immigration problems, miscarriages and illnesses' through blaming the position that they find themselves in on the possession of their children by spirits (AFRUCA 2020: 3). This is a situation then that can be dealt with through 'deliverance' rituals that may involve emotional, physical and sexual abuse of children by faith leaders.

Spiritual Abuse Within the Family

Simonic et al. (2013) explore religious-related abuse in the family, which often overlaps with and reinforces spiritual abuse in faith settings, outlining two main types. The first type is where the abuser 'turns to theological explanations and reasoning as grounds for physical abuse of their partner or punishment of their children' (2013: 349). The second type is where religion can be used as a form of

[6] https://afruca.org/.

emotional abuse, 'whereby spreading fear instilling religious beliefs triggers feelings of fear, guilt and shame in the abused individuals, ultimately making them feel alone, distressed, worthless, neglected or even cursed' (2013: 349). Often it is the case that these forms of violence have a gender dimension, and a number of publications focus specifically on the links between religion and GBV in the family (e.g. Nienhuis and Kienzle 2018; Davis and Johnson 2021; Cares and Cusick 2012; Dorff 2015; Dehan and Levi 2009), while others draw attention to the important role that religious leaders and faith communities can play in addressing GBV, particularly when it has religious underpinnings (Roux et al. 2016; Oakley and Kinmond 2016).

A specific example of spiritual abuse in the family is found in cases of the so-called forced marriage, where religion/spirituality is used to coerce individuals into marriages that they otherwise would not have consented to. Forced marriage is not the same as arranged marriage, as by definition the latter is considered to be freely consented to. The pressure to marry can include physical threats and violence as well as emotional and psychological manipulation to make people feel that, by not consenting, they are letting their family or community down. As Klug (2019) notes, LGBTQI+ people can also be vulnerable to forced marriage where heteronormativity dominates in religious families and communities. Forced marriage was made illegal in the UK in 2014, and the government is currently debating raising the legal age of marriage from 16 to 18, to avoid the forced marriage of younger people (Price 2021). However, given the thin line between forced and arranged marriages, the law can be difficult to enforce. While forced marriage is often seen as a harmful traditional or cultural practice that mainly impacts communities who follow Hinduism, Islam and Sikhism, it is also found across other faith traditions, including Christianity, particularly branches of evangelicalism and within Orthodox Jewish communities (Anitha and Gill 2009; Kuruvilla 2017; Rocker 2021). However, in the case of forced marriage, it is not that act per se that is sanctioned by the religious tradition, but instead recourse to religion is used to bring about compliance. Given the gender imbalance within religions, women and girls find that challenging this is particularly hard.

Spiritual Abuse Within the Public Sphere

The final category of spiritual abuse that I will address occurs within the public sphere carried out by the state, public and private institutions and individual perpetrators. First, it is not uncommon for national governments to discriminate against people because of their religion, including implementing laws that curtail religious freedom. One example of this are laws banning Muslim women wearing the veil in public, currently the case in France, for instance (Pahl 2019). Although I have not so far encountered this being described as a form of spiritual abuse, to deny people the right to fully practice their religion amounts to this. This case of spiritual abuse affects women and can exacerbate against women in minority faith communities in settings already wrought with religio-racial tensions. As Pahl writes, 'anti-hijab laws … share one consequence: stoking public animosity against Muslim women …

headscarf bans stigmatize and potentially even stoke violence as a form of discrimination against women' (2019: 728). Conversely, however, states that make wearing the veil a legal requirement are also guilty of spiritual abuse in using where 'coercive … to enforce specific standards of dress and conduct for women' (2019: 728).

Second, there are examples where people experience spiritual abuse within public and private institutions, including schools, prisons and workplaces, with equalities and human rights legislation often being ineffective. For instance, writing about spiritual/religious abuse at the Guantinamo Bay detention centre towards Muslim men, Anderson quotes from a 2003 Washington Post article that 'some … complained that American soldiers insulted Islam by sitting on the Koran or dumping their sacred text into a toilet to taunt them' (2011: 759). This abuse was perpetrated by both male and female soldiers, who also used forms of sexual humiliation that went against international human rights guidelines in violating 'fundamental cultural and religious taboos against public nudity' (Fletcher and Stover 2008: 76).

A third type of spiritual abuse within the public sphere is where individual perpetrators use faith to coerce people to engage in activities. Heil (2017) explores how human traffickers use religion as a tool of coercion through 'spiritual abuse'. One of her examples involves a 12-year-old girl from Niger who 'was subjected to both labor and sex trafficking, which was legitimized through culture intertwined with religion' (2017: 52). Although the girl was theoretically protected by law from slavery, Heil suggests that 'regional interpretations of the teachings of Islam' play a role where it is believed that slavery is consistent with Islamic teachings and traffickers assert control through 'transcendental threats of not obeying the master' (2017: 53, 54). Heil also writes about the use of witchcraft and *juju* rituals as a tool to traffic women from Nigeria and other African countries where they are 'forced to take oaths, with body hair, nails, and underwear left on shrines to remind the victims that if they run away, the gods will cause them harm' (2017: 58). In these cases, the 'trafficker has completely stripped the victim of free will when the threat is religious in nature, for the victim already is in a position of unconditional compliance to their belief system. The victim truly believes that it is God's will for them to obey his/her oppressor' (2017: 60).

The above three sections examine spiritual abuse in faith settings, the family and the public sphere, against the backdrop of the absence of the recognition of 'spiritual abuse' as a distinctive form of violence by third sector and statutory bodies in the UK and internationally.

Summary

- Spiritual abuse occurs within faith settings and the family and the wider public sphere.
- Spiritual abuse is identical to GBV since it is mostly perpetrated by men taking advantage of the patriarchy and heteronormativity of religious traditions to suit their interests. Women can also carry out spiritual abuse, but even in these cases, the vulnerability of survivors is compounded by gender inequality.

- The term spiritual abuse is viewed by some as controversial and potentially damaging and that to single out some forms in this way risks reinforcing existing racial and cultural bias (Evangelical Alliance 2018). At the same time, others argue that without such a category, some forms of abuse may be missed, and therefore specialist strategies and solutions to deal with them overlooked (Davis and Johnson 2021).
- When adopting this label, scholars and practitioners need to be reflexive and cautious but that naming some forms of abuse as spiritual or religious is a helpful strategy that will promote a wider consideration of the context for abuse that leads to GBV. This will increase understanding of the motivations and means of perpetrators as well as how abuse is experienced and challenged from the perspective of survivors.

References

Anderson MS (2011) Free exercise, establishment and statutory provisions at guantanamo. Columbia J. Transnatl. Law 49(3):755–783

Anitha S, Gill A (2009) Coercion, consent and the forced marriage debate in the UK. Fem Leg Stud 17:165–184

AFRUCA (2020) Exploring Child Witchcraft Abuse In BME Families Before and During COVID 19 Pandemic. AFRUCA Briefing Paper 4: COVID 19. https://afruca.org/briefing2

Barker E (1986) Religious movements: cult and anticult since Jonestown. Annu Rev Sociol 12(1):329–346

Blue KM (1993) Healing spiritual abuse: how to break free from bad church experiences. IVP Books, Downers Grove, IL

Cares AC, Cusick GR (2012) Risks and opportunities of faith and culture: the case of abused Jewish women. J Fam Violence 27:427–435

Chandler C (2019) Enthralled: the Guru Cult of Tibetan Buddhism. Bookbaby, North Charleston, SC

Craig SL, Austin A, Rashidi M, Adams A (2017) Fighting for survival: the experiences of lesbian, gay, bisexual, transgender, and questioning students in religious colleges and universities. J Gay Lesbian Soc Serv 29(1):1–24

Davis M, Johnson M (2021) Exploring black clergy perspectives on religious/spiritual related domestic violence: first steps in facing those who wield the sword abusively. J. Aggress. Maltreatment Trauma 30:7;950–971. https://doi.org/10.1080/10926771.2020.1738615

Dehan N, Levi Z (2009) Spiritual abuse: an additional dimension of abuse experienced by Abused Haredi (Ultraorthodox) Jewish Wives. Viol Against Women 15(11):1294–1310

Delaney B (2019) He made a fortune from his trademarked Bikram yoga, but now his empire is in tatters. Guardian. https://www.theguardian.com/tv-and-radio/2019/dec/03/he-made-a-fortune-from-his-trademarked-bikram-yoga-but-now-his-empire-is-in-tatters#:~:text=From%20his%20base%20in%20Los,of%20rape%20and%20sexual%20assault.&text=Choudhury%20was%20sued%20by%20former,against%20racial%20and%20sexual%20minorities

Diederich FR (2017) Broken Trust: a practical guide to identify and recover from toxic faith, toxic church, and spiritual abuse, vol 4. CreateSpace Independent Publishing Platform, Scotts Valley, CA

Dorff EN (2015) A conservative Jewish approach to family violence. In: Johnson AJ (ed) Religion and men's violence against women. Springer, New York, NY, pp 117–132

Dyson PS (2020) Premka: white bird in a golden cage: my life with Yogi Bhajan. Eyes Wide Publishing, Maui, Hawaii

Ellis-Petersen H (2018) 'Under Swami's spell': 14 tourists claim sexual assault by guru at Thai yoga retreat. Guardian. https://www.theguardian.com/world/2018/sep/07/under-swamis-spell-14-tourists-claim-sexual-assault-by-guru-at-thai-yoga-retreat

Evangelical Alliance (2018) Reviewing the discourse of 'spiritual abuse' logical problems & unintended consequences. A report. Evangelical Alliance Theology Advisory Group. https://www.eauk.org/current-affairs/media/press-releases/upload/Reviewing-the-Discourse-of-Spiritual-Abuse.pdf

Finnigan M, Hogendoorn R (2019) Sex and violence in Tibetan Buddhism: the rise and fall of Sogyal Rinpoche. Jorvik Press, Portland, OR

Fletcher LE, Stover E (2008) Guantánamo and Its Aftermath: detention and interrogation practices and their impact on former detainees. Human Rights Center and International Human Rights Law Clinic, University of California, Berkeley, CA. https://www.law.berkeley.edu/files/IHRLC/Guantanamo_and_Its_Aftermath.pdf

Gatiss L (2019) What is spiritual abuse? Anglican Link. https://anglican.ink/2019/07/23/what-is-spiritual-abuse/

Goodwin M (2020) Abusing religion: literary persecution, sex scandals, and American Minority Religions. Rutgers University Press, New Brunswick, NJ

Greenough C (2018) Some Christian groups still promote 'gay conversion therapy' – but their influence is waning. The Conversation. https://theconversation.com/some-christian-groups-still-promote-gay-conversion-therapy-but-their-influence-is-waning-91523

Harrison G (2016) Why no one should ever use the word "cult". Psychol Today. https://www.psychologytoday.com/gb/blog/about-thinking/201607/why-no-one-should-ever-use-the-word-cult

Heil EC (2017) It is God's will: exploiting religious beliefs as a means of human trafficking. Crit Res Relig 5(1):48–61

Johnson D, VanVonderen J (2005 [1991]) Subtle power of spiritual abuse, the: recognizing and escaping spiritual manipulation and false spiritual authority within the church. Bethany House Publishers, Minneapolis, MN, Repackaged edition.

Klug P (2019) Early or forced marriages at the intersection of religion, gender and the state. The Woolf Institute, Cambridge. https://www.woolf.cam.ac.uk/blog/early-or-forced-marriages-at-the-intersection-of-religion-gender-and-the-state

Kuruvilla C (2017) In some evangelical circles, grown men pursuing teens isn't all that unusual. HuffPost. https://www.huffpost.com/entry/roy-moore-evangelicalism_n_5a05f4f8e4b0e37d2f37573d

Langone MD (1995) Recovery from cults: help for victims of psychological and spiritual abuse. W. W. Norton & Company, New York, NY

McPhillips K (2020) Religion after the royal commission: challenges to religion state relations. Religions 11:1–13

Nagle LE, Owasanoye B (2016) Fearing the Dark: the use of witchcraft to control human trafficking victims and sustain vulnerability. Southw Law Rev 45:561–593

Nienhuis N, Kienzle BM (2018) Saintly women: medieval saints, modern women, and intimate partner violence. Routledge, London; New York, NY

Oakley L, Kinmond K (2016) The relationship between spiritual abuse and domestic violence and abuse in faith-based communities. In: Hilder S, Bettinson V. (eds) DomesticViolence. Palgrave Macmillan, London, pp. 203–225. https://doi.org/10.1057/978-1-137-52452-2_10

Oakley L, Humphreys J (2019) Escaping the maze of spiritual abuse: creating healthy Christian cultures. SPCK, London

Oakley LR, Kinmond K (2013) Breaking the silence on spiritual abuse. Palgrave, Basingstoke

Oakley LR, Kinmond KS (2014) Developing safeguarding policy and practice for spiritual abuse. J Adult Protect 16(2):87–95

Oakley LR, Kinmond KS, Humphreys J (2018) Spiritual abuse in Christian faith settings: definition, policy and practice guidance. J Adult Protect 20(3/4):144–154

Orlowski BM (2010) Spiritual abuse recovery: dynamic research on finding a place of wholeness. Wipf and Stock, Eugene, OR

Pahl JE (2019) Violence implicit in hijab suppression laws in Uzbekistan, Tajikistan, and France under the CEDAW framework. Wash Law Rev 28(3):727–762

Parker J, Lawrie W (2021) Conversion therapy ban: campaigners dismayed over delay. BBC News. https://www.bbc.co.uk/news/health-57059459. Accessed 30 Jun 2021

Plowman EE (1975) The deepening rift in the charismatic movement. Christ Today:65–66

Price E (2021) Under-18 marriages "thriving" in UK and should be banned, say charities. BBC News. https://www.bbc.co.uk/news/uk-56982309

Reader IJ (2000) Religious violence in contemporary Japan: the case of Aum Shinrikyo. Curzon Press, Richmond

Rocker S (2021) Call to stop forced marriages in the Jewish community. The Jewish Chronicle. https://www.thejc.com/news/uk/call-to-stop-forced-marriages-in-the-jewish-community-1.511606

Rogers C (2011) African children trafficked to UK for blood rituals. BBC News. https://www.bbc.co.uk/news/uk-15280776

Roux E, Kramm N, Scott N, Sandilands M, Loots L, Olivier J, Arango D, O'Sullivan V (2016) Getting dirty: working with faith leaders to prevent and respond to gender-based violence. Rev Faith Int Affairs 14:22–35

Scott S (2001) The politics and experience of ritual abuse: beyond disbelief. Open University Press, Buckingham

Simonic B, Mandelj TR, Novsak R (2013) Religious-related abuse in the family. J Fam Violence 28:339–349

Smith M, Pazder L (1980) Michelle remembers. Congdon & Lattes, New York, NY

Swindle PJ (2017) A twisting of the sacred: the lived experience of religious abuse. PhD thesis. The University of North Carolina at Greensboro (UNCG). https://libres.uncg.edu/ir/uncg/f/Swindle_uncg_0154D_12186.pdf

Waterhouse RT (2014) Satanic abuse, false memories, weird beliefs and moral panics. PhD thesis. City University London. https://core.ac.uk/download/pdf/42628845.pdf

Yates J, Snodgrass JL (2019) The religious locations of LGBTQ+ survivors: survivors of Christian nonsexual spiritual abuse. In: Snodgrass JL (ed) Navigating religious difference in spiritual care and counseling, essays in honor of Kathleen J. Greider. Claremont Press, Claremont, CA, pp 251–280

Emma Tomalin is Professor of Religion and Public Life at the University of Leeds. Her research focuses on the role of religion in society, including how it impacts gender inequality in both the public and private spheres.

Wartime Violence and Intimate Partner Violence

Romina Istratii

Learning Objectives
Having read this chapter, you should be able to understand:

- The relationship between wartime violence and intimate partner violence.
- Explanatory theories, prevalence rates, and risk factors.
- Women's perceptions and experiences of intimate partner violence and their responses to it in conflict and post-conflict time and in displaced contexts.
- How interventions may be designed to respond to partner abuse in conflict and post-conflict time.

Introduction

This chapter discusses the relationship between wartime and intimate partner violence (IPV), focusing on women's perspectives and experiences of the effects of war on their partners and the family context (see Box 1 for definitions). The chapter draws heavily from a recent review that examined the international evidence on the relationship between wartime violence, including sexual and gender-based violence

R. Istratii (✉)
School of History, Religions and Philosophies, SOAS University of London, London, UK
e-mail: ri5@soas.ac.uk

P. Ali, M. M. Rogers (eds.), *Gender-Based Violence: A Comprehensive Guide*,
https://doi.org/10.1007/978-3-031-05640-6_25

(SGBV), and IPV to inform responses in the humanitarian sector (see Box 2).[1] Violence affecting women in wartime and in post-conflict includes (a) violence from strangers and militant elements, including sexual violence, abduction, sexual exploitation, and torture, (b) violence from spouses or intimate romantic partners, and (c) violence from the community, such as when a person's wartime victimisation is not recognised by others in their surroundings causing their re-traumatisation or interfering with their rehabilitation in post-conflict society.

While the evidence review on which this chapter is based was limited to IPV to exclude parent-child or child-parent violence and violence from other relatives, studies that referred to effects on children through war-related partner violence were included. The review engaged only with studies in English and examined IPV within military populations (soldiers and veterans); civilian populations affected by war, including ex-combatants; and refugee and displaced populations. Studies were drawn primarily from North America, Africa, Latin America, the Levant, and South Asia and areas of the world that have documented conflict in recent decades, such as Northern Ireland. The large majority were quantitative cross-sectional studies, population surveys, and statistical and econometric analyses. A relatively lower number were qualitative and ethnographic studies that incorporated women's perspectives and providers' experiences of supporting victims and survivors of war-related violence, which this chapter has placed emphasis on.

Box 1 Definitions of Key Terms

Definition: Wartime Violence

Wartime violence refers to violence experienced or witnessed during war or conflict and could be perpetrated by militant elements from any of the warring sides and combatants recruited from the general population. War violence may include physical violence and injury, torture, death, abduction, sexual and gender-based violence (SGBV), genocidal violence, as well as witnessing any of these forms of violence with implications for one's psychological wellbeing.

Alternative Terminology

War violence, Conflict violence, Political violence.

Definition: Intimate Partner Violence

Intimate partner violence (IPV) is violence experienced between intimate romantic partners who cohabitate either under a formal marital union or a more irregular union arrangement. It can include various forms of violence, such as physical, psychological, emotional, financial, and spiritual violence.

Alternative Terminology

Spousal violence, Conjugal violence, Marital violence.

[1] This essay repeats some of the content of the working paper 'War and domestic violence: A rapid scoping of the international literature to understand the relationship and to inform current responses in the Tigray humanitarian crisis' authored by Dr. Romina Istratii and published by project dldl/ድልድል. The content is reproduced with permission of the author and the original publisher, https://projectdldl.org/.

Box 2 Geographical Focus of Previous Studies

Study Locations

Rwanda, Uganda, Liberia, Sierra Leone, Democratic Republic of the Congo (DRC), South Africa, Timor-Leste, Cote d'Ivoire, Papua New Guinea, Sri Lanka, Afghanistan, occupied Palestinian territory, Lebanon, Colombia, Peru, Northern Ireland, former Yugoslavia.

Historical Context

While the relationship between wartime violence and IPV received limited attention historically, this has changed in recent decades as new evidence emerged to establish close associations between different forms of violence. This evidence documents direct associations between exposure to political violence (either directly as a perpetrator or victim or indirectly as a witness of violence or loss of relatives) and an increased likelihood of victims, survivors, and perpetrators experiencing or resorting to violence in the domestic sphere as a consequence of their exposure to wartime violence. The review pointed to four types of studies comprising the current evidence:

1. Studies that explored the relationship of war and IPV within military and civilian populations.
2. Studies that related SGBV to IPV in refugee camps, displaced contexts, and refugee populations.
3. Studies that applied a gender-sensitive or feminist lens to conflict and post-conflict violence.
4. Studies that examined the consequences of war on family violence and children's wellbeing.

Reviewing the available evidence suggested that interest in the sector transitioned from a focus on IPV in military populations to looking at the effects of war violence in civilian populations and wider communities. Studies on SGBV distinguish themselves by drawing attention to the interlinkages between wartime violence, and specifically conflict-related SGBV, and society-wide gender norms and violence existing prior to conflict.

Explanatory Approaches

The existing scholarship points to a multi-dimensional mechanism that connects political violence to violence committed by intimate partners, such as through:

- Mental health trauma affecting victims, survivors, or perpetrators of war-related violence, which can influence their behaviour with intimate partners.

- Direct effects on the behaviour of soldiers and veterans, including abusing alcohol and substances or reduced ability to regulate emotions in situations of stress that include situations of conflict with their intimate partners.
- Socio-cultural influences and normative frameworks contributing to further the abuse of war victims and survivors in post-conflict.
- The breakdown of structures, support systems, and community solidarity that would be available to victims and survivors of domestic or other forms of violence in peacetime.

Feminist perspectives distinguish themselves by seeing violence as a continuum, with war-related sexual violence and its consequences on the domestic sphere being thought to be exacerbated by pre-existing socio-cultural ideals of sexuality and gendered standards of behaviour within marriage, the breakdown of law fostering impunity, and the militarisation of the private sphere in post-conflict contexts (Davies and True 2015). Moreover, conflict-related violence is seen as being interlinked with SGBV and the vulnerabilities women and girls experience during flight from a conflict zone and during displacement, reinforcing an understanding of violence as a continuous threat (Krause 2015).

Prevalence Rates

Military Populations

The general evidence shows that IPV in military populations is higher than in the civilian population, although this evidence is disproportionately informed by research with western populations. The most recent systematic review of studies that measured IPV in military populations reported that all studies had been conducted in the USA, with one being from Canada (Kwan et al. 2020). Thirty of a total of 42 studies reported prevalence of physical IPV ranging between 5% and 57.6%. Fifteen studies were included in a meta-analysis, resulting in a pooled prevalence rate of 26%, which was higher than the reported prevalence rates for US civilians (between 4% and 15%). A study that explored the relationship between a soldier's length of deployment and the probability of spousal violence during a 1-year period found that the probability of self-reporting severe aggressive behaviour was more significant for soldiers who had been deployed in the past year than those who had not (McCarroll et al. 2010). Moreover, the length of deployment seemed to have a small, but statistically significant, effect on severe spousal abuse.

Civilian Populations

In general, studies report a significant positive relationship between IPV frequency and exposure to war-related violence. A study that tested the relationship involving multiple sub-Saharan African countries established an independent and significant effect of conflict and a woman's risk of IPV and other forms of SGBV in her home region (Østby 2016).

Reports from studies on individual countries in other parts of the world reinforce these findings. A study from the occupied Palestinian territory reported that women whose partners were exposed to political violence were nearly twice as likely to experience physical and sexual violence compared with those whose partners were not directly exposed (Clark et al. 2010). A study from Colombia reinforced these findings and furthermore found that the intensity of war-related violence increased the risk of women being abused by partners, with the highest estimates showing over 12 percentage points of higher incidence in an intensely conflict-affected environment (Noe and Rieckmann 2013).

Displaced Populations

A systematic review on prevalence rates of sexual and gender-based violence in complex emergency contexts found that IPV rates ranged between 3% and 52%, which were higher than most of the reported rates of wartime rape and sexual violence perpetrated by strangers (Stark and Ager 2011). A study that measured SGBV incidence rates in camps hosting internally displaced persons in Northern Uganda estimated an overall incidence of IPV in the past year of 51.7% (based on respondents' estimates), 44% (based on respondents' sisters' estimates), and 36.5% (based on respondents' neighbours' estimates) (Stark et al. 2010). The study also found a high incidence of forced sex by husbands, but relatively fewer incidents of stranger rape. This evidenced that IPV combined with other forms of violence, but was a considerably more prevalent problem to address.

A study that assessed the magnitude of intimate partner physical violence and associated factors among women in Shimelba refugee camp, Northern Ethiopia, found that the prevalence of physical violence in the last 12 months and lifetime was 25.5% and 31%, respectively (Feseha et al. 2012). In terms of risks factors, the authors reported that the likelihood of experiencing intimate partner physical violence was higher in Muslim and Catholic followers than among Christian Orthodox adherents. Similarly, a study with refugee women affected by the conflict in Burma (Myanmar) at the Thai-Burma border found that women who experienced conflict victimisation were 5.9 times more likely to report past-year partner abuse than women who had not experienced victimisation (Falb et al. 2013).

Gender Differentials

While many studies with military populations investigated IPV odds for both female and male soldiers, the evidence in the civilian population and displaced contexts has focused on female victims, with few studies attempting to investigate female-to-male abuse. Within military populations, a systematic review reported higher levels of past-year IPV for males than for females (Kwan et al. 2020). However, six studies in the sample reported higher levels of physical IPV for females than males, although for severe IPV perpetration gender differences were minimal.

In the civilian population, two studies were inclusive of both males and females. A cross-sectional study from Liberia found that men were more likely to have experienced severe beating by a spouse or partner if they had direct exposure to war-related events, while women were more likely to have experienced severe beating if they had direct exposure to war-related events, exposure to crime, having participated in the conflict, and having higher income (Vinck and Pham 2013). Additionally, women were found to have higher prevalence rates of post-traumatic stress disorder (PTSD) and depression, which could be associated with differences in conflict-related experience of violence, different coping mechanisms, and differences in women's sense of control in their lives (Cloitre et al. 2002 and Tolin and Foa 2002 cited in Vinck and Pham 2013, 47).

A study that explored the association between IPV and common mental health disorders among inhabitants of post-genocide Rwanda is also distinctive as it considered the possibility of IPV being mutual in some couples (Verduin et al. 2013). The study found that participants who reported IPV had higher odds of health disorders. Interestingly, this association was not found for victims of IPV only, but found for those who reported being both a victim and a perpetrator in their relationship. None of these associations were significant, but they suggest that perpetrators of IPV may experience more mental health problems than victims in post-genocide Rwanda, which would need special attention in treatment programmes.

Aetiologies, Risk Factors, and Predictors

Numerous aetiologies (the cause or manner of causation) have been proposed or established to explain the higher frequency of IPV within military populations. Service men and women and veterans were found to be more likely to be affected by war trauma, including post-traumatic stress disorder (PTSD) symptomatology, which could consequently influence relationships with intimate partners and family members. Service personnel and veterans often manifested a reduced ability to adjust feelings and emotions in marital relationships, as well as hyper-sensitivity as a result of stressors faced in combat. These findings suggest that standard treatment programmes for perpetrators of IPV might be ineffective for military populations if they do not take into account and address war trauma (Love et al. 2015) and that there may be a need for pre-deployment and post-deployment specific programmes to support service personnel with stage-specific stressors and to effectively prevent relationship problems that can foster partner abuse (Schmaling et al. 2011).

Studies examining IPV within civilian populations affected by war have proposed that violence may render men powerless, who can then seek to re-assert their power by using abuse with partners (Clark et al. 2010; Kohli et al. 2015). Moreover, violence can foster humiliation, stress, mental ill health, and substance and alcohol abuse in men that can manifest as aggression (Clark et al. 2010; Mannell et al. 2020) (Box 3). Additional causal mechanisms may include a higher normalisation of

Box 3 Case Study Describing the Impact of Conflict-Related Experiences on Combatants and Civilians

Case Study

In 2017, Rachel Jewkes, Nwabisa Jama-Shai, and Yandisa Sikweyiya published a study from Bougainville, Papua New Guinea, that described the conflict-related experiences of former combatants and civilians, the long-term impact of these experiences, and associations with mental health problems about 14 years after the end of civil war. Data collection was achieved through a household survey involving 864 men and 879 women. According to the questionnaire analysis, 29.2% of male respondents had been combatants, and about 20% had beaten, raped, or forced a woman into marriage during the conflict. A portion (6.7%) disclosed having been the victims of rape themselves. About one fourth of the female respondents (23.3%) had been raped in the previous year, and over one third (33.3%) had been the victim of physical or sexual partner violence. The findings overall showed high prevalence of

violence for both men and women (Guruge et al. 2017) and a victim's heightened hesitation to leave an abusive environment in fear of losing the protection it offers (Noe and Rieckmann 2013).

As an especially pernicious form of war violence, sexual violence experienced during conflict can cause physical disability, health problems, unwanted pregnancies, and dysregulated affect in females, interfering with healthy intimate relationships in post-conflict times (Josse 2010). Moreover, exposure to war-related SGBV may make women and girls more vulnerable to prostitution, sexual exploitation, and human trafficking (Handrahan 2004). In many societies, rape victims may face challenges to be accepted as brides or may be divorced if already married (Manjoo and McRaith 2011).

Studies in refugee camps and displaced contexts described IPV to be the result of emotional distress, changes in gender roles, shifts in family power structures, and male unemployment (Meffert and Marmar 2009). Victims of partner abuse were also reported to be reluctant to leave their abusive husbands, to report the abuse, and to use humanitarian services. Reasons included perceived and experienced stigma, reliance on the social or economic security support from husbands, lack of awareness of services, and a fear that children will be kidnaped while mothers sought services (Al-Natour et al. 2019; Horn 2010).

Lastly, studies on war violence and family violence established that violence against children in post-conflict is often an extension of political violence and a consequence of domestic violence perpetrated by family members (Catani et al. 2009). Intimate partner abuse can interfere with parenting skills, which can lead to child abuse or affect children's psychological state and wellbeing, as well as affect children's behaviour in future adult relationships (Dalgaard et al. 2020). Furthermore, perpetration of violence against children has been associated with PTSD symptoms among veterans (Sullivan and Elbogen 2014).

mental ill health, including high depressive symptomatology among both women and men, substance and alcohol abuse among men, and PTSD symptoms in both women and men. Respondents' answers about long-term impact revealed negative effects on employment and societal peace, as well as challenges to control aggression and build trust with others.

Severe partner violence and non-partner rape and war trauma were associated with PTSD symptoms among women. Among men, PTSD symptoms were associated with war trauma. Severe partner violence and non-partner rape were also associated with depressive symptoms and alcohol abuse among women. Among men, depressive symptoms and drug abuse were associated with conflict impact. Moreover, enduring conflict impact was associated with perpetrating past-year rape and physical and/or sexual partner violence. The overall analysis pointed to multiple effect pathways, with exposure to war increasing the risk of PTSD symptoms, and depressive symptomatology being associated with intimate partner violence. Moreover, the enduring impact of conflict increased the risk of perpetrating rape and physical and/or partner abuse.

Women's Perceptions and Experiences

Intimate Partner Violence in the Civilian Population

Horn and co-authors previously explored women's perceptions of the causes of IPV in Sierra Leone and Liberia (Horn et al. 2014). The study consisted of 14 focus group discussions and 20 individual interviews in two locations in Sierra Leone and two locations in Liberia. Women generally felt that men who had committed violence, which included assaulting women sexually, were more likely to become violent and be disrespectful to women in their personal lives. Respondents spoke about men abusing drugs during and after the war, which they linked to some violent behaviour. Traditionally in both societies, men were expected to be breadwinners, but the war had resulted in many women's economic independence, which some respondents thought had reduced violence at home because it took some stress off men's shoulders. Overall, the study found that while no individual woman considered the war to be the direct cause for her spouse's violence, it was unanimously agreed that the war had impacted on intimate relationships and the likelihood of abuse.

A study that examined risk factors, individual and family consequences, and community-driven responses to IPV in the eastern Democratic Republic of Congo following a conflict that had lasted over 18 years provides further insight into women's perspectives (Kohli et al. 2015). The qualitative study involved 13 female survivors and 5 male perpetrators of IPV in South Kivu Province. As in other studies, some female participants reported men's problems with alcohol abuse, which they thought was encouraged through peer pressure in the post-conflict environment. Women also spoke about men judging women as disobedient and men needing to reaffirm control in the household. The participants of the study spoke extensively about the breakdown of traditional, community institutions and support systems, economic deprivation, and financial stresses resulting from the war and a lack of local leadership that made difficult alleviation of the problem.

Research from Sri Lanka on women's experiences of and responses to IPV at the end of the 30-year civil war pointed in turn to important gender dynamics (Guruge et al. 2017). The study consisted of qualitative interviews with 15 women who had experienced partner abuse and 15 service providers. In addition to finding that physical, sexual, and psychological partner violence were pervasive, the authors reported that IPV was a 'hidden' problem. While women of all backgrounds were affected, the perception was that Tamil and Muslim women were disproportionately affected due to war dynamics and trauma and restrictions experienced by women under Muslim laws (e.g. concerning marriage). Some providers thought that perpetrators may have become used to violence because of the war, while some women considered that men's inability to provide as breadwinners caused conflict, leading to violence. It also emerged that women hesitated to leave abusive relationships due to the risk of community violence, for fear of becoming outcasts if they separated or divorced and due to a lack of support systems.

A more recent study examined Afghan women's experiences of domestic violence and relationship to conflict based on semi-structured interviews with 20 women living in safe houses (Mannell et al. 2020). The authors identified three themes in the interviews that suggested possible connections between conflict and violence at home: violence from loss of male support, violence due to men's substance use under the booming drug trade during the conflict, and violence due to women's increased vulnerability due to poverty. As a result of conflict, women lost male relatives and consequently the protection of male guardians, which overall made them more vulnerable to forced marriages, partner abuse, neglect, and psychological or other forms of abuse. The study demonstrated the interdependent nature of the public and private sphere, with women's lived experiences of partner abuse being directly informed by society-wide conflict, poverty, and other changes caused by war.

Intimate Partner Violence in Displaced Populations

Recent studies have explored Syrian refugee women's experiences of violence in Lebanon (Usta et al. 2019) and in displacement centres in Jordan (Al-Natour et al. 2019). The former study, which consisted of focus group discussions with 29 Syrian women in NGO community centres in Lebanon, reported important partner violence, which women associated with men's increased stress in the host environment, harassment, and community violence. The women spoke about difficult living conditions due to crowding and a lack of privacy, unemployment, and poverty. They also found their children harder to manage, particularly as they needed to be constrained from playing outside due to safety risks, or they faced harassment in the host society, making the children stressed and irritable. Numerous coping strategies were reported by the women, such as not speaking back and keeping a low profile, letting go of partner abuse-related stress by beating their children, or finding solidarity in other members of the community. The women also referred to problems regarding the aid they received from humanitarian services, expressing beliefs that these provided help haphazardly or with discrimination that reinforced or created new power hierarchies in the community or divided people by religious affiliation.

The latter study described the lived experience of Syrian refugee women with marital violence during the Syrian civil war relying on data from 16 semi-structured interviews with women in displacement centres in Jordan (Al-Natour et al. 2019). Participants were aged between 22 and 68 years old, were financially dependent on their spouses, and identified with the Islamic faith. The authors found that women felt loss and insecurity and experienced many stressors and hardships as a result of the flight from Syria and the resettlement in the refugee camps. The women spoke about their husbands' changed behaviour following the war and them becoming easily irritable, nervous, or verbally abusive. Women often responded to abuse by being silent or endured in the hope that their husbands might change, because of their children or because they needed the social support of their husbands and family relatives in the refugee community. As coping strategies, women also found recourse to their faith, tried to appease their husbands, or focused on protecting their children from marital conflict.

The Importance of Religious and Cultural Parameters

While religious affiliation, faith, and spiritual parameters emerged to be salient in many of the reviewed studies, these factors have received minimal attention in the humanitarian sector and need to be better integrated when appraising alleviation strategies in conflict and post-conflict contexts and among refugee and displaced populations. The influence of clergy, which has been postulated in studies on religion and domestic violence more generally, could also be further explored.

The aforementioned study with Syrian female victims of IPV found that coping strategies included reading the Quran, fasting, and offering prayers of forgiveness to avoid conflict (Al-Natour et al. 2019). Studies that have examined domestic violence in religious communities have found that female victims may resort to religious beliefs to condemn the abuse and through their ordeals may acquire a more justice-oriented understanding of their faith, helping them to address the harmful situation (see detailed literature review in Istratii 2020). Anthropological research from Ethiopia that analysed conjugal abuse through the religio-cultural framework of the Ethiopian Orthodox *Täwahədo* population found that faith helped women to face and overcome painful marital experiences and was never openly used to justify intimate partner abuse, which the faith clearly taught against (Istratii 2020). Moreover, the clergy were found to be directly involved in the mediation of conjugal problems, and despite some lacking awareness of the extent of the problem in their societies or not responding to victims with the utmost sensitivity of risks involved, the majority prioritised the victimised party and often supported them in ways that secular institutions did not (ibid).

A study by Saile and colleagues that sought to identify the prevalence and predictors of partner violence in Northern Uganda also made reference to culture-specific beliefs about spiritual activity, suggesting more pernicious implications (Saile et al. 2013). The authors related the problem of women's isolation to beliefs in the local society that the re-traumatisation symptoms they experienced, such as flashbacks, were due to evil spirits called 'cen'. They explained that members of the local communities believed that those who had committed atrocities during conflict were possessed and, subsequently, those who manifested symptoms could be perceived as 'murderers' and could be abused, isolated, or mistreated by people in their surroundings. The study also suggested that women identified with 'cen' possession could be abused by partners who might fear them and employ aggression to control them.

A longitudinal study by Doyle and McWilliams that summarised women's experiences of IPV in the conflict in Northern Ireland reported important culture-specific religious influences (Doyle and McWilliams 2018). In 1992, as opposed to 2016, victims of partner abuse were more concerned about the reactions of the Catholic clergy, and their responses to the abuse they faced were more directly shaped by how they perceived religious standards and expectations upheld in the wider society. Despite such attitudes having weakened by 2016, victims of partner violence still experienced consequences that were underpinned by rigid religious standards, such as stigma or the fear of being judged for being a single parent, divorcing their (abusive) spouses, or having children from different fathers. According to the authors, 45% of interviewed women in the 2016 cohort expressed such concerns and attitudes, which seemed to interfere with them reporting the abuse or seeking to exit their harmful situations.

A Case Study with Policy Implications

In a study published in 2018, Mootz and colleagues conducted research with women to determine their level of exposure to alcohol misuse, low socioeconomic status, gender (in)equitable decision-making, intimate partner violence, and armed conflict and to test how these different indicators related to each other. The study was motivated by a recognition that oftentimes multiple issues combined to perpetuate problematic trends. Alcohol misuse could be an important indicator, but the mechanism relating exposure to conflict, IPV, and alcohol misuse needed to be established further.

The study involved 605 women aged 13 to 49 randomly selected through multistage sampling across three districts in Northeastern Uganda in 2016. The study found that 88.8% of the respondents experienced conflict-related violence and that 30.7% of the respondents' partners consumed alcohol daily. The lifetime and past 12-month prevalence of experiencing IPV was 65.3% and 50.9% for psychological abuse and 59.9% and 43.8% for physical abuse. The authors found that the partner alcohol misuse pathway was significant for women who made healthcare decisions alone and not for women who decided jointly with their partners. However, IPV was significantly associated with socioeconomic status for those respondents who made healthcare decisions jointly. These findings implied that interventions to address partner violence and alcohol misuse in humanitarian settings should consider exposure to armed conflict and gender dynamics within couples, which could serve as important mediating factors.

Directions for Research and Practice

Victim support services in conflict and post-conflict time need to consider the multifaceted effects of conflict-related violence that make women, and often men, vulnerable to abuse. These require research-intensive approaches that engage with individuals directly, especially in view of the fact that humanitarian responses have often been guided by top-down recommendations (Horn 2010). Moreover, these have not substantively engaged with religious beliefs and spiritual aspects of life that may be salient in tradition-oriented religious communities, which may have interfered with a proper understanding of local gender normative frameworks, but also with leveraging on the resourcefulness of religious beliefs (Istratii 2020). Numerous studies found that faith could serve as coping mechanisms and as a source of improved mental health (e.g. Al-Natour et al. 2019), suggesting that religious beliefs, faith, and the clergy need to be better integrated in psychosocial responses.

For psychosocial services to be effective in diverse humanitarian settings, the distinct understandings and aetiologies of different forms of violence need to be understood and researched thoroughly. Responding to different aetiologies may require a combination of community-wide measures with more individual psychological or clinical support. To facilitate such efforts, the meaning and usage of the term 'psychosocial' needs to be revisited (Miller et al. 2021). As opposed to its broad and sometimes vague usage in humanitarian discourse, Miller and co-authors have proposed classifying psychosocial services as socio-environmental and clinical to evidence the different types of needs, aetiologies for the problem, or causal mechanisms and specialisations involved. These distinct remedies should be ideally delivered in parallel informed by expert diagnoses and data collected through rigorous research.

Summary

- The relationship between wartime violence and domestic violence has been extensively documented, with the frequency and intensity of violence being associated with a higher likelihood of intimate partner abuse.
- The existing scholarship points to a multi-dimensional mechanism that connects political violence to intimate partner violence, such as through mental health

trauma and behavioural change, socio-cultural parameters contributing to the further abuse of war survivors, or the breakdown of support systems and community solidarity that would be available to victims in peacetime.

- Individuals affected by conflict continue to face trauma-related consequences for many years following conflict, which are defined within wider gender and marriage normative frameworks and material realities, as well as individual histories of trauma.
- It is important to prioritise aetiologies of violence as upheld by victims and survivors themselves and to embed these and attitudes around them in wider socio-cultural and material realities.
- Responses to conflict-related IPV must consider how political violence may intersect with pre-existing forms of domestic or societal violence and seek to support affected groups in ways that can prevent further abuse in domestic and communal life.
- Any intervention or response needs to be contextualised in communities' beliefs systems and normative frameworks and to consider how religious and cultural parameters can interfere with or facilitate effective responses to IPV in conflict and post-conflict times.

References

Al-Natour A, Al-Ostaz SM, Morris EJ (2019) Marital violence during war conflict: the lived experience of Syrian refugee women. J Transcult Nurs 30:32–38. https://doi.org/10.1177/1043659618783842

Catani C, Schauer E, Elbert T, Missmahl I, Bette J-P, Neuner F (2009) War trauma, child labor, and family violence: life adversities and PTSD in a sample of school children in Kabul. J Trauma Stress 22:163–171. https://doi.org/10.1002/jts.20415

Clark CJ, Everson-Rose SA, Suglia SF, Btoush R, Alonso A, Haj-Yahia MM (2010) Association between exposure to political violence and intimate-partner violence in the occupied Palestinian territory: a cross-sectional study. Lancet 375:310–316. https://doi.org/10.1016/S0140-6736(09)61827-4

Cloitre M, Koenen KC, Gratz KL, Jakupcak M (2002) Differential diagnosis of PTSD in women R. Kimerling, P. Ouimette, J. Wolfe (Eds.), Gender and PTSD, The Guilford Press, New York 117–149

Dalgaard NT, Thøgersen MH, Væver MS, Montgomery E (2020) Family violence in traumatized refugee families: a mixed methods study of mother/child dyadic functioning, parental symptom levels and children's psychosocial adjustment. Nord Psychol 72:83–104

Davies SE, True J (2015) Reframing conflict-related sexual and gender-based violence: bringing gender analysis back in. Secur Dialogue 46(6):495–512. https://doi.org/10.1177/0967010615601389

Doyle J, McWilliams M (2018) Intimate partner violence in conflict and post-conflict societies: insights and lessons from Northern Ireland. Political Settlements Research Programme. https://pure.ulster.ac.uk/en/publications/intimate-partner-violence-in-conflict-and-post-conflict-societies

Falb KL, McCormick MC, Hemenway D, Anfinson K, Silverman JG (2013) Violence against refugee women along the Thai-Burma border. Int J Gynecol Obstet 120:279–283. https://doi.org/10.1016/j.ijgo.2012.10.015

Feseha G, G/mariam A, Gerbaba M (2012) Intimate partner physical violence among women in Shimelba refugee camp, northern Ethiopia. BMC Public Health 12:125. https://doi.org/10.1186/1471-2458-12-125

Guruge S, Ford-Gilboe M, Varcoe C, Jayasuriya-Illesinghe V, Ganesan M, Sivayogan S, Kanthasamy P, Shanmugalingam P, Vithanarachchi H (2017) Intimate partner violence in the post-war context: Women's experiences and community leaders' perceptions in the Eastern Province of Sri Lanka. PLoS One 12(3):e0174801. https://doi.org/10.1371/journal.pone.0174801

Handrahan L (2004) Conflict, gender, ethnicity and post-conflict reconstruction. Secur Dialogue 35:429–445. https://doi.org/10.1177/0967010604049521

Horn R (2010) Responses to intimate partner violence in Kakuma refugee camp: refugee interactions with agency systems. Soc Sci Med 70:160–168. https://doi.org/10.1016/j.socscimed.2009.09.036

Horn R, Puffer ES, Roesch E, Lehmann H (2014) Women's perceptions of effects of war on intimate partner violence and gender roles in two post-conflict West African countries: consequences and unexpected opportunities. Confl Heal 8(12). https://doi.org/10.1186/1752-1505-8-12

Istratii R (2020) Adapting gender and development to local religious contexts: a decolonial approach to domestic violence in Ethiopia. Routledge, London. https://doi.org/10.4324/9781003006992

Jewkes R, Jama-Shai N, Sikweyiya Y (2017) Enduring impact of conflict on mental health and gender-based violence perpetration in Bougainville, Papua New Guinea: a cross-sectional study. PLoS One 12(10):e0186062. https://doi.org/10.1371/journal.pone.0186062

Josse E (2010) They came with two guns: the consequences of sexual violence for the mental health of women in armed conflicts. Int Rev Red Cross 92:177

Kohli A, Perrin N, Mpanano RM, Banywesize L, Mirindi AB, Banywesize JH, Mitima CM, Binkurhorhwa AK, Bufole NM, Glass N (2015) Family and community driven response to intimate partner violence in post-conflict settings. Soc Sci Med 146:276–284. https://doi.org/10.1016/j.socscimed.2015.10.011

Krause U (2015) A continuum of violence? Linking sexual and gender-based violence during conflict, flight, and encampment. Refug Surv Q 34(4):1–19. https://doi.org/10.1093/rsq/hdv014

Kwan J, Sparrow K, Facer-Irwin E, Thandi G, Fear NT, MacManus D (2020) Prevalence of intimate partner violence perpetration among military populations: a systematic review and meta-analysis. Aggress Violent Behav 53:101419. https://doi.org/10.1016/j.avb.2020.101419

Love AR, Morland LA, Menez U, Taft C, MacDonald A, Mackintosh M-A (2015) 'Strength at home' intervention for male veterans perpetrating intimate partner aggression: perceived needs survey of therapists and pilot effectiveness study. J Interpers Violence 30:2344–2362. https://doi.org/10.1177/0886260514552445

Manjoo R, McRaith C (2011) Gender-based violence and justice in conflict and post-conflict areas 44 CORNELL INT'L L J 1

Mannell J, Grewal G, Ahmad L, Ahmad A (2020) A qualitative study of women's lived experiences of conflict and domestic violence in Afghanistan. Violence Against Women 27(11):1862–1878. https://doi.org/10.1177/1077801220935191

McCarroll JE, Ursano RJ, Liu X, Thayer LE, Newby JH, Norwood CAE, Usa M, Fullerton CS (2010) Deployment and the probability of spousal aggression by U.S. army soldiers. Mil Med 175:5

Meffert SM, Marmar CR (2009) Darfur refugees in Cairo: mental health and interpersonal conflict in the aftermath of genocide. J Interpers Violence 24:1835–1848. https://doi.org/10.1177/0886260508325491

Miller KE, Jordans MJD, Tol WA, Galappatti A (2021) A call for greater conceptual clarity in the field of mental health and psychosocial support in humanitarian settings. Epidemiol Psychiatr Sci 30:e5. https://doi.org/10.1017/S2045796020001110

Mootz JJ, Muhanguzi FK, Panko P, Mangen PO, Wainberg ML, Pinsky I, Khoshnood K (2018) Armed conflict, alcohol misuse, decision-making, and intimate partner violence among women in Northeastern Uganda: a population level study. Confl Heal 12(1):37. https://doi.org/10.1186/s13031-018-0173-x

Noe D, Rieckmann J (2013) Violent behaviour: the effect of civil conflict on domestic violence in Colombia. Working Paper No. 136

Østby G (2016) Violence begets violence: armed conflict and domestic sexual violence in sub-Saharan Africa. No. 233; HiCN working papers. Households in conflict network. https://ideas.repec.org/p/hic/wpaper/233.html

Saile R, Neuner F, Ertl V, Catani C (2013) Prevalence and predictors of partner violence against women in the aftermath of war: a survey among couples in Northern Uganda. Soc Sci Med 86:17–25. https://doi.org/10.1016/j.socscimed.2013.02.046

Schmaling KB, Blume AW, Russell ML (2011) Intimate partner violence and relationship dissolution among reserve soldiers. Mil Psychol 23:685–699. https://doi.org/10.1080/08995605.2011.616821

Stark L, Ager A (2011) A systematic review of prevalence studies of gender-based violence in complex emergencies. Trauma Violence Abuse 12(3):127–134. https://doi.org/10.1177/1524838011404252

Stark L, Roberts L, Wheaton W, Acham A, Boothby N, Ager A (2010) Measuring violence against women amidst war and displacement in northern Uganda using the "neighbourhood method". J Epidemiol Community Health 64:1056–1061. https://doi.org/10.1136/jech.2009.093799

Sullivan CP, Elbogen EB (2014) PTSD symptoms and family versus stranger violence in Iraq and Afghanistan veterans. Law Hum Behav 38:1–9. https://doi.org/10.1037/lhb0000035

Tolin DF, Foa EB (2002) Gender and PTSD: a cognitive model R. Kimerling, P. Ouimette, J. Wolfe (Eds.), Gender and PTSD, The Guilford Press, New York 76–97

Usta J, Masterson AR, Farver JM (2019) Violence against displaced Syrian women in Lebanon. J Interpers Violence 34:3767–3779. https://doi.org/10.1177/0886260516670881

Verduin F, Engelhard EAN, Rutayisire T, Stronks K, Scholte WF (2013) Intimate partner violence in Rwanda: the mental health of victims and perpetrators. J Interpers Violence 28(9):1839–1858. https://doi.org/10.1177/0886260512469106

Vinck P, Pham PN (2013) Association of exposure to intimate-partner physical violence and potentially traumatic war-related events with mental health in Liberia. Soc Sci Med 77:41–49. https://doi.org/10.1016/j.socscimed.2012.10.026

Romina Istratii, PhD is UKRI Future Leaders Fellow at the School of History, Religions and Philosophies at SOAS University of London. Her research lies at the intersection of gender, religious and development studies and is orientated towards identifying culture-sensitive and faith-based responses to domestic violence, including in conflict and emergency situations.

Part VI

Human Trafficking

Abuses Against Female Migrant Domestic Workers in the UK: An Intersectional Approach

Joyce Jiang

Learning Objectives

Having read this chapter, you should be able understand.

1. The notion of 'intersectionality' and apply an intersectional approach to the study of gender-based violence.
2. The intersected structural causes of abuses against female migrant domestic workers.
3. The nature and scale of abuses against female migrant domestic workers in the UK.

Introduction

Domestic work remains a female-dominated sector, employing 57.7 million women, who account for 76.2% of domestic workers worldwide (ILO 2021). Women domestic workers outnumber men domestic workers in nearly all countries and regions except the Arab States, with the highest share being in the Americas at 89% (ILO 2021). Domestic work also remains an important source of employment among migrant women workers. It is estimated that migrants made up 54.6% of domestic workers in Northern, Southern and Western Europe (ILO 2015). Migrant women workers are particularly vulnerable as the intersection of race, migrant status, work sector, caste, class, gender and other social dynamics might amplify the discrimination and marginalisation faced by them. Female migrant domestic workers (MDWs)

J. Jiang (✉)
University of York, York, UK
e-mail: joyce.jiang@york.ac.uk

P. Ali, M. M. Rogers (eds.), *Gender-Based Violence: A Comprehensive Guide*,
https://doi.org/10.1007/978-3-031-05640-6_26

face a continuum of violence and abuses ranging from verbal, psychological abuse to severe physical abuse, sexual assault and rape (Jiang 2019). They also suffer from poor working conditions, long working hours, low pay and racism (Jiang 2019). This chapter focuses on MDWs who are mostly women in the UK. In order to understand the nature of abuses against female MDWs, this chapter emphasises the importance of adopting an intersectional approach that considers how gender intersects with other sources of inequalities and oppressions to produce unique experiences of violence. The chapter argues that gender-based violence (GBV) cannot be considered in isolation from the patriarchal, capitalist and racist system in which that violence is perpetrated.

With a focus on female MDWs, the chapter does not naturally associate 'gender' with women and ignores the role of male domestic workers in global care chains. However, there is limited existing data about the abuse and violence against male MDWs, and further research is needed to investigate male MDWs. The chapter first introduces the context of MDWs. The second part explains the notion of intersectionality and why an intersectional approach is particularly important for studying female MDWs. The third part focuses on intersected abuses against female MDWs in the UK by drawing on the interview data from the author's two research projects on MDWs[1] and the survey data from two major organisations – The Voice of Domestic Workers (VoDW)[2] and Kalayaan[3] which provide support and advocacy to MDWs in the UK.

Context

The concept of MDW is intrinsically connected to the wider concept of the 'global care chain' (Hochschild 2000:131) which describes the phenomenon of domestic work (see Box 1) in middle- or high-income host countries being fulfilled by migrant women workers from lower-income countries. With increasing gaps in care provision, paid care work has become one of the main migrant occupations in high-income countries in Europe and the world (Lutz 2008; Yeates 2009). Domestic workers are over-represented in upper-middle-income countries: 53.1% of all domestic workers are in upper-middle-income countries (ILO 2021). Domestic work remains a female-dominated sector. According to recent ILO estimates, there are 75.6 million domestic workers in the world, of whom approximately 76.2 are women (ILO 2021). There is also a historical and international pattern of domestic

[1] The interview data in this chapter comes from the author's two research projects on MDWs in the UK. The first one is the author's PhD project – an ethnographic study of MDWs in the UK conducted between 2009 and 2013. The second one is a participatory video project conducted with 12 MDWs from VoDW between 2018 and 2019. Some interviewees are anonymous, while others do not use their real names in this chapter.

[2] The Voice of Domestic Workers is an advocacy and campaign group led by MDWs themselves. It is based in London and provides education, advocacy and support to MDWs across the UK.

[3] Kalayaan is a London-based charity organisation led by professionals which provides support and advocacy to MDWs across the UK.

workers stemming from disadvantaged racial and ethnic groups. In the UK, 31.2% of the workforce in domestic personnel are migrant workers (Jiang and Korczynski 2016).

Box 1
Definition

Domestic worker is 'work performed for a household or households, within an employment relationship and on an occupational basis' (ILO 2021).

Domestic workers means 'any person engaged in domestic work within an employment relationship' (ILO 2021).

MDWs in this chapter refer to domestic workers who enter the UK with the Overseas Domestic Worker (ODW) visa. Each year the Home Office issues approximately 19,000 ODW visas under its 'domestic workers in private households' scheme, which allows employers to bring domestic workers to the UK (Jiang et al. 2020). Domestic workers include cleaners, chauffeurs, cooks, nannies and those providing personal care for the employer and their family. ODWs are only authorised to come to work in the UK if their overseas-based employers are present, and they therefore do not have an independent route of entry. The majority of these MDWs are women from the Philippines, India, Pakistan, Indonesia, Sri Lanka, Morocco, Nigeria, Ghana, Uganda and other Asian and African countries (Jiang 2021).

Understanding Abuses Against Female MDWs: An Intersectional Approach

Intersectionality is a feminist theory that recognises gender-based inequalities intersect with other sources of oppression. The term was initially coined by Crenshaw (1989, 1991) to capture the multiple and compounded layers of oppression faced by women of colour in the United States. Broadly speaking, the concept directs our focus away from essentialized identities and experiences based on single-axis social categories, towards the multiplicity of differences, power relations and subsequent subordinations. Since then the term 'intersectionality' has been used to understand women's experiences at the intersection of multiple sources of oppression including (but not limited to) race, class, caste, gender, ethnicity, sexuality, disability, nationality, immigration status, geographical location, religion and so on. It is important to apply the intersectionality lens to the study of lived experiences of female MDWs because they are embedded in multiple social structures. They are workers, migrants, women as well as ethnic minorities. Consequently an analysis of their disadvantages, discrimination and marginalisation requires an intersectional framework which recognises the multi-layer sources of oppression, such as class, ethnicity, gender and legal status (Box 2).

Box 2

Definition

Intersectionality is a term coined by Crenshaw (1989, 1991) to capture the multiple and compounded layers of oppression faced by women of colour in the United States.

The domestic worker sector is identified as vulnerable by the International Labour Organization (ILO) (Piper 2013) because it is the sector where migrant workers are concentrated and labour relations are mostly unregulated; it involves largely individualised forms of employment relations; and the temporary nature of their residential/employment status makes political activism by migrant workers a risky undertaking. There is a vast body of research on paid domestic work in high-income countries around the world (Anderson 2000; Cox 2004; Lutz 2008; Yeates 2009). Domestic work is distinctive in that it trespasses the boundaries between the informal and formal economy, between market work and family work and between public and private spaces (Fudge 2012). Domestic work is often delineated as a separate area of work when productive and reproductive work is separated. Domestic workers have traditionally lacked recognition as 'real' workers, and this is deeply rooted in the perceptions and behaviour of employing households and society at large. ILO characterises the employee status of domestic workers as 'invisible because they work inside the household' (ILO 2010: 2).

There is also a widespread tendency among employers across different countries to claim that domestic workers are their 'family members' (Fish 2006; Lan 2006). These familial dynamics tend to obscure the labour relation and aggravate power inequalities, fostering often exploitative and abusive conditions (Anderson 2000; Jiang and Korczynski 2016). According to the UK employment law, if one is a member of his/her employer's family, living in their home and helping to run family business or household chores, one is not entitled to the National Minimum Wage. This blurs the status of MDWs as 'workers' and allows some employers to solicit unpaid services (Jiang 2013). The non-compliance of the National Minimum Wage and harsh working conditions are prevailing in the domestic worker sector. Globally, about 42.5% of the world's domestic workers do not enjoy minimum wage coverage despite the fact that in the countries in which they work minimum wages are set for other types of workers (ILO 2013). Domestic workers frequently report long working hours, substandard living and working conditions and insufficient food. Many work all week, without a day off, and have to continue working even when they are sick (GAATW 2019). In some countries, domestic workers are not allowed to join trade unions, such as in Malaysia, Thailand and the United States (HRW et al. 2013). Even where they are, established unions generally have not prioritised the rights of domestic workers because they are invisible and the employment relationship in this sector is highly fragmented. Barriers to freedom of association and collective bargaining pose challenges for MDWs to collectively respond to abuses and exploitations.

Apart from the nature of the domestic worker sector, the situation of MDWs is compounded by the gendered and racialised nature of the MDW group. Domestic work is gendered and mostly done by women (Albin and Mantouvalou 2012). Female MDWs experience a continuum of GBV, ranging from psychological abuse and bullying to severe physical abuse, rape and sexual assault throughout their migration (GAATW 2019). Female MDWs often describe being pushed into overseas domestic work because of a lack of employment opportunities in their countries of origin, debt, economic hardship and the breadwinner role falling to women (Jiang and Korczynski 2016). In spite of the breadwinner role falling on women, decision-making power is still heavily patriarchal. Female MDWs are not only seen by states as a source of remittances, but by families, in such a way that their acceptance and love by family and community was heavily dependent on their 'success' in migration (GAATW 2019). Many female MDWs also cite violence and abuses from husbands and male family members at home as a major push factor for their migration (GAATW 2019).

The GBV often continues once they arrive in the country of destination. It is widely reported that employers throw things at them, slap, pull their hair, punch, kick, beat and burn them, along with insults telling them they are stupid, lazy, dirty, an idiot, a flirt, a bitch and a liar (HRW 2016). Many female MDWs report stories of sexual violence, often perpetrated by male employers including sons, brothers, uncles, fathers and grandfathers living in the house (GAATW 2019). Female domestic workers are also commonly found to be paid less than male domestic workers (HRW 2016). In spite of the significant scale of gender-based abuse against MDWs, many feminist movements have not prioritised the rights of paid domestic workers. Scholars argue that despite some individual efforts, most feminist organisations have not focused on domestic worker rights; indeed, many middle-class feminists rely on MDWs as well (Blofield 2012; De Santana Pinho and Silva 2010). The status of MDWs as ethnic minorities further makes them more vulnerable to discrimination and violence. It is commonly reported by MDWs that their employers abuse them because of their skin colour (HRW 2016). They may experience institutional racism when they seek help in the country of destination. Ullman and Filipas' (2001) study suggests that ethnic minority women, including migrant women, are more likely to report negative experiences of seeking help from police and to experience negative social reactions such as racial stereotyping and victim blaming.

Furthermore, scholars have widely discussed the historical and international practices of excluding domestic workers from legislative protection in many countries. This is described as the 'legislative precariousness' for domestic workers (Albin and Mantouvalou 2012:4), which refers to the special vulnerability faced by domestic workers because of their partial or complete exclusion from protective laws or the lower degrees of legal protection they are eligible for in comparison to other workers. MDWs, in particular, suffer from 'legal precariousness' in relation to immigration policies and employment laws. The ILO report reveals that gaps in national legislation were particularly frequent with regard to the coverage of domestic workers by minimum wages, limitation of working hours, inclusion in social security schemes and measures to ensure occupational safety and health (ILO 2010).

An estimated 21.5 million domestic workers have no minimum wage that is applicable to them, although they exist for other types of workers. Among those who are covered, many are entitled to a rate that is lower than the minimum wage for other workers (ibid). In the UK, domestic workers are excluded from working time regulation and health and safety legislation and can be paid less than the minimum wage when they receive accommodation, and if treated as family members, domestic workers are exempted from the minimum wage Act (Albin and Mantouvalou 2012). In Asia, MDWs are particularly exposed to the lack of legal protection under the labour laws of host countries. Similarly, labour laws in Arab states largely exclude domestic workers who are mostly migrant women from Asia and Africa (ILO 2013). After the sustained activism of women's groups, domestic workers NGOs, trade unions and internal support within the ILO, the tripartite ILO conference (national employer bodies, unions and governments) voted overwhelmingly to adopt the ILO Convention concerning Decent Work for Domestic Workers (Domestic Workers Convention, No. 189) in 2011. Under the Convention, domestic workers are entitled to the same basic rights as those available to other types of workers, including weekly days off, limits to hours of work, minimum wage, overtime compensation, safety, social security and clear information on the terms and conditions of employment. The new convention was embraced worldwide while underrated in some countries, such as the UK (Jiang 2020).

In addition to labour legislation that excludes domestic workers from its scope, further legal precariousness is created by the UK immigration policies which treat MDWs differently. Up until April 2012, provided a domestic worker had worked in the employer's household for at least a year and the employer decided to bring the domestic worker to the UK, the domestic worker could obtain an Overseas Domestic Worker (ODW) visa. The ODW visa can be renewed as long as the domestic worker would be employed continuously on full-time basis in private households. MDWs were also allowed to change employers when they were in the UK, as long as they remained a domestic worker. Once the ODW visa holders had worked in the UK for 5 years, they could apply for indefinite leave to remain and further citizenship 1 year after the permanent settlement. The pre-2012 ODW visa clearly identified MDWs as workers who could enjoy the similar employment and legal rights as those available to other types of migrant workers in the UK. However, in 2012, the government imposed restrictions on the ODW visa which removed MDWs' right to renew visa. Under the current ODW visa regime, unless MDWs are identified as victims of human trafficking through the National Referral Mechanism (NRM), they have to leave the UK or become undocumented after their 6-month ODW visa expires.

Evidence suggests that the non-renewable ODW visa has worsened MDW's vulnerable position in the labour market (Jiang 2019). The non-renewable visa has created enormous difficulties for the workers to change employers when MDWs are subject to abuses. Without recourse to public funds and without the right to work, undocumented MDWs often have to accept any work offered to them or to face destitution. Some employers exploit their vulnerability and set them up in exploitative work conditions by telling workers they are taking a risk in hiring them (Kalayaan 2019). If they report abuses to the authorities, they might face imprisonment and deportation. Some employers refuse to hire with the introduction of the offence of illegal working in the Immigration Act 2016. The non-renewable ODW visa has also made it difficult for MDWs to be protected by the UK employment law in practice. MDWs are entitled to the National Minimum Wage and have the right to make claims against their employers to the Employment Tribunal. However, the average waiting time towards a hearing stood at 207 days in the 12 months to 31 March 2018, compared with 204 days in 2016/2017 and 195 days in 2015/2016, shows Ministry of Justice's data obtained by the law firm GQ Littler (Webber 2018). This means that MDWs who have been suffering from abusive employers will not have enough time to complete the Employment Tribunal process before their 6-month ODW visa expires. The only support mechanism available to MDWs – the NRM – treats MDWs as victims who can only get access to support when they have been condemned to modern slaves. Those who are in danger of the potentially severe abuse are excluded from the NRM framework.

The Intersectional Abuses Against Female MDWs: The UK Case

Being enmeshed in class relations integrated with gendered, racialised and legal structures of oppression, MDWs experience greater exploitation than do workers in most occupations. They are not only subject to non-compliance of the National Minimum Wage and long working hours, but also to verbal, physical and sexual abuses in the UK.

Labour Exploitation

MDWs are entitled to the National Minimum Wage in the UK. However, the non-compliance with the National Minimum Wage is prevalent in the domestic work industry. According to a survey completed by 539 MDWs (VODW 2019), 82.3% of survey participants reported they held an employment contract. Contracts regularly stated a 40–72-hour working week and either 1 or 2 days off. However, their working realities were very different from the contractual terms and conditions. Their average weekly working hours was 91 ranging from 40 to 154. The corresponding weekly salary level was between £250 and £450. During a discussion with 12 MDWs in an employment advice session, the lowest salary reported was £100 per month before tax (Jiang 2013: 164). Some MDWs did not receive any salary as described here:

> My next employers were doctors. I worked as a nanny and a housekeeper, a live-out job from 7:00 am to 7:30 pm excluding travelling time. I was allowed no food and worked from Monday to Saturday. I have been cheated on my wages. I wasn't paid 4 months' salary and deductions were made from my wages supposedly for tax and NI when the employer just pocketed this money. (Indian domestic worker Nancy).

Kalayaan's (2018) annual report also shows that among 50 MDWs who entered the UK with the ODW visa after April 2016, 32% reported they had not received any salary.

Overworking is a common issue among MDWs. Some workers are required to be ready to serve their employers at any time of the day for all tasks including bringing a cup of juice to their employer. Kalayaan's (2018) annual report suggests that the majority of MDWs (ranging from 50% to 87% depending on their visa status) were expected to be 'on call' for 24 hours and more than half of the surveyed MDWs (ranging from 59% to 88% depending on their visa status) had no days off. Their employers also threatened to make MDWs redundant when they made complaints.

> At night, I had to wait for my employer to open the door even at midnight though she had a key. Everyday was like a torture. So I tried to ask for days off. 'I am very tired. I need a day off. Please let me have a day off on Sunday', I told my employer, but she asked me to get off of her life. 'Don't wait for Sunday. You can go now!', she told me. (Nigerian domestic worker)

Many MDWs suffered from health problems due to the heavy workload:

> Normally start to work at 7 am–10.30 pm, Monday to Saturday. It was hard work and salary was only 150 pounds a week. I became very ill and the doctor said that I was overwork and advised me to rest, but how could I rest? I had to work even if I was very ill. (Moroccan domestic worker)

Withholding of Passports

The withholding of passports by employers is a major problem for MDWs in the UK. It is common for employers to detain the passports of MDWs in order to prevent them from escaping the house. Kalayaan's (2018) annual survey with 94 MDWs shows that more than 75% (ranging from 75% to 93% depending on their visa status) of MDWs' passports were kept by their employers. As a Filipino domestic worker Lily described,

> One day, she asked me to bring a spoon in Hyde Park and said that I shouldn't come back to our flat until she rings me, which I can't help but wonder why. When I came back at night, I noticed that my suitcase was open. My stuff was not in the right order anymore. My identification card in my wallet was outside my suitcase. I already knew that something's going on. (Filipino domestic worker Lily).

Consequently, many MDWs feel fearful of leaving employers without documents to prove their immigration status. Abusive employers exploit this fear to enforce harsh working conditions, long hours and other forms of mistreatment. If MDWs decide to leave employers, they are often left in an immigration limbo and are forced to embark on the time-consuming, expensive and difficult task of obtaining new documents from embassies or the Home Office. As Mary shared her experience of escaping her abusive employer,

> In 2013 I escaped when I left my employer. I felt for the reason that I think it's too much for me because of the way they treated me. When the first time when I came here, I thought I would work in only one family, but they let me work in three families. I woke up in the morning at 6 am, until I slept at 1 or 2 o'clock. I don't have a day off. I also don't have

> proper accommodation. I work 7 days a week. They don't give my salary. That's why I can't take it anymore. I left them...without my passport, without anything. (Filipino domestic worker Mary)

The UK Visas and Immigration information sheet for overseas domestic workers clearly states that MDWs instead of employers should retain their passports, but it does not provide any information as to what MDWs can do if their employers withhold their passports against their will.[4] In the UK, the problem is compounded due to the issue concerning the ownership of passports. The passport belongs to the government which has issued the document, and thus the police are not legally obliged to intervene if an employer takes a passport from a worker. The withholding of passports is not classified as 'theft' either. In practice, therefore, there is no legal framework which prevents employers withholding MDWs' passports or assists MDWs in retrieving their passports.

Forced Confinement and Social Isolation

As MDWs come to the UK with their employers, they have limited social networks available to them in the receiving society upon their arrival. It is commonly reported that MDWs are not allowed to go out without being accompanied or supervised by their employers. Kalayaan's (2018) annual report suggests that more than half of MDWs (ranging from 53% to 93% depending on their visa status) were not allowed out. Some MDWs were even locked against their will.

> We live on the third floor. So I climb there because the door is closed and locked. I take my courage to get down. I don't know what is going to happen to me if I fall down. I'm just thinking I want to send money to my daughter. I just get down without anything happening to me because one of the cleaners (she is a foreigner) helped me and gave me a ladder to get down, but my boss saw me on camera and they told me that if I do that, they going to send me to police station and they will say that I am a thief inside the house. (Filipino domestic worker Grace)

Many MDWs were under nearly surveillance almost 24 h a day by the CCTV camera installed by employers:

> There's CCTV. We can't go out. We can't buy our personal stuff. We will just make a list and give it to the driver, and the driver will buy those for us. (Filipino domestic worker Lucy).

MDWs also reported that they were not allowed to use Wi-Fi to contact their family members or friends and some employers imposed a 'no friend policy' which meant that MDWs could not bring any friends home even when their employers were away (Jiang 2013).

[4] UK Visas and Immigration, 'Overseas domestic worker information sheet', https://www.gov.uk/government/uploads/system/uploads/attachment_data/file/265823/dworkers-informationsheet.pdf (accessed June 5, 2021).

Physical and Sexual Abuse

A survey with 539 MDWs conducted by VoDW (2019) reveals that 76.5% of respondents had experienced abuse at work, including verbal (54.4%), physical (18.9%) and sexual (7%) abuse (VoDW 2019). Many MDWs reported that they had been slapped and kicked by their employers for no good reasons.

> I told her I cannot work like this because in my contract I have only one employer. So how come I have two employers for one day? I told her I want to go back. Then she called her husband and her husband knocking my head… she slaps me because me and my colleague couldn't find the medicine. I told her I am not the one who arrange all the things of your daughter. She slaps me again then she told if you do not find the medicine, go out form my house. Because we are in the Berkeley hotel at that time, she says you sleep outside in the Berkeley hotel. I said ok I can sleep in the lobby and she hit my head. (Filipino domestic worker Jane)

VoDW's (2019) report also reveals that 69% of MDWs did not have their own room in employers' houses and only 49.4% had enough food to eat. Some MDWs were often forced to sleep on the sofa, floor or table. As a Filipino domestic worker Grace described,

> I just sleep in the library. I don't have a proper bed, just a sofa. So I sleep there and then if they are going to call me anytime, I need to answer them. (Filipino domestic worker Grace)

Some employers also imposed hygiene rules on MDWs. For example, some workers were asked not to cook strong-smelling food.

> They said I could cook whatever food I want, but they also said they didn't like any smell in the house. How can I cook, then no smell? So I could just put rice in the boiling water and eat it. Sometimes I put some food into the microwave. (Indian domestic worker Alice)

There were some extreme cases where MDWs were raped and burnt. As the chair of VoDW Marissa commented,

> Some have been raped. I've seen the bruises in the body, the hot water and oil that the employer had poured on the body. I know how it is when they talk to me about rape because I had that employer as well. He gave me this massage book that I know is not part of my work, but I had to do it because I needed the work and I needed the money for my children. Private household should be the safest and happiest space, but for many domestic workers it's not. We had to be a self defence expert. So I said, 'Sir, I read in the book this is the best massage ever'. So I karate him so hard and he said 'get off'. I was really strong because I was angry because they look at us like we are sex objects.

Verbal and Physiological Abuse

Verbal insults are common. This not only comes from their employers, but also sometimes from their employers' young children. It is commonly reported by MDWs that their employers would shout at them and call them abusive names such as 'dog', 'monkey', 'witch', 'idiot' and 'bitch'.

> The lady accused me that I am a witch. She got ill and she accused me that I am a witch. She told me that I will pay everything when we get back to the UAE. (Filipino domestic worker Lucy).
>
> I came to the UK to work for a famous British actress who had previously employed me in India. I started working at 7:00 am until 3:00 am often having to cater big parties. She would call me 'stupid Indian'. (Indian domestic worker Nancy)
>
> My employer and daughter is spitting on my face, knocking my head, calling me 'donkey', 'monkey'. She did not call my name. We are four Filipinos there, but she's calling us 'monkey', 'donkey' like that. She calls me 'dog'. She will not call our names. (Filipino domestic worker Rose)

Many MDWs reported that they were not trusted by their employers and would be accused of being thieves when items are lost or misplaced.

> I found another employer but she accused me of stealing £225 and very expensive leather jacket. But she found the money in her wallet and the jacket was just in the dressing room. (Moroccan domestic worker)

When some MDWs made complaints or took resistive actions against this abuse, their employers threatened them with groundless charges.

> I have been sexually abused. I was threatened if ever I told anyone about this, I would be accused of hurting their child, the baby that I adored like mine. I had to put up with this abuse and torture. (Filipino domestic worker Ruby)

Summary

- Intersectionality is a feminist theory that recognises gender-based inequalities intersect with other sources of oppression. It directs our focus towards the multiplicity of differences, power relations and subsequent subordinations.
- As migrant domestic workers are embedded in multiple social structures, an analysis of their disadvantages, discrimination and marginalisation requires an intersectional framework which recognises the multi-layer sources of oppression, such as class, ethnicity, gender and legal status.
- Being enmeshed in class relations integrated with gendered, racialised and legal structures of oppression, migrant domestic workers are not only subject to non-compliance of the National Minimum Wage, long working hours and harsh working conditions, but also to verbal, psychological, physical and sexual abuses in the UK.
- An intersectional approach is necessary in all areas of work relating to ending violence against women and girls as violence is contingent on the various social structures in which women are embedded in and their individual attributes.

References

Albin E, Mantouvalou A (2012) The ILO convention on domestic workers: from the shadows to the light. Ind Law J 41(1):67–78

Anderson B (2000) Doing the dirty work? The global politics of domestic labour. Zed Books, London

Blofield M (2012) Care work and class: domestic workers' struggle for equal rights in Latin America. Pennsylvania State University Press, College Park

Cox R (2004) The servant problem: domestic employment in a global economy. IB, Tauris, London

Crenshaw K (1989) Demarginalizing the intersection of race and sex: a black feminist critique of antidiscrimination doctrine, feminist theory and antiracist politics. University of Chicago Legal Forum. Issue 1, Article 8. http://chicagounbound.uchicago.edu/uclf/vol1989/iss1/8

Crenshaw K (1991) Mapping the margins: intersectionality, identity politics, and violence against women of colour. Stanford Law Rev 43(6):1241–1299

De Santana Pinho P, Silva E (2010) Domestic relations in Brazil: legacies and horizons. Lat Am Res Rev 45(2):90–113

Fish JN (2006) Domestic democracy: at home in South Africa. Routledge, New York

Fudge J (2012) Global care chains: transnational migrant care workers. Int J Comp Labour Law Ind Relat 28(1):63–70

GAATW (2019) Demanding justice: women migrant workers fighting gender-based violence. https://www.gaatw.org/publications/Demanding_Justice_complete.pdf. Accessed 5 June 2021

Hochschild AR (2000) Global care chains and emotional surplus value. In: Hutton W, Giddens A (eds) On the edge: living with global capitalism. Jonathan Cape, London

HRW (2016) "I was sold": abuse and exploitation of migrant domestic workers in Oman. https://www.hrw.org/report/2016/07/13/i-was-sold/abuse-and-exploitation-migrant-domestic-workers-oman. Accessed 6 June 2021

HRW, ITUC, IDWN (2013) Claiming rights: domestic workers' movements and global advances for labor reform. https://www.hrw.org/sites/default/files/related_material/2013_Global_DomesticWorkers.pdf. Accessed 6 June 2021

ILO (2010) Decent work for domestic workers. International Labour Conference, 99th session, 2010. Report IV (1). ILO, Geneva

ILO (2013) Domestic workers across the world: global and regional statistics and the extent of legal protection. Geneva, ILO. https://www.ilo.org/wcmsp5/groups/public/%2D%2D-dgreports/%2D%2D-dcomm/%2D%2D-publ/documents/publication/wcms_173363.pdf. Accessed 5 June 2021

ILO (2015) ILO global estimates on migrant workers: results and methodology-special focus on migrant domestic workers. https://www.ilo.org/wcmsp5/groups/public/%2D%2D-dgreports/%2D%2D-dcomm/documents/publication/wcms_436343.pdf. Accessed 22 Apr 2020

ILO (2021) Making decent work a reality for domestic workers: Progress and prospects ten years after the adoption of the Domestic Workers Convention, 2011 (No. 189). https://www.ilo.org/wcmsp5/groups/public/%2D%2D-dgreports/%2D%2D-dcomm/%2D%2D-publ/documents/publication/wcms_802551.pdf. Accessed 23 Sept 2021

Jiang Z (2013) Collective mobilisations among immigrant workers in low-skilled sectors: a study of community Organising of immigrant workers in the UK. Unpublished PhD thesis

Jiang Z (2019) A special vulnerability: migrant domestic workers enslaved by the non-renewable six-month overseas domestic worker visa in the UK. Policy report for The Voice of Domestic Workers, London. https://16fae8ab-6f0a-412c-b753-4986ecc84967.filesusr.com/ugd/6608f3_39dcbbd4f03245a7b795dc4c40a890d6.pdf. Accessed 5 June 2021

Jiang Z (2020) Migrant domestic workers in the UK: struggle and resistance. In: Leal Filho W, Azul A, Brandli L, Lange Salvia A, Wall T (eds) Decent work and economic growth. Encyclopedia of the UN sustainable development goals. Springer, Cham

Jiang Z (2021) A manual for organising migrant domestic workers: lessons from The Voice of Domestic Workers in London, tools to transform. https://toolstotransform.net/portfolio/joyce-jiang-20210521-a-manual-for-organising-migrant-domestic-workers-lessons-from-the-voice-of-domestic-workers-in-london/. Accessed 5 June 2021

Jiang Z, Korczynski M (2016) When the 'unorganisable' organise: collective mobilisation of migrant domestic workers in London. Hum Relat 69(3):813–838

Jiang Z, Kobylinska T, VoDW (2020) Art with marginalised communities: participatory video as a tool of empowerment and resistance for migrant domestic workers in London. City 24:348. https://doi.org/10.1080/13604813.2020.1739460

Kalayaan (2018) Kalayaan annual report and financial statements. http://www.kalayaan.org.uk/wp-content/uploads/2019/07/Annual-report-17-18.pdf. Accessed 6 June 2021

Kalayaan (2019) Briefing on overseas domestic workers for the Modern Slavery Strategy and Implementation Group (MSSIG) prevent meeting. http://www.kalayaan.org.uk/wp-content/uploads/2019/10/Kalayaan_report_October2019.pdf. Accessed 5 June 2021

Lan PC (2006) Global cinderellas: migrant domestics and newly rich employers in Taiwan. Duke University Press, Durham, NC

Lutz H (2008) Introduction: migrant domestic workers in Europe. In: Lutz H (ed) Migration and domestic work: a European perspective on a global theme. Ashgate, Aldershot

Piper N (2013) Resisting inequality: the rise of global migrant rights movement. In: Bastia T (ed) Migration and inequality. Routledge, Abingdon

Ullman S, Filipas HH (2001) Correlates of formal and informal support seeking in sexual assault victims. J Interpersonal Violence 16(10):1028–1047

VoDW (2019) Understanding our members' working conditions. The Voice of Domestic Workers, London

Webber A (2018) Employment tribunal hearing delays rise to seven months. Personnel Today. https://www.personneltoday.com/hr/employment-tribunal-hearing-delays-rise-to-seven-months/. Accessed 6 June 2021

Yeates N (2009) Globalising care economies and migrant workers: explorations in global care chains. Macmillan, Basingstoke

Joyce Jiang, PhD, is a Senior Lecturer in Human Resource Management in The York Management School, University of York, UK. Her main research areas include migrant labour (migrant domestic workers in particular), labour organising and art activism.

Human Trafficking

Judit Montenegro Sebastian

Learning Objectives

Having read this chapter, you should be able to understand:

- How human trafficking is defined in international law.
- The gendered nature of trafficking within the global political economy of migration.
- Some of the limitations of existing transnational mechanisms to protect victims and prevent the crime and alternative survivor-led initiatives.

Introduction

Human trafficking is thought to be one of the most widespread crimes in the world. In 2016, there were an estimated 40.3 million victims of human trafficking and modern slavery globally (ILO and Walk Free Foundation 2017; see Box 1). And while testimonies of victims have exposed the horrifying exploitation behind it, their identification and protection remain a challenge for anti-trafficking efforts (Aronowitz 2009). This chapter explores, on the one hand, how the scope provided by the international anti-trafficking Protocol (UN 2000) supports the current understanding of the forms in which trafficking is perpetrated. On the other hand, it studies the gendered nature of this crime (Kempadoo 2005; Sullivan 2015) and how some of the most invisible victims continue to be left behind in transnational approaches against trafficking.

J. Montenegro Sebastian (✉)
Survivors' Network, Sussex, UK
e-mail: judit@survivorsnetwork.org.uk

P. Ali, M. M. Rogers (eds.), *Gender-Based Violence: A Comprehensive Guide*,
https://doi.org/10.1007/978-3-031-05640-6_27

The chapter first introduces the international definition of trafficking and analyses what the latest global data (UNODC 2021b) on the issue tells us while exposing how it affects different genders. Drawing attention to the gaps in international figures and one of the most hidden forms of trafficking (domestic servitude), the chapter continues by studying how trafficking occurs within the global political economy of migration (Pettman and Hall 2015) and the causes behind it. The testimonies of survivors of domestic servitude in Peru and the UK from my various research projects on modern slavery and trafficking[1] provide a valuable insight into the complexity of the crime and the needs of victims. The chapter concludes with an overview of the limitations of international anti-trafficking efforts and strategies and some impactful survivor-led alternatives and interventions to protect and support victims.

Defining Human Trafficking in International Law

In recent years, we have seen human trafficking emerging as a priority concern in the global politics agenda. The initial debates and international efforts on the issue focused on addressing the crime within wider concerns about prostitution. At the beginning of the twentieth century, conversations considered trafficking to occur solely within prostitution and had an abolitionist agenda, which regarded prostitution as rape and an abuse of women's rights (Doezema 2002; see 1933 International Convention for the Suppression of the Traffic in Women 1933). These views concentrated, particularly, on the abduction of European women and their transportation to be forced into prostitution with non-white men (Doezema 2002; Sullivan 2015).

These arguments, firstly, failed to recognise trafficking as a crime affecting all regions and most countries in the world (UNODC 2021b), committed by a complex range of organised and individual traffickers.[2] As some academics in the field have highlighted, initial views emerged from a 'racialized social panic' in which women

[1] The survivors' testimonies in this chapter come, firstly, from the author's research project on the trafficking of domestic workers and child domestic exploitation in Peru. This project is the result of the qualitative primary research work conducted by the author during her collaboration with the third sector organisation AGTR-La Casa de Panchita in Lima (Peru) in 2016.

Secondly, some of the testimonies of survivors of trafficking have been reproduced with the consent of the survivors from the book *Our Journey. Standing up for Our Rights* (VoDW 2020). The book consists of interview data and the firsthand written testimonies of over 40 MDWs members of the grassroots charity VoDW in London, in which the author was the primary researcher and editor. The disclosure of identity has been consented by testimonies and withheld by mutual agreement in the requested cases, in which a fictitious name has been used.

[2] While most persons investigated, arrested, prosecuted, and/or convicted of trafficking continue to be male (over 60% of the totals in the three categories), studies show that women traffickers may be particularly active in the recruitment phase of human trafficking. Women also represent a higher share for those convicted compared to males (See pp. 37–40 of the UNODC *Global Report on Trafficking in Persons 2020*, 'Profile of offenders' (United Nations publication, Sales No. E.20. IV.3.)).

were thought to have a 'vulnerable sexuality' at risk of being exploited by non-white men (Kempadoo 2005). And secondly, as Sullivan (2015: 87) points out, the issue of consent was not considered within the discussions, and international agreements did not envisage 'the possibility of women being active agents in their own lives, for example by migrating to undertake lucrative paid work in the sex trade'.

The input of sex workers and their allies in the 1980s and 1990s, arguing that prostitution should be regarded as a form of labour—sex work—(Sullivan 2015), started to draw distinctions in the debate. Trafficking began to be considered to involve forced labour, while sex work to be undertaken voluntarily[3] (Saunders 2005). Experts also pointed out that literature and efforts having a sole focus on sex trafficking in the debate were unhelpful, as they lacked insight into many other forms in which trafficking occurs (Aronowitz 2009).

These perspectives eventually led to the first agreed international definition of human trafficking, with the ratification of the *Protocol to Prevent Suppress and Punish Trafficking of Persons, Especially Women and Children* (UN 2000),[4] which provided a definition that was considered to represent a 'compromise' between the above opposing views (Sullivan 2015). In it, human trafficking is defined as:

> The recruitment, transportation, transfer, harbouring or receipt of persons, by means of the threat or use of force or other forms of coercion, of abduction, of fraud, of deception, of the abuse of power or of a position of vulnerability or of the giving or receiving of payments or benefits to achieve the consent of a person having control over another person, for the purpose of exploitation.
>
> Exploitation shall include, at a minimum, the exploitation of the prostitution of others or other forms of sexual exploitation, forced labour or services, slavery, or practices similar to slavery, servitude or removal of organs. (UN Protocol, Article 3 (a)).

As illustrated in Fig. 1, the United Nations Office of Drugs and Crime (UNODC), responsible for the Protocol, establishes that trafficking has occurred if three core elements are present:

1. The action of recruiting, transporting, transferring, harbouring, moving, or receiving someone across borders or within a single country.
2. The means by which those actions are carried out (threat or use of force, coercion, abduction, fraud, deception, abuse of power or vulnerability, or giving payments or benefits to a person in control of the victim).
3. The purpose of exploitation or enslavement, for financial or personal gain.

[3] These views considered sex work to be carried out through an informed decision about how to best earn a living and considering that not all migration for sex would necessarily involve violence, coercion, and trafficking (Saunders 2005).

[4] As of May 2020, the protocol has been ratified by 178 countries, and it entails states to make a commitment to adopt a range of measures to prevent and combat trafficking in persons, protecting and assisting victims of trafficking, and promoting cooperation among states in order to meet those objectives.

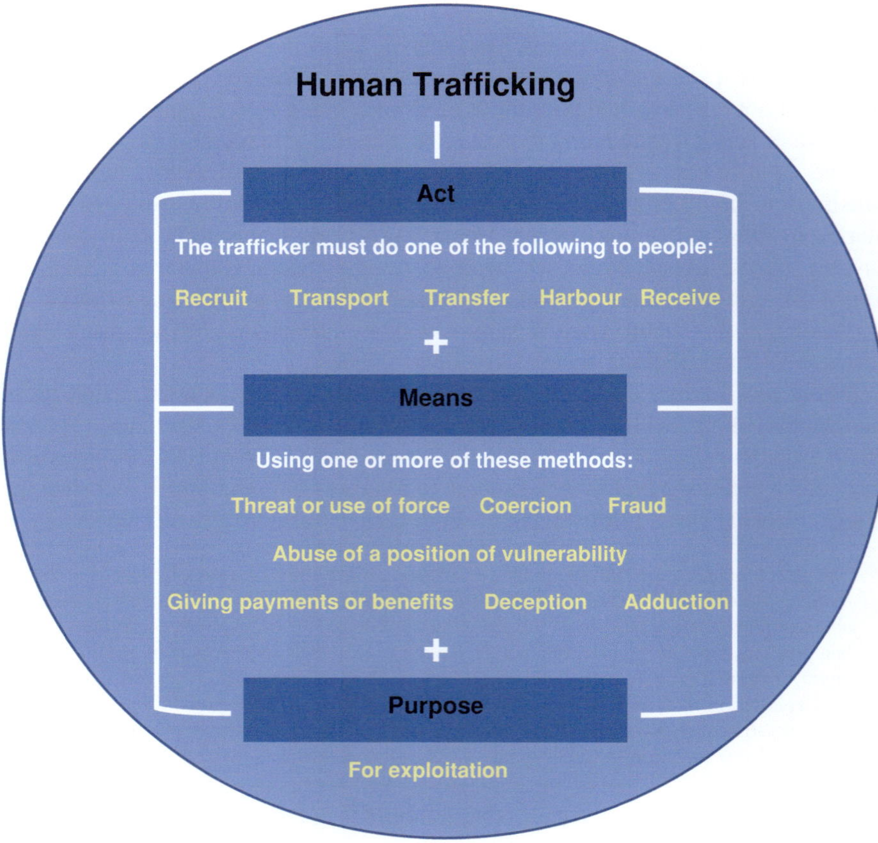

Fig. 1 The criminal elements of human trafficking. Own graphic. (Source: UNODC (2021a). 'Human trafficking. The Crime'. Available at: https://www.unodc.org/unodc/en/human-trafficking/crime.html (Accessed: 20 April 2021))

This international framework also extends special protection to children under the age of 18. For this age group, it considers that a crime of trafficking has taken place if there is at least one of the above actions and the purpose of exploitation, even if it does not involve any of the means set forth above. The recognition in the protocol that trafficking encompasses many diverse forms of exploitation was also a first step to recognise some of the most invisible and under-detected victims (Aronowitz 2009).

International Context

According to the latest report on forced labour by the International Labour Organization (ILO) and the Walk Free Foundation (2017), in 2016 there were an estimated 40.3 million victims of human trafficking and modern slavery globally. Yet, as experts in the field highlight, achieving an accurate picture of human trafficking remains a difficult task (Aronowitz 2009; Shelley 2010). There still exists a huge disparity between estimated numbers and actual numbers of trafficking victims who reach out for help and have been identified by authorities and relevant organisations (UNODC 2021b).

Box 1 Modern Slavery Definition

Modern slavery is the illegal exploitation of people for personal or commercial gain. It is an umbrella term which covers a wide range of abuse and exploitation and includes holding a person in a position of slavery, forced servitude or compulsory labour, or facilitating their travel with the intention of exploiting them soon after (Such et al. 2020).

Human trafficking is a form of modern slavery which is defined by the movement and transportation of the victims for the purpose of exploitation and slavery.

Alternative terminology

Exploitation, Modern-day slavery, Enslavement, Servitude, Subjugation, Serfdom, Thrall.

The UNODC, the body responsible for collecting data on human trafficking globally, recognises that people of all ages and backgrounds can become victims of trafficking. The identification of victims and global data on the crime is crucial (UNODC 2018) to, firstly, gain knowledge of changing trends and prevalence of trafficking; secondly, to tailor how effective the efforts and commitments in the fight against the crime are; and finally, to support decision-making in improving policy responses and develop effective anti-trafficking programmes.

Yet, while data is crucial in the trafficking issue, its current coverage is still limited. The information collected globally is disaggregated by few characteristics (for example, form of exploitation or sex of victims), while others are not contemplated (UNODC 2021b). This might often leave many trafficking trends and victims unidentified and unreported. For instance, as the latest UNODC (2021b) highlights, a growing body of research shows that lesbian, gay, bisexual, transgender, queer and intersex (LGBTQI+) individuals[5] are at higher risk of becoming victims of trafficking (Martinez and Kelle 2013). Studies show that LGBTQI+ identity increases the vulnerability of children and young adults to trafficking (U.S. Department of State 2016), 'as they are often marginalised in society and ostracised by friends and relatives who may force them out of their home' (UNODC 2021b: 38). Moreover, strong social stigma or severe laws criminalising same-sex relationships and/or transgender identities might make persons like the LGBTQI+ community more vulnerable to exploitation.

[5] Persons who are lesbian, gay, bisexual, transgender, queer, or have other sexual orientations or gender identities

Traffickers particularly target persons who are at the margins of societies and less protected and seek to exploit these oppressive circumstances (U.S. Department of State 2016). Still, the UNODC (2021b: 38) recognises that 'administrative records reported by most governments are not often helpful in understanding how LGBTQI+ individuals […] are vulnerable to trafficking in persons'. There is, indeed, a need for further research and improvement for data collection on the issue.

While acknowledging these limitations and the challenges they present, global available data on trafficking exposes patterns on the profile of victims and the gendered nature of this crime.

The UNODC's (2021b) latest report, based on official figures from over 148 countries, shows that:

- Female victims continue to be the primary targets and particularly affected by human trafficking.
- In 2018, for every ten victims detected globally, about five were adult women and two were girls.
- Approximately one third of the overall detected victims were children, with girls representing 19% and boys 15%, while 20% were adult men.
- Sexual exploitation[6] continued to be the most prevalent form of trafficking (the 50% of the total detected victims), followed by labour exploitation (38%).

As Fig. 2 shows, in 2018 sexual exploitation was, disproportionately, the most predominant form of trafficking for females.

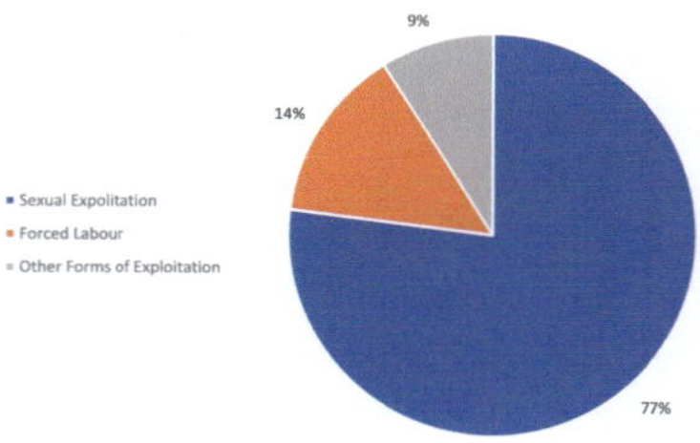

Forms of exploitation among detected adult women victims of trafficking in person 2018 (or most recent) 106 countries (n=12162 victims whose age, sex and form of exploitation was reported

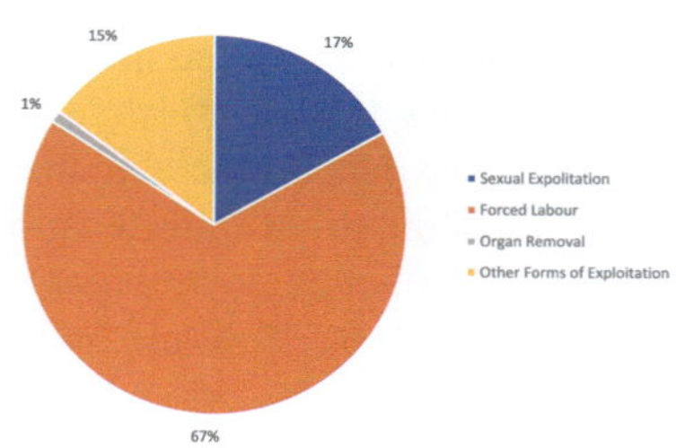

Forms of exploitation among detected adult women victims of trafficking in person 2018 (or most recent) 106 countries (n=3762 victims whose age, sex and form of exploitation was reported

Fig. 2 Shares of forms of exploitation globally in 2018 by sex. Own graphic. (Adapted from UNODC (2021b). 'Global Report on Trafficking in Persons 2020', Vienna, January 2021. United Nations publication, Sales No. E.20.IV.3: pp. 33)

[6] The World Health Organization (WHO) provides the used definition of sexual exploitation within the UN and defines it as the 'Actual or attempted abuse of a position of vulnerability, power, or trust, for sexual purposes, including, but not limited to, profiting monetarily, socially or politically from the sexual exploitation of another' (WHO 2017, pp. 4).

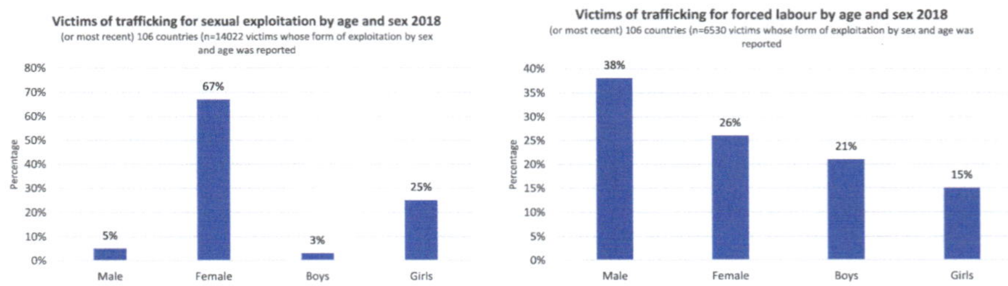

Fig. 3 Shares of detected victims for sexual exploitation and forced labour in 2018, by age and sex. Own graphic. (Adapted from UNODC (2021b). 'Global Report on Trafficking in Persons 2020', Vienna, January 2021. United Nations publication, Sales No. E.20.IV.3: pp. 36)

Comparatively, as Fig. 3 illustrates, while females represent the 92% of detected victims for sexual exploitation and forced labour was most common among men and boys, the sex and age profiles for forced labour is more diverse (UNODC 2021b).

The global data on trafficking for forced labour (UNODC 2021b, pp. 96) evidences how sex and age of detected victims are 'connected to the types of employment where victims are exploited'. As the feminist GCC/GVC[7] literature documents (Lebaron and Gore 2020), gender is directly linked with the type of profession women carry out in supply chains (Barrientos 2019). Authors in the field argue that gender norms and relations may influence the fact that certain groups of workers concentrate in certain parts of a chain, 'for example, in sections that are predominantly feminised or masculinised' (Lebaron and Gore 2020: 1099).

Indeed, available figures on forced labour show that females predominate in domestic servitude (representing 88% of total victims of this form of trafficking). On the other hand, more adult men are detected on large construction sites or in the fishing industry (UNODC 2021b). Studies in the cocoa industry in Ghana, for example, show that the preference for male workers 'was attributed to the perception that men will be able to undertake more arduous physical labour on the farm' (Lebaron and Gore 2020: 1109).

Similarly, other forms of exploitation are rooted in unequal gender status and power relations (OHCHR 2014). For instance, albeit in smaller numbers:

- Adult females and girl victims are also trafficked for the purpose of forced marriages, and a few cases of trafficking of pregnant women and/or trafficking of infants, both for the purpose of illegal adoption, were also reported in multiple countries.
- Boys are more commonly targeted for trafficking for forced criminal activity.

[7] GCC stands for global commodity chain and GVC for global value chain.

Although the United Nations (UN) Protocol brought the recognition of other forms of exploitation, as Sullivan (2015: 93) argues, most anti-trafficking efforts 'continue to focus on sex trafficking' and pay far less attention to mixed forms of exploitation or other forms of trafficking, such as the 'situation of women and girls trafficked for forced labour outside prostitution (for example, domestic labour) or to the trafficking of men and boys'.

Drawing attention to the available evidence on some of the most invisible forms of trafficking, like domestic servitude, provides unique learnings about the process and causes of trafficking. This can help improve anti-trafficking and victim detention efforts.

The Journey into Trafficking and Causation

Domestic work,[8] carried out in the private sphere, encompasses chores that have historically been strongly associated with *femininity* and as 'women's work' or even 'women's natural duty' (Pettman and Hall 2015). Experts have argued that this belief contributes to wider societal views attributing a lesser value to this profession (Drobnič and Treas 2010) and a significant prevalence of informality in the sector (ILO 2020).

The deterioration of labour rights and work conditions is a common pattern encountered in trafficking for forced labour (UNODC 2021b) and can often set a foundation for potential exploitation in domestic work. In regions like Latin America and the Caribbean, domestic work represents between 10.5% and 14.3% of women's employment, and it commonly entails precarious conditions and limited access to social protection (ILO 2020).

While male victims of domestic servitude remain a minority within detected victims, it is recognised that stigma and many other factors (Hestia 2018) might contribute to males being unidentified in this form of trafficking. Similarly, research on the experiences of male victims of domestic servitude is still limited (UNODC 2021b). Although further research and efforts to identify male victims are crucial, some studies (Awumbila et al. 2017) suggest that male workers 'tend to have clearer duties and job descriptions than female domestic workers', providing them with 'greater grounds for, and legitimacy in, challenging unfair treatment', for example, being asked to work additional hours (Lebaron and Gore 2020: 1101). Female domestic workers, on the other hand, often have no contract or job description (Awumbila et al. 2017).

Several factors are recognised as key to increasing the vulnerability of victims to become trapped in various forms of trafficking, like domestic servitude. Compounded by gender norms (Awumbila et al. 2017), these include gender inequality, the feminization of poverty, and migration (Osezua 2016), as well as 'patriarchal social structures (limiting the economic opportunities of women), social and economic

[8] Women represent over 80% of the 67.1 million domestic workers worldwide. In some regions, like Latin America and the Caribbean, women represent 93% of people engaged in domestic work (ILO 2020).

marginalisation, failed and corrupt governments, family breakdown, and historical precedents of bonded labour' (Sullivan 2015: 90). Yet, many scholars and international bodies identify poverty as the main cause of trafficking (Aronowitz 2009; ILO 2016).

The Peruvian Ombudsman report on domestic workers (Defensoría del Pueblo 2016) exposes that in Peru, this profession is almost exclusively carried out by women (95.8%) who are, generally, in poverty situations without a complete access to education and often migrants from the province areas who migrate to the Peruvian capital or abroad. Indeed, research shows that victims of domestic servitude come from some of the most impoverished areas of the world and are, in many cases, national or international migrants (ILO 2016).[9] Poverty 'pushes' them away from their communities in order to survive (Sullivan 2015; UNODC 2008), and this is the starting point of their journey.

The ILO (2013) reports that high income countries[10] are the major destination for migrant workers globally, accounting for more than 90 million of the 150 million migrant workers globally and 80% of the migrant domestic workers (MDWs) worldwide. Thus, these regions play a key role in this global political economy with the 'transnational reproductive labour' (Pettman and Hall 2015: 292).

Sullivan (2015: 90) suggests that it is 'not surprising that the main "trafficking flows" in the world today follow general migration paths': between poorer and wealthier regions of the world, developing and wealthier countries, and from rural or marginalised areas to the cities. The increasing demand and supply for people (particularly in a globalised world) flourishes the business for transnational criminals (Aronowitz 2009; Shelley 2010).

As Kempadoo (2005: ix) highlights 'women are disproportionately represented among the poor, the debt-bonded, and the international migrant workforce', and migrating becomes an escape and opportunity. Yet, 'most legal migration channels are strongly biased toward work that is traditionally done by men, while two very common areas of migration for women, domestic and entertainment work, have very little protection under labour laws' (Marshall and Thatun 2005: 52).

Experts and international bodies recognise that the 'combination of informality, precarity, gender inequality, and a lack of legal rights and access to justice' increases female domestic worker's vulnerability to be exploited by traffickers (Lebaron and Gore 2020: 1100). The Peruvian Ombudsman highlights that domestic worker's condition as migrant aggravates the special situation of vulnerability these workers already experience due to their sex, gender identity, ethnic background, economic situation and age, and how these factors make them 'exposed to situations of multiple discriminations' (Defensoría del Pueblo 2016, pp. 38). Due to the nature of the work, especially for migrants, domestic workers are often isolated and segregated from wider society.

[9] The latest data from the ILO shows that one in every five domestic workers is an international migrant—this is 11.5 million migrant domestic workers (MDWs) (ILO 2016).

[10] Together, the Arab states, North America, and northern, southern and Western Europe account for about 52% of the 11.5 million domestic workers worldwide.

In my research work in Peru (2016), I interviewed children and adult domestic workers who had migrated to Lima (Peru's capital) with the hope of moving away from situations of poverty and extreme poverty, violence, grief, or family conflicts. My work within the charity AGTR-La Casa de Panchita included listening to over 30 domestic workers and professionals working with survivors. They explained that victims, like many young people living in the rural areas of the country, migrated to Lima by themselves as children. They did this, firstly, to overcome struggle by finding better opportunities, through work and ensuring access to education, and secondly, to earn money to support their families back home. Some made this decision by themselves, while others were sent to work for someone by their families.

Most testimonies from domestic workers explained having had experiences of abuse from *employers*[11] who made them work over 14 hours per day. Similar to the findings of available research (AGTR 2004; Defensoría del Pueblo 2016), psychological abuse was the most common form of abuse amongst these workers, followed by physical, sexual, and financial abuse. Some workers had also had *employers* who made them work for no pay and for extended family and did not allow them to study.

These testimonies illustrate how the need to move from poverty-ridden rural areas to cities creates opportunities for trafficking and modern slavery (Kempadoo 2005; Sullivan 2015).

It also exposes how children are particularly vulnerable and easy targets for traffickers (UNODC 2021a), as their work is often critical for poor households (Thorsen 2012). The decision from parents to send their children away, to work for relatives or unknown employers, is reported to be a 'coping mechanism for families to survive in conditions of extreme poverty' (Psacharopoulos 1997) and seen by parents as an opportunity for their children to access education.

Similarly, those with fewer income and migration options 'are less able to negotiate or challenge oppressive work conditions' (Sullivan 2015: 90–91). Thus, workers with a conditional or illegal status also 'compounds the vulnerabilities they already experience as poorer, less protected workers, and often as women' (Pettman and Hall 2015: 291).

As the UNODC (2021: 10) exposes, migrants make up a significant share of the detected victims in most regions of the world,[12] and victims 'who do not have permission to work or stay in the country of exploitation face an extra layer of

[11] The term 'employer' was used by domestic workers during interviews to refer to their abusers, and it is used in this chapter with the aim to differentiate the different parties perpetuating modern slavery and trafficking (agencies, perpetrators of the exploitation and violence, other agents facilitating the transportation of victims and the exploitation). Yet, it is relevant to note these 'employers' refer to the people victims are forced to work for.

[12] Migrant victims of trafficking represent the '65 per cent in Western and Southern Europe, 60 per cent in the Middle East, 55 per cent in East Asia and the Pacific, 50 per cent in Central and South-Eastern Europe, and 25 per cent in North America' (UNODC 2021b, p. 10).

vulnerability'. Traffickers might trick victims into illegal migration routes or exploit their fear of being exposed as an irregular migrant to authorities (Aronowitz 2009; UNODC 2021b).

Criminals might use binding visas (frequently tied to an individual employer), victim's isolation, or victims being unaware of their rights to exploit them (UNODC 2021b). Threats, debt bondage, false promises, coercion, and limitation to movement are also common techniques to exploit workers and create dependency (UNODC 2021b).

Box 2 Lyann's Case (Survivor of Domestic Servitude)[13]

'I applied to work abroad through an agency in Manila in May 2014. I was immediately deployed to Qatar. I was picked up by an employee of an agency. My passport and documents were taken from me the moment I arrived. [...] I couldn't complain, because the agency would ask me to pay 10,000 Riyal (£2227) to allow me to go home. One of the employers [...] brought me to London with the agreement of the agency. This wasn't even discussed with me, and I wasn't given a copy of their agreement. This employer's employee brought me to the British Embassy to apply for my visa. I signed the papers without properly seeing the documents[...].

I arrived in London [...] and I was threatened by this employer that if I escape, she would kill me. My employer is powerful in Qatar. I knew she could kill me. [...] I was heavily guarded all the time by their two staff members. The whole house had CCTV inside and outside.

[...] My agency then sold me to this employer for 100,000 Riyal (£22,278), [...] [who] promised me that she would treat me well, help me buy my own house and increase my salary if I returned to them from my holiday [back home]. [...] My nightmares began the moment I returned to the UK. [...] I worked straight away with no rest and no food. I looked after the baby for 24 hours because I slept in the same room. I had no proper bed, I slept on the floor.

[...] My employer had a bad temper [...]. Her shouting has caused me nervous breakdowns. She would tell me that she could afford to buy my life. It was so painful to hear this most of the time, as if I was nothing and no one.'

Victims of domestic servitude are exposed to multiple forms of exploitation and violence 'that is rarely seen in other forms of trafficking' (UNODC 2021b: 12), including sexual, physical, and psychological abuse. Experiences of victims like Lyann's (see Box 2), however, often go undetected, taking place in households 'which are largely unregulated or hard to monitor or organise' (Pettman and Hall 2015: 292). Although efforts from the international community have increased since the UN Protocol, the identification and protection of victims and the prevention of trafficking remain challenging tasks.

[13]The Voice of Domestic Workers (2020). 'Our Journey, Standing up for our rights', p. 101

Limitations of Anti-trafficking Strategies

Immigration Restrictions Facilitating Trafficking

Some authors argue one of the greatest challenges governments face is the protection of trafficked persons and, at the same time, enforcing immigration restrictions (Aronowitz 2009). Empirical evidence has demonstrated that efforts from governments to restrict immigration assist trafficking, rather than block and prevent it (Marshall and Thatun 2005). Strategies to combat the crime are compromised, in countries like the UK, 'hostile environments' for migrant victims with an irregular status.

The creation of the Immigration Enforcement Competent Authority (IECA) by the UK government and the Nationality and Borders bill faced criticisms by experts, the Independent Anti-Slavery Commissioner (IASC) and NGOs for increasing the burden of proof to identify victims of trafficking and disqualifying some victims, including children, who were compelled by traffickers to commit unlawful acts (U.S. Department of State 2022). Moreover, as latest reports on the issue highlight (U.S. Department of State 2022), a minority of foreign trafficking victims evaluated for discretionary leave were granted this immigration status in the UK. Due to this context, observers raised concerns that some victims may not engage with official mechanisms to identify victims due to fear of deportation. In the UK, migrant victims of domestic servitude who escape their traffickers often find that their visa has expired, leaving them undocumented and subject to arrest and deportation (VoDW 2020). This fear is significant as protection and assistance for victims are often conditional on cooperation with law enforcement officials (Sullivan 2015). Similarly, as the ILO (2016) and experts have pointed out, MDWs in the UK are at an increased risk of trafficking, abuse, and slavery due to being restricted to a non-renewable six-month visa that binds them to live in their employer's household.

The case of Lyann (see Box 2) demonstrates how this crime is meticulously perpetrated and the difficulty of gathering evidence. The fear of deportation if victims are not able to provide enough evidence of their experiences stops them from seeking support (VoDW 2020). Thus, tight immigration rules become a significant barrier for victims in need of support from official bodies, while those who manage to escape their traffickers become at risk of ongoing cycles of exploitation due to their undocumented status.

Protecting Worker's Rights

Ensuring the protection of labour rights and decent working conditions is key to reducing the vulnerability of workers to forced labour (Nishimoto 2018; ILO 2013), especially for those employed precariously in sectors like domestic work, the agriculture and fishing sectors, and other informal work.

The ILO recognises some of the essential measures to facilitate this might be (Nishimoto 2018):

- Tackling discriminatory treatment, particularly for women and migrant workers.
- Extending social protection schemes so that all workers can benefit.
- Broadening the mandate and resources of labour inspectorates to enforce labour laws.
- Facilitating access to complaint mechanisms through outreach and legal assistance.
- Guaranteeing freedom of association for workers to organise and bargain collectively.

These measures, among further recommendations to improve worker's rights, are collected in the ILO's Domestic Workers Convention Number 189. Yet, to this date only 29 (out of the 195 countries) have ratified this convention globally. While the UK is not on this list of countries, Peru ratified the convention in 2018, and this led to the modification of the national domestic workers legislation in 2020. The new Peruvian legislation (*Ley de los Trabajadores del Hogar, Act 27986, 2020*) equated domestic worker's rights to the ones of workers in other sectors; among other measures, it established that their salary must not be under the national minimum wage and contracts to mandatorily be written.[14]

The Root Causes of Trafficking

Addressing the socio-economic factors that create an environment susceptible to be exploited by traffickers is essential to address the crime. Particularly considering the impact of the COVID-19 pandemic, as the UNODC (2021b) recognises, strategies to prevent trafficking need to focus on marginalised communities and groups (UNODC 2008). Some of these measures might include addressing poverty and precarity (Aronowitz 2009), economic inequalities resulting from gender discrimination, and 'reinforcing social ties and safety nets for households in economic need' (UNODC 2021b: 19). This must consider long-term sustainable strategies, particularly in key countries and areas of origin (Aronowitz 2009).

Engagement with local grassroots organisations constitutes a building block for anti-trafficking strategies. As the UNODC's (2021b: 19) trafficking report concludes, community-led 'interventions aimed at creating new sustainable livelihood' for populations at risk and victims are crucial, and 'increasing awareness of the risks of irregular migration or child labour should be promoted'. For instance, the grassroots NGO AGTR-La Casa de Panchita in Peru implements various community programmes to prevent trafficking and exploitation. Their project *Empowering*

[14] The previous legislation established domestic worker's contracts could be either written or verbal. This was recognised to greater the vulnerability of workers to abuse and exploitation whilst making it difficult for victims to demonstrate the agreed conditions between the parties, but also that the agreement happened at all – a great barrier to prosecute perpetrators and traffickers (Carla Villarreal López, Commissioner and Manager of the Women's Rights Department for the Ombudsman of Peru, Interview by Judit Montenegro Sebastian, Lima, Peru, 13 May 2016).

Child Domestic Workers (CDWs) in Peru (AGTR 2017) resulted in 502 families becoming aware of the risks for CDWs and protecting their children by withdrawing them from work or taking measures to improve their situation. Other outcomes of this programme included reducing isolation for 638 teenagers in domestic work, who lived with their employers, through their teacher's support to maintain communication with their families. Similarly, providing emergency accommodation for survivors escaping their traffickers and delivering projects to empower women and adult migrant domestic workers are essential (VoDW 2020). Education on workers' rights is also fundamental to prevent the risk of forced labour and provide workers with the tools to negotiate and challenge oppressive practices (Nishimoto 2018).

Impunity

Despite the existing legal framework on combating trafficking, impunity for traffickers prevails globally (UNODC 2021b) and becomes a great stimulant for trafficking. Data collected over the past 3 years 'shows a steep decline' and extremely low number of prosecution and convictions,[15] while the number of identified victims grows (OSCE 2020: 2020). As Shelley (2010: 2–3) states, traffickers choose to trade in humans 'because there are low start-up costs, minimal risks, high profits, and large demand', as there appears to be a small risk for traffickers to face justice.

The OSCE[16] (2020: 2) argues that this is due to the criminal justice sector suffering from a number of challenges, 'including lack of resources, insufficient training and innovation, and limited political will'. Yet, there will be nothing deterring traffickers from further offending if perpetrators do not face a credible risk of being proportionally convicted and sentenced for their crimes.

Thus, transnational criminals exploit the vulnerabilities of victims and obtain high profits at a very minimal risk – a reality which presents great barriers to preventing the crime and protecting victims.

Summary

- Human trafficking affects every region of the world and is one of the fastest-growing crimes globally.
- Trafficking is a gendered crime. Female victims continue to be the primary targets and are particularly affected by the crime. Male victims are mostly affected by forced labour, while sexual exploitation is the most predominant form of trafficking for females.

[15] The '2019 Trafficking in Persons Report' in the USA shows a 52% decrease in prosecutions between 2015 and 2018 within Europe, while the number of trafficking victims identified within the area increased by over 51% (U.S. Department of State 2019).

[16] The Organisation for Security and Co-operation in Europe.

- Poverty is the main cause of trafficking. Transnational criminals exploit the political economy of migration and the growing demand for people in wealthier regions of the world and urban sites.
- Attempts to restrict immigration facilitate trafficking, rather than preventing or stopping it.
- Anti-trafficking efforts must focus on strengthening labour protections and rights, tackle the root causes of trafficking, and work towards ending impunity for criminals. Further research and improving data collection and mechanisms to identify victims are also crucial.

References

1933 International Convention for the Suppression of the Traffic in Women (1933) 11 October, Geneva

Aronowitz AA (2009) Human trafficking, human misery. The Global Trade in Human Beings. United Stated, Praeger

Asociación Grupo De Trabajo Redes (AGTR) (2004) De la sierra a la capital. Trabajadoras del hogar Lima - Perú. AGTR, Lima

Asociación Grupo De Trabajo Redes (AGTR) (2017) AGTR Memoria Anual 2017. Lima (Peru), AGTR

Awumbila M, Teye JK, Yaro JA (2017) Of silent maids, skilled gardeners and careful madams: gendered dynamics and strategies of migrant domestic workers in Accra, Ghana. GeoJournal 82(5):957–970

Barrientos S (2019) Gender and work in global value chains: capturing the gains? Cambridge University Press, Cambridge

Defensoría del Pueblo (2016) Las Trabajadoras del Hogar en Perú. Balance sobre el cumplimiento de las recomendaciones defensoriales. Serie Informes de Adjuntía – Informe N° 001–2016-DP/ADM

Doezema J (2002) Who gets to choose? Coercion, consent, and the UN trafficking protocol. Gend Dev 10(1):20–27

Drobnič S, Treas J (eds) (2010) Dividing the domestic: men, women, and household work in cross-national perspective. Stanford University Press, Stanford, CA

Hestia (2018) Underground lives. Male victims of modern slavery. https://www.hestia.org/Handlers/Download.ashx?IDMF=60de8cf2-497f-4c80-8831-f35b335ae6b1. Accessed 6 Nov 2021

International Labour Organisation (ILO) (2013) Domestic workers across the world: global and regional statistics and the extent of legal protection. International Labour Office, Geneva

International Labour Organisation (ILO) (2016) Migrant domestic workers across the world: global and regional estimates. Research series. Global action programme on migrant domestic workers and their families, labour migration branch (MIGRANT). ILO, Geneva

International Labour Organisation (ILO) (2020) Domestic Workers in Latin America and the Caribbean during the COVID-19 Crisis. ILO, 12 June, Brief vol. 1.1

International Labour Organisation (ILO), Walk Free Foundation (2017) Global estimates of modern slavery: forced labour and forced marriage. ILO, Geneva

Kempadoo K (2005) Introduction. From moral panic to global justice: changing perspectives on trafficking. In: Kempadoo K (ed) Trafficking and prostitution reconsidered: new perspectives on migration, sex work and human rights. Paradigm Publishers, Boulder, CO

Lebaron G, Gore E (2020) Gender and forced labour: understanding the links in global cocoa supply chains. J Dev Stud 56(6):1095–1117

Marshall P, Thatun S (2005) Miles away. The trouble with prevention in the greater Mekong subregion. In: Kempadoo K (ed) Trafficking and prostitution reconsidered: new perspectives on migration, sex work and human rights. Paradigm Publishers, Boulder, CO

Martinez O, Kelle G (2013) Sex trafficking of LGBT individuals: a call for service provision, research, and action. Int Law News 42(4):21–24

Nishimoto T (2018) Labour rights: the means to tackle human trafficking'. International Labour Organisation (ILO) News, 27 July. https://www.ilo.org/asia/media-centre/news/WCMS_635351/lang%2D%2Den/index.htm. Accessed 2 June 2021

Office of the High Commissioner for Human Rights (OHCHR) (2014) Child and forced marriage - manifestation of gender discrimination. OHCHR, 11 July. https://www.ohchr.org/en/newsevents/pages/childandforcedmarriagemanifestationofgenderdiscrimination.aspx. Accessed 5 Oct 2021

Organization For Security and Co-Operation in Europe (OSCE) (2020) Ending impunity, delivering justice through prosecuting trafficking in human beings. 20th conference of the alliance against trafficking in persons. Office of the Special Representative and Co-ordinator for Combating Trafficking in Human Beings, Conference 30–31 March, Hofburg, Vienna. https://www.osce.org/files/f/documents/c/5/447646.pdf. Accessed 1 June 2021

Osezua C (2016) Gender issues in human trafficking in Edo State, Nigeria. Afr Sociol Rev 36(20):36–66

Pettman J, Hall L (2015) Migration. In: Shepherd LJ (ed) Gender matters in global politics. A feminist introduction to international relations. Routledge, Abingdon

Psacharopoulos G (1997) Child labor versus educational attainment some evidence from Latin America. J Popul Econ 10:377–386

Saunders P (2005) Traffic violations. Determining the meaning of violence in sexual trafficking versus sex work. J Interpers Violence 20(3):343–360

Shelley L (2010) Human trafficking: a global perspective. Cambridge University Press, New York

Such E, Laurent C, Salway S (2020) Modern slavery and public health: a rapid evidence assessment and an emergent public health approach. Public Health 180:168–179

Sullivan B (2015) Trafficking in human beings. In: Shepherd LJ (ed) Gender matters in global politics. A feminist introduction to international relations. Routledge, Abingdon

The Voice of Domestic Workers (VoDW) (2020) Our journey. Standing up for our rights. The Voice of Domestic Workers, London

Thorsen D (2012) Children Working in Mines and Quarries, Evidence from West and Central Africa. Dakar: UNICEF, Briefing Paper No. 4

United Nations General Assembly (2000) Protocol to prevent, suppress and punish trafficking in persons, especially women and children, supplementing the United Nations Convention against transnational organized crime, 15 November. https://www.ohchr.org/en/professionalinterest/pages/protocoltraffickinginpersons.aspx. Accessed 15 Apr 2021

United Nations Office on Drugs and Crime (UNODC) (2008) Toolkit to combat trafficking in persons. Global programme against trafficking in human beings. United Nations, New York

United Nations Office on Drugs and Crime (UNODC) (2018). 'Why is it so important to have comprehensive data in the fight against trafficking in persons?', Pretoria (South Africa), 21 May. https://www.unodc.org/unodc/en/human-trafficking/glo-act/why-is-it-so-important-to-have-comprehensive-data-in-the-fight-against-trafficking-in-persons.html. Accessed 15 Sept 2021

United Nations Office on Drugs and Crime (UNODC) (2021a) Human trafficking. The crime. https://www.unodc.org/unodc/en/human-trafficking/crime.html. Accessed 20 Apr 2021

United Nations Office on Drugs and Crime (UNODC) (2021b) Global report on trafficking in persons 2020', Vienna, January 2021. United Nations publication, Sales No. E.20.IV.3

US Department of State (2016) Trafficking in persons report 2016. US Department of State, Washington, DC

U.S. Department of State (2019) Trafficking in persons report. June, Department of State, United States of America

U.S. Department of State (2022) Trafficking in Persons Report: United Kingdom. July, Department of State, Office to Monitor And Combat Trafficking In Persons. United States of America

World Health Organization (WHO) (2017) Sexual exploitation and abuse prevention and response. Policy and procedures March 2017'. WHO, Office of Compliance, Risk Management and Ethics, March 2017

Judit Montenegro Sebastian is a journalist, social researcher and data professional with a decade of experience in the non-profit sector in the UK, Spain and Peru. She has dedicated her career to supporting survivors of, and researching issues related to, Modern Slavery, Human Trafficking (with a focus on domestic work), sexual violence and gender-based violence.

Migration and Gender-Based Violence

Rachel Alsop

Learning Objectives
Having read this chapter, you should be able to understand

- The interconnections between migration and gender-based violence (GBV).
- Risk factors that increase the likelihood of GBV within migrant communities.
- How violence is perpetrated on structural as well as interpersonal levels.

Introduction

Migration operates as an umbrella term to encompass a range of mobilities and lived experiences (see Box 1). While the focus of this chapter will be on international migration, which involves the crossing of national borders, migration can also be domestic and refer to internal relocation within a nation's borders. In 2021, it is estimated that there are 281 million international and 763 million internal migrants worldwide. This means that one seventh of the global population is a migrant.[1] A range of push and pull factors shape migration—poverty, lack of economic opportunities, war, conflict, persecution as well as natural disasters (or often a combination thereof) are key drivers for people to leave their home countries in the hope of greater prosperity and/or safer, more secure lives. Specific pull factors towards destination countries include job opportunities, higher wages, more developed welfare

[1] https://www.iom.sk/en/migration/migration-in-the-world.html.

R. Alsop (✉)
Centre for Women's Studies at the University of York, York, UK
e-mail: rachel.alsop@york.ac.uk

P. Ali, M. M. Rogers (eds.), *Gender-Based Violence: A Comprehensive Guide*,
https://doi.org/10.1007/978-3-031-05640-6_28

and healthcare systems, liberal democratic governance, humanitarian assistance and diasporic links (Castelli 2018), with social, familial and national networks playing a pivotal part in shaping migratory routes. As Lutz and Palenga-Möllenbeck (2012) explain in relation to transnational care, migration is informed by a complex entanglement of macro-, meso- and micro-level factors.

Defining Migration

Migration research increasingly recognises that drawing a boundary between voluntary migration (often equated with economic migration) and forced migration (in response to humanitarian crises, persecution or conflict) is too simplistic (Freedman 2015) and that instead both should be considered as existing on a continuum. As Erdal and Oeppen (2018: 981) argue in relation to the forced-voluntary distinction, 'whilst there may be identifiable extreme cases, most migrants' experiences of the degree of volition in their migration decisions means that they fall somewhere in the blurry middle of the forced-voluntary spectrum'. Furthermore, within this continuum, the legal and political rights granted to migrants vary. Some may receive legal authorisation from their destination nation for permanent or temporary residence (with or without full citizenship). Some remain (or become) undocumented or irregular migrants because of arriving through irregular means, visa overstay, breach of visa regulations, being born to parents who are themselves irregular migrants or staying after an asylum application is refused. Others sit in limbo, awaiting, for example, decisions on asylum claims.

While countries may adhere in principle to international legal frameworks intended to protect migrants' human rights, the recognition and implementation of migrants' rights, in practice, differs (Migration Data Portal 2021) creating contexts 'where sovereign prerogatives continue to resist human rights claims' (Mullaly 2014:146). As Taran (2000: 7) notes 'in many States, legal application of human rights norms to non-citizens is inadequate or seriously deficient, especially regarding irregular migrants'. Mullaly (2014: 145) argues that gender 'plays a key role in [...] determining the terms of belonging imposed by states', with presumptions of migrant women's vulnerability (see chapter on trafficking for the purposes of sexual exploitation) used to manage migration, close down safe routes of passage and justify the 'coercive interventions of the state' (Mullaly 2014: 146).

Migration and Violence

Analyses of migration are entwined with analyses of the structural violence perpetrated by states and institutions towards migrants 'that is built into practices, policies, institutional and legal frameworks', which 'manifests itself as discrimination resulting in social exclusion from protection and/or support [...] and increases the likelihood/reproduction of interpersonal gender based violence' (Tastsoglou et al. 2021: n.p). Phillimore et al. (2021) point to three interrelated types of structural violence constructing the lived experiences of migrants: violent abandonment, slow violence and the violence of uncertainty. Violent abandonment refers to the multiple ways in which states fail to act to protect migrants—this could be through the lack of intervention to provide safe migratory routes or the failure to provide services in destination countries to adequately support migrants to live with dignity and safety (what they describe as 'inaction as action'). Migrants seeking asylum, for example, have to endure the slow violence that occurs trying to survive with minimal resources, often in poor accommodation with insufficient means to meet daily needs. In turn, material deprivation compounds psychological stress and the risk of interpersonal violence. The violence of uncertainty is (re)produced through the lengthy delays within asylum systems, the lack of clarity in processes and decisions and the inability to move on with one's life while waiting. The violence here is slow and also can result in instances of violent abandonment if claims are unsuccessful and migrants are repatriated or forced to go underground. 'Uncertainty and fear are said to have a greater impact on asylum seekers than premigration trauma [...] and result in wide-ranging mental health problems such as depression, anxiety, psychosocial distress, and suicide ideation' (Phillimore et al. 2021: 8).

Feminist Interventions in Migration Scholarship

An early contribution by feminist migration scholars was to challenge the androcentric bias of mainstream migration research which foregrounded the experiences of male workers and then made generalising statements about migration from these findings (Nawyn 2010). The male migrant worker had historically been constructed as the norm in migration studies, with women's migration considered on a secondary basis in relation to male kin—'the trailing spouse' syndrome (Izaguirre and Walsham 2021: 8). Feminist scholarship has been crucial in demonstrating 'how gender shapes the size, destination and composition of migration flows' (Izaguirre and Walsham 2021: 9) and how migration both informs, and is informed by, gender relations.

While there has been increased attention to the 'feminisation of migration' in recent decades, there is debate as to whether greater visibility of women in migration studies necessarily means the greater feminisation of migration itself (Piper 2003; Russell 2014). Feminist migration scholarship points out that women have always migrated, sometimes as dependents but also as independent transnational migrants for work, education or as heads of households (Freedman 2015). However, women's migration, it is argued, has been less visible in studies because of a lack of disaggregated data and a male bias within research. Nonetheless, there is acknowledgement by some scholars that rates of women migrating independently of family members have been on the increase (Russell 2014), particularly in certain migratory routes. In the early part of the twenty-first century, women made up half of all international migrants, compared to around 47 per cent in the 1960s, an increase in the overall share of migration, albeit relatively small (Brettell 2016).

Feminist analyses have moved on from early interventions to make women visible in migration studies—the 'add women and stir' model which deployed a 'binary variable of male versus female' (Nawyn 2010: 750)—to more complex analyses of migration as a 'gendered process' (Hondagneu-Sotelo 2011). Feminist research has destabilised gendered binaries and extended migration research into new fields, for example, transnational care, gendered labour markets, migrant masculinities, sexuality, love and intimacy, health and disability and, importantly for this chapter, the study of GBV (including trafficking for the purposed of sexual exploitation as discussed in Chap. 27). Within research there is increasing attention to gendered migration from an intersectional perspective (Izaguirre and Walsham 2021) to unpack the multiple and intersecting inequalities and forms of discrimination that migrants face and how these render migrants more at risk of violence (Menjivar and Salcido 2002).

Moreover, feminist scholars have highlighted ways in which discourses of equal rights pertaining to gender and sexuality have been co-opted by western states to forward anti-immigration agenda (Voegele 2019) in which concepts of equality are manipulated to serve wider nationalist objectives. Here immigration is framed primarily as a security issue which 'shifts the narrative away from responsibility to support those fleeing war, terror and poverty, towards needing protecting from them' (Voegele 2019: 17). Within these narratives the migrant male is constructed as the dangerous, violent, predatory 'other' who places (white) women and nation at risk. The migrant woman's position here is more ambivalent—constructed as passive and without active agency, yet not always deserving of protection by the state.

Feminist debates on migration counter the reproduction of narratives of female passivity which serves to negate the agency of migrant women (Russell 2014; Freedman 2015; Andrijasevic and Mai 2016) However, as Tyszler (2019) in a discussion of migrant women in Morocco argues, some research also repeats 'the predominant figure of the migrant-woman-victim with no agency, found in the political media discourse' (n.p.). In humanitarian and other discourses, women and children are lumped together as vulnerable refugees—and while the precarity of migrants' lives remains real—such depictions of migrant women seek to both infantilise women and deny them as active, agentic subjects. As Freedman (2015:116–117) notes: 'These unequal power relationships within which refugees are constructed as 'vulnerable' or 'helpless' victims may have particular resonance in the case of women refugees, reinforcing gendered constructions of women's powerlessness and lack of agency in certain societies'. However, migrant women may also exercise agency in re-appropriating these stereotypes of vulnerability as a strategy for survival (Russell 2014; Freedman 2015).

Box 1 Definitions

Migrant – There is no international legal definition of a migrant. According to the International Organization for Migration (IOM), a **migrant** is 'any person who is moving or has moved across an international border or within a State away from his/her habitual place of residence, regardless of the person's legal status; whether the movement is voluntary or involuntary; what the causes for the movement are; or what the length of stay is'.

Irregular migrant—A person who lacks legal status in host or transit country because of irregular entry, breach of condition of entry or expiry of their legal basis for entering and residing.

Asylum seeker—'a person who has left their country and is seeking protection from persecution {…] but who hasn't yet been legally recognized as a refugee […] Seeking asylum is a human right' (Amnesty International).

Refugees—In legal terms, refugees are people who have fled war, violence, conflict or persecution and have crossed an international border to find safety in another country (UNICEF). Refugees are defined and protected in International law. The 1951 Refugee Convention defines a refugee as 'someone who is unable or unwilling to return to their country of origin owing to a well-founded fear of being persecuted for reasons of race, religion, nationality, membership of a particular social group, or political opinion'.

Gender-Based Violence and Migration

Research suggests a strong correlation between migration and GBV, indicating that migrant, asylum-seeking and refugee women are at particular risk of GBV (Pillai 2001; Menjivar and Salcido 2002; Anitha 2010; Rights of Women 2011; Calderón Jaramillo et al. 2020). In the UK, for example, asylum-seeking and refugee women are more likely to be victims of rape and sexual assault, more prone to domestic violence and less able to access services and support (Refugee Council 2009; Anitha 2011). Hubbard et al.'s (2013: 8) analysis of GBV in Wales notes that 'asylum seeking, migrant and refugee women face higher levels of violence than native-born women due to a variety of factors, such as age, language barriers, vulnerability, isolation, and poverty'. These patterns are replicated across the globe. Calderon-Jaramillo et al. (2020: n.p.) in their exploration of sexual and GBV at the Colombia-Venezuelan border illustrate how female migrants and refugees are 'exposed to many forms of SGBV and also face challenges in the access to essential healthcare for many reasons, including legal status, language barriers, discrimination, misinformation on the availability of SRH services, and the growing spread of conservative views on sexual and reproductive health and rights (SRHR) which pose a considerable threat to human rights'. The UN acknowledges that migrant women are more susceptible to GBV because of 'the multiple and intersecting forms of discrimination they face' (von Hase et al. 2021) and urges for the wider collection of intersectional disaggregated data in order to adequately and appropriately inform policy.

Migration research also recognises that GBV is prevalent at all stages of the migratory journey—in the country of origin (GBV may be a mitigating factor in outward migration) in-transit, in the destination country and on return to country of origin (Rights of Women 2011) within 'an accumulation of inequalities and disadvantages that occur over time and place' (Phillimore et al. 2021: 6). Violence is perpetrated both structurally and on an interpersonal level, i.e. on the micro-level by partners, family members, other migrants, smugglers and traffickers, police and border guards, as well as at the macro-level, where violence is exercised 'structurally by institutions, laws, policies and practices relating to migration governance that either directly generate violence or fail to protect from it' (Tastsoglou et al. 2021: n.p).

Thus, it is widely recognised in feminist migration research that any analysis of the prevalence of GBV in migrant communities requires attention to the ways in which violence is exercised both structurally and on an interpersonal level as well as to how these violences interconnect (Menjivar and Salcido 2002; Sokoloff and Dupont 2005; Sokoloff 2008). Research shows how structural violences are exercised – through not enabling safe routes of passage, of cumbersome bureaucratic immigration systems enforcing a hostile environment towards migrants that is focused on reducing immigration rather than attending to humanitarian need and of welfare policies that exclude migrants or reduce access to support—all facilitate the perpetration of interpersonal acts of violence (Phillimore et al. 2019).

Risk Factors

Across research, a number of intersecting risk factors are identified as 'intensifying' the risk of migrant, refugee and asylum-seeking women to GBV (Rights of Women 2011: 5) rendering them also less able to access protective legal and social support systems to end that violence. These 'intensifiers' include:

Language, Communication and Cultural Knowledge

Language barriers can prevent migrant, asylum-seeking and refugee women from being able to access support (in destination countries or in-transit), restrict knowledge of available services (Graca 2017), limit employment opportunities, compound social isolation and thereby keep women in abusive situations (Phillimore et al. 2019). As Menjivar and Salcido (2002: 903) note, 'for many immigrant women language is a barrier in accessing and communicating their needs to community-service providers and in seeking protection from their abusers through the criminal justice system'. Preventing women from accessing language classes can be used by perpetrators as a further form of coercive control. Gaining language skills challenges the power of the perpetrator, in some cases, leading to an escalation of violence (Menjivar and Salcido 2002).

While learning the language of the host country is regarded as a key enabler to women's longer-term integration and empowerment (Burman and Chantler 2005; Family Violence Prevention Fund 2009), the provision of specialist support services that provide support to migrant women in their own languages and with relevant cultural knowledge is often pivotal in enabling migrant, asylum-seeking and refugee women access support services and the interventions they need (Imkaan 2016; Mcilwaine et al. 2019). Algaggia et al. (2017:472) note that in the violence against women sector '[n]ewcomer and immigrant clients with limited language abilities face serious communication barriers that can leave them compromised in informed decision-making about their lives, and the lives of their children and families'.

Limited host language is a major impediment when communicating with immigration authorities, at border crossings, transit locations and asylum interviews. Research suggests that sharing experiences of violence and abuse via interpreters can also be fraught with difficulties, with interpreters usually not having specialist training in GBV and bringing their own values and biases to bear on their translation (Menjivar and Salcido 2002; Algaggia et al. 2017). Moreover, trauma inhibits the ability of migrant victims/survivors of violence to recount experiences. The demand from authorities to re-tell stories of violence and abuse during the asylum process (usually multiple times) is retraumatizing and demonstrates a failure on the part of authorities to adequately protect those who have been subject to GBV and is itself a form of structural GBV perpetrated by the state. Research by the London School of Hygiene and Tropical Medicine and Scottish Refugee Council (2009) emphasised how PTSD was high among migrant victims/survivors of violence and compromised their ability to communicate their experiences in asylum interviews: 'Difficulty remembering is a common symptom among individuals suffering PTSD. This has serious implications for women's asylum testimonies and consideration of their initial asylum applications and appeals, particularly with regards to possible adverse credibility findings on the basis of narrative inconsistencies' (London School of Hygiene and Tropical Medicine and Scottish Refugee Council (2009: 28).

Social Isolation, Shame and Stigma

Social isolation intensifies women's experiences of GBV (Rana 2012; Phillimore et al. 2019). If migrant, refugee and asylum-seeking women are cut off from extended networks of family, friends and other forms of social support, this can amplify vulnerability to violence and make accessing support, both informally and formally, harder. Social isolation is often exploited by perpetrators to exercise violence, either as a means to further perpetrate violence within pre-existing abusive relations or within new encounters and relationships (Hubbard et al. 2013).

However, research also indicates that having family and friendship networks in place does not preclude social isolation and can also act as a barrier to seeking help (Phillimore et al. 2019). Families may blame victims for their abuse or prevent them from seeking help for fear of bringing shame on the family or community. Migrant women who are victims of GBV are therefore silenced through fear of marginalisation, retaliation or rejection and compelled to stay in abusive relationships (Pillai 2001; Ben-Porat 2010; Hubbard et al. 2013). As discussed in Chap. 27, many women and girls who have been trafficked for sexual exploitation are unable to return to their family of origin because of the shame and stigma associated with their trafficking. Trafficked women who are returned to their home countries are therefore particularly vulnerable to re-trafficking because of the absence of familial and social networks of support (Corrin 2005; Tahiraj 2017).

During the COVID-19 pandemic, victims of GBV were subjected to further social isolation through mandates to lockdown, the withdrawal of support services, the disruption of social networks as well as decreased opportunities to make money. Phillimore et al. (2021: 18) point to the interlocking of structural and interpersonal violence during the pandemic, in which the 'loss of escape mechanisms gave women no choice but to endure interpersonal violence and exploitation'. They argue that there was a direct relationship between structural and interpersonal violence during the pandemic, with the violent abandonment by states enacted by the withdrawal or lack of extension of support for vulnerable and marginalised communities—their 'active inaction'—increasing risks of sexual and gendered-based violence. Von Hase et al. (2021) likewise conclude that the 'Covid-19 pandemic has exacerbated women's risk of GBV at all stages of migration, particularly those with irregular immigration status or those who are sexual and gender minorities' (n.p.).

Insecure Immigration Status

Insecure immigration status can intensify women's risk of GBV (Anitha 2010; Anitha 2011; Mullaly 2011; Rana 2012; Girishkumar 2014; Mcilwaine et al. 2019). Firstly, the threat of deportation, whether that is a real threat or imagined, can be used to isolate victims and prevent them seeking external help. Research in the UK by Mcilwaine et al. (2019) notes that such psychological abuse where perpetrators threaten to report women to immigration authorities is often compounded by bureaucratic abuse where abusers withhold immigration papers or passports and exclude women from other formal documents, like tenancy agreements or bank accounts. Secondly, women may lack knowledge of their legal rights and be reluctant to make contact with services for fear of being believed, fear of having their children taken away (if they are mothers) and/or fear of deportation (Mcilwaine et al. 2019). Thirdly, the law itself may bring 'added risks and vulnerability' (Mullaly 2011: 462), especially for women with uncertain or dependent migration status. As Burman and Chantler (2005: 66) assert: 'Women who may want to access support to help them escape domestic violence may in effect be replacing domestic violence with potential state violence through deportation'. Indeed, there is widespread consensus within feminist migration research that immigration policy and processes compound violence and fail to adequately address the lived realities of women with insecure immigration status who are experiencing GBV (Burman and Chantler 2005; Anitha 2010; Anitha 2011; Mullaly 2011; Hubbard et al. 2013; Girishkumar 2014; Graca 2017). If women's residency is dependent on their partners, women are reluctant to report intimate partner/domestic violence because of deportation risk (von Hase et al. 2021). In instances where residency is dependent on a work visa, again reporting GBV in the workplace could also result in loss of job and loss of residency – a particular issue for migrant domestic workers who may also reside in their place of work and who are in many instances female migrant workers (Kouta et al. 2021).

Poverty

Research demonstrates that migration is both a cause and consequence of poverty. Poverty acts as a catalyst to migration (Corrin 2005), but migration does not necessarily alleviate poverty, with the result that many migrants continue to live in disadvantaged material circumstances post-migration. Data from the EU indicates that in general non-EU citizens were twice as likely to live in severe material deprivation than EU citizens and that migrant women were at most risk of poverty.

Poverty, migration and GBV are inter-linked in a number of ways. For example:

- Economic hardship makes migrants, particularly (although not exclusively) women and girls, targets of trafficking and sexual exploitation. Research in Albania, for example, indicates that 'the majority of identified victims of trafficking (62%) lived in poverty prior to being trafficked' (Tahiraj 2017:11). Smugglers and traffickers prey on the economic vulnerability of migrants who are dependent on unsafe, irregular routes of migration or unable to find regular, well-paid forms of employment in their destination countries. This can result in debt slavery or coercion into transactional sex (Freedman 2015). Research with migrant, asylum-seeking and refugee women in Wales notes that many women 'were living in poverty or destitution, which makes them vulnerable to various forms of violence, from forced labour to prostitution' (Hubbard et al. 2013: 3–4).
- Within destination countries migrant women, especially those who are undocumented, are more likely to work in the informal economy, for poor wages and no labour protection, which exacerbates risks of GBV within the workplace and curtails options to escape violence (von Hase et al. 2021).
- Within families and households, perpetrators may control household finances and limit women's access to earnings and household resources as a form of abuse and control (Anitha 2011; Rana 2012).

- Immigration policies may compound migrant poverty and risks of GBV. If women's immigration status is dependent upon their spouses, or if welfare support is unavailable to certain categories of migrants, victims of GBV may have the stark choice of staying with partners, risk deportation or face destitution (Anitha 2011; Hubbard et al. 2013).

Inadequate GBV Services

Research recognises that the violence experienced by migrant, asylum-seeking and refugee women may be intensified by a lack of appropriate services in place to meet their particular needs. There are three key issues identified.

Firstly, there is an overall lack of services to help all victims of GBV (Towers and Walby 2012; Corry 2018). During the pandemic, UNICEF reports that face-to-face access to services was further restricted, as GBV services were often not considered by governments as essential services. Moreover, money for GBV services was redirected towards other health services considered more vital (UNICEF 2021).

Secondly, mainstream services may lack the 'cultural competence' to address the particular needs of migrant, refugee and asylum-seeking women. Cultural competence here is defined as 'an understanding of the cultural differences of clients as well as the particular cultural and structural needs that different communities have—including language specialism; immigration expertise' (Sokoloff and Dupont 2005: 51; see also Menjivar and Salcido 2002; Ben-Porat 2010; Larasi 2013). As a result, migrant women often lack confidence in the systems in place to assist them and protect them from violence (Rodella Sapia et al. 2020).

Thirdly, there is huge shortage of specialist services that can attend to the particular needs of migrant, asylum-seeking and refugee women in relation to issues of violence (Hubbard et al. 2013; Larasi 2013; Women's Aid 2017) in destination countries and in refugee camps (see Box 2). For example, in the UK there is limited provision for Black and Minority Ethnic women outside London. In the South West, for example, there are no refuges specifically for BME women (Women's Aid 2017). Examples of specialist services in the UK include a Vietnamese outreach programme set up by the NGO Refuge that works specifically with Vietnamese women who 'have experienced—or at risk of—multiple types of violence including human trafficking and modern slavery'[2] and the Empower Women project, a joint initiative between the Shpresa Programme (a charity supporting the Albanian-speaking refugees, asylum seekers and migrants in UK) and Solace Women's Aid (a third sector organization tackling violence against women and girls) to support women in the Albanian-speaking community in London affected by violence.[3]

[2] https://www.refuge.org.uk/our-work/our-services/culturally-specific-services/ accessed 7 November 2021

[3] https://shpresaprogramme.org/projects/empower-women/ accessed 7 November 2021

Box 2 Case Study: GBV in the Dadaab Refugee Settlement

The Dadaad Refugee Settlement in Kenya is one of the largest in the world, with an estimated ¼ million inhabitants in 2018. Originally set up to respond to the conflict in Somalia, the camp now includes many fleeing conflict, famine and drought in other parts of Africa too. Research by Muuo et al. (2020) found that gender-based violence is prevalent in the camp. 'Young, single, or unmarried women, girls, and newly arrived refugees (who are often assigned to less secure housing structures and have fewer social networks) are often at elevated risk of violence' (n.p. section on background). Women and girls adopt individual strategies to protect themselves from violence, including limiting their movements around the camp (for example, not going out after dark and avoiding certain places). GBV care provided on the camp was limited, and while those taking part in the research 'considered it responsive to their needs', most women and girls did not feel able to report gender and sexual violence because of shame, stigma and fear of reprisals or being denied access to provisions by guards. The study highlighted some success in raising awareness of GBV through campaigns in the camp and highlighted the importance of education programmes to challenge social norms and improve knowledge of health and violence. However, it also emphasised the importance of tackling the structural barriers to accessing help and of building up trust between survivors and service providers.

Wider research points to high levels of IPV and other forms of sexual and gender violence in refugee camps in part because of extreme poverty but also because of the erosion of social structures, family fragmentation and a lack of social cohesion overall (Wachter et al. 2018). Crowded conditions, inadequate or absent toilet facilities, precarious living and sleeping arrangements increase women's risk of violence (Freedman 2015). Women and girls are at risk of violence not only from families and other migrants but also from humanitarian aid workers with reported cases of women and children being coerced for sex in exchange for food or medical help (Ferris 2007).

Summary

- Migrant, asylum-seeking and refugee women and girls are at particular risk of GBV because of the multiple and intersectional inequalities and discriminations they face.
- Migrant, asylum-seeking and refugee women face multiple barriers to accessing support services.
- GBV against migrants is systemic. It is exercised structurally (for example, through anti-immigration policies, inequalities in the labour market, exclusionary welfare systems, as well as lack of action). This produces and exacerbates interpersonal GBV.

- Boundaries between forced and voluntary migration distinction are blurred. GBV cross-cuts all forms of migration.
- More research is needed to produce both intersectional statistical data on migration and GBV and qualitative data that foregrounds the lived experiences of migrant, refugee and asylum-seeking victims/survivors of GBV.

References

Algaggia R, Maiter S, Jenney A (2017) In whose words? Struggles and strategies of service providers working with immigrant clients with limited language abilities in the violence against women sector and child protection services. Child Family Social Work 22(1):472–481

Andrijasevic R, Mai N (2016) Editorial: trafficking (in) representations: understanding the recurring appeal of victimhood and slavery in neoliberal times. Anti-Trafficking Review 7:1–10

Anitha S (2010) No recourse, no support: state policy and practice towards South Asian women facing domestic violence in the UK. Br J Social Work 40:462–479

Anitha S (2011) Legislating gender inequalities: the nature and patterns of domestic violence experienced by South Asian women with insecure immigration status in the United Kingdom. Violence Against Women 17(10):1260–1285

Bell H (2003) Cycles within cycles. Violence Against Women 9:1245–1262

Ben-Porat A (2010) Connecting two worlds: training social workers to deal with domestic violence against women in the Ethiopian community. Br J Soc Work 40(8):2485–2501

Brettell CB (2016) Gender and migration. Polity, Cambridge

Burman E, Chantler K (2005) Domestic violence and minoritisation: legal and policy barriers facing minoritized women leaving violent relationships. Int J Law Psychiatry 28:59–74

Calderón Jaramillo M, Parra D, Royo M, Rivillas J, Forero L (2020) Migrant women and sexual and gender-based violence at the Colombia-Venezuela border: a qualitative study 1-2:100003. https://doi.org/10.1016/j.jmh.2020.100003

Castelli F (2018) Drivers of migration: why do people move? J Travel Med 25(1):tay040. https://doi.org/10.1093/jtm/tay040

Corrin C (2005) Transitional road for traffic: analysing trafficking in women from and through central and Eastern Europe. Eur Asia Stud 57(4):543–560

Corry D (2018) Hearing women's voices: why women 2018. Women Resource Centre, London

Erdal MB, Oeppen C (2018) Forced to leave? The discursive and analytical significance of describing migration as forced and voluntary. J Ethn Migr Stud 44(6):981–998. https://doi.org/10.1080/1369183X.2017.1384149

Family Violence Prevention Fund (2009) Intimate partner violence in immigrant and refugee communities: challenges, promising practices and recommendations. Robert Wood Johnson Foundation, Princeton

Ferris EG (2007) Abuse of power: sexual exploitation of refugee women and girls. Signs 32(3):584–591. https://doi.org/10.1086/510338

Freedman J (2015) Gendering the international asylum and refugee debate. Palgrave Macmillan, Basingstoke

Girishkumar D (2014) From multi- to interculturalism? Domestic violence and British South Asian women. Human Welfare 3:53–70

Graca S (2017) Domestic violence policy and legislation in the UK: a discussion of women's vulnerabilities. Eur J Curr Leg Issues 23(1)

Hondagneu-Sotelo P (2011) Gender and migration scholarship: an overview from a 21st century perspective. Migraciones internacionales 6(1):219–233. http://www.scielo.org.mx/scielo.php?script=sci_arttext&pid=S1665-89062011000100008&lng=es&tlng=en. Accessed 6 Nov 2021

Hubbard A, Payton J, Robinson A (2013) Uncharted territory: violence against migrant, refugee and asylum-seeking women in Wales, Home Office/Wales Migration Partnership

Imkaan (2016) Capital losses: the state of the specialist BME ending violence against women and girls sector in London. Imkaan, London

Izaguirre L, Walsham M (2021) South-south migration from a gender and intersectional perspective: an overview, MIDEQ Working Paper, MIDEQ

Kouta C, Pithara C, Apostolidou Z, Zobnina A, Christodoulou J, Papadakaki M, Chliaoutakis J (2021) A qualitative study of female migrant domestic workers' experiences of and responses to work-based sexual violence in Cyprus. Theol Sex 2:315–330. https://doi.org/10.3390/sexes2030025

Larasi M (2013) A fuss about nothing?: delivering services to black and minority ethnic survivors of gender violence – the role of the specialist black and minority ethnic women's sector. In: Rehman Y, Kelly L, Siddiqui H (eds) Moving in the shadows. Violence in the lives of minority women and children. Routledge, London

London School of Hygiene and Tropical Medicine and Scottish Refugee Council (2009) Asylum-seeking women, violence and health: results from a pilot study in Scotland and Belgium. https://www.scottishrefugeecouncil.org.uk/wp-content/uploads/2019/10/Asylum-seeking-women-violence-and-health.pdf. Accessed 6 Nov 2021

Lutz H, Palenga-Möllenbeck E (2012) Care workers, care drain, and care chains: reflections on care, migration, and citizenship. Soc Polit Int Stud Gend State Soc 19(1):15–37

Mai N (2016) Too much suffering: understanding the interplay between migration, bounded exploitation and trafficking trough Nigerian sex workers' experiences. Sociological Research Online 21(4):159

Mcilwaine C, Granada L, Valenzuela-Oblitas I (2019) The right to be believed: migrant women facing violence against women and girls (VAWG) in the 'hostile immigration environment' in London. https://doi.org/10.13140/RG.2.2.31107.35367

Menjivar C, Salcido O (2002) Immigrant women and domestic violence: common experiences in different countries. Gend Soc 16(6):898–920

Migration Data Portal (2021) Migrant rights. https://www.migrationdataportal.org/themes/migrant-rights. Accessed 6 Nov 2021

Mullaly S (2011) Domestic violence asylum claims and recent developments in international human rights law: a Progress narrative? Int Comparative Law Q 60(2):459–484

Mullaly S (2014) Migration, gender, and the limits of rights. In: Rubio-Marín R (ed) Human rights and immigration. Oxford University Press, Oxford, pp 145–176. https://ssrn.com/abstract=2574197

Muuo S, Muthuri SK, McAlpine A, Bacchus LJ, Ogego H, Bangha M, Hossain M, Izugbara C (2020) Barriers and facilitators to care-seeking among survivors of gender-based violence in the Dadaab refugee complex. Sex Reprod Health Matters 28(1):1722404. https://doi.org/10.1080/26410397.2020.1722404

Nawyn S (2010) Gender and migration. Integrating feminist theory into migration studies. Sociology Compass 4(9):749–765

Phillimore J, Brand T, Bradby H, Padilla B (2019) Healthcare bricolage in Europe's superdiverse neighbourhoods: a mixed methods study. BMC Public Health. 9(1):1325

Phillimore J, Pertek S, Akyuz S, Hoayda D, Hourani J, McKnight, P, Ozcurumez, Taal S (2021) "We are forgotten": forced migration, sexual and gender-based violence, and coronavirus disease-2019. Violence Against Women 28:2204. https://doi.org/10.1177/10778012211030943

Pillai S (2001) Domestic violence in New Zealand: an Asian immigrant perspective. Econ Polit Wkly 36(11):965–974

Piper N (2003) Feminization of labor migration as violence against women: international, regional, and local nongovernmental organization responses in Asia. Violence Against Women 9(6):723–745. https://doi.org/10.1177/1077801203009006006

Rana S (2012) Addressing domestic violence in immigrant communities: critical issues for culturally competent services. VAWnet, a project of the National Resource Center on Domestic Violence, Harrisburg, PA

Refugee Council (2009) The vulnerable Women's project. Refugee ad asylum seeking women affected by rape or sexual violence. Literature review. Refugee Council, London

Rights of Women (2011) Silenced voices speak: strategies for protecting migrant women from violence and abuse. Rights of Women, London

Rodella Sapia MD, Wangmo T, Dagron S, Elger B (2020) Understanding access to professional healthcare among asylum seekers facing gender-based violence: a qualitative study from a stakeholder perspective. BMC Int Health Hum Rights 20:25. https://doi.org/10.1186/s12914-020-00244-w

Russell AM (2014) "Victims of trafficking": the feminisation of poverty and migration in the gendered narratives of human trafficking. Societies 4:532–548

Sokoloff NJ (2008) The intersectional paradigm and alternative visions to stopping domestic violence: what poor women, women of colour, and immigrant women are teaching us about violence in the family. Int J Sociol Fam 34(2):153–185

Sokoloff NJ, Dupont I (2005) Domestic violence and the intersections of race, class, and gender: challenges and contributions to understanding violence against marginalized women in diverse communities. Violence Against Women 11:38–64

Tahiraj E (2017) Understanding trafficking girls and women from Albania. Working paper, Shpresa Programme. London

Taran PA (2000) Human rights and migrants: challenges of the decade. Int Migr 38(6):7–51

Tastsoglou E, Petrinioti X, Karagiannopoulou C (2021) The gender-based violence and precarity nexus: asylum-seeking women in the Eastern Mediterranean. Front Hum Dyn 3:660682. https://doi.org/10.3389/fhumd.2021.660682

Towers J, Walby S (2012) Measuring the impact of cuts in public expenditure on the provision of services to prevent violence against women and girls, Northern Rock Foundation and Trust for London

Tyszler E (2019) From controlling mobilities to control over women's bodies: gendered effects of EU border externalization in Morocco. Comparative Migration Stud 7:25. https://doi.org/10.1186/s40878-019-0128-4

Unicef (2021) Impact of Covid-19 on Gender-based Violence Refugee and Migrant Response. https://www.unicef.org/eca/media/15751/file (also https://www.unicef.org/media/68086/file/GBV%20Service%20Provision%20During%20COVID-19.pdf)

Voegele H (2019) Precarious borders: frames of (im)migration and the potentiality of affect. Raisons Politiques 76:121–143. https://doi.org/10.3917/rai.076.0121

Von Hase I, Stewart-Evans M, Volpe V, Kuschminder K (2021) From evidence to action. Tackling gender-based violence against migrant women and girls. Policy Brief, UN Women, New York. https://www.unwomen.org/-/media/headquarters/attachments/sections/library/publications/2021/policy-brief-from-evidence-to-action-tackling-gbv-againstmigrant-women-and-girls-en.pdf?la=en&vs=2606. Accessed 6 Nov 2021

Wachter K, Horn R, Friis E, Falb K, Ward L, Apio C, Wanjiku S, Puffer E (2018) Drivers of intimate partner violence against women in three refugee camps. Violence Against Women 24(3):286–306. https://doi.org/10.1177/1077801216689163

Women's Aid (2017) Nowhere to turn. Findings from the first year of the no woman turned away project. Women's Aid, Bristol

Rachel Alsop is a Lecturer in the Centre for Women's Studies at the University of York. Her key areas of research expertise are in the fields of gender and migration and gender theory, with a particular interest in young people's experiences of seeking asylum.

Sex Work and Sex Trafficking

Laura Connelly

> **Learning Objectives**
> Having read this chapter, you should be able to understand:
>
> - How choice and coercion exist within the sex industry.
> - The importance of avoiding the conflation of sex work and trafficking.
> - The feminist debates around sex work and trafficking and their influence on the key international regulatory models that govern the sex industry.

Introduction

There are few feminist debates as fiercely contested as those that occur around the topics of sex work and sex trafficking. Although the ferocity of these debates reached a zenith during the so-called sex wars of the 1980s and 1990s, they continue to fundamentally shape academic discourse, policy and practice across the world. On the one hand, second wave feminism gave rise to the view that prostitution is itself violence against women, 'paid rape', a form of sexual slavery to which no woman would consent. This radical feminist perspective still carries much weight today, as exemplified by the increasing number of countries introducing policies that criminalise the purchase of sex. On the other hand, the sex-positive defence of sex work (and pornography) that arose in response to radical feminism was initially founded on notions of sexual liberation and non-conformism.

L. Connelly (✉)
Department of Sociological Studies, The University of Sheffield, Sheffield, UK
e-mail: l.j.connelly@salford.ac.uk

P. Ali, M. M. Rogers (eds.), *Gender-Based Violence: A Comprehensive Guide*,
https://doi.org/10.1007/978-3-031-05640-6_29

More recently, however, there has been a 'significant shift in the sex worker movement away from protective "Happy Hooker" myths, towards a Marxist-feminist, labour-centred analysis' (Mac and Smith 2018: 13). Those adopting this latter position call for sex work to be understood as a form of labour and for sex workers to be granted the rights afforded to those working in other sectors as a way of protecting against violence, exploitation, stigmatisation and marginalisation. This perspective moves us away from the problematic coercion-choice binary that has historically dominated discussions of sex work and sex trafficking—a binary that has functioned to gloss over the complexities and ambivalences of lived experience. It is in the spirit of this latter position—referred to as the *sex work as work* perspective—that this chapter is written.

This chapter does not argue that sex work is inherently violent but nor does it suggest that violence, exploitation and trafficking do not exist within the sex industry. Instead, the chapter shows that States can give rise to, or offer rights and protections against, a whole range of harms (including but not limited to trafficking) via the regulatory model that they adopt. The chapter begins with some initial background context: exploring what is meant by sex work and trafficking and the importance of not conflating the two phenomena, whilst simultaneously avoiding the binarization of coercion and choice. Next, it outlines two key positions—radical feminist anti-prostitutionism and the sex work as work perspective—not because these are the *only* feminist voices in this arena but because they are the most dominant positions in academic scholarship on, and policy and practice within, the sex industry. The final part of the chapter examines the influence of radical feminism and the sex work as work perspective on two regulatory approaches: end-demand criminalisation and decriminalisation. As the chapter progresses, it should become clear that by bolstering sex workers' demands for improved rights and safety, we can better support sex workers to resist the interpersonal and structural harms present within the sex industry.

Background

The sex industry encompasses a vast range of sexual services, which are bought and sold usually in return for monetary remuneration. Involving both physical contact and indirect sexual stimulation, these services include stripping, webcamming, live sex shows, phone sex, pornography and prostitution. It is not uncommon for sex workers to work across multiple aspects of the sex industry, to work a non-sex work job alongside their sex work and/or to move in and out of the sex industry in quite fluid ways over time (Bowen 2021; Sanders et al. 2016). The term 'sex worker'—first coined by Carol Leigh (aka Scarlot Harlot)—is used to recast sex work as a form of work and, as Leigh (2003) explains, helps to 'unify peep show dancers, strippers, and prostitutes'. Although the terms 'sex work' (see Box 1) and 'sex worker' are now fairly common parlance, at their origin they represented a political intervention to reduce the negative connotations ascribed to 'the prostitute' and align the sex industry with other service industries.

Box 1
Definitions

Sex work is a term used to describe a wide range of direct and indirect activities, in which sexual services are negotiated and performed, either regularly or occasionally, in exchange for (usually) monetary remuneration.

Sex trafficking is the recruitment, transportation, transfer, harbouring or receipt of persons through force or other forms of coercion or deception, with the aim of sexually exploiting them for profit.

Although sex has been sold throughout human history, the advent of the internet has dramatically reshaped the ways in which sex work is negotiated and performed. The outdoor sex market—the historic focus of academic enquiry—has shrunk, along with managed premises for selling sex in the form of brothels, saunas and parlours. Commercial sexual services are now largely marketed through web-based advertising and facilitated through technology, such as forums, review sites, email, social media, phone and webcam (Sanders et al. 2016). The move indoors and online has enabled independent sex workers to implement a range of technologically mediated strategies to improve their safety, such as the screening and vetting of clients using reviews and number checking tools (Sanders et al. 2018). These safety strategies are used alongside those sex workers have employed for a long time, such as working with other sex workers or with maids and other third-parties for protection (although, all of these things are criminalised in the UK context). Rates of violence within the sex industry are nonetheless high, with 45–75% of sex workers reporting workplace violence globally (Deering et al. 2014). Violence is not, however, equally distributed across the aforementioned sex markets. The outdoor sex market—albeit the smallest in the UK—has much higher rates of violence than both indoor premises (brothels, sauna and parlours) and escorting either independently or through an agency (Connelly et al. 2018).

Whilst there is overwhelming evidence that the vast majority of people selling sex have made a rational choice to do so, there is no denying that a range of harms exist within the sex industry. Some migrant women are made false job offers in hospitality and domestic labour and then forced to pay off large debt bondages by selling sex. Others have sold sex in other parts of the world and migrate to the UK to earn a better income through sex work, only to find the conditions under which they will sell sex are not as they agreed (Mai 2011). Both of these scenarios meet the definition of trafficking outlined under the United Nations Trafficking Protocol. Yet the stereotypical victims of sex trafficking perpetuated in populist discourse—abducted from her family and locked away by her trafficker—are very few and far between, and sensationalist depictions of this nature only obscure the complex realities of harm within the sex industry. Indeed, in addition to sex trafficking, harms are created, maintained and perpetuated through domestic policies that criminalise sex work, functioning to deter sex workers from reporting victimisation to the police for fear of arrest (Connelly et al. 2018; Klambauer 2018) and, in turn, enabling dangerous clients and unscrupulous managers to act with impunity. Anti-immigration policy and practice compels people who migrate to pursue illegal mechanisms of entry and unregulated forms of labour, such as sex work, both of which leave them at greater risk of exploitation and human trafficking (Mai 2011). Furthermore, the COVID-19 pandemic has rendered an already marginalised social group all the more vulnerable. Whilst many sex workers were compelled to stop direct (physical contact) sex work, a lack of financial support meant that others simply cannot afford to stop. Stigma and criminalisation serve as barriers to sex workers' ability to access economic protections and/or health services, barriers that are all the greater for sex workers who are homeless or are undocumented migrants (Platt et al. 2020).

Feminist Theorical Perspectives

Now that some background context has been established, this chapter explores two dominant feminist positions in relation to sex work and trafficking. As noted in the introduction, the debates around sex work and trafficking that grew out of the feminist 'sex wars' remain fiercely contested today. Although the key principles of the radical feminists' vehemently anti-prostitution position have changed little since the 1980s and 1990s, the initial sex-radical opposition—which viewed sex work as empowering—has recently given way to a more Marxist-inflected, labour-based analysis. In that respect, the key theoretical tenets of the radical feminism and the sex work as work perspective are outlined here.

Radical feminists make little or no distinction between forced and voluntary prostitution. In this respect, prostitution and trafficking are viewed as inseparable (Jeffreys 1997: 10), for no woman would choose to sell sex. It is from this position that the Coalition Against Trafficking in Women, an international non-governmental organisation aligned with the radical feminist perspective, argues that prostitution is a violation of women's human rights regardless of consent. In this light, they 'reject the very concept of benign migration for the purpose of sex work', and instead the term sex trafficking 'is applied to every instance of relocation to a destination where an individual sells sex' (Weitzer 2007: 453). Radical feminists view 'prostituted women and girls' as victims of circumstance—victims of men who are empowered by sex, race and class-based inequalities (Moran and Farley 2019). For Pateman (1988: 204), prostitution cannot be viewed simply as a job like any other since it involves the sale of women's bodies, and 'to have bodies for sale in the market, as bodies, looks very like slavery'. In this respect, radical feminists typically reject the language of 'sex worker' and 'sex work' and instead refer to those who sell sex as 'prostituted women' or 'survivors' through discourses of 'sexual exploitation', 'modern slavery' and 'paid rape'.

For radical feminists, the sex industry is not only deeply harmful for women who sell sex but is emblematic of, and operates to sustain, violence against *all* women. From this position, prostitution is regarded as 'the absolute embodiment of patriarchal male privilege' (Kelser 2002: 19). It is demonstrative of the inferior socio-political status of women relative to men, and, in that respect, the 'prostitute' becomes that paradigmatic image of women's economic, sexual and social repression in society as a whole. As Giobbe (1990: 77) puts it, 'her status is the basic unit by which all women's value is measured and to which all women can be reduced' (Giobbe 1990: 77). Key to radical feminist understandings of prostitution and trafficking, therefore, is the notion that the 'sex trade' 'perpetuates the objectification and sexualisation of *all* women and girls' (CATW 2021). Considered incompatible with the promotion of gender equality, the sex industry is understood to be a male-driven market. As Moran and Farley (2019: 1947) argue, 'prostitution exists because of the male demand for it'. It exists because 'users' or 'perpetrators' of prostitution gain gratification from objectifying, subjugating and exploiting women and girls. It is the male demand for the purchase of sex that is thus considered to be the root cause of trafficking for sexual exploitation.

Critics of the radical feminist perspective argue that by conflating the phenomena of sex work and trafficking, the diversity of lived experience within the sex industry becomes totalised. Variability in levels of personal autonomy are ignored in favour of an essentialist victimising narrative (Connelly et al. 2015). In light of these critiques, sex-radical narratives—prominent particularly in the 1990s and early 2000s—framed sex work as a 'potentially liberating terrain' (Chapkis 1997): one that allows women to exert their sexual autonomy and foregrounds pleasure and freedom of (sexual and financial) expression. As the sex workers and authors Mac and Smith (2018) suggest, although this position is an understandable response to a radical feminist narrative that frames sex workers as 'damaged, an animal or piece of meat', it operates to elide the harms present within the sex industry. In this respect, in seeking to oppose the radical feminist viewpoint, sex-radicalism contributes to a simplified debate that promotes one-dimensional and essentialist understandings—a deeply polarised debate that binarizes 'choice' in relation to the radical feminist emphasis on 'coercion' (Scoular 2016). This binary has become so deeply instilled within debates around sex work and trafficking that, as Chapkis (1997) notes, scholars have faced pressure to align themselves with one of the two perspectives: 'the certainty and conviction of those who disagree with me make my own enthusiasm for partial and contradictory truths feel inadequate'. Yet, in recent years, the sex workers' rights movement has increasingly called for debates to move beyond the coercion-choice dichotomy to take better account of how structural factors act to mediate the levels of exploitation and violence sex workers experience, with non-citizens, the poor and women of colour more likely to experience abuse, whilst middle- and upper-class white women remain better able to obtain high remuneration in the course of their sex working.

This more nuanced position, moving beyond a simplistic binary, foregrounds a labour-based analysis that recognises sex work, first and foremost, as *work*. This position fundamentally opposes the conflation of sex work and trafficking that underpins radical feminist scholarship and instead recognises them as different phenomena. Sex work as work advocates point to evidence that most sex workers—including migrant sex workers—make conscious choices to enter the sex industry (Weitzer 2007; Mai 2011). In this respect, sex work is regarded as an understandable response to socio-economic constraint, a way for people—women, men, transgender and non-binary folx—to make a living under white supremacist capitalist heteronormative patriarchy. In particular, sex work may offer a viable and flexible labour option to those who migrate to a new country, especially from the global South to the global North, in a context where access to formal labour markets may be restricted by repressive immigration policies and racist nativism (Mai 2011). For those adopting a sex work as work perspective, sex workers should be afforded the same basic human, legal, political and worker's rights as those in other professions.

Proponents of the sex work as work position also argue that the sex industry is not inherently exploitative or violent but, rather, exploitation and violence are facilitated by poor working conditions, societal stigma and processes of criminalisation. Indeed, in countries where sex work is criminalised (or quasi-criminalised such as in the UK), sex workers are deterred from reporting victimisation to the police for fear of arrest (Klambauer 2018). This enables violent clients and other perpetrators to act with impunity, shifting the balance of power away from sex workers. The effects of criminalisation are compounded for migrant sex workers, who are made susceptible to violence and exploitation by the vulnerabilities that emerge through precarious immigration status. Indeed despite experiencing increased violence, xenophobia and racism post-EU Referendum, migrant sex workers report being unable to rely on the police for support and having to compromise on their safety in order to avoid arrest, detention and deportation (Connelly and English Collective of Prostitutes 2021). To critique working conditions should not be taken to imply that sex work is inherently problematic but, rather, as further evidence that sex workers need the labour protections fought for and, in some cases, won in other sectors of work (Mac and Smith 2018) in order to keep themselves safe.

International Contexts: Policy and Practice

The radical feminist and sex work as work perspectives have not only occupied a central space within scholarly literature on sex work and trafficking but influence policy debates that occur at the local, national and global levels too. This part of the chapter offers some brief analysis of two key regulatory systems—end-demand criminalisation and decriminalisation—that are informed by radical feminist and sex work as work positions, respectively. It focuses in particular on the implementation of end-demand criminalisation in Sweden and decriminalisation in New Zealand.

End-demand criminalisation—the radical feminist gold standard—appears, at present, to be the *en vogue* model of regulation. In the last couple of decades, an increasing number of countries have adopted what is variously known as end-demand criminalisation, neo-abolitionism, the 'Swedish Model' or the 'Nordic Model': a regulatory approach that criminalises the purchase but not the sale of sex. First implemented in Sweden in 1999, end-demand criminalisation has since been successfully marketed, with Finland (2006), Iceland (2009), Norway, Canada

(2014), Northern Ireland (2015), France (2016), Ireland (2017) and Israel (2018) all having since adopted the approach. In Sweden, the sex purchase law passed with little opposition. Its stated aims were to combat prostitution, which was regarded as not only harmful to those directly involved but also oppositional to gender equality more broadly, and to reduce incidents of sex trafficking (Government of Sweden 2010). Ultimately, end-demand criminalisation seeks to eradicate the sex industry by ending the demand for prostitution through penalising the client.

Although proponents of end-demand criminalisation in Sweden hail it a success, there is a burgeoning body of evidence to the contrary. For example, advocates claim the sex purchase law has achieved a key aim of reducing the size of the sex industry, with a 50% reduction in outdoor prostitution (Government of Sweden 2010). Yet, critical analysis indicates that the decline in outdoor prostitution was only a short-term result of displacement as sex workers moved indoors in order to avoid detection (Levy and Jakobsson 2014). Furthermore, whilst a government evaluation claims that fears around the negative impact that the purchase ban would have on sex workers 'have not been realised' (Government of Sweden 2010: 37–38), sex workers report a whole range of harmful consequence of the law. Far from keeping sex workers safe, the Swedish model has increased the stigma experienced by sex workers (Dodillet and Östergrem 2011)—a stigma that manifests in interactions with clients, deters sex workers from engaging with health and support services and is present in media and public discourse (Fuckförbundet 2019).

Criminalising the client also reduces sex workers' ability to manage risk. As clients are fearful of arrest, outdoor sex workers are compelled to solicit in secluded areas where the risk of violence is greater and to hurry the screening of clients (Krüsi et al. 2021; Global Network of Sex Work Projects 2015; Levy and Jakobsson 2014). Fewer clients has meant that there is increased competition (Dodillet and Östergrem 2011; Levy 2014), and, in turn, prices are driven down (Global Network of Sex Work Projects 2015). As such, sex workers are compelled to accept clients they would previously have rejected or provide services they are not comfortable with in order to make a living. Therefore, whilst the Swedish model purports to target the client, it is clear that, in practice, it empowers the client to the detriment of the sex worker.

Although advocates claim that the Swedish model protects sex workers from criminalisation, we once again see that in practice the evidence suggests otherwise. It is clear that 'there *are* laws and polices used directly to destabilise the lives of sex workers themselves' (Levy and Jakobsson 2014: 603). Sex workers in Sweden are, for example, being harmed through the enforcement of brothel-keeping laws that prevent sex workers working in groups for safety (Fuckförbundet 2019), and the police are reporting sex workers to landlords in order to force an eviction (Global Network of Sex Work Projects 2015). There is also evidence of sex workers losing custody of their children due to their sex working status (Global Network of Sex Work Projects 2015), including in the case of Petite Jasmine (see Box 2). Furthermore, whilst proponents claim that the Swedish model curtails sex trafficking (Government of Sweden 2010), there is little supporting evidence.

On the contrary, there is evidence that criminalisation has led sex work to be driven underground thereby enhancing risk of exploitation, which is likely to make victims of trafficking even more reluctant to reach out to authorities (Healy et al. 2020). There is also evidence that trafficking and voluntary sex work are being conflated under the new category of 'trafficking-like prostitution' introduced by the National Police Board in Sweden 2006. This new category is defined as 'foreign women who during a temporary visit to Sweden, offer sexual services' (cited in Wagenaar et al. 2013) and leaves no room for migrant sex workers who travel to Sweden to sell sex of their own volition. What is abundantly clear, therefore, is that without addressing the reasons why people (need to) sell sex, criminalising the client does little to reduce demand and simply creates further harm to sex workers. These harms are felt greatest by those who are already most vulnerable and those engaged in 'survival' sex (Levy and Jakobsson 2014).

Although the radical feminist informed approach (end-demand criminalisation) has gained significant traction across the globe, it is the decriminalisation model that is preferred by the vast majority of sex workers and their allies within the sex workers' rights movement. Whilst sex work was decriminalised in the state of New South Wales, Australia, in 1995, New Zealand remains the only country to have implemented the decriminalisation model of regulation, passing the Prostitution Reform Act (PRA) in 2003. Although frequently conflated in popular discourse with legalisation—a model that sees the State regulation of particular aspects of the sex industry, 'legalising *some* sex work in *some* contexts' (Mac and Smith 2018: 176)—decriminalisation involves the removal of all laws that criminalise consensual sex work. This means that whilst buying and selling sex is legal indoors and outdoors and so too is operating a brothel (in accordance with local bylaws), sex trafficking remains criminalised and it is against the law to compel anyone to sex work or for a third party to facilitate anyone under the age of 18 years old into the sex industry. The key aims of the PRA are to safeguard the human rights of sex workers, offer protection from exploitation and promote the welfare, and health and safety of sex workers, as well as wider public health.

Box 2

Case study: Petite Jasmine

Eva Marree Kullander Smith (27), otherwise known as Petite Jasmine, was a Swedish national who lost custody of her two children after a family member informed the Swedish authorities that she had been selling sex. Eva had only been selling sex for 2 weeks, following her separation from an abusive partner. Social services removed Eva's two young children and placed them in the care of their father, her abusive ex-partner. They told Eva that she was suffering from false consciousness: that she did not realise that her sex work was a form of self-harm. She was not permitted to see her children.

Appalled at her treatment and the State's stigmatization of sex workers, Eva became a sex worker rights' activist organising with the Rose Alliance.

After four trials, she also successfully secured visitation rights to see her children. On 11 July 2013, at one such parental visit, her ex-partner brutally murdered her and injured the social workers present. He has threatened and stalked her on numerous occasions in the leadup to her murder. Yet, despite asking for State protection, Eva never received it.

Eva's case is widely seen as emblematic of the structural harms and stigma that is (re)produced by the Swedish Model.

Evaluations of decriminalisation have shown the PRA to be successful in meeting these aims. Indeed, in a context where sex workers report often feeling spoken over and on behalf of in radical feminist narratives (ICRSE 2015), the PRA Bill was drafted in collaboration with the New Zealand Prostitutes' Collective (Abel et al. 2007), functioning to ensure that sex workers' needs and experiential knowledge were at its heart. As the New Zealand Prostitutes' Collective reports, one of the key advantages of the PRA is that it has encouraged discourses surrounding law enforcement to shift from those of punitiveness to protection, which operates in practice to better enable sex workers to report victimisation to the police without fear of negative repercussions (Healy et al. 2020). In turn, sex workers are more likely to report suspicions around trafficking and are less tolerant of poor working conditions. An initial government-commissioned evaluation of the PRA found that 90% of a sample of sex workers felt that they had improved rights, and 65% felt that they were better able to refuse clients (Abel et al. 2007). The same evaluation also found that post-decriminalisation, sex workers are better able to negotiate safer sex practices with clients (Abel et al. 2007). Furthermore, contrary to the situation in countries that have adopted end-demand criminalisation, sex workers have noted that they are better able to vet clients in the outdoor market without fear that spending time engaging in a vetting process leaves them more susceptible to arrest (Armstrong and Abel 2020).

The decriminalisation model adopted in New Zealand is, however, imperfect. Although it offers improved safety and workers' rights for New Zealand national sex workers and those with permanent resident status, it does little to improve conditions for undocumented migrant sex workers. Indeed, it 'explicitly prohibits temporary migrants from working in the sex industry' (Armstrong and Abel 2020: 6). In this respect, the most marginalised and precarious sex workers remain under-protected by the State. The stigma that surrounds sex work has not dissipated. Indeed, a hierarchy of respectability continues to exist in New Zealand, with so-called high-end workers experiencing greater social acceptance than so-called low-end workers (Easterbrook-Smith 2020a). There is also evidence of sustained surveillance and harassment of trans sex workers, particularly trans women of colour, by self-appointed 'community representatives' (Easterbrook-Smith 2020b).

Although there are necessary improvements that can be made to the PRA, decriminalisation remains the preferred model for those adopting the sex work as work perspective. In the UK, key sex worker-led collectives, the English Collective of Prostitutes and SWARM, are leading the fight for decriminalisation and are joined by a burgeoning group of academics and practitioners. In recognition of the enhanced rights and safety of sex workers under decriminalisation, a large number of non-government organisations have also publicly supported sex workers' demands for decriminalisation, from the World Health Organization, to Amnesty International, Human Rights Watch and the United Nations Entity for Gender Equality and the Empowerment of Women. Decriminalisation has also been supported by the Global Alliance Against Traffic in Women and La Strada International, two key anti-trafficking organisations (ICRSE 2015).

Summary

- The radical feminist anti-prostitution position dominates State responses to sex work and trafficking, despite there being overwhelming evidence that end-demand criminalisation does little to protect sex workers.
- There is little doubt that human trafficking, exploitation and victimisation occur within the sex industry. Yet, international evidence indicates that the solution does not lie with criminalising the client.
- Instead, it should be recognised that trafficking is but one of many harmful consequences that arise both from the criminalisation and stigmatisation of the sex industry and anti-immigration policy and practice.
- To reduce the incidences and effects of these harms, we must support sex workers' demands to improve rights and safety. Sex work is work and, like other industries, requires the legal protections that help to curtail interpersonal and structural abuses and harms.

References

Abel G, Fitzgerald L, Brunton C (2007) The impact of the prostitution reform act on the health and safety practices of sex workers. University of Otago, Christchurch

Armstrong L, Abel G (2020) Introduction. In: Armstrong L, Abel G (eds) Sex work and the New Zealand model: decriminalisation and social change. Bristol University Press, Bristol, pp 1–14

Bowen R (2021) Work, money and duality: trading sex as a side hustle. Polity, Bristol

CATW (2021) The sex trade. https://catwinternational.org/the-challenge/the-sex-trade/

Chapkis W (1997) Live sex acts: women performing erotic labor. Routledge, New York

Connelly L, English Collective of Prostitutes (2021) EU migrant sex work in the UK post-referendum. ECP, London. https://prostitutescollective.net/eu-migrant-sex-work-in-the-uk-post-referendum/

Connelly L, Jarvis-King L, Ahearne G (2015) Editorial: blurred lines – the contested nature of sex work in a changing social landscape. Grad J Soc Sci 11(2):4–20

Connelly L, Kamerade D, Sanders T (2018) Violent and non-violent crimes against sex workers: the influence of the sex market on reporting practices in the United Kingdom. J Interpers Violence 36(7):3938–3963

Deering K, Amin A, Shoveller J et al (2014) A systematic review of the correlates of violence against sex workers. Am J Public Health 104(5):42–54

Dodillet S, Östergrem P (2011) The Swedish sex purchase act: claimed success and documented effects. Paper presented at decriminalizing prostitution and beyond: practical experiences and challenges, The Hague, 3–4 March 2011

Easterbrook-Smith G (2020a) 'Genuinely keen to work': sex work, emotional labour, and the news media. In: Armstrong L, Abel G (eds) Sex work and the New Zealand model: decriminalisation and social change. Bristol University Press, Bristol, pp 157–176

Easterbrook-Smith G (2020b) 'Not on the street where we live': walking while trans under a model of sex work decriminalisation. Fem Media Stud 20(7):1013–1028
Fuckförbundet (2019) Twenty years of failing sex workers: a community report on the impact of the 1999 Swedish sex purchase act. https://www.nswp.org/sites/nswp.org/files/20_years_of_failing_sex_workers.pdf
Giobbe E (1990) Confronting the liberal lies about prostitution. In: Leidholdt D, Raymond J (eds) The sexual liberals and the attack on feminism. Pergamon Press, London
Global Network of Sex Work Projects (2015) Community guide: The real impact of the Swedish model on sex workers. https://www.nswp.org/resource/the-real-impact-the-swedish-model-sex-workers-advocacy-toolkit
Government of Sweden (2010) Evaluation of the prohibition of the purchase of sexual service: English summary. Ministry of Justice, Sweden
Healy C, Drewery T, Sweetman B (2020) Decriminalise sex work to prevent trafficking and abuse. Open Democracy, 11 January 2020. https://www.opendemocracy.net/en/beyond-trafficking-and-slavery/decriminalise-sex-work-prevent-trafficking-and-abuse/
ICRSE (2015) Nothing about us without us! Ten years of sex workers' rights activism and advocacy in Europe. https://ruj.uj.edu.pl/xmlui/bitstream/handle/item/30042/dziuban_stevenson_nothing_about_us_without_us.pdf?sequence=1&isAllowed=y
Jeffreys S (1997) The idea of prostitution. Spinifex, North Melbourne
Kelser K (2002) Is a feminist stance in support of prostitution possible? An exploration of current trends. Sexualities 5(2):219–235
Klambauer E (2018) Policing roulette: sex workers' perception of encounters with police officers in the indoor and outdoor sector in England. Criminol Crim Just 18(3):255–272
Krüsi A, D'Adamo K, Sernick A (2021) Criminalised interactions with law enforcement and impacts on health and safety in the context of differing legislative frameworks governing sex work globally. In: Goldenberg SM, Thomas RM, Forbes A et al (eds) Sex work, health and human rights: global inequities, challenges, and opportunities for action. Springer, Cham
Leigh C (2003) Unrepentant whore: the collected works of Scarlot Harlot. Last Gasp, San Francisco
Levy J (2014) Criminalising the purchase of sex: lessons from Sweden. Routledge, London
Levy J, Jakobsson P (2014) Sweden's abolitionist discourse and law: effects on the dynamics of Swedish sex work and on the lives of Sweden's sex workers. Criminol Crim Just 14(5):593–607
Mac J, Smith M (2018) Revolting prostitutes: the fight for sex workers' rights. Verso, London
Mai N (2011) In whose name? Migration and trafficking in the UK sex industry: delivering social interventions between myths and reality. ESRC, London
Moran R, Farley M (2019) Consent, coercion, and culpability: is prostitution stigmatized work or an exploitative and violent practice rooted in sex, race and class inequality? Arch Sex Behav 48:1947–1953
Pateman C (1988) The sexual contract. Stanford University Press, Stanford
Platt L, Elmes J, Stevenson L et al (2020) Sex workers must not be forgotten in the Covid-19 response. Lancet 396:9–11
Sanders T, Connelly L, Jarvis-King L (2016) On our own terms: the working conditions of internet-based sex workers in the UK. Sociol Res Online 21(4):133–146
Sanders T, Scoular J, Campbell R et al (2018) Internet sex work: beyond the gaze. Palgrave, London
Scoular J (2016) The subject of prostitution: sex work, law and social theory. Routledge, London
Wagenaar H, Altink S, Amesberger H (2013) Final report on the international comparative study of prostitution policy. https://issuu.com/platform31/docs/p31_prostitution_policy_report/121
Weitzer R (2007) The social construction of sex trafficking: ideology and institutionalization of a moral crusade. Polit Soc 35(3):447–475

Laura Connelly, PhD, is a Lecturer in Criminology in the Department of Sociological Studies at the University of Sheffield. Her research sits at the intersections of race, gender and migration, and she often explores these issues within the context of the sex industry.

Part VII

Institutional Violence

Obstetric Violence

Rodante van der Waal and Kaveri Mayra

Learning Objectives
Having read this chapter, you should be able to understand:

- Obstetric violence as a form of racialised gender-based violence specific to the nature of the obstetric institution in which healthcare is provided.
- The different forms of obstetric violence and the extent and impact of this issue.
- The history of obstetric violence and its intersection with global structures of suppression.
- The systemic nature of obstetric violence.

Introduction

Obstetric violence is a form of gender-based violence (GBV) that happens within an obstetric environment during pregnancy, childbirth, and/or the postpartum period. It consists of several specific forms of physical, verbal, structural, and epistemological violence. Examples of obstetric violence are unconsented procedures, neglect, gas-lighting, shaming, discrimination, unwanted episiotomies, vaginal examinations,

R. van der Waal (✉)
Care Ethics Department, University for Humanistic Studies, Utrecht, The Netherlands
e-mail: Rodante.vanderwaal@phd.uvh.nl

K. Mayra
Birth Place Lab, University of British Columbia and a Subject Matter Expert at the WHO HQ, Vancouver, BC, Canada

Global Health, Obstetric Violence in India, University of Southampton, Southampton, UK

P. Ali, M. M. Rogers (eds.), *Gender-Based Violence: A Comprehensive Guide*,
https://doi.org/10.1007/978-3-031-05640-6_30

and the exaggeration of risks to the baby's life to obtain consent for interventions (Bohren et al. 2015; Cohen Shabot 2019; Shabot and Korem 2018; Villarmea and Fernández Guillén 2011; Morton et al. 2018) (see Table 1).

Table 1 Typology of mistreatment of women during childbirth

Domains	Sub-domains	Indicators
Physical abuse	Use of force	Patients beaten, slapped, kicked, or pinched during childbirth
	Physical restraint	Patients physically restrained to the bed or gagged during childbirth
Sexual abuse	Sexual abuse	Sexual abuse and rape
Verbal abuse	Harsh language	Harsh or rude language
		Judgemental or accusatory comments
	Threats and blaming	Threats of withholding treatment or threats that poor outcomes will ensue
		Blaming women for poor outcomes
Stigma and discrimination	Discrimination based on socio-demographic characteristics	Discrimination based on ethnicity/race/religion
		Discrimination based on age
		Discrimination based on socioeconomic status
		Discrimination based on parity
	Discrimination based on medical conditions	Discrimination based on HIV status
		Discrimination based on disability
Failure to meet professional standards of care	Lack of informed consent	Lack of informed consent process
		Breaches of confidentiality
	Physical examinations and procedures	Unnecessarily painful vaginal examinations
		Refusal to provide pain relief
		Performance of unconsented surgical operations
	Neglect and abandonment	Neglect, abandonment, or long delays
		Skilled attendant absent at time of delivery
Poor support between patients and providers	Ineffective communication	Poor communication
		Dismissal of patient's concerns
		Language and interpretation issues
		Poor staff attitudes
	Lack of supportive care	Lack of supportive care from health workers
		Denial or lack of health companions
	Loss of autonomy	Patients treated as passive participants during childbirth
		Denial of food, fluids, or mobility
		Lack of respect of women's preferred birth positions
		Denial of safe traditional practices
		Objectification of women
		Detainment in facilities

Table 1 (continued)

Domains	Sub-domains	Indicators
Health system conditions and constraints	Lack of resources	Physical condition of facilities
		Staffing constraints
		Staffing shortages
		Supply constraints
		Lack of privacy
	Lack of policies	Lack of redress
	Facility culture	Unclear fee structure
		Unreasonable requests of women by health workers
		Bribery and extortion

Obstetric violence has an extensive history that pre-dates the founding of formalised obstetric institutions. It is a highly complex form of violence that is expressed in the specific techniques and power relations of obstetrics, simultaneously reflecting the vectors of oppression particular to the geo-political region in which any given obstetric institution is situated. It is perpetrated and perpetuated by obstetricians, obstetric nurses, midwives, and other formal and informal healthcare providers. The term obstetric violence refers to violence within obstetrics as an institution and does not aim to accuse individual birth workers of violence. The critique of obstetric violence addresses problems endemic to institutions of care and is grounded in the presupposition—shared by the World Health Organization (WHO)—that a good birth goes beyond good outcomes and supports the elimination of all forms of mistreatment and abuse during childbirth (WHO 2014).

Definition and Terminology

Obstetric violence is a relatively new term that was introduced by South American activists in the early 2000s to raise awareness about violence against people during childbirth. This violence includes sexist attitudes and remarks; verbal, physical, and sexual abuse; manipulation; and unconsented or unnecessary medical procedures (Sadler et al. 2016; Williams et al. 2018; Villarmea 2015). Over the last two decades, researchers and activists have identified obstetric violence as a form of GBV that is endemic to maternity care in countries around the world. This greater awareness has recently culminated in a report by the United Nations' rapporteur on violence against women, entitled 'A human rights-based approach to mistreatment and violence against women in reproductive health services with a focus on childbirth and obstetric violence' (Šimonović and UNHCR 2019). Among many other forms of abuse, the report details testimonies of 'profound humiliation, verbal abuse and sexist remarks during childbirth' (11). Women in Honduras reported the following comments from healthcare workers attending their births: 'You didn't shout when the penis was inside you, why do you shout now?' In another case, a woman giving birth was told: 'You didn't cry when you did it, open your legs or your baby will die, and it will be your fault' (11). In these cases, sexist verbal abuse, sexual assault, and manipulation in the form of accusations of infanticide (or playing the 'dead baby card', a specific form of shroud waving in obstetrics when the risk to the baby's life is exaggerated to make the mother comply with hospital policy) are concurrent. This is referred to as 'obstetric mistreatment', 'disrespect and abuse', 'obstetric violence', or, seen from the opposite direction, as a lack of 'respectful maternity care' (Sen et al. 2018; Chadwick 2017; Freedman et al. 2014) (Box 1).

Box 1 Alternative and Related Terminology to *Obstetric Violence*

Alternative terms:	Related terms:
Disrespect; abuse; mistreatment; violence during childbirth; reproductive injustice/ violence; birth rape; dehumanised birth; birth violence	Humanising childbirth; respectful maternity care; human rights in childbirth; birth justice; reproductive justice

The terminology of obstetric violence is territorialised by politics and power. Terminologies which are more gentle and subtle such as 'mistreatment', 'disrespect', and 'misbehaviour' are used by development organisations such as the WHO and the United Nations (UN). The term 'obstetric violence', however, is valuable since it derives from activists who have experienced this violence themselves. Importantly, contrary to the other, milder, terms, 'obstetric violence' can address the structural and institutionalised nature of this form of GBV, rather than framing it as a problem of good or bad intentions of individual healthcare workers. By underscoring the term *obstetric*, it is clear at first sight that it is a specific form of violence inherent to the obstetric institution (Van der Waal et al. 2023; Van der Waal et al. 2021).

Impact of Obstetric Violence

A systemic consequence of obstetric violence is that the midwife or obstetrician becomes the active agent of birth, instead of the person in labour. An example of this is the English verb 'delivering'. In English, the doctor or midwife *delivers* the mother *of* her baby. This is symptomatic of how the obstetrician is constructed as the active subject of childbirth, while the labouring person is constructed as the object of birth.

Specific consequences for parents are trauma, post-traumatic stress disorder (PTSD), tokophobia (fear of childbirth), and postpartum depression (Beck et al. 2013; Kitzinger 1992; Scotland 2020; Pickles and Herring 2020). Women find it difficult to describe their experience and often use the language of their oppressor, in this case the medical terminologies that the care providers tell them were necessary for the survival of the baby and woman. A study by Kitzinger reports that victims of violence during childbirth tend to avoid sharing their experiences. They have feelings of depersonalisation that lead to fear, pain, and distress; experience denial and feelings of isolation, they feel helpless and think no one would understand, and experience self-disgust and self-blame (Kitzinger 1992). When they do find the words to share their experience, they draw parallels with feeling raped, and the language includes being 'stripped off', 'tethered', 'forcibly exposed', 'sexual organs put on display', 'disempowered', 'shocked', 'numb', and 'feeling like being a slab of meat being butchered'. Victims remember details of the trauma for decades (Kitzinger 1992).

Studies in India have found that obstetric violence during childbirth leads to a fear of birth that can discourage women from seeking care (Mayra and Kumar 2017; Jha et al. 2017), even when complications arise (Bhattacharya et al. 2013). This in turn results in women avoiding facility-based birth during complications, threatening progress towards reductions in maternal mortality (Bohren et al. 2014; Bohren et al. 2015). Lack of privacy is a commonly reported factor causing women to decide against institutional birth (Afsana and Rashid 2001; Otis and Brett 2008; Sorensen et al. 2011; Mrisho et al. 2017; Hadwinger and Hadwinger 2012; Bhattacharya et al. 2013).

Observing traumatic births, working in a traumatic environment, and being pressured to participate in obstetric violence and racism also have consequences for midwives, obstetric nurses, obstetricians, and gynaecologists, including relatively high numbers of secondary trauma, PTSD, and tokophobia (Van der Waal et al. 2021; Mayra et al. 2021b). Often, care for pregnant people is understood to be secondary to the safety of the foetus during childbirth, even in midwifery, which is oriented to support people's ability to give birth. Birth workers have a displaced sense of responsibility which is exacerbated and reinforced by fear and trauma that prioritises the foetus over the mother and reduces the mother to a complicating rather than enabling factor in childbirth, reinforcing an image of the mother as merely being a 'fetal container' (Kingma 2015; Shabot and Korem 2018; De Vries 2017; Newnham and Kirkham 2019; Fontein-Kuipers et al. 2018; Chadwick 2018).

Types and Scope of Obstetric Violence

In order to highlight the structural dimension of obstetric violence and its connection to hierarchy, power, status, and control, obstetric violence has been theorised as structural violence (Miltenburg et al. 2018), normalised violence (Chadwick 2018), birth abuse (Hill 2019), a structural form of separation of pregnant people from their children and/or reproductive capacities (Van der Waal and Van Nistelrooij 2022), a philosophical form of violence based on a diminishing of subjectivity and rationality in the case of pregnancy and childbirth (Villarmea 2020; 2021; Villarmea & Kelly 2020), and symbolic violence (Morgan and Thapar-Björkert 2006) (see Box 2). Both Chadwick and Shabot theorise obstetric violence as a form of epistemic violence and/or injustice. Shabot identifies hermeneutic and testimonial epistemic injustice, as well as gaslighting, as forms of obstetric violence. She defined obstetric violence as GBV that functions to reproduce feminised gender identities through shame, gaslighting, and epistemic injustice (2020, 2018, 2016). Chadwick (2021) conceptualises silencing as well as a form of epistemic violence. Some countries have defined obstetric violence in law, mainly recognising over-medicalisation as a key form of obstetric violence. For instance, in Venezuelan criminal law, obstetric violence is one of 19 punishable acts of violence against women and is defined as:

> The appropriation of the body and reproductive processes of women by health personnel, which is expressed as dehumanized treatment, an abuse of medication, and to convert the natural processes into pathological ones, bringing with it loss of autonomy and the ability to decide freely about their bodies and sexuality, negatively impacting the quality of life of women. (Pe′rez D'Gregorio 2010: 201).

Sadler et al. (2016) expanded this definition by theorising the relation of obstetric violence to women's marginalisation within the larger political economy. Sadler et al. (2016) defines obstetric violence as 'a form of violence deployed during childbirth against women, reflective of other forms of marginalisation, contingent on their location within the larger political economy'. Similarly, Chadwick (2018) refers to the shaping of obstetric violence by gendered, racialised, medicalised, and classed norms. Chadwick (2017) describes obstetric violence as 'an assemblage of disciplinary, bodily and material relations that are shaped by racialised, medicalised and classed norms about "good patients", "good women" and "good birthing bodies"'. Researching obstetric violence experienced by privileged white women in private hospitals and marginalised Black women in public hospitals in South Africa, Chadwick points out that obstetric violence in the former context mostly takes the form of medicalisation of the birth process, while in the latter obstetric violence often expresses itself in a lack of access to high-quality care and neglect during childbirth resulting in giving birth alone (Chadwick 2018). Not only over-medicalisation but also neglect and abandonment are clear cases of obstetric violence and have negative medical outcomes for pregnant people and their babies, as reported in the Dominican Republic, where in one case the missing heartbeat of an infant and the ruptured uterus of a woman went unnoticed (Miller and Lalonde 2015). As such, obstetric violence cuts across the ideological discussion regarding natural or normal versus medicalised childbirth (Chadwick 2021).

Davis (2019a) established that obstetric violence is not merely GBV, but race-based as well, coining the term 'obstetric racism'. Davis defines obstetric racism as 'the intersection between obstetric violence and medical racism' consisting of diagnostic lapses, neglect, dismissiveness or disrespect, intentionally causing pain, coercion, ceremonies of degradation, medical abuse, and racial reconnaissance (Davis 2019a; Davis 2019b). In India, intersections of oppression, such as lower levels of education, skin colour, caste, religion, gender, socioeconomic status, and other social determinants of health, increase people's vulnerability to obstetric violence, which is embedded in India's post-colonial patriarchal context (Mayra et al. 2021b). Obstetric violence and racism can also be understood as consisting of forms of medical apartheid, such as a lack of access to good quality obstetric care, differentiation in the quality of care based on race or class, or when racialised people are used as bodies for education and experimentation (Bridges 2011; Washington 2006).

Studies also report the presence of different forms of obstetric violence embedded in medical education, and hence part of care providers' learned behaviour, such as being pressured to perform vaginal examinations without consent, practising on people of colour without their consent, and instrumentalising labouring people's bodies to tick off lists of mandatory numbers of practised procedures (Sen et al. 2018; Nayak and Nath 2018; Diniz et al. 2018; Mayra 2020b; Srivastava and Sivakami 2019; Van der Waal et al. 2021, 2023). This leads to particularly extreme cases of disrespect and abuse in the tertiary level teaching hospitals, where attention is given to medical student's practice, at the expense of attention to labouring people, making labouring people more vulnerable to obstetric violence when experiencing and receiving care related to complications (Srivastava and Sivakami 2019). In Brazil, a study reported a case in 2014 where a Black woman was reportedly given two episiotomy cuts during her labour, on the right and left, so that two medical students could practice episiotomy and suturing on the same woman (Diniz et al. 2018).

Bowser and Hill (2010) categorised mistreatment during childbirth into (1) physical abuse, (2) non-consented care, (3) non-confidential care, (4) non-dignified care,

Box 2 Case Study: Obstetric Violence

Case Study.

Forced episiotomy: Kelly's story.

A famous case study from the United States details how Kelly had a forced episiotomy in 2013 that was documented on video. The case was pursued by the organisation Human Rights in Childbirth (HRIC) by the lawyer Hermine Hayes-Klein.

In the video, we see Kelly lying with her legs in the stirrups, pushing with every contraction. Then, another contraction comes. The nurse directs Kelly to 'push, push, push, go, go, go'. In the foreground, the doctor bustles with scissors and a medical cloth. He throws the cloth over Kelly's lower belly, exposing her perineum below it, and approaches with the scissors. Panting with the contraction, Kelly calls out desperately, 'No, don't cut me!' Kelly begs, 'No! Why? Why can't we try?' The doctor's voice is authoritative, even angry, as he responds: 'What do you mean, "Why?" That's my reason. Listen: I am the expert here'. Kelly pleads, 'But why can't I try?' The doctor answers, '"Why can't I try?" You can go home and do it. You go to Kentucky'.

The nurse and Kelly's mother urge her to agree with the doctor. Kelly's mother says, 'Dear, you can't argue with the doctor. Doctor, do your job'. The nurse adds, 'If the baby rips you, it will be more than just a cut and you will feel much more pain. The doctor said it will be only an inch. It isn't that bad'. Another contraction follows. Kelly tries to push and keeps silent. Her mother repeated, 'Do it, doctor'. The doctor starts cutting the young woman with the scissors. We hear the scissors cut her 12 times. After a while, he pulls the baby out of Kelly. Everybody cheers throughout this event. But Kelly remains silent. The nurse gives her baby to the woman. She tries to smile.

After giving birth, Kelly wrote in her letter to the hospital: 'The doctor cut my vagina 12 times! Before the procedure the nurse assured me it's only going to be an inch cut. This "little cut" turned into the doctor's rage against his patient. I wanted to cry and I was so scared while the doctor was cutting me. I could not imagine that I would have to experience "Birth Rape" at your hospital'.

She never received a response.

For the video, see: https://www.youtube.com/watch?v=lCfXxtoAN-I.

The case was picked up by the activist movement https://improvingbirth.org/2014/08/vid/ and by human rights in childbirth http://humanrightsinchildbirth.com/kellys-story.

Hayes-Klein (2014). Forced episiotomy: Kelly's story. Human Rights in Childbirth. http://humanrightsinchildbirth.com/kellys-story.

(5) discrimination based on specific patient attributes, (6) abandonment of care, and (7) detention in facilities. Bohren et al. (2015) differentiated three domains, subdomains, and specific indicators. The domains include (1) physical abuse, (2) sexual abuse, (3) verbal abuse, (4) stigma and discrimination, (5) failure to meet professional standards, (6) poor support between women and providers, and (7) health system conditions and constraints Bohren et al. (2015). This typology breaks the categories down to the specific actions and hence is easy to identify in healthcare facilities. Table 1 presents an adaptation of the original typology by Bohren et al. (2015) with some additions added by Mayra et al. 2021 based on her research in India. A typology of the mistreatment of newborn babies was also published in 2018 in line with Bohren's typology but adapted for newborns, based on a systematic literature review (Sacks 2017).

Obstetric violence is prevalent globally, with scientific evidence from at least 75 countries (Šimonović and UNHCR 2019; Drandic et al. 2022). Literature suggests an underreporting of obstetric violence during childbirth. This can be a result of women's low expectations or not knowing what to expect during childbirth; experiencing disrespect and abuse but considering it a part of care provision; being aware of the experience of disrespect and abuse during childbirth but considering it women's fault due to their fear of the consequences of speaking out; and fear of speaking against the only care provider in the area or fear of not being heard and taken seriously (Kitzinger 1992; Cleghorn 2021). In Ethiopia, 78.6% of women in a study reportedly experienced obstetric violence during childbirth, but only 16.2% reported it (Asefa and Bekele 2015). This changed when the 'What Women Want' campaign reached out to 1.2 million women in 114 countries asking their one demand for quality reproductive and maternal healthcare. The top ranking 'want' was respectful maternity care (White Ribbon Alliance 2019).

Obstetric violence is reported to be most prevalent in post-colonial countries (Davis 2019a; Davis 2019b; Bohren et al. 2015, 2019; Sen et al. 2018; Betron et al. 2018; Miltenburg et al. 2018; Mayra et al. 2021b). Colonial violence results in high mortality rates among indigenous populations, where midwives were expropriated from their traditional practices, and people are prevented from birthing on their indigenous land within their communities. Medical colonialism has robbed many countries of the evolution of traditional midwives, even in countries with a strong history of midwifery (Vega 2018). This is a form of epistemic and cultural obstetric violence that has uprooted midwifery practices from their position in the cultural traditions of the community, where they were intimately connected to rituals, beliefs, and norms. The expropriation of traditional midwives of childbirth is a dehumanisation and a deculturalisation of birth, forcing it into a purely biological paradigm (Wynter 2015). Beyond addressing the problem of physical violation and harm, the call for the humanisation of birth is hence also a call for emotional, psychological, spiritual, and cultural safety.

Historical Causes of Obstetric Violence

Obstetric violence is a complicated global problem, one that we frame as structural and institutional, driven by racial capitalism, rather than consisting of individual perpetrators and victims. The history of obstetrics reveals a constitutive entwinement with oppressive structures such as capitalism, eugenics, colonialism, and slavery, as well as a role in the reproduction and maintenance of structures of racialised and misogynous violence. After the closing of the Trans-Atlantic slave trade in the United States in 1808, doctors and plantation owners worked together to better the reproductive health of enslaved Black women for 'breeding' purposes, in order to increase labour power (Owens 2018; Davis 2019a). It is here that modern obstetrics was born—through experiments on enslaved women (Owens 2018). This history still expresses itself in the higher maternal and neonatal mortality rates for Black people, 3–7 times higher in the United States and the UK (Petersen et al. 2019; Knight et al. 2019); the higher prevalence of premature birth for Black people in the United States (Davis 2019b); and in ongoing practices globally where students 'practice' on people of colour (Washington 2006; Van der Waal et al. 2021). Similarly, the witch-hunts in pre-modern Europe were essential in establishing primordial state-control over reproduction necessary for the constitution of the modern biopolitical institution of obstetrics (Federici 2004). Fear and paranoia of infanticidal witchcraft practices led to the construction of maternal subjectivity and autonomous midwifery practices as dangerous and the subjection of reproduction to state-control. Suspicion of pregnant people, midwives, doula's, and other autonomous independent birthers and birthworkers is still highly present in state-policy and the obstetric institution. Obstetric violence is hence racialised institutional GBV that comes forth out of the history of the institution wherein multiple axes of oppression intersect. It has historical, structural, global, and intersectional causes and cannot be reduced to bad intentions or a failure of evidence-based practice.

Summary

- Obstetric violence is systemic institutional violence.
- Obstetric violence happens globally within the obstetric institution.
- Obstetric violence is co-constituted by structural forms of violence and suppression such as misogyny, slavery, racism, coloniality, and racial capitalism.

References

Afsana K, Rashid SF (2001) The challenges of meeting rural Bangladeshi women's needs in delivery care. Reprod Health Matters 9(18):79–89

Asefa A, Bekele D (2015) Status of respectful and non abusive care during facility based childbirth in a hospital and health centers in Addis Ababa, Ethiopia. Reprod Health 12:33. https://doi.org/10.1186/s12978-015-0024-9

Beck CT, Driscoll JW, Watson S (2013) Traumatic childbirth. Routledge, New York

Betron M, McClair T, Currie S, Banerjee J (2018) Expanding the agenda for addressing mistreatment in maternity care: a mapping review and gender analysis. Reproductive Health 15:143. https://doi.org/10.1186/s12978-018-0584-6

Bhattacharya S, Srivastava A, Avan BI (2013) Delivery should happen soon and my pain will be reduced: understanding women's perception of good delivery care in India. Glob Health Action 6:22635. https://doi.org/10.3402/gha.v6i0.22635

Bohren MA, Hunter EC, Munthe-Kaas HM, Souza JP, Vogel JP, Gülmezoglu AM (2014) Facilitators and barriers to facility based delivery in low and middle income countries: a qualitative evidence synthesis. Reprod Health 11:71

Bohren MA, Vogel JP, Hunter EC, Lutsiv O, Makh SK, et al. (2015) The Mistreatment of Women during Childbirth in Health Facilities Globally: A Mixed-Methods Systematic Review. PLOS Medicine 12(6): e1001847. https://doi.org/10.1371/journal.pmed.1001847

Bohren MA, Mehrtash H, Fawole B, Maung TM, Balde MD, et al. (2019). How women are treated during facility-based childbirth in four countries: a cross-sectional study with labour observations and community-based surveys. The Lancet 394(10210)1750–1763, https://doi.org/10.1016/S0140-6736(19)31992-0

Bowser D, Hill K (2010) Exploring evidence for disrespect and abuse in facility-based childbirth: report of a landscape analysis. USAID-TRAction Project (Harvard School of Public Health)

Bridges KM (2011) Reproducing race. An ethnography of pregnancy as a site of racialization. University California Press, Berkeley, CA

Chadwick R (2017) Ambiguous subjects: obstetric violence, assemblage and South African birth narratives. Fem Psychol 27(4):489–509

Chadwick R (2018) Bodies that birth: vitalizing birth politics. Routledge, New York

Chadwick R (2021) Breaking the frame: obstetric violence and epistemic rupture. Agenda 35(3):104–115. https://doi.org/10.1080/10130950.2021.1958554

Cleghorn E (2021) Unwell women. Penguin Random House, London

Cohen Shabot S (2019) Amigas, sisters, we are being gaslighted in: Childbirth, vulnerability, and Law ed. Camilla Pickles and Jonathan Herring. New York: Routledge

D'Gregorio P (2010) Obstetric violence a new legal term introduced in Venezuela. Int J Gynaecol Obstet 111(3):201–202. https://doi.org/10.1016/j.ijgo.2010.09.002

Davis DA (2019a) Obstetric racism: the racial politics of pregnancy, labor, and birthing. Med Anthropol 38(7):560–573. https://doi.org/10.1080/01459740.2018.1549389

Davis D (2019b) Reproductive injustice: racism, pregnancy and premature birth. New York University Press, New York

De Vries R (2017) Obstetric ethics and the invisible mother. Narrat Inq Bioethics 7(3):215–220. https://doi.org/10.1353/nib.2017.0068

Diniz C, Rattner D, Lucas d'Oliveira A, Marques de Aguiar J, Niy D (2018) Disrespect and abuse in childbirth in Brazil: social activism, public policies and providers' training. Reprod Health Matters 26(53):19–35. https://doi.org/10.1080/09688080.2018.1502019

Drandić D, Drglin Z, Mihevc B, et al (2022) Women's perspectives on the quality of hospital maternal and newborn care around the time of childbirth during the COVID-19 pandemic: Results from the IMAgiNE EURO study in Slovenia, Croatia, Serbia, and Bosnia-Herzegovina. Int J Gynecol Obstet. 159(Suppl. 1):54–69. https://doi.org/10.1002/ijgo.14457

Federici S (2004) Caliban and the witch. Women, the body, and primitive accumulation. Autonomedia, New York

Fontein-Kuipers Y, Romijn C, Sakko E, Stam C, Steenhuis N, de Vries D, van Willigen I, Koster D (2018) Women's traumatic childbirth experiences: reflections and implications for practice. J Pregnancy Child Care

Freedman LP, Ramsey K, Abuya T et al (2014) Defining disrespect and abuse of women in childbirth: a research, policy and rights agenda. Bull World Health Organ 92:915–917

Hadwinger MC, Hadwinger SC (2012) Filipina mothers' perceptions about childbirth at home. Int Nurs Rev 59(1):125–131

Hayes-Klein H (2014) Forced episiotomy: Kelly's story. Human rights in childbirth. http://humanrightsinchildbirth.com/kellys-story

Hill M (2019) Give birth like a feminist. HarperCollins Publishers, London

Jha P, Larsson M, Christensson K, Skoog Svanberg A (2017) Satisfaction with childbirth services provided in public health facilities: results from a cross- sectional survey among postnatal women in Chhattisgarh, India. Glob Health Action 10(1):1386932. https://doi.org/10.1080/16549716.2017.1386932

Kingma E (2015) Better understanding the metaphysics of pregnancy: organisms, identity, personhood & persistence. ERC Starting Grant, Research proposal

Kitzinger S (1992) Birth and violence against women: generating hypotheses from women's accounts of unhappiness after childbirth. Routledge, New York

Knight M, Bunch K, Kenyon S et al (2019) A national population-based cohort study to investigate inequalities in maternal mortality in the United Kingdom, 2009-17. Paediatr Perinat Epidemiol 34:392–398

Mayra K (2020b) A starched cotton fluorescent-yellow saree, khopa, belly button and safety pins: decoding the 'dignified Indian nurse-midwife'. Pract Midwife J 23(6)

Mayra K, Kumar AIK (2017) Perceptions of antenatal women, husbands and health care providers on husband being birth companion during childbirth: a qualitative study. Public Health 1(1)

Mayra K, Matthews Z, Padmadas SS (2021b) Why do some care providers disrespect and abuse women during childbirth? Women Birth

Mayra K, Matthews Z, Sandall J (2021) 'Surrogate decision-making' in India for women competent to consent and choose during childbirth, Agenda, 35(3) 92–103. https://doi.org/10.1080/10130950.2021.1958549.

Miller S, Lalonde A (2015) The global epidemic of abuse and disrespect during childbirth: history, evidence, interventions and FIGO's mother-baby friendly birthing facilities initiative. Int J Gynecol Obstet 131:549–552

Miltenburg AS, van Pelt S, Meguid T, Sundby J (2018) Disrespect and abuse in maternity care: individual consequences of structural violence. Reprod Health Matters 26(53):88–106. https://doi.org/10.1080/09688080.2018.1502023

Morgan K, Thapar-Björkert S (2006) "I'd rather you'd lay me on the floor and start kicking me": understanding symbolic violence in everyday life. Women's Stud Int Forum 29:451–452. https://doi.org/10.1016/j.wsif.2006.07.002

Morton C, Henley M, Seacrist M, Roth L (2018) Bearing Witness: United States and Canadian maternity support in workers' observations of disrespectful care in childbirth. Birth: Issues in Perinatal Care 45, https://doi.org/10.1111/birt.12373

Mrisho M, Schellenberg JA, Mushi AK, Obrist B, Mshinda H, Tanner M, Schellenberg D (2017) Factors affecting home delivery in rural Tanzania. Tropical Med Int Health 12(7):862–872. https://doi.org/10.1111/j.1365-3156.2007.01855.x

Nayak AK, Nath A (2018) There is an urgent need to humanize childbirth in India. Econ Polit Wkly 53(2)

Newnham E, Kirkham M (2019) Beyond autonomy: care ethics for midwifery and the humanization of birth. Nurs Ethics 26(7-8):2147–2157. https://doi.org/10.1177/0969733018819119

Otis KE, Brett JA (2008) Barriers to hospital births: why do Bolivian women give birth at home? Rev Paman Salud Publica 24(1):46–53

Owens DC (2018) Medical bondage. Race, gender, and the origins of American gynecology. University of Georgia Press, Athens, GA

Petersen EE, Davis NL, Goodman D et al (2019) Racial/ethnic disparities in pregnancy-related deaths — United States, 2007–2016. MMWR Morb Mortal Wkly Rep 68:762–765. https://doi.org/10.15585/mmwr.mm6835a3

Pickles C, Herring J (2020) Women's birthing bodies and the law. Unauthorised intimate examinations, power and vulnerability. Hart, Oxford

Sacks E (2017) Defining disrespect and abuse of newborns: a review of the evidence and an expanded typology of respectful maternity care. Reprod Health 14:66. https://doi.org/10.1186/s12978-017-0326-1

Sadler M, Santos MJDS, Ruiz-Berdun D et al (2016) Moving beyond disrespect and abuse: addressing the structural dimensions of obstetric violence. Reprod Health Matters 24:47–55

Scotland M (2020) Birth shock. Pinter and Martin, London

Sen G, Reddy B, Iyer A (2018) Beyond measurement: the drivers of disrespect and abuse in obstetric care. Reprod Health Matters 26(53):6–18

Shabot S, Korem K (2018) Domesticating bodies: the role of shame in obstetric violence. Hypatia 33(3):384–401. https://doi.org/10.1111/hypa.12428.

Šimonović D, UNHCR (2019) A human rights-based approach to mistreatment and violence against women in reproductive health services with a focus on childbirth and obstetric violence. Note by the Secretary-General. Report of the Special rapporteur on violence against women. 74th session on Advancement of women. A/74/137. https://digitallibrary.un.org/record/3823698. Accessed 29 May 2021

Sorensen BL et al (2011) User and provider perspectives on emergency obstetric care in a Tanzanian rural setting: a qualitative analysis of the three delays model in a field study. Afr J Reprod Health 15(2)

Srivastava S, Sivakami M (2019) Evidence of 'obstetric violence' in India: an integrative review. J Biosoc Sci 52(4):610–628. https://doi.org/10.1017/S0021932019000695

Van der Waal R, Mitchell V, van Nistelrooij I, Bozalek V (2021) Obstetric violence as students' rite of passage. The relation of the obstetric subject and its racialized (m)other. Agenda 33

van der Waal R, Mayra K, Horn A, Chadwick R (2023) Obstetric Violence: An Intersectional Refraction through Abolition Feminism. Feminist Anthropology. https://doi.org/10.1002/fea2.12097

van der Waal R, van Nistelrooij I (2022) Reimagining relationality for reproductive care: Understanding obstetric violence as "separation." Nursing Ethics 29(5):1186–1197. https://doi.org/10.1177/09697330211051000

Vega R (2018) No alternative: childbirth, citizenship and indigenous culture in Mexico. University of Texas Press, Austin, TX

Villarmea S (2015) On obstetrical controversies: refocalization as conceptual innovation. In: Perona A (ed) Normativity and praxis. Remarks on controversies – philosophy 13. Mimesis International

Villarmea S (2020) When a uterus enters the room, reason goes out the window. In: Pickles C, Herring J (eds) Women's birthing bodies and the law: unauthorised medical examinations, power and vulnerability. Hart, Oxford, pp 63–78

Villarmea S (2021) Reasoning from the uterus: Casanova, women's agency, and philosophy of birth. Hypatia 36:1

Villarmea S, Fernández Guillén F (2011) Fully entitled subjects: birth as a philosophical topic. Ontol Stud 211–230

Villarmea S, Kelly B (2020) Barriers to establishing shared decision-making in childbirth: unveiling epistemic stereotypes about women in labour. J Eval Clin Pract 26:515–519

Washington HA (2006) Medical apartheid. The dark history of medical experimentation on black Americans from colonial times to the present. Harlem Moon, New York

White Ribbon Alliance (2019) Respectful maternity care: the universal rights of childbearing women

WHO (2014) Defining disrespect and abuse of women in childbirth: a research,policy and rights agenda. Bulletin World Health Organ 92:915–917

Williams CR, Jerez C, Klein K, Correa M, Belizan JM, Gormick C (2018) Obstetric violence: a Latin American legal response to mistreatment during childbirth. BJOG 125(10):1208–1211. https://doi.org/10.1111/1471-0528.15270

Wynter S (2015) Unparalleled catastrophe for our species? Or, to give humanness a different future: conversations. In: McKrittick K (ed) Sylvia Wynter, on being human as praxis. Duke University Press, London

Rodante van der Waal, MA is a PhD-candidate in Care Ethics at the University for Humanistic Studies. She works on obstetric violence, reproductive justice, and the philosophy of pregnancy. She studied philosophy, BA and MA (cum laude) at the university of Amsterdam. She is also an independent midwife working in Amsterdam

Kaveri Mayra, PhD is a Postdoctoral researcher at the Birth Place Lab, University of British Columbia and a Subject Matter Expert at the WHO HQ. She has qualifications in Nursing, Midwifery and Public Health from India. She has recently acquired a PhD in Global Health where she specifically focussed on the drivers of Obstetric Violence in India, from the University of Southampton.

Pornography

Chris Waugh

> **Learning Objectives**
> Having read this chapter, you should be able to understand:
>
> - The distinction between pornography and erotica.
> - How pornography functions as a form of work.
> - How pornography is consumed.
> - Sociological and critical approaches to pornography.

Introduction

Pornography (often referred to as porn) can be defined simply as the portrayal of sexual subject matter (including, but not limited to, depicting sexual acts) for the purposes of sexual arousal (Seltzer 2011). The word 'pornography' originates from the Greek word 'pornographos', meaning 'writing about prostitutes', though the term 'pornography' itself is first recorded in the 1840 as the French 'pornographie' (Anon 2021). The term pornography is generally used to refer to presentations within media of such material, including videos, film, writing, magazines and via social media. Pornography is subject to a variety of legal restrictions around the world, and understandings of what is, and what is not, pornographic vary across historical and cultural contexts (Johnson 2012).

C. Waugh (✉)
Department of Sociology, The University of Manchester, Manchester, UK

Department of Strategy, Enterprise and Sustainability, Manchester Metropolitan University, Manchester, UK

University of Law, Manchester, UK
e-mail: chris.waugh-2@manchester.ac.uk

P. Ali, M. M. Rogers (eds.), *Gender-Based Violence: A comprehensive guide*,
https://doi.org/10.1007/978-3-031-05640-6_31

Erotic or sexual forms of art have a long history: sexual art has been discovered from prehistoric times, and archaeological findings suggest art depicting heterosexual sex was popular in ancient Mesopotamia (Rudgley 2000). However, pornography has evolved with the development of the internet and virtual reality; concurrently, the mode of production of pornography has shifted in recent years, with a move away from major studio productions to platform labour websites such as OnlyFans (Lines 2020). With the development of the internet, pornographic films and materials in general became much more widely available than in previous decades. In 2019, the pornographic website Pornhub received 42 billion visits, or around 115 million per day, with a selection of 1.36 million hours of pornographic videos available to visitors (Pornhub 2019). Estimates of the revenue of the porn industry vary between $6 billion and $97 billion dollars (Benes 2018). While data suggests that only 911 individuals formally work in the US porn industry (Anon 2020), the true figures is harder to say, given the significant amount of 'amateur' pornography and amateur porn actors, as well as the varied forms of the medium itself.

Pornography must be understood in several different ways: as a form of cultural production, as a form of consumer product, as a form of work and labour and also as a more nebulous conception referring to the ways in which elements of culture adopt the style and sometimes content of pornography—a process often referred to as 'pornification' (Paasonen 2016). This chapter provides an overview of considerations of pornography as a form of work and as a form of product. Subsequently, critical perspectives within sociological literature on pornography are provided. For alternative terms used to describe pornography see Box 1.

Box 1 Alternative Terminology

Amateur porn, erotica, obscenity, pornography, porn, sex work

Pornography as Work

In considering pornography as work, it is important to take into account some variations among the kinds of workers, and the kinds of work, within that industry. It is important to acknowledge the distinctions between 'professional' porn actors and actresses (who in general are represented by an agent and contracted—either short or long term—to a pornography studio) and 'amateur' porn actors and actresses, who are more likely to exist within the industry as platform labourers and to generate income from websites such as OnlyFans, ManyVids and AdmireMe. In addition, within professional pornography, there will be cameramen, producers, directors, make-up artists, etc. In amateur pornography, these roles are usually conducted by the performer themselves.

What does unite professional and amateur porn performers is that both groups are considered to be sex workers. Sex work is defined as 'the exchange of sexual services, performances or products for material compensation' (Lutnick and Cohan 2009: 38). Sex work is a broad term which covers pornographic performers, erotic dancers, escorts, prostitutes, phone sex operators and webcam models, among others (Harcourt and Donovan 2005). Generally speaking, sex work is not easy; despite the size of the sex industry, and the evident demand by the consumers, sex workers often face discrimination, stigma and in some cases violence or repression.[1] While some sex workers achieve significant financial security, fame and sometimes mainstream popularity outside of the world of sex work, it remains the case that for many sex workers—including pornographic performers—their work is risky and precarious. This section of the chapter attempts to bear in mind the disparity of sex workers' lived experience and conditions in the subsequent discussion of porn as a form of work.

Pay for porn performers can vary wildly; for example, within heterosexual pornography, professional female performers tend to earn the highest wages. A female performer in a 'boy/girl' scene can expect to earn between $800 and $1000 (£500 to £700), while a top-tier female performer would be paid between $1500 and $2000 per scene (£1096 to £1460), with an average of four scenes per day (Morris 2016). Male performers, on the other hand, can expect around $500–$600 per day (£360–£430), meaning that—on paper at least—professional pornography is one of the few industries where the gender wage gap benefits women (Stanger 2016). Newcomers of both genders might expect to be paid as little as $300 per scene (£220) (Morris 2016). However, women generally spend less time in the industry than their male counterparts. The average female performer spends 3 years in the industry, while male performers stay for an average of 9 years (Millward 2013). Despite the gender pay gap, even successful female porn performers can face inconsistent pay: Lebanese-American former porn star Mia Khalifa spent 3 months in professional porn in 2014. Despite her short tenure, she became extremely popular, becoming the top-ranked pornstar on Pornhub (Saul 2015), and remains one of the most watched performers on the site. However, Khalifa revealed that she only made $12,000 by the time she left the industry and received no money since then, as residuals for her videos went to BangBros (the company she was contracted to) and not to her (Horton 2019).

Porn performers also face health and safety risks within their work. In both heterosexual and homosexual pornography, the majority of sexual acts are unprotected (that is, condoms are not used); within gay porn, 'barebacking' (penetrative anal sex without a condom) is its own 'unique identity' (Birkhold 2012, p. 2). However, unprotected sex does place pornographic performers at increased risk of diseases such as chlamydia, gonorrhoea, syphilis and HIV/AIDS (Rodriguez-Hart et al.

[1] A full analysis of sex workers' lived experience is sadly beyond the scope of this chapter. In addition, until recently, the voices of sex workers were often marginalised within the academic literature. For a source that provide an academic analysis of sex work and sex workers (which is also authored by sex workers), the author recommends Smith, M., and Mac, J., 2018. Revolting prostitutes: The fight for sex workers' rights. Verso Trade.

2012). Though most porn studios require that performers are screened for sexually transmitted infections every 2 weeks, there have been numerous outbreaks of STIs among pornographic performer communities—in 2004, performer Darren James tested positive for HIV, resulting in a 60-day shutdown of the American porn industry, and five other performers were found to have contracted the virus (Madigan 2004). As a result, California introduced Measure B, a law requiring the use of condoms in all vaginal and anal sex filmed in Los Angeles County, though the measure was opposed by numerous porn performers (B VYo 2012; Kernes 2012).

However, the ease of access to testing can vary from country to country. In the UK, where sex work is often associated with criminalisation (despite being legal, especially pornography), sex workers reported discrimination and stigma in seeking support for their sexual health (Trust 2020). In addition, porn performers face other health and safety concerns, ranging from pressure to engage in acts they might be uncomfortable with, to poor mental health support (Webber 2019), and an apparent failure to respond to serious allegations of sexual violence (see Case Study 1). As Sullivan and McKee (2015) point out, it is often in smaller and lower budget porn studios where health and safety risks are at their worst. As a result, many newer and less well-known professional porn performers find themselves in 'a vicious cycle stigmatisation whereby individuals working in porn are assumed to tolerate high risk and get what they bargained for' (Sullivan and McKee 2015: 34).

Pay, conditions and safety within amateur pornography is somewhat harder to analyse, as academic work has in general not paid sufficient attention to online sex work (Ruberg 2016). Amateur porn performers do not have the backing of studios, and as such films are made via phone cameras or commercially available film cameras and usually uploaded to YouTube-style porn websites such as Pornhub. For some individuals, this is not done primarily for monetary gain, but as a form of sexual self-expression, much like the writing and sharing of free erotica or nude images via social networking sites such as Reddit (Paasonen 2007). However, there is often a blurring of the boundaries between professional and amateur pornography—the so-called reality porn is produced by a professional studio, but aims to emulate the low-budget, candid style and supposed authenticity of amateur porn (Allen and Hill 2004).

In a sense, the idea of freely shared sexual expression which is often associated with amateur pornography is commodified, suggesting that content is produced for pleasure and not profit, and articulates a broad cultural anxiety about connecting sex with money which is often at the heart of much of the discrimination faced by sex workers (Ruberg 2016). While the professional porn performer, who's paid labour is sex, is degraded, the amateur porn performer somehow exists outside of the capitalist system, sexually self-actualised rather than sexually commodified. However, this utopian conception of sexual labour is divorced from the lived reality of both amateur porn performers and the nature of digital labour more broadly.

Case Study 1 James Deen

James Deen (born Bryan Sevilla) is an American pornographic actor who rose to prominence in the early 2000s. Deen was especially popular with both male and female consumers of pornography due to his slender build, everyman persona and approachable attitude, bucking the trend of hypermasculinity often shown in heterosexual pornography (Hess and Grover 2012). Deen himself claimed to be feminist and worked with the non-profit Project Consent, which sought to combat rape culture (Wiseman 2015). Deen starred in over 3000 pornographic films and starred in mainstream cinema as well (IAFD 2021). However, in 2015, pornographic actress Stoya (who had dated Deen between 2012 and 2014) alleged that Deen had repeatedly sexually abused her during their relationship. Another ex of Deen's, pornographic actress Joanna Angel, also alleged that Deen had raped and beaten her; Angel and Stoya were later joined by two more adult actresses who made similar allegations; allegations also emerged that Deen was unnecessarily rough when filming scenes with younger female stars (Hanson 2015). In the aftermath, Deen was dropped by three major porn companies (Kink.com, Evil Angel and HardX.com), and he was dropped from numerous journalistic projects (Carroll 2015) Deen himself seemingly announced his retirement from porn in 2018 (Deen 2018).

However, the allegations appear to have done little to impact on Deen's appeal or monetary earnings from the pornographic industry. At time of writing, Deen continues to make videos (having starred in 21 alone in 2020 (AFD 2021)) and is ranked as the 66th most popular porn star on Pornhub (based on views and revenue (Pornhub 2021)). Deen's continued success in the porn world, despite the severity of the allegation against him, raises questions around accountability processes within the industry. Innes, writing in 2020, saw Deen's case indicative that the porn industry was insulated from the ramifications of the #MeToo movement, compounding issues around ongoing concerns around consent and abusive practises within the field (Innes 2020).

A lack of meaningful revenue from YouTube-style porn sites resulted in an almost mass migration of amateur porn performers to platform labour websites such as OnlyFans and AdmireMe. Platform labour refers to when work is outsourced via a web-based platform (usually a website or a mobile phone app) to a dispersed and flexible workforce. Workers will match their skills to their customers via the platform, and customers can request the services of a worker who is either chronologically or geographically available to them at any given time (FR et al. 2019). Examples of platform labour include Uber drivers, freelancers on Fiverr, bar staff via apps such as HAP or Hyr, etc. (Posada and Shade 2020). While platform labour offers flexibility for the workers and convenience for the consumer, it can also produce precarious working conditions, with an absence of normal working benefits such as sick pay or holiday pay and (in many cases) an inability to unionise and safeguard labour rights (Katta et al. 2020).

For porn performers, the most ubiquitous platform is (for now at least) OnlyFans. OnlyFans was founded in 2016 as a content subscription service, connecting users (fans) to content creators. Revenue is generated via a monthly fee (from which OnlyFans takes a cut) and one-time tips and pay-per-view features, which are paid directly to the content creator (Dickson 2020a). OnlyFans was not originally intended to be a platform for sex workers, though the website became famous for, and most heavily populated by, amateur sex workers who used the platform to receive regular payments for their labours (Hall 2018). OnlyFans swiftly gained a popular culture reputation for being a platform of sexual content and pornography; Beyonce referred to the website in her remix of Megan Thee Stallion's 'Savage'; a number of prominent YouTubers posted videos drawing attention to the website's sexual content; TikTok (which bans explicit content) hosted a significant number of videos, framing OnlyFans and the 'OnlyFans girl life' as a means by which young women could achieve both financial gain and sexual self-empowerment (Sung 2020).

Case Study 2: Bella Thorne and the 'Gentrification' of OnlyFans

Actress Bella Thorne is one of numerous celebrities who started an OnlyFans page. Thorne was not completely new to the adult industry, having directed a well-received pornographic film in 2019; however, her entry to OnlyFans was not without controversy. Thorne announced that her OnlyFans page would contain with the promise of nudes and sexual content for $200 per post, significantly more than the majority of sex workers charged for PPV content. Within 24 h, she had made over $1 million, purely from monthly subscription fees, despite having uploaded no content.

However, Thorne's content was non-nude and non-sexually explicit, leading to a record demand for refunds and allegations of scamming. In response, OnlyFans changed the way content creators were paid from weekly to monthly and placed limits on how much they could charge for their PPV posts, which many sex workers rely on to supplement their income from subscription fees (Donaldson 2020). For many amateur sex workers, who did not have the public profile of Thorne, the effect of this was financial hardship and a negative association with online sex work as. Thorne caused more consternation among sex workers after she claimed (in response to criticism of her actions) that her OnlyFans page was actually research for an upcoming film project with director Sean Baker, though Baker denied that he had any upcoming projects with Thorne; Baker claimed that he had in fact urged Thorne to consult and listen to sex workers before she decided to join OnlyFans (Noor 2020). As sex worker Aussia Rachel put it, Thorne and other celebrities were 'gentrifying a platform and making obscene amount of money without acknowledging the plight of sex workers' (Dickson 2020b).

The year 2020 proved to be a pivotal year for OnlyFans for two reasons; firstly, the website gained even more public attention after American sex worker Kaylen Ward offered both nude images and sexual content via her OnlyFans page to subscribers who could prove that they had donated to efforts to combat the Australian wildfires of January 2020. Ward raised over $1 million, and OnlyFans supported her work and offered their own donations (Nguyen 2020). Secondly, as COVID-19 put the majority of the world's nations into strict lockdown, limiting the ability of sex workers to engage in person to person work, numerous sex workers (including both amateurs and professionals) flocked to OnlyFans to supplement their income. As a result, by December 2020, OnlyFans hosted more than 1 million content creators (the majority sex workers) and paid out $2 billion in revenues to creators (Boseley 2020). However, a number of recent developments appear to be about to force sex workers (especially amateurs) back into precarity. As the site became more popular, a number of celebrities and influencers opened their OnlyFans pages, leading to concerns that the platform is experiencing a form of gentrification (see Case Study 2).

In 2021, OnlyFans abruptly announced that it would ban pornographic content, citing pressure from credit card companies such as Mastercard to move away from adult content (Fung 2021). Mary Moody (a sex worker and representative of the Adult Industry Laborers and Artists union) articulated the anxiety of many amateur sex workers after the decision, 'what happens is the privileged few are able to move and adapt, while more marginalized workers, who may have worked in riskier street-based sex work prior to OnlyFans are pushed offline, and into the streets' (Solis 2021).

Pornography as Consumer Product

Concerns around the impacts of pornography consumption pertain to both the mind and body. Scientific research into pornography has also highlighted concerns about health impacts; several studies suggested a link between excessive porn consumption and desensitisation towards the victims of sexual violence, as well as a connection between increased porn usage and the propensity to commit sexual crimes (Koop 1987). Other studies have highlighted the addictive elements of pornography which can affect the brain of the user over time, resulting in impulsiveness and dysfunctional anxiety response and, in male users, increased risk of erectile dysfunction (Kraus et al. 2016; Foubert 2017). Similarly, research suggests that even irregular use of pornography can have impacts on sexual self-esteem, satisfaction with one's own body and other body image issues (Kvalem et al. 2014; Griffith et al. 2012). Pornography use has also been connected to rape culture and the blaming of (especially female) victims of sexual violence (Makin and Morczek 2015). However, researchers often struggle with sampling bias and the fact that specific issues might actually be features of wider pathologies, rather than simply problems in themselves (that is, porn addiction as a feature of a wider sex addiction and so on) (de Alarcón et al. 2019; Fidgen 2013).

The methodological issues around research into porn consumption means that comparatively little rigorous research has been done on the impacts of porn consumption on children, despite a widely held societal belief that minors should be shielded from explicit content. As Heins points out, there is little empirical research on porn and children because no university or research team would ethically approve such research, either from a moral standpoint or for fear of negative headlines (Heins 2007). As a result, what research exists is generally based on self-reporting by children, which can be problematic due to the stigma of admitting to accessing adult content (Dawson and O'Higgins 2019). The consistent weakness of sex education in schools has contributed to increasing numbers of children accessing porn via smartphones (Mowlabocus and Wood 2015). Research from 2011 suggested that 57% of 9–19-year-olds in the UK accessed pornography at least once a week (Tsaliki 2011). Even if children do not seek out pornography deliberately, children are more likely to be unintentionally exposed to pornographic content via spam or via illicit materials on mainstream social media sites such as Facebook, TikTok, Twitter and so on (Horvath et al. 2013).

Technological developments had led to similar concerns surrounding what is known as 'deepfake porn'. 'Deepfake' software allows for a person with an existing image or video to be replaced with another person's likeness, usually when another person's face is superimposed onto a different body and their new likeness mimics the mannerisms and movements of the original subject (Westerlund 2019). Deepfake porn involves applying the different faces onto the bodies of pornographic performers, usually those of female celebrities (Öhman 2020). *Star Wars* star Daisy Ridley and *Avengers* star Scarlett Johansson are common targets of non-consensual deepfake pornography (Roegetters 2018), but deepfake porn can also be made of non-celebrity women (and men) for the purposes of blackmail, humiliation and intimidation (Maddocks 2020). Deepfakes can also be used to easily make intimate image abuse, also known as 'revenge porn' (Delfino 2020), especially due to the relative ease of access to technologies such as DeepNude, an app that allowed users to create deepfakes of their contacts on social media from either their laptop or phone (Greengard 2019). While some social media sites such as Reddit and Discord have outright banned deepfake content from their servers, deepfake pornography falls into a legal loophole in most countries; as only a person's face is used by the deepfaker, an individual often has little recourse to legal action under existing laws against intimate image abuse, as what is shared non consensually is not (in isolation) intimate or explicit (Harris 2018).

Theoretical Perspectives

Critical perspectives on pornography can broadly be divided between antipornography perspectives and pro-pornography perspectives. However, as this section demonstrates, the 'lines' in the debate around pornography are blurred by intersecting debates about sex work, censorship and freedom of expression.

Feminist perspectives on pornography are most commonly associated with the anti-porn camp, largely as a result of the vocal presence of feminist writers in what is now called the 'feminist sex wars'—a series of collective debates among feminist groups (predominantly in the USA and UK) around issues relating to sex and sexuality, including abortion, prostitution, BDSM, transgender identity and pornography (Duggan and Hunter 2006). Notable in these debates were the works of Andrea Dworkin and Catherine Mackinnon, who's work defined the anti-porn side. Dworkin argued that pornography as an industry inherently hated and dehumanised women. Porn represented violence against women in both its production (through the treatment of female porn producers) and also through its consumption by eroticising the humiliation and dehumanisation of women (Dworkin 1981). For Dworkin, pornography was just one axis of the means of male power over women; women existed in a world where male patriarchy defined the nature of life, the nature of value and interpersonal dynamics on every level and where porn, along with male literature, science, and philosophy, was the discourse of male truth and antithetical to women (Dworkin 2006).

Mackinnon made a similar argument in her work; based on a number of empirical studies, Mackinnon concluded that pornography was not just a form of entertainment, but instead was the contributing force behind attitudes and behaviours of discrimination which defined the treatment and status of all women, by all men (MacKinnon 1989). Jointly, Mackinnon and Dworkin proposed the Antipornography Civil Rights Ordinance, which sought to classify pornography in all its forms as a violation of women's civil and human rights and allow for women to seek compensation for damages caused to them by pornography (West 2004). Contrastingly, sex-positive feminists hold less antipathy towards porn. Ellen Willis (who coined the term 'sex-positive feminism') argued that anti-porn feminism reinforced Victorian ideas around sex, where men want sex and women merely endure it, whereby erasing women's sexual agency (Willis 1981). Gayle Rubin, in her influential essay *Thinking Sex*, took issue with the pervasive attitude in society of sex negativity, which framed sex as a dangerous and destructive force. She proposed the idea of a 'charmed circle' of sex, that is, the sexual acts and conducts seemed legitimate by society (that is, heterosexual sex, sex within marriage, sex within monogamy and so on) which existed in a binary with 'illegitimate' sexual practises (non-monogamy, pornography, BDSM and so on). By drawing a delineation between 'good sex' and 'bad sex' (the charmed circle and its opposites), sexual behaviour was both grossly simplified and also given an excess of significance, and the rejection of 'bad sex' in principle was a dangerous and discriminatory practise (Rubin 2007). To this day, pornography (and sex work in general) remains a hotly contested issue within feminist discourse.

Outside of feminism, Michel Foucault offered ways of theorising pornography which both supported and critiqued various aspects of the feminist porn debate (Kurylo 2017). While Mackinnon and Dworkin saw pornography as an aspect of patriarchal male power over women, Foucault argued that power was not overarching and top-down, but was instead constructed from disparate and dynamic relations between individuals and institutions that varied across history. As history progressed from the mediaeval period to the early modern capitalist state, power began to manifest most commonly through the administration and control of the individual body. The so-called disciplinary power allowed for the precise monitoring and 'disciplining' of individual bodies (how we walk, talk, interact with others, have sex and so on) which allowed for the state to control a whole population on an individual level. Foucault referred to this form of power as 'bio power' (Foucault 1990), which ensures that 'the administration of population is ensured on the individual and social level' (Kurylo 2017). As Foucault argues in *The History of Sexuality*, the deployment of power begins in regulating an individual's body, namely beginning with their reproductive conduct—in short, how they had sex, with whom and what they thought about sex in all its forms. Sex and power, therefore, have a symbiotic relationship. However, as Foucault argued elsewhere, where there is power, there is resistance (Foucault 1990).

Against the idea of the 'repressive hypothesis' (the commonly held idea that prudish eighteenth-century societies silenced and eradicated discussions of sex and sexuality), Foucault contends that repression caused the bodies of the subjects within those societies to revolt: repression caused the forbidden to be created, new forms of sexuality and new forms of experiencing sexual pleasure (including pornography). The more subjects were repressed, the more they rebelled. However, Foucault was not arguing that this era produced a kind of sexual revolution as seen in the 1960s (a revolution of which Foucault was deeply sceptical). Dominant powers and institutions were not usurped by the sudden rise of pornography; the growth of lesbian, gay, bisexual and transgender (LGBT) rights movements; and the increasing acceptance of sexual fetishes within the mainstream; instead, power morphed and manifested as new strategies of controlling the body through the stimulation of sexual desire—being gay, watching porn and engaging in kink, all were acceptable *if done the right way*, that is, in a way which supported the dominant order. One thinks of the pornification of profitable popular culture, the commercialisation of Pride (divorced now from its roots of radical protest) or the financial success of kink-influenced writing such as *Fifty Shades of Grey*—all co-opting resistance to repression into a profitable, neoliberal order. In short, Foucault's line of thinking is not dissimilar to Gayle Rubin—the concept of good sex (that which is profitable and passive) conflicts in modern discourse with bad sex (that which is subversive, insurrectionary and calls dominant ways of thinking in question).

Summary

- Pornography has a long history, and while pornography is legal in many parts of the world, it remains heavily regulated.
- Both professional and amateur porn performers are sex workers, and their working conditions, pay and safety can vary wildly. The recent growth of platform labour porn (facilitated by websites such as OnlyFans) has granted some sex workers stability, though such labour is not without risks.
- While porn is regularly consumed, there are significant health concerns about the impacts of its consumption, especially for minors. Similarly, the distressing growth of non-consensual pornography has not yet been effectively tackled by lawmakers and policymakers.
- Pornography has divided theorists, especially those within feminism, and there are contentious debates ongoing around power, money and sex within porn.

References

AFD (2021) James Deen Filmography. https://www.adultfilmdatabase.com/actor/james-deen-36326/. Accessed 22 Aug

Allen RC, Hill A (2004) The television studies reader. Psychology Press

Anon (2020) Adult & pornographic websites in the US - employment statistics 2005–2026. https://www.ibisworld.com/industry-statistics/employment/adult-pornographic-websites-united-states/#:~:text=There%20are%20911%20people%20employed,the%20US%20as%20of%202021. Accessed 11 Aug

Anon (2021) Pornography (n.). https://www.etymonline.com/word/pornography. Accessed 12 Aug

B VYo (2012) The Los Angeles County Medical Association says vote yes on B. https://web.archive.org/web/20121029100926/http://www.yesonb.info/. Accessed 23 Aug

Benes R (2018) Porn could have a bigger economic influence on the US than Netflix. Quartz. Accessed 20 June 2018

Birkhold AS (2012) Poking holes in LA's new condom requirement: pornography, barebacking, and speech. Wash UL Rev 90:1819

Boseley M (2020) 'Everyone and their mum is on it': OnlyFans booms in popularity during the pandemic. The Guardian. Accessed 22 Dec 2020

Carroll R (2015) Porn industry groups cut ties to star James Deen amid sexual assault claims. The Guardian

Dawson K, O'Higgins S (2019) The porn identity: overcoming cultural barriers and designing effective interventions in 21st century Ireland. Sex education*:* global perspectives, effective programs and socio-cultural challenges. p 121

de Alarcón R, de la Iglesia JI, Casado NM et al (2019) Online porn addiction: what we know and what we don't—a systematic review. J Clin Med 8(1):91

Deen J (2018) I think I'm...peace out y'all. In: James Deen Blog http://jamesdeenblog.com/2018/06/27/porn-star-james-deen-goodbye-public/. Accessed 2021

Delfino RA (2020) Pornographic Deepfakes: the case for Federal Criminalization of revenge Porn's next tragic act. Actual Probs Econ L 105

Dickson E (2020a) Sex workers built OnlyFans. Now they say they're getting kicked off. Rolling Stone. Accessed 18 May 2020

Dickson E (2020b) Sex workers worry Bella Thorne's $2 million payday could ruin OnlyFans. https://www.rollingstone.com/culture/culture-news/bella-thorne-onlyfans-sex-workers-1050102/. Accessed 24 Aug

Donaldson K (2020) Bella Thorne OnlyFans controversy explained. https://screenrant.com/bella-thorne-onlyfans-controversy-scam-explained/. Accessed 24 Aug

Duggan L, Hunter ND (2006) Sex wars: sexual dissent and political culture. Taylor & Francis

Dworkin A (1981) Men possessing women. Perigee, New York

Dworkin A (2006) Intercourse. Basic Books (AZ)

Fidgen J (2013) Do we know whether pornography harms people? https://www.bbc.co.uk/news/magazine-22987051. Accessed 25 Aug

Foubert JD (2017) The public health harms of pornography: the brain, erectile dysfunction, and sexual violence. Dignity 2(3):6

Foucault M (1990) The history of sexuality: an introduction, vol I. Trans. Robert Hurley. Vintage, New York, p 95

FR L, DNK N, PRT G (2019) 6.6 Platform-mediated workers

Fung B (2021) Why did OnlyFans ban sexually explicit content? It says it's the credit card companies. https://edition.cnn.com/2021/08/20/tech/onlyfans-explicit-content-ban-payment/index.html. Accessed 24 Aug

Greengard S (2019) Will deepfakes do deep damage? Commun ACM 63(1):17–19

Griffith JD, Mitchell S, Hammond B et al (2012) A comparison of sexual behaviors and attitudes, self-esteem, quality of life, and drug use among pornography actors and a matched sample. Int J Sex Health 24(4):254–266

Hall J (2018) OnlyFans is the site where porn is more intimate than ever. https://www.dazeddigital.com/science-tech/article/38717/1/onlyfans-is-the-site-where-porn-is-more-intimate-than-ever. Accessed 24 Aug

Hanson H (2015) Two more adult actresses accuse James Deen of sexual assault. The Huffington Post. Accessed 30 Nov 2015

Harcourt C, Donovan B (2005) The many faces of sex work. Sex Transm Infect 81(3):201–206

Harris D (2018) Deepfakes: false pornography is here and the law cannot protect you. Duke L Tech Rev 17:99

Heins M (2007) Not in front of the children. Rutgers University Press

Hess A, Grover S (2012) 'What women want: Porn and the frontier of female sexuality', Good: A Magazine for the global citizen. Available at: https://web.archive.org/web/20160125115839/https://magazine.good.is/articles/what-women-want

Horton A (2019) Mia Khalifa is among the world's most-watched women. Yet the porn industry is keeping the profits. The Washington Post. Accessed 16 Aug 2019

Horvath MA, Alys L, Massey K, et al. (2013) Basically... porn is everywhere: a rapid evidence assessment on the effects that access and exposure to pornography has on children and young people

IAFD (2021) James Deen. https://www.iafd.com/person.rme/perfid=jamesdeen/gender=m. Accessed 22 Aug

Innes C (2020) Why did we ignore porn's #MeToo?. Cosmopolitan. Accessed 17 Feb 2020

Johnson Z (2012) Lindsay Lohan, Porn Star James Deen costarring in The Canyons. Us Magazine. Accessed 13 June 2012

Katta S, Badger A, Graham M et al (2020) (Dis) embeddedness and (de) commodification: COVID-19, Uber, and the unravelling logics of the gig economy. Dialogues Hum Geogr 10(2):203–207

Kernes M (2012) 'No on Government Waste' Committee holds 1st press conference. https://avn.com/business/articles/legal/no-on-government-waste-committee-holds-1st-press-conference-488400.html. Accessed 23 Aug

Koop CE (1987) Report of the Surgeon General's workshop on pornography and public health. Am Psychol 42(10):944

Kraus SW, Voon V, Potenza MN (2016) Should compulsive sexual behavior be considered an addiction? Addiction 111(12):2097–2106

Kurylo B (2017) Pornography and power in Michel Foucault's thought. J Polit Power 10(1):71–84

Kvalem IL, Træen B, Lewin B et al (2014) Self-perceived effects of internet pornography use, genital appearance satisfaction, and sexual self-esteem among young Scandinavian adults. Cyberpsychology 8(4)

Lines BWG (2020) You can see me naked (after the paywall): how OnlyFans transforms the online sex industry

Lutnick A, Cohan D (2009) Criminalization, legalization or decriminalization of sex work: what female sex workers say in San Francisco, USA. Reprod Health Matters 17(34):38–46

MacKinnon C (1989) Towards a Feminist Theory of the State (Harvard University Press 1989) and Victor Tadros, 'Rape Without Consent' (2006). Oxf J Leg Stud 26:515

Maddocks S (2020) 'A Deepfake porn plot intended to silence me': exploring continuities between pornographic and 'political'deep fakes. Porn Studies 7(4):415–423

Madigan N (2004) Voice of Health in a Pornographic World. The New York Times. Accessed 10 May 2004

Makin DA, Morczek AL (2015) The dark side of internet searches: a macro level assessment of rape culture. Int J Cyber Criminol 9(1):1

Millward J (2013) Deep inside: a study of 10,000 porn stars and their careers. Jon Millward, Data Journalist

Morris C (2016) Porn's dirtiest secret: what everyone get's paid. CNBC. Accessed 21 Jan 2016

Mowlabocus S, Wood R (2015) Introduction: audiences and consumers of porn. Taylor & Francis

Nguyen T (2020) Nude photos raised over $1 million for the Australia fires. https://www.vox.com/the-goods/2020/1/8/21056863/australia-fires-nudes-charity-porn. Accessed 24 Aug

Noor P (2020) A Thorne in the site: the Bella Thorne and OnlyFans controversy explained. The Guardian. Accessed 31 Aug 2020

Öhman C (2020) Introducing the pervert's dilemma: a contribution to the critique of Deepfake pornography. Ethics Inf Technol 22(2):133–140

Paasonen S (2007) Epilogue: porn futures. Pornification: sex and sexuality in media culture. 161–170

Paasonen S (2016) Pornification and the mainstreaming of sex. Oxford research encyclopedia of criminology and criminal justice

Pornhub (2019) The 2019 year in review. https://www.pornhub.com/insights/2019-year-in-review. Accessed 11 Aug 2021

Pornhub (2021) James Deen. https://www.pornhub.com/pornstar/james-deen. Accessed 22 Aug

Posada J, Shade LR (2020) Platform labour discourse: how Hyr targets the "bucket list generation". Democratic Communiqué 29(1):78–96

Rodriguez-Hart C, Chitale RA, Rigg R et al (2012) Sexually transmitted infection testing of adult film performers: is disease being missed? Sex Transm Dis 39(12):989–994

Roegetters J (2018) Porn producers offer to help Hollywood take down deepfake videos. https://variety.com/2018/digital/news/deepfakes-porn-adult-industry-1202705749/. Accessed 27 Aug

Ruberg B (2016) Doing it for free: digital labour and the fantasy of amateur online pornography. Porn Studies 3(2):147–159

Rubin GS (2007) Thinking sex: notes for a radical theory of the politics of sexuality. Routledge

Rudgley R (2000) The lost civilizations of the stone age. Simon and Schuster

Saul H (2015) Pornhub star Mia Khalifa received death threats after being ranked the site's top adult actress. The Independent. Accessed 7 Jan 2015

Seltzer LF (2011) What distinguishes erotica from pornography. Psychol Today 6

Solis M (2021) Sex workers made OnlyFans valuable - then it sold them out. https://www.theverge.com/2021/8/23/22638310/onlyfans-ban-explicit-content-payment-processing-visa. Accessed 24 Aug

Stanger M (2016) Here's what the gender pay gap looks like in the porn industry. https://www.revelist.com/career/average-porn-salaries/851. Accessed 23 August

Sullivan R, McKee A (2015) Pornography: structures, agency and performance. Wiley

Sung M (2020) Influencers are flocking to OnlyFans but not everyone is happy. https://mashable.com/article/influencer-onlyfans-sex-work. Accessed 24 Aug

Trust TTH (2020) The state of the nation: sexually transmitted infections in England. Reportno. Report Number, Date. Place Published: Institution

Tsaliki L (2011) Playing with porn: Greek children's explorations in pornography. Sex Education 11(3):293–302

Webber V (2019) Occupational health in porn production: new frameworks. In: Impact ethics. https://impactethics.ca/2019/11/06/occupational-health-in-porn-production-new-frameworks/. Accessed 2021

West C (2004) Pornography and censorship

Westerlund M (2019) The emergence of deepfake technology: a review. Technol Innov Manag Rev 9(11)

Willis E (1981) Lust horizons: is the women's movement pro-sex. Village Voice 26:36–37

Wiseman E (2015) James Deen, the porn star who failed as a feminist fantasy. The Guardian. Accessed 13 Dec 2012

Chris Waugh is a doctoral researcher at the University of Manchester. His research areas include masculinities, affect, radical left wing social movements and the politics of authenticity.

Reproductive Coercion and Abuse

Sam Rowlands and Susan Walker

Learning Objectives
Having read this chapter, you should be able to understand:

- Interference with women's reproductive autonomy by sexual partners or the wider family is common.
- Coercion or abuse relating to choices about use of contraception or about an established pregnancy comes in various forms and degrees of severity.
- Contraceptive sabotage is deliberate interference with agreed use of contraception, with the intent to cause pregnancy, so invalidating consent to sex.
- Non-consensual condom removal is a separate entity with a hallmark of disrespect and lack of consent—there is not necessarily any intent to promote pregnancy.

Introduction

A framework of reproductive justice stipulates that women should have the right to have children, the right not to have children and the right to parent children in a safe and healthy environment. In other words, women should have *reproductive*

S. Rowlands (✉)
Department of Medical Science & Public Health, Bournemouth University, Bournemouth, UK
e-mail: srowlands@bournemouth.ac.uk

S. Walker
School of Nursing & Midwifery, Anglia Ruskin University, Chelmsford, UK
e-mail: susan.walker@aru.ac.uk

P. Ali, M. M. Rogers (eds.), *Gender-Based Violence: A Comprehensive Guide*,
https://doi.org/10.1007/978-3-031-05640-6_32

autonomy—this entails being free from coercion and violence. Unfortunately, many women have their reproductive autonomy compromised. Behaviours which are used to influence or control a woman's reproductive decision-making and reduce or remove her reproductive autonomy can include economic control; threats and intimidation; isolation from friends, family and from sources of support; and emotional and physical abuse. These constitute reproductive coercion and abuse (RCA). This topic is generally limited to 1:1 relationships and wider family groupings. This chapter adopts this approach and does not extend to reproductive coercion/violence by state actors or in the context of conflict nor criminal sex-trafficking activity.

RCA is a construct distinct from intimate partner violence (IPV) but shares some associations. Whilst RCA and IPV can occur between same-sex couples and can be perpetrated by women upon men, the focus of this chapter is RCA in which women–or any people who have female reproductive capacity–are the coerced party. As with other types of gender-based violence (GBV), RCA arises from misogyny and gender inequality and is both a consequence of and a means of perpetuating patriarchal values and domination. The authors have previously referred to this phenomenon as reproductive control but, in light of further evidence from qualitative studies of the presence of violence in these complex relationships and behaviours, they have adopted the terminology reproductive coercion and abuse favoured by Tarzia (Tarzia and Hegarty 2021).

RCA is common, and many women presenting to health and counselling services may be currently subject to it, may have experienced it in the past or may be at risk of experiencing it. It is therefore important that those caring for women in these services are aware of RCA and the differing forms it can take. RCA may be a factor in contraceptive 'failure' or non-adherence, frequent requests for emergency contraception, for pregnancy or sexually transmitted infection (STI) testing or in having more than one abortion. This chapter seeks to clarify the various manifestations of RCA and outlines possible means of prevention.

What Is Reproductive Coercion and Abuse?

Definition

Reproductive coercion and abuse comprises a wide range of behaviours, from psychological pressure such as emotional blackmail, societal or family expectations through to threats of, and actual, physical and sexual violence. It can be defined as any *deliberate* attempt to dictate a woman's reproductive choices or interfere with her reproductive autonomy. It can include physical, psychological or sexual tactics and occurs in a context of fear and/or control in an interpersonal relationship (Tarzia and Hegarty 2021). RCA can be viewed as sitting on the intersection between sexual violence, domestic violence and IPV (Tarzia and Hegarty 2021). RCA fundamentally interferes with women's reproductive autonomy generally and with their autonomous sexual decision-making more specifically (Katz et al. 2017; Rowlands and Walker 2019). RCA is mediated through the decisions around whether or not to start, continue or terminate a pregnancy, including whether or not to use contraception. It may be exercised in relation to intercourse, conception, gestation or delivery.

Perpetrators of Reproductive Coercion and Abuse

Perpetrators of RCA are most often intimate partners but can include wider family members, acting alone or together. Misogynist cultural and social norms in society can reinforce RCA and may link individual and family behaviour. Controlling behaviours and attitudes need to be recognised and confronted at different levels by bystanders, be they family members, peers, professionals or wider society (Levy-Peck 2017). Healthcare settings need to have clear protocols that take into account the privacy of potential/actual survivors and bar access to certain parts of consultations to potential/actual perpetrators. Treatment programmes for perpetrators must develop ways of reducing RCA behaviours (Levy-Peck 2017).

Prevalence of and Associations with RCA

A lack of definitional clarity around RCA in the past has resulted in widely varying prevalence estimates for RCA, a poor understanding of risk factors and difficulty in demonstrating the effectiveness of interventions (Tarzia and Hegarty 2021). Nonetheless, estimates of the extent of RCA are disturbingly high in varied global settings. In studies of the prevalence of RCA among women of reproductive age attending health services in the USA, between 8% and 30% of women reported ever having suffered RCA (Rowlands and Walker 2019). One-third of heterosexual women surveyed in an Australian sexual health clinic reported having experienced non-consensual condom removal (Latimer et al. 2019). In a large population-based study of RCA in India, 12% of women of reproductive age reported ever having experienced RCA from their current husband or their in-laws (Silverman et al. 2019).

RCA is associated with other indicators of poor sexual wellbeing. Those experiencing RCA are less likely to have contraceptive and sexual self-efficacy and less likely to take responsibility for the direction of sexual activity and for contraceptive use (Katz et al. 2017).

Several studies have shown a positive association between RCA and unintended pregnancy. It has also been shown that the risk of unintended pregnancy doubles in those who suffer both IPV and RCA. Reproductive coercion and abuse and other forms of sexual violence, marginalisation and sexual ill-health coincide. Experience of contraceptive sabotage is positively correlated with ever having an STI, ever engaging in transactional sex (exchange of sex for money or drugs) and having multiple sexual partners in the previous six months (Willie et al. 2021). In a study of US college students, experiences of RCA co-occurred with experience of other forms of sexual violence such as stalking, sexual harassment and sexual assault (Swan et al. 2020).

These associations are found across the world. In India, women experiencing RCA are much less likely to use modern contraceptive methods (Tomar et al. 2020). In South Africa, RCA is positively associated with becoming HIV positive (McCloskey et al. 2020). In a study from Kenya, it was found that the intersection of IPV and high rates of unintended pregnancy might be explained by reproductive coercion, including, in that context, the threat by a partner to take another wife/have a child with another woman (Boyce et al. 2020). RCA is an important factor when considering pregnancy intention (Borrero et al. 2015). There is a strong but complex association between RCA and IPV. Women experiencing IPV are more likely to have a male partner who refuses to use contraception, to experience unwanted pregnancy and to give birth during adolescence, compared to those not experiencing such violence.

Whilst any woman can experience RCA, there is some evidence that younger women are more frequent victims. Women who have recently experienced RCA are more likely to request pregnancy testing and STI testing and to seek emergency contraception—this should be borne in mind in the face of multiple requests for these services (Kazmerski et al. 2015).

Forms of Reproductive Coercion and Abuse Perpetrated by Intimate Partners

RCA may manifest itself across a range of behaviours from pregnancy pressure to contraceptive sabotage or pregnancy outcome control. Various forms of RCA perpetrated by intimate partners are considered below.

Preventing Use of Contraception

In a study of college women in the USA, 8% had experienced RCA, and the commonest form, reported by nearly 7%, was for male partners to tell women not to use contraception (Sutherland et al. 2015). Some women may be prevented from obtaining supplies of contraception. Partners themselves may also refuse to use condoms or exhibit various degrees of condom use resistance.

Contraceptive Sabotage

Intimate partners may deliberately sabotage or interfere with a woman's attempts to use contraception. The commonest means of contraceptive sabotage are failure to practise withdrawal, as previously agreed, or non-use of condoms. Deceptive behaviour may extend to a male partner falsely stating that he has had a vasectomy (see the case study in Box 1). Contraceptive sabotage also includes various actions including piercing condoms or other barrier methods, tampering with or throwing away supplies of oral contraceptives or forcibly removing transdermal patches, vaginal rings or intrauterine devices (Rowlands and Walker 2019).

Contraceptive sabotage interacts and overlaps with sexual coercion and violence. In such cases, consent to sex has been given on the understanding that contraception will be used. Contraceptive sabotage thus invalidates consent—but there are complicated arguments as to how any legal redress would be sought against saboteurs. The criminalisation of contraceptive sabotage has been strongly supported by scholars (Chesser and Zahra 2019). Singapore has amended its Penal Code so that consent to sex obtained by deception or false representation is criminalised and specifically mentions this in relation to the use of contraception (Republic of Singapore 2019). A Canadian court convicted a man who pierced holes in a condom before having sex with a woman who subsequently conceived. It was found that the consent was invalidated by fraud/deception and that the increased risk of pregnancy constituted a risk of 'serious bodily harm'. The perpetrator received an 18-month custodial sentence (Supreme Court of Canada 2014). In many other jurisdictions, cases are not litigated, or those that are result in no conviction being made. A Court of Appeal case in the UK has clarified the concept of 'conditional consent' and what types of deception are considered sufficient to invalidate consent—see Box 1.

Box 1 Case Study: R v Lawrance

Jason Lawrance linked up with Ms. A via a dating website in the UK. They met up and, prior to sex, JL assured Ms A. that he had a vasectomy. Later, he admitted he had lied about his fertility. Ms. A became pregnant and had an abortion. JL was convicted of rape under the Sexual Offences Act 2003 at a Crown Court. JL appealed against his conviction and was successful (UK Court of Appeal 2020).

The judgement considered the circumstances in which deception by an accused man was capable of invalidating ostensible consent. Only deception that is 'closely connected' to the nature or purpose of sexual intercourse was deemed to invalidate consent. Lying about whether a condom would be worn or whether the penis would be withdrawn prior to ejaculation were both considered by the court to be sufficiently closely connected to sex because they physically change the nature of penetration. In contrast, a lie about fertility is not, because it is not related to the performance of the sexual act. In other words, everything hinges on the fact of ejaculation in the woman's body rather than the quality of the ejaculate.

Non-consensual Condom Removal

Contraceptive sabotage includes non-consensual condom removal (NCCR), known informally as 'stealthing' and first expounded on by Alexandra Brodsky (Brodsky 2017). NCCR is defined as the non-consensual, surreptitious removal of a condom before or during penetrative sex, when consent has been given specifically for condom-protected sex, i.e. it is done without knowledge or consent (Czechowski et al. 2019). NCCR has features that differentiate it from contraceptive sabotage in general. The perpetrator is motivated primarily by dislike of condoms rather than by seeking to promote pregnancy (Tarzia et al. 2020). It appears that NCCR is more commonly seen in the context of short-term or casual encounters without the dependency characteristic of RCA (Tarzia et al. 2020).

NCCR as a form of sexual violence has been shown to be associated with sexual aggression, hostility towards women, adversarial heterosexual beliefs and rape myth acceptance (Davis 2019). Perhaps unsurprisingly, perpetrators are more likely to have ever been diagnosed with an STI and more likely to have had a partner with an unplanned pregnancy than other men (Davis 2019).

NCCR is a legal grey area in many jurisdictions, perhaps because it does not fit neatly into existing frameworks of crimes of a sexual nature (Chesser and Zahra 2019). A Swiss Court convicted a man who removed a condom during sex of rape; at the Court of Appeal, the verdict was changed to a 'sex act with a person incapable of resistance', and he received a 12-month suspended sentence (Criminal Court of Appeal - Vaud Canton 2017).

Women's Actions to Reassert Reproductive Autonomy by Contraceptive Use

Women's attempts to reassert reproductive autonomy in the face of RCA include seeking contraceptive methods that can be used covertly (Boyce et al. 2020; Kibira et al. 2020). It has been reported that covert use of contraception is a widespread practice to resist RCA in Africa in response to the gender power dynamics in patriarchal settings and in the context of pronatalist norms and policies (Kibira et al. 2020; Silverman et al. 2020). Contraceptive concealment may be difficult and, in some situations, dangerous. Unfortunately, some women in violent relationships may risk an escalation of violence if they try to negotiate contraceptive use. If an intimate partner is likely to discover contraceptive supplies, other forms of contraception may provide a greater chance of concealability. Intrauterine devices with the threads cut shorter are one option. Injectables are 'invisible', but when a woman is in a situation of intimate partner control, leaving the home to obtain contraception may be difficult. Healthcare professionals may need to be alert to the woman's need to conceal contraception when discussing contraceptive methods, especially in situations where her choice seems difficult to understand or after a disclosure of IPV and/or RCA. Survivors of RCA may request access to contraceptive services in places, during times and with people that avoid the intimate partner's knowledge and involvement. Telehealth and self-administration of injectable contraception are important options here.

Reproductive Coercion During Pregnancy

Once a pregnancy has become established, RCA can take the form either of forced continuation or forced termination of a pregnancy, against the woman's wishes.

Coerced Continuation of a Pregnancy

RCA can include insistence on continuation of a pregnancy which the woman regards as unintended or unwanted. Attempts to access surgical abortion may be sabotaged by preventing a woman accessing a clinic. In these circumstances, medical abortion may be more accessible than surgical abortion to a woman being subjected to RCA, especially if performed according to a no-test, telemedical protocol. This is an aspect of a woman's choice of methods which providers of abortion need to be aware of.

Forced or Perpetrator-Induced Termination of a Pregnancy

Reproductive coercion may also involve forced termination of a pregnancy. Partners may coerce a woman into having a therapeutic abortion, or a woman may be assaulted with the intention of causing a miscarriage. Covert administration of abortifacients to terminate a pregnancy has been reported and prosecuted (Rowlands and Walker 2019).

Reproductive Coercion and Abuse Beyond the Intimate Partner

Perpetration of RCA may extend beyond a single intimate partner and may be part of a pattern of wider family abuse.

Control over Family Size by the Wider Family

In some cultural settings, the wider family—and in particular older female relatives—may have societally endorsed control over reproductive decision-making. Mothers-in-law in patrilineal societies may strongly influence reproductive decisions on the composition of the family (Char et al. 2010), although this need not necessarily be coercive. Family-based RCA is often linked with the status of women and how this is affected by their ability to reproduce (Boyce et al. 2020; Gupta et al. 2012). Links between IPV and wider family abuse during pregnancy, at delivery and postpartum have been reported in two studies of IPV in India (Raj et al. 2011; Silverman et al. 2019).

Impact

There is some overlap between the impact of RCA on mental and physical health and the impact of IPV, which is covered elsewhere in this book. So far, little is known about the impact of RCA. Associations have been found specifically between RCA and negative mental health outcomes in the general population in Côte d'Ivoire (McCauley et al. 2014), in women attending for counselling about pregnancy options in Australia (Price et al. 2022) and in women continuing their pregnancies in Liberia (Willie and Callands 2018).

Prevention, Detection, Education and Harm Reduction

Recognising the existence and extent of RCA provides opportunities for prevention and harm reduction. Prevention and intervention can be complicated by the fact that women subjected to RCA may not necessarily view their relationship as unhealthy or abusive, especially if there is no physical violence. The degree of control that a male partner can exert will vary.

Considering RCA as a public health problem allows prevention to be conceptualised in terms of primary, secondary and tertiary prevention. Primary (universal/population level) prevention at its most ambitious would depend on societal modification of attitudes and behaviour. An overall approach is needed to enhance gender equity, non-violent and non-coercive conflict resolution and respect for reproductive autonomy within intimate relationships (Levy-Peck 2017). It may include enabling women to acquire the necessary skills and education to avoid entrapment in coercive relationships and, crucially, to provide early assistance to women seeking to exit such relationships. Secondary prevention would identify existing cases of RCA using standardised questions concerning risk factors (see below). Appropriate health service settings for secondary prevention are maternity, early pregnancy, sexual assault, SRH and abortion services and in general practice. Ethically, a prerequisite to the identification of cases is the capacity to provide effective interventions, including harm reduction. Tertiary prevention would involve support to individuals and families that cannot extricate themselves from the RCA, to minimise harm and to provide support for survivors.

Screening questions have been formulated to help healthcare professionals identify women who are subject to RCA—see Box 2 (Rowlands et al. 2022).

Box 2 Standardised Questions for Identification of Cases of RCA

Does your partner support your decisions about when or if you want to become pregnant?

If not pregnant:

Is your partner supportive of your ongoing use of contraception?

If not trying to become pregnant:

Has your partner ever tried to get you pregnant, when you did not want to be pregnant?

Has your partner ever interfered with the contraceptive method you were using?

If already pregnant:

Do you and your partner agree on what you should do about your pregnancy?

Are you worried your partner will hurt you if you do not do what he wants regarding the pregnancy?

If RCA is detected, a range of support may be offered, tailored to the woman's needs at the time. Advice about contraception should take place within the wider context of helping women minimise or escape from situations of domestic violence and abuse. Help with negotiating condom use may be useful. When necessary, concealable methods may be offered, if a woman is unable to escape the abuse at that time. Healthcare professionals can also ensure that women know how to access emergency contraception.

Providers themselves are likely to need training in responding to RCA. There are examples of educational materials on RCA that have been developed for provider and advocate training (Burton and Carlyle 2015; Cappelletti et al. 2014). An educational intervention in sexual and reproductive health clinics, which comprised enhanced screening, assisting the client to access local services and sexual assault resources, combined with tailored harm reduction strategies, such as concealable contraceptive methods, was found to reduce the odds of pregnancy coercion by 71% and to significantly increase the odds of ending a relationship due to perceptions that it was unhealthy (Miller et al. 2011).

The 'Addressing Reproductive Coercion in Health Settings (ARCHES)' intervention study was a cluster randomised controlled trial evaluating the effectiveness of a brief, clinician-delivered universal education and counselling intervention to reduce IPV, RCA and unintended pregnancy compared to standard-of-care in family planning clinic settings (Tancredi et al. 2015). As well as education for healthcare professionals, it supplied palm-sized brochures for clients, which described healthy and unhealthy relationships, and offered information about harm reduction and IPV-related resources. The trial did not show a reduction in RCA or IPV, but participants reported that they had improved knowledge of IPV resources such as a domestic violence hotline and felt more able to enact harm reduction behaviours (Miller et al. 2016).

There is scope for addressing wider cultural gender relationships in schools and a need for the development and evaluation of specific educational materials around reproductive autonomy for students in secondary or tertiary education, as part of relationships and sex education.

Implications for Service Providers and Policymakers

Those working in health and social care specialties relating to women's health, and in general practice, should be aware of RCA. Healthcare professionals should be alert to RCA in consultations with women who are displaying behavioural patterns such as persistent lack of use of contraception (despite not wishing to become pregnant), frequent requests for emergency contraception, frequent attendances for pregnancy testing or STI testing and requests for more than one abortion. Women attending health services with escorts should, at some stage, be seen alone so that these sensitive issues can be raised and, if necessary, explored.

Despite the benefits and acceptability of screening for IPV and abuse, fewer than half of healthcare providers routinely do so (Alvarez et al. 2017). Factors that may motivate healthcare professionals to identify more cases have been described and are complex. They include a greater willingness to screen very young women, or in cases where children are at risk, and motivation to screen where harm has been noted or the provider perceives the woman to be 'at risk'. The experience or perception of being able to make a difference or improve the situation and the importance of routinising such enquiry have also been found to be motivating factors (Burton and Carlyle 2020).

There are now standardised questions for RCA detection (Box 2) and interventions that can assist in reducing its harms. Pathways and mechanisms of referral to other agencies need to be available to staff, as a matter of routine clinical policy, to enable them to respond appropriately if RCA is disclosed. Information may need to be shared with safeguarding agencies, especially with respect to younger women or those who lack mental capacity.

Policy must be underpinned by comprehensive, multi-sectoral and rights-based approaches. Public health policymakers need to take account of RCA as a causative factor in unintended pregnancy. Research findings reinforce the importance of relationships and sex education, including respect for partners and open communication about contraceptive use. Practical advice can focus on strengthening conflict resolution, skill building and awareness.

Future Research

There remains much to be learnt about RCA and NCCR and how they affect women (Fay and Yee 2018; Rowlands and Walker 2019). Qualitative research has given a particularly rich insight into the subject, and more is needed, for example, relating to intent, fear and control (Tarzia and Hegarty 2021). More focus is needed on the non-physical elements of abusive relationships and to survivors' voices, coping methods and resistance strategies. Also, more needs to be understood about whether RCA relates to a particular partner or whether RCA experiences with one partner negatively impact future sexual relationships.

More understanding of perpetrators' motivations for engaging in RCA is needed. Further research should be conducted into the reasons why partners engage in RCA behaviours, as well as women's perceptions of partner intent. Young people are especially vulnerable to RCA, and research is needed which focuses on their dating relationships.

Research is also needed on the effectiveness of primary, secondary and tertiary prevention measures for RCA. So far, there are no robust evaluations of collaborative models of care or referral pathways. As always, in an era of overstretched healthcare professionals working with limited resources, the most efficient and effective means of using routine consultations to identify and reduce the harms of RCA need to be identified and disseminated. Evidence-based guidelines and training are currently lacking (Tarzia et al. 2019).

Summary

- RCA is any deliberate attempt to interfere with a woman's reproductive autonomy—it infringes women's reproductive rights.
- RCA is common but may not be revealed.
- RCA is primarily carried out by intimate partners but is also perpetrated by the wider family.
- RCA may consist of pregnancy pressure, contraceptive sabotage or pregnancy outcome control.
- RCA is associated with poor use of contraception. Past experience of RCA adversely affects women's feelings of agency during sexual and contraceptive interactions.
- Contraceptive sabotage invalidates consent, but its definition as a crime is legally complex, and very few jurisdictions have developed a meaningful approach to prosecuting it.
- Non-consensual condom removal is a type of contraceptive sabotage but is not necessarily related to pregnancy promotion. It is primarily a form of sexual violence, often with disrespect and selfishness underlying it. As a general rule, NCCR is seen in the context of short-term relationships, in contrast to RCA in longer-term relationships.
- Women exposed to RCA may seek out concealable methods of contraception, although they risk possible retaliation if this were to be discovered.
- Few strategies for prevention of RCA have, so far, been developed.
- Professionals working in a range of women's services should be aware of the existence of RCA and equipped to detect it.

References

Alvarez C, Fedock G, Trister K, Campbell J (2017) Provider screening and counseling for intimate partner violence: a systematic review of practices and influencing factors. Trauma Violence Abuse 18(5):479–495. https://doi.org/10.1177/1524838016637080

Borrero S, Nikolajski C, Steinberg JR, Freedman L, Akers AY, Ibrahim S, Schwarz EB (2015) "It just happens": a qualitative study exploring low-income women's perspectives on pregnancy intention and planning. Contraception 91:150–156. https://doi.org/10.1016/j.contraception.2014.09.014

Boyce SC, Uysal J, DeLong SM, Carter N, Undie C, Liambila W, Wendoh S, Silverman JG (2020) Women's and girl's experiences of reproductive coercion and opportunities for intervention in family planning clinics in Nairobi, Kenya: a qualitative study. Reprod Health 17:96. https://doi.org/10.1186/s12978-020-00942-7

Brodsky A (2017) "Rape-adjacent": imagining legal responses to nonconsensual condom removal. Columbia J Gender Law 32:183–210. https://doi.org/10.7916/D8708D06

Burton CW, Carlyle KE (2015) Screening and intervening: evaluating a training program on intimate partner violence and reproductive coercion for family planning and home visiting providers. Fam Community Health 38(3):227–239. https://doi.org/10.1097/fch.0000000000000076

Burton CW, Carlyle KE (2020) Increasing screening for intimate partner violence and reproductive coercion: understanding provider motivations. Violence Against Women 27(11):1913–1929. https://doi.org/10.1177/1077801220969875

Cappelletti M, Gatimu J, Shaw G (2014) Exposing reproductive coercion: a toolkit for awareness raising, assessment, and intervention. FWHC, NCADV, NOMAS. https://www.communitysolutionsva.org/files/RCtoolkit%281%29.pdf

Char A, Saavala M, Kulmala T (2010) Influence of mothers-in-law on young couples' family planning decisions in rural India. Reprod Health Matters 18(35):154–162. https://doi.org/10.1016/S0968-8080(10)35497-8

Chesser B, Zahra A (2019) Stealthing: a criminal offence? Curr Issues Crim Justice 31(2):217–235. https://doi.org/10.1080/10345329.2019.1604474

Criminal Court of Appeal - Vaud Canton (2017) Decision no. 145 of 8 May 2017. www.findinfo-tc.vd.ch

Czechowski K, Courtice EL, Samosh J, Davies J, Shaughnessy K (2019) "That's not what was originally agreed to": perceptions, outcomes, and legal contextualization of non-consensual condom removal in a Canadian sample. PLoS One 14(7):e0219297. https://doi.org/10.1371/journal.pone.0219297

Davis KC (2019) "Stealthing": factors associated with young men's nonconsensual condom removal. Health Psychol 38(11):997–1000. https://doi.org/10.1037/hea0000779

Fay K, Yee L (2018) Reproductive coercion and women's health. J Midwifery Womens Health 63(5):518–525. https://doi.org/10.1111/jmwh.12885

Gupta J, Falb K, Kpebo D, Annan J (2012) Abuse from in-laws and associations with attempts to control reproductive decisions among rural women in Côte d'Ivoire: a cross-sectional study. BJOG 119(9):1058–1066. https://doi.org/10.1111/j.1471-0528.2012.03401

Katz J, Poleshuck EL, Beach B, Olin R (2017) Reproductive coercion by male sexual partners: associations with partner violence and college women's sexual health. J Interpers Violence 32(21):3301–3320. https://doi.org/10.1177/0886260515597441

Kazmerski T, McCauley HL, Jones K, Borrero S, Silverman JG, Decker MR, Tancredi D, Miller E (2015) Use of reproductive and sexual health services among family planning clinic clients exposed to partner violence and reproductive coercion. Matern Child Health J 19(7):1490–1496. https://doi.org/10.1007/s10995-014-1653-2

Kibira SPS, Karp C, Wood SN, Desta S, Galadanci H, Makumbi FE, Omoluabi E, Shiferaw S, Seme A, Tsui A, Moreau C (2020) Covert use of contraception in three sub-Saharan African countries: a qualitative exploration of motivations and challenges. BMC Public Health 20:865. https://doi.org/10.1186/s12889-020-08977-y

Latimer RL, Vodstrcil LA, Fairley CK, Cornelisse VJ, Chow EPF, Read TRH, Bradshaw CS (2019) Non-consensual condom removal, reported by patients at a sexual health clinic in Melbourne, Australia. PLoS One 13(12):e0209779. https://doi.org/10.1371/journal.pone.0209779

Levy-Peck JY (2017) Perpetrators and reproductive coercion. In: McOrmond-Plummer P, Easteal P, Levy-Peck JY (eds) Perpetrators of intimate partner sexual violence, a multidisciplinary approach to. Jessica Kingsley, pp 112–122

McCauley HL, Falb KL, Streich-Tilles T, Kpebo D, Gupta J (2014) Mental health impacts of reproductive coercion among women in Côte d'Ivoire. Int J Gynecol Obstet 127(1):55–59. https://doi.org/10.1016/j.ijgo.2014.04.011

McCloskey LA, Hitchcock S, Eloff I, Dinh P, Masemola K (2020) The role of reproductive coercion in women's risk for HIV: a case-control study of outpatients in Gauteng, South Africa. Int J Gynecol Obstet 151(3):377–382. https://doi.org/10.1002/ijgo.13373

Miller E, Decker MR, McCauley HL, Tancredi DJ, Levenson RR, Waldman J, Schoenwald P, Silverman JG (2011) A family planning clinic partner violence intervention to reduce risk associated with reproductive coercion. Contraception 83(3):274–280. https://doi.org/10.1016/j.contraception.2010.07.013

Miller E, Tancredi DJ, Decker MR, McCauley HL, Jones KA, Anderson H, James L, Silverman JG (2016) A family planning clinic-based intervention to address reproductive coercion: a cluster randomized trial. Contraception 94(1):58–67. https://doi.org/10.1016/j.contraception.2016.02.009

Price E, Sharman LS, Douglas HA, Sheeran N, Dingle GA (2022) Experiences of reproductive coercion in Queensland women. J Interpers Violence 37(5-6):NP2823–NP2843. https://doi.org/10.1177/0886260519846851

Raj A, Sabarwal S, Decker MR, Nair S, Jethva M, Krishnan S, Donta B, Saggurti N, Silverman JG (2011) Abuse from in-laws during pregnancy and post-partum: qualitative and quantitative findings from low-income mothers of infants in Mumbai, India. Matern Child Health J 15(6):700–712. https://doi.org/10.1007/s10995-010-0651-2

Republic of Singapore (2019) Criminal Law Reform Act 2019 s 376H. www.sso.agc.gov.sg/Acts-Supp/15-2019/

Rowlands S, Holdsworth R, Sowemimo A (2022) How to recognise and respond to reproductive coercion. BMJ 378:e069043. https://doi.org/10.1136/bmj-2021-069043

Rowlands S, Walker S (2019) Reproductive control by others: means, perpetrators and effects. BMJ Sex Reprod Health 45(1):61–67. https://doi.org/10.1136/bmjsrh-2018-200156

Silverman JG, Boyce SC, Dehingia N, Rao N, Chandurkar D, Nanda P, Hay K, Atmavilas Y, Saggurti N, Raj A (2019) Reproductive coercion in Uttar Pradesh, India: prevalence and associations with partner violence and reproductive health. SSM Popul Health 9:100484. https://doi.org/10.1016/j.ssmph.2019.100484

Silverman JG, Challa S, Boyce SC, Averbach S, Raj A (2020) Associations of reproductive coercion and intimate partner violence with overt and covert family planning use among married adolescent girls in Niger. EClinicalMedicine 22:100359. https://doi.org/10.1016/j.eclinm.2020.100359

Supreme Court of Canada (2014) R v Hutchinson [2014] 1 SCR 346 (Can). https://scc-csc.lexum.com/scc-csc/scc-csc/en/item/13511/index.do

Sutherland MA, Fantasia HC, Fontenot H (2015) Reproductive coercion and partner violence among college women. JOGNN 44:218–227. https://doi.org/10.1111/1552-6909.12625

Swan LET, Mennicke A, Kim Y (2020) Reproductive coercion and interpersonal violence victimization experiences among college students. J Interpers Violence 36(23-24):11281–11303. https://doi.org/10.1177/0886260519898424

Tancredi DJ, Silverman JG, Decker MR, McCauley HL, Anderson HA, Jones KA, Ciaravino S, Hicks A, Raible C, Zelany S, James L, Miller E (2015) Cluster randomized controlled trial protocol: addressing reproductive coercion in health settings (ARCHES). BMC Womens Health 15:57. https://doi.org/10.1186/s12905-015-0216-z

Tarzia L, Hegarty K (2021) A conceptual re-evaluation of reproductive coercion: centring intent, fear and control. Reprod Health 18:87. https://doi.org/10.1186/s12978-021-01143-6

Tarzia L, Wellington M, Marino J, Hegarty K (2019) How do health practitioners in a large Australian public hospital identify and respond to reproductive abuse? A qualitative study. Aust N Z J Public Health 43(5):457–463. https://doi.org/10.1111/1753-6405.12923

Tarzia L, Srinivasan S, Marion J, Hegarty K (2020) Exploring the gray areas between "stealthing" and reproductive coercion and abuse. Women Health 60(10):1174–1184. https://doi.org/10.1080/03630242.2020.1804517

Tomar S, Dehingia N, Dey AK, Chandurkar D, Raj A, Silverman JG (2020) Associations of intimate partner violence and reproductive coercion with contraceptive use in Uttar Pradesh, India: how associations differ across contraceptive methods. PLoS One 15(10):e0241008. https://doi.org/10.1371/journal.pone.0241008

UK Court of Appeal (2020) R v Lawrance [2020] EWCA Crim 971. https://www.bailii.org/ew/cases/EWCA/Crim/2020/971.html

Willie TC, Callands TA (2018) Reproductive coercion and prenatal distress among young pregnant women in Monrovia, Liberia. Health Care Women Int 39(9):968–974. https://doi.org/10.1080/07399332.2018.1490740

Willie TC, Alexander KA, Caplon A, Kershaw TS, Safon CB, Galvao RW, Kaplan C, Caldwell A, Calabrese SK (2021) Birth control sabotage as a correlate of women's sexual health risk: an exploratory study. Womens Health Issues 31(2):157–163. https://doi.org/10.1016/j.whi.2020.10.003

Sam Rowlands, LLM, MD, FRCGP, FFSRH is a Visiting Professor at Bournemouth University. He has researched and published widely on emergency contraception, long-acting reversible contraception, abortion, sterilisation, reproductive ethics and medicolegal issues.

Susan Walker, PhD is an Associate Professor of Contraception, Sexual and Reproductive Health at Anglia Ruskin University. Her research areas include contraceptive and reproductive health behaviour with an interest in health inequalities, and the effect of gender and sexuality on health behaviour.

Workplace Harassment

Chris Waugh

Learning Objectives
Having read this chapter, you should be able to understand:

- Key terms in the study of workplace harassment and some of the consequences of workplace harassment for individuals and organisations.
- Theoretical ideas about the causes and impacts of workplace harassment.
- The legal framework around workplace harassment in the UK.

Introduction

The purpose of this chapter is to introduce the concept of workplace harassment; it draws on both legal and sociological work in order to do so. The following sections will help you understand some of the key terms and language used around workplace harassment and the impacts of workplace harassment and consider which demographics are most likely to be at risk of harassment in the workplaces. Thereafter, an overview of the history of workplace harassment (that is, how we came to understand it as a social phenomenon) is provided followed by an exploration of some of the theoretical frameworks for understanding and explaining how

C. Waugh (✉)
Department of Sociology, The University of Manchester, Manchester, UK

Department of Strategy, Enterprise and Sustainability, Manchester Metropolitan University, Manchester, UK

University of Law, Manchester, UK
e-mail: chris.waugh-2@manchester.ac.uk

P. Ali, M. M. Rogers (eds.), *Gender-Based Violence: A Comprehensive Guide*,
https://doi.org/10.1007/978-3-031-05640-6_33

and why workplace harassment occurs. Lastly, existing laws around harassment in the UK are discussed. Several case studies are presented to illustrate some of the theoretical, sociological, and political concepts.

Defining and Explaining Workplace Harassment

The term 'workplace harassment' is commonly used in journalistic, professional, and academic writing; however, trying to pin down a concrete definition is harder than it would initially seem. This is in large part because there is no one definitive definition of workplace harassment (Ehrenreich 1999). In many cases, especially in media discussions, workplace harassment is a term often used to refer to sexual harassment or unwanted sexual attention in the workplace—this conflation of the two is, perhaps, more prevalent in recent years due to the cultural and social impact of the #MeToo movement, though as demonstrated in the following section, much academic attention has been given to sexual harassment in the workplace. However, while sexual harassment is a form of workplace harassment, workplace harassment itself is a much broader phenomenon, and some studies suggest that non-sexual forms of workplace harassment are more common than sexual harassment (Richman et al. 1999).

There are a few things to note before reading further—many of the examples and laws discussed in this chapter originate from the UK since this is the framework most familiar to the author. To fully cover the nuances of laws and policies around workplace harassment around the world would be beyond the scope of this chapter. Additionally, while much of the harassment discussed in this chapter will relate to sex and gender (as befits the overall volume in which this chapter is situated), it will be situated in a broader understanding that harassment can occur which does not have a direct connection to sex or gender; equally, this chapter will try to highlight how workplace harassment affects men, women, and transgender people in the examples it provides.

Understanding the Key Terms

If you read any academic text, article, or even a news article about workplace harassment, you will immediately notice that a lot of the terminology within the topic is used interchangeably. Terms like 'harassment', 'bullying', and 'mobbing' will often appear in accounts of inappropriate behaviour in the workplace, but it is important to understand that there are subtle differences between all of these concepts, both in terms of their definitions, but also, importantly, in terms of the legal implications of each action or set of actions.

Bullying refers to an act, or series of acts, which can be perpetrated by an individual or group of individuals, which intimidates, dominates, or threatens the victim (Juvonen and Graham 2014). Bullying is most commonly understood as a phenomenon in school children, though there has been a lot of work done on bullying in the workplace. A few key features of 'bullying' are important to bear in mind: firstly, 'bullying' implies a direct and vicious intent to harm—as discussed below, this can cause difficulties with dealing with workplace harassment as malicious intent can be tricky to prove. As Einarsen notes, only a perpetrator can verify their intent, and intentions can change throughout a series of actions (Zapf and Einarsen 2001). Secondly, bullying tends to be seen as an individualised phenomenon—while the reasons for bullying may link to concepts of structural oppressions (i.e. racism, sexism, homophobia, etc.) bullying implies that harmful actions are conducted by individuals or small groups of individuals, rather than tied to institutional practises (Besag 1989). It is, however, worth nuancing this claim slightly, as there is a concept called 'bullying culture' which is explored more in Case study 1.

Mobbing overlaps with bullying to an extent; put simply, mobbing refers to the bullying of an individual by a group, be that in a school environment, a family, or a workplace. Originating from studies of animal behaviour (Lorenz 2002), it has been used in the context of the workplace to describe situations where an individual is 'ganged up on' by other employees/their employers (Leymann 1996). Mobbing comes with the clear implication of a kind of mindless, animalistic aggression, a collective burst of violence or will to harm. Some theorists argue that this suggests a total *lack* of intention, which, again, provides difficulties in trying to tackle workplace harassment (Davenport et al. 1999).

Harassment is a rather nebulous concept, and there is no one set definition of harassment. As feminist theorist Catharine Mackinnon (speaking specifically of sexual harassment) remarked in 1979, 'it is not surprising…that women would not complain of an experience for which there has been no name' (MacKinnon 1979, p. 27). Within the UK, harassment is broadly defined as when 'someone behaves in a way which makes you feel distressed, humiliated or threatened'; this behaviour can be from someone you know or a total stranger (Bureau 2021). A slightly more concrete definition of workplace harassment, from the non-governmental public body Advisory, Conciliation and Arbitration Service (ACAS), goes as follows:

> [Harassment is] …Spreading malicious rumours, exclusion or victimisation, unfair treatment, overbearing supervision, misuse of power and position, unwelcome sexual advances, making threats and comments about job security without foundation, deliberately undermining a competent worker, preventing individuals from progressing by intentionally blocking promotion or training opportunities. (Leaver 2019)

Harassment is often seen as a sustained series of actions or conduct and can include online as well as offline conduct. Harassment in the UK is most commonly associated with the targeting of someone with 'protected characteristics' under the Equality Act 2010, yet overall harassment remains something of a vague term, as we will discuss in more detail in the section on Workplace Harassment and the Law.

There are a few unifying features of these various terms—firstly, there is a power imbalance between the perpetrator and victim (Juvonen and Graham 2014). However, the exact nature of that power imbalance can be difficult to pin down. As

Leaver, and others, argue, most legalistic and academic frameworks for understanding workplace harassment tend to focus on the individual dynamic between the harasser and the harassed, without always tying said harassment to structural oppressions such as sexism, racism, and so on (Leaver 2019).

> **Alternative Terminology: Workplace Harassment**
> Bullying, mobbing, bashing, hounding, intimidation, persecution, bullying culture, workplace abuse, workplace molestation, workplace aggression, workplace mistreatment, discrimination at work.

Impacts of Workplace Bullying

It will come as little surprise that workplace bullying and harassment have profoundly negative impacts on the victims. Workplace bullying and harassment can affect the victim's mental health, resulting in depression, anxiety, and in some cases, post-traumatic stress disorder or suicide (Bartlett and Bartlett 2011). Victims can also suffer significant physical health impacts, including cardiovascular disease, weight gain, and a decline in overall physical health (Johnson and Rea 2009). In addition, victims are more likely to develop issues around alcohol and drug misuse as a coping mechanism, sleep disruption, and high use of sleep medication (Yildiz 2007). Furthermore, existing physical and mental health conditions increase the risk that an individual will be subject to workplace bullying or harassment (Nielsen et al. 2014). As well as the health impacts, victims of workplace bullying/harassment can suffer negative career prospects, such as absenteeism or quitting work, which can have an impact on future employability (Gardner and Johnson 2001; Yildiz 2007).

Conversely, it remains the case that despite legal and policy frameworks (which are discussed in more detail below), the perpetrators of workplace harassment rarely lose their jobs (Glambek et al. 2016). Especially around sexual harassment, there exists a culture of silencing, whereby victims often feel unable to speak out for fear of losing their jobs—a 2018 survey of 4000 women found that 16% had experienced sexual harassment but not reported it due to fear of being sacked or having hours reduced (Trust 2018). According to a 2017 report, in France individuals who made a complaint of sexual harassment at work were either reprimanded or fired in 40% of cases (Rubin 2017). More broadly, many workplaces require the signing of non-disclosure agreements as a condition of employment (despite this practice being illegal in the UK, USA, and most of Europe), which makes complaints of workplace harassment, especially sexual harassment, difficult or impossible for the victims. While some high-profile perpetrators of sexual harassment have lost their jobs, more often than not, perpetrators of harassment will face lesser penalties—see the Avital Ronel case study later in this chapter for an example.

Workplace bullying/harassment can have considerable consequences for the organisation, as well as the individual. Consequences can include missed deadlines, lower morale among staff, a breakdown in relationships between supervisors and peers, and if allegations become public, potential loss of reputation with customer bases and clients (Bartlett and Bartlett 2011) or even the collapse of the organisation. Notably, the online content service UNILAD suffered a major crisis after considerable evidence of historic misconduct on the part of managers against employees (including, but not limited to, sexual harassment) was made public, leading to a loss of advert revenue, a sharp decline in readership, and eventual collapse into administration (Kale 2020). Even if allegations of workplace bullying/harassment do not result in the collapse of a company, it can result in damning and often fatal consequences (see Box 1).

Box 1 The Francis Report

Case study #1—the Francis Report

The 2013 Francis Report exposed serious concerns about workplace culture and bullying within the National Health Service in the UK (Francis 2013). Focussing on Stafford Hospital, the report noted the shocking figure of between 400 and 1200 unnecessary patient deaths between 2005 and 2008. The report attributed this state of affairs to two factors: firstly, a preoccupation among management with national targets at the expense of quality of care (Leaver 2019), and secondly, a 'culture of secrecy, where problems in maintaining the quality of patient care were caused by front-line staff working within an "endemic culture of bullying"' (Francis 2013). Staff members would be bullied into remaining silent about the diminishing quality of care, for fear of being victimised if they spoke up. The report went on to conclude that the culture within Stafford Hospital was mirrored in other areas of the NHS (Francis 2013).

Three important points can be drawn from this case study: first, that workplace cultures that sustain harassment can have real, and often tragic, impacts on service delivery for an organisation; second, that harassment can arise without direct malice aimed at the victims of that harassment (the Francis Report notes that the management of Stafford Hospital did not intend to harm patients or staff, instead believing their actions were helping the hospital fit statistical and target-based goals); and, third, that both workplace bullying and workplace harassment are systemic issues, rather than simply being the malicious action of an individual or group of individuals against a worker or group of workers.

Who Are the Targets of Workplace Harassment?

In theory, anyone can be subject to harassment in the workplace, regardless of age, religion, gender, sexuality, etc. However, statistical evidence suggests that certain groups are more likely to be targeted within the workplace than others. Data from

2019 suggests that 54% of women experience sexual harassment in the workplace, ranging from inappropriate comments and messages to unwanted touching and pressuring into sexual favours, with a further 20% reporting that the harassment was perpetrated by a manager or senior colleague (Government Equalities Office 2019). According to the trade union Unison, some 50% of transgender people have reported harassment at work (Unison 2019). While the majority of those affected by sexual harassment identify as women, this is by no means to suggest that men are not victims of such harassment. A 2018 survey by the BBC found that 20% of men in the workforce had experienced some form of sexual harassment, ranging from inappropriate comments to sexual assaults; the same survey found that 79% of those men had not reported their experiences of harassment due to shame, fear of ridicule, or that aspersions would be cast on their masculinity (Charles 2018). Indeed, some researchers have argued that men who oppose other men's sexual harassment can sometimes become the targets of sexual harassment themselves (Holland et al. 2016). Again, this suggests that the current understanding of sexual harassment among working people tends to be closely tied to power dynamics around gender.

Workplace Harassment: A Brief History

The following section provides a history of the concept of workplace harassment in both academic and legal literature. It is meant to provide an overview, rather than a comprehensive summary, and it is worth remembering that this draws on literature and law predominantly from the Anglosphere (i.e. the English-speaking and developed world). The need for further analysis of definitions and understandings of workplace harassment from outside of this sphere is apparent.

The concept of 'bullying' or 'mobbing' (as it is sometimes referred to) within organisations finds its roots in work on bullying in schools conducted in schools in Scandinavia (Olweus 1987). Though this research was in schools, academics involved in organisational studies noted its implications for improper conduct in the workplace (Zapf and Einarsen 2001). However, before this, there was a growing acknowledgement of the issue of harassment within feminist theory (which is discussed in more detail below). Feminist legal scholar Catherine Mackinnon was among the first to draw on legal and theoretical frameworks to discuss the concept of sexual harassment of women in the workplace (MacKinnon 1979). Around the same time, Brodsky's *The Harassed Worker* defined five distinct kinds of harassment—sexual harassment, name-calling, work pressure, physical abuse, and scapegoating (Brodsky 1976). While Brodsky's work offered a more nuanced and detailed take on workplace harassment, it was largely overlooked until the 2000s, and as a result, early work on workplace harassment was somewhat disjointed.

However, within the UK, there was a growing awareness of the problem. Crawford and Adams's book, *Bullying in the Workplace* (which was subsequently followed by a popular BBC Radio 4 programme) proved pivotal in drawing more public attention to the prevalence of the problem (Adams 2014; Zapf and Einarsen 2001). The popularity of the book and radio show led to developments in the law—while racial and sexual discrimination was already illegal, harassment became illegal under the Protection from Harassment Act 1997, following the Disability Discrimination Act of 1995. At the time of writing, the current UK government framework for dealing with workplace harassment is enshrined in the Equality Act 2010—discussed in more detail below.

This brief history highlights a few key points; first, that academic, and often activist, literature has been a driving force for legal changes in the UK—it is a 'bottom-up' rather than 'top-down' approach to legislation. This is especially true for sexual harassment, as Wise and Stanley note, there was: 'no mention of any such animal as "sexual harassment" in the English press, certainly none that we could find, before the reporting of American sexual harassment cases and the review of feminist and feminist-influenced books on the subject at the end of 1979'. (Wise and Stanley 1987, p. 30). Secondly, while legal frameworks exist, cultural and theoretical understandings of workplace harassment have pointed towards some gaps in existing laws.

One such gap is the concept of a 'bullying culture' (Leaver 2019)—this can refer to the idea that within certain workplaces, there exists a culture that either directly encourages, or turns a blind eye to, the harassment of certain workers or certain groups of workers (Williams 2011). In part, this is due to how research (and, to an extent, law) has focussed on the problem and its impacts, the individual harasser and the harassed, at the expense of developing a conceptual framework for understanding workplace harassment as a social phenomenon (Keashly and Harvey 2005). As a result, this might explain the limited ability of the law, policy, and academia to respond to examples of systemic or structural workplace harassment (See Box 2).

Case study #2: #MeToo and its consequences.

The #MeToo movement is one of the most prolific and recognisable social movements in recent times, seeking to draw attention to sexual harassment—many of which take place in work environments. The term 'MeToo' originates from a 2006 blog post by activist and sexual assault survivor Tarana Burke (Ohlheiser 2017), though it came to more public attention via allegations of sexual abuse of actresses by former Hollywood producer Harvey Weinstein in 2017 around what was called quid pro quo harassment (i.e. the exchanging of sexual favours for job security or advancement) and in particular from an October 2017 tweet by Alyssa Milano concerning Weinstein's behaviour (Milano 2017). The trend spread virally on social media and led to a number of high profile firings in Hollywood and eventual criminal convictions against Weinstein (Pierson 2020). Though the majority of accusers were women, some high-profile men also used the movement to highlight their own experiences of sexual harassment at work, notably *Brooklyn 99* actor Terry Crews. While much media attention focussed on #MeToo in the film industry, and within the United States, the movement had profound impacts internationally (see (Green 2021) and in other sectors, including with churches, schools and universities, the military, and government (Hillstrom 2018). While some countries made small legal reforms in response to the movement (Caldwell 2018), the MeToo movement had mixed impacts on general workplace culture, with 58% of American workers surveyed by SurveyMonkey reporting that they did not feel that the movement had improved their workplace, even though 24% of respondents felt that their workplace could have a 'MeToo' situation (Gitlin 2018). This is indicative of some of the criticisms of MeToo [footnote], namely, that the movement's overall goals are not clear and as a result do not have consistent legal or policy aims (Wilhelm 2017). Equally, the movement has been accused of ignoring the risks of sexual harassment for certain demographics of worker, specifically workers in the sex industry (Thrasher 2019).

Power, Privilege, and Posturing: Theories of Workplace Harassment

Thus far, this chapter has explored what workplace harassment is, what its consequences are, and how our understanding of the concept has developed in both legal and academic terms. However, one key question remains: *why* are people harassed at work?

There are various theoretical models of workplace harassment, and a detailed definition of all of these would be outside of the scope of this chapter. What follows is a very brief overview of the major trends in research into workplace harassment up to the present. Subsequently, this chapter will focus on two major frameworks that are most relevant to current discussions around workplace harassment: feminist frameworks and Michel Foucault's work around power and its relationship to knowledge.

Feminist approaches to workplace harassment have largely focused on understandings of sexual harassment and harassment related to gender and have had considerable impacts on modern academic and organisational understandings of the topic. As Wise and Stanley note, the very term 'sexual harassment' had no real use in the English language before early feminist work on the subject in the 1970s (Wise and Stanley 1987). Feminist frameworks on workplace harassment tried to shift the focus away from the idea that harassment is in any sense a one-off, individualised set of actions, but needs to be seen in the light of patriarchy and patriarchal power structures (Wood 1994). Gutek explains the harassment of women in the workplace as the result of when the patriarchal idea of women as a sex object spills over into the workplace (Gutek 1985). In other words, ideas about women's value, informed by patriarchal culture, lead to women being harassed at work, especially, as Gutek (1985) argues, if a role normally occupied by a man is occupied by a woman, thus making her gender more noticeable. Other feminist writers, such as Paglia, argue that harassment is driven by an innate issue with male sexual desire, which is always 'hunting and scanning….Everywhere the beautiful woman is scrutinized and harassed' (Paglia 1992).

Feminist theorising has informed organisational studies into harassment as well—Hearn and Parkin, for example, argue that sexuality pervades the workplace, impacting the roles individuals hold, the relationships between employees, and how they communicate with one another. They write that 'Organizations construct sexuality and yet contradictorily sexuality constructs organizations' (Hearn and Parkin 1987, p. 3). In this sense, harassment can occur as an extension of human sexuality under patriarchy, but also because organisations enable the perpetuation of normative gender and power relations, thus employees can be harassed for sexual favours, etc. Cockburn, in her study of three workplaces, argues that harassment arises from a patriarchal backlash against efforts to get more women into the workplace, similar to how women would often be excluded or sidelined from networking and social events in bigger organisations; as a result 'heterosexual and sexist culture generated by men within the workplace…this culture includes women but marginalizes and controls them' (Cockburn 2018, p. 142).

Key Concept: Patriarchy

Patriarchy refers to a social system where men hold a disproportionate amount of power and occupy the majority of positions of intellectual, political, and social influence. As a result of this, men tend to have power over women and have access to certain privileges that women cannot.

What unites these various feminist approaches is the appreciation of power dynamics within workplaces under patriarchy. As Mackinnon writes: 'The way the sexual subordination of women interacts with other forms of social power men have can now be more precisely delineated. Economic power is to sexual harassment as physical force is to rape' (MacKinnon 1979, p. 217). At this stage, it is worth trying to pin down a more precise understanding of the meaning of power. A simplistic understanding of power would be that a person (A) has the power over another person (B) to the extent that A can get B to do something that B would otherwise not do out of their own free choice (Dahl 1957). In this sense, power is something that can be gained by an individual and wielded like a tool or a weapon against another person.

For French philosopher Michel Foucault, this understanding of power was far too limited and only really tried to explain how power functioned on the micro-level—that is, how power might function between two individuals. It failed to address how power worked on the macro-level (i.e. at the level of institutions and national policy) and what later theorists have called the meso-level (i.e. within the workplace) (Messner 2009). According to Foucault, power is also not the homogeneous domination of one person, group, or class over another. Power circulates; it is discontinuous and uneven. The individual, says Foucault, is, in fact, an effect of power, rather than either the starting point or something that is dominated by power (Foucault 1980).

According to Foucault, not only is power nebulous, and fluid, but there are multiple different forms of power. In *Discipline and Punish*, Foucault maps out the development of various forms of power over the ages. In older forms of society, power mainly took the form of spectacle power—grand, public shows of strength or might, which Foucault calls 'sovereign power'. However, as society progressed, and capitalism developed, a new form of power emerged, which Foucault called 'disciplinary power'. Using the transition from the spectacle of public executions to the heavily regimented lives of prisoners as his example, Foucault argues that discipline—the intense monitoring and regulation of activities, spaces, behaviours, and so on—coerced the bodies of individuals and divorced power from the body, turning that individual into a relation of strict subjugation (Foucault 2012). In simple terms, when an individual finds themselves within an institution with strict regulation (such as a prison, a school, or a workplace), they are either encouraged or coerced into becoming compliant—they become what Foucault calls 'docile bodies', ideal productive and compliant units.

As Leaver puts it, disciplinary power functions when 'institutions are rigidly organised, to encourage workers to be separated from each other rather than form together as a collective' (Leaver 2019, p. 27). It is important to understand that this form of power does not rely so much on laws as it does on normalisation and also on surveillance. In modern society, we are not always under literal surveillance (though there are many workplaces where literal surveillance is very prominent, such as call centres), but we fear that we *might* be under surveillance at any given moment—in the same way as the prisoner in the Panopticon fear that they *might* be being watched by the guards and thus will behave themselves. The individual internalises the idea that they are under surveillance and thus engages in a process of self-regulation—and becomes a docile body. Importantly, this functioning of power fitted within a regime of discourse, a historically contingent social system that produces knowledge and meaning. Dominant discourses produce regimes of truth that regulate how and why people are classified and controlled. Those whose behaviour falls outside of the acceptable boundaries of behaviour are subjected to a process of othering, perceived as deviant and, more often than not, ostracised (Fahie 2014).

Foucault's work, and his understanding of power, can provide a useful framework for understanding workplace harassment. Leaver has drawn on Foucault's understanding of power to explore and explain bullying within the NHS (Leaver 2019); in her study, she identifies how women of colour became targets for harassment due to their visibility within the organisation, echoing Foucault's sentiment that 'discipline and the control of the subject could be pursued through compulsory visibility on its subjects' (Foucault 2012, p. 778). Fahie, in their analysis of workplace harassment within school settings, draws on Foucault to explain how bullying and harassment can involve creating discourses around the victim—that they are a 'troublemaker' or 'lazy', for example; such discourses come with expectations of (a) how the employee will behave (even if this is based on a prejudice) and (b) justifies a process of othering and ostracism (Fahie 2014). Seen through a Foucauldian lens, workplace harassment can also be seen as a mean of enforcing the 'docility' or productivity of workers—where a worker might be seen to not being sufficiently docile (say, for example, as a female worker who takes time off for caring responsibilities or a Muslim employee who requests time to pray during Ramadan), this becomes more visible; they defy a dominant discourse and become subjected to harassment and ostracism if they do not conform.

Another use of Foucault for the study of workplace harassment is that he offers a framework for critiquing how we think and gain knowledge about workplace harassment. Since Foucault argues that we are subject to, and made by, discourse, we are also complicit in reproducing discourse and the expectations that come with it. Put simply, we reproduce various discourses (and the knowledge and expected behaviours connected to them) as if they are true because we believe them to be true. The job of intellectuals, according to Foucault, is not to reveal the truth, but to challenge established truth and critically consider what aspects of it might connect to power and assumption (Foucault 1980; Foucault 1982). Some academics, such as Brewis, draw on Foucault, to argue that a prevailing attitude in feminist work on sexual harassment suggests that thinkers such as Mackinnon claimed to have 'revealed' the truth about gender roles in the workplace to the world and that sexual harassment, in particular, is a form of 'bad' sex based on an abuse of power, distinct from 'good' sex which is based on mutual attraction (Brewis 2001). Such an attitude also ties the roles of victim and perpetrator to specific genders (man = perpetrator, woman = victim); while this is often the case, it means that when a case arises that conflicts with this knowledge, our responses can often be messy and incoherent, as we will see in the case study below:

Case Study Three: Avital Ronnell

Avital Ronnell, a highly respect American academic in the humanities, was accused by Nimrod Reitman (one of her former PhD students) of sexual harassment in 2018. Reitman's claim alleged that Professor Ronnell had subjected him to sexual harassment over a period of 3 years, including inappropriate touching and name calling to abusing her power as his advisor (Greenberg 2018).

The case provoked fervent debate about gender, power, and harassment in the higher education sector. Liu and Bailey argued that Ronnell's action were enabled by power she wielded as a 'theory star' within the humanities (Liu and Bailey 2018), while others highlighted the prevalence of sexual harassment within universities, with data from 2018 suggesting that 89% of harassers, and Ronnell belonged to the 5% of female harassers (Pitchford et al. 2020). Perhaps the most controversial response was a draft letter—signed by prominent 'celebrity' academics such as Judith Butler and Slavoj Zizek—alleged that the allegations against Ronnell were 'malicious intention' and not actual evidence (despite the fact that the signatories had not seen the 'confidential dossier' of evidence presented to NYU) (Leiter 2018).

The case raises complex questions about workplace harassment in academia—both in terms of defining harassment (both Ronnell and her defenders argued that her conduct fitted in with the dynamics of 'a penchant for florid and campy communications arising from our common academic backgrounds and sensibilities' (Greenberg 2018)) and a departure from 'traditional' power dynamics in circumstances of sexual harassment (the female the aggressor, the male the victim, and both parties identifying as gay)—and also raises questions about the ability, or inability, to achieve justice in matters of sexual harassment (Gessen 2018).

Workplace Harassment and the Law in the UK

Broadly, the UK Government defines workplace harassment as 'behaviour that makes someone feel intimidated or offended' within the workplace; within the UK, harassment is illegal under the Equality Act 2010, if such harassment relates to what UK law defines as 'protected characteristics' of an individual, that is, age, sex, disability, gender reassignment, marriage and civil partnership, pregnancy and maternity, race, religion or belief, and sexual orientation (Government 2021).

Within the UK, behaviour that can be perceived as harassment is regulated under several acts of parliament. The 1997 Protection from Harassment Act prohibits conduct and behaviour which amounts to the harassment of another and where the individual concerned knows or should know that their behaviour constitutes harassment. This covers physical actions and verbal and non-verbal actions (Government 1997). UK Legislation was expanded by the Equality Act 2010, which outlined the protected characteristics mentioned above.

One immediate element that is apparent in UK harassment law is that it is broad and laws do not explicitly forbid explicit forms of harassment. For example, sexual harassment is not formally against UK Law; a UK court would instead interpret sexual harassment as breaching the Equality Act, as it constitutes an individual being treated negatively because of their sex (Clarke 2007). While this broadness of existing law, in theory, makes legislation adaptable, it can raise some issues. For instance, the above way of understanding sexual harassment equates 'sex' with 'sexual'—that is to say, it presumes a sexual element in sex discrimination. As Franke argues, this results in courts sometimes focussing on the sexual elements of a case (i.e. was there evidence that the perpetrator was sexually attracted to the victim) at the expense of the sex discrimination element (i.e. was the perpetrators harassing behaviour motivated by wanting to subjugate the victim because of their sex or sexuality) (Franke 1997). As such, potential power dynamics and patterns of discrimination can, potentially, be overlooked, and a perpetrator could potentially avoid consequences by claiming that there was a lack of sexual desire underpinning their actions. This vagueness as well, it could be argued, raises for employers a concern that the presence of sexual expression can open a company to risk of enable sexual harassment; as Schultz puts it, 'if the presence of sex is a problem, then one way to deal with it is to segregate "the sexes"' (Schultz 2003, p.2134). As a result, some companies can engage in a process of informal segregation of sexes in the workplace, which prevents women (and other minorities) from achieving equity in work (Clarke 2007).[1]

Similarly, other elements of vagueness in the law present challenges for both UK workers and UK employers. This is particularly prescient for the rights of transgender workers. According to research conducted by Crossland Solicitors, around 74% of employers claim to have never knowingly worked with a transgender person, suggesting that many transgender workers will conceal their gender identity from their employer. Similarly, 23% of employers were unaware of laws that protected transgender workers; in part, this could be a result of the ambiguity of the Equality Act, which prohibits discrimination on grounds of gender reassignment—thus implying (falsely) that only transgender workers who have gone through gender reassignment surgery are protected (Solictors 2018). It is worth remembering that while the aforementioned legislation does put a duty on employers to safeguard the rights of employees with protected characteristics, this does not often equate to workplace policies to achieve those aims being put into place. Only 12% of UK workplaces reported having a specific policy around transgender rights in the workplace, and in certain UK sectors, such as the tech sector, only 7% of employers reported having such policies (Ibid). This is not just a matter of concern for transgender individuals, as many workplaces, especially universities, tend to opt towards catch-all policies such as Dignity at Work, rather than specific policies to tackle expressions of harassment.[2] This raises the question of how effective any macro-level anti-harassment legislation can be if there is an absence of policies that empower workers at the meso-level. The building of a strong workers' rights or trade union presence, along with collaborative approaches by management, could go some way towards addressing these issues (Carbo 2009).

Summary

- While there is a history of work that has tried to explain and understand the causes of workplace harassment, it remains a real and lived phenomena for many individuals and groups within the workforce—and, more often than not, the existence of workplace harassment links to existing hierarchies of oppression around gender.

[1]Here, it's worth thinking back to where we discussed Foucault earlier—the various practises outlined here are based upon a kind of discourse around sex and the expectations that are attached to that discourse. You may find it peculiar that sexual harassment laws presume that there is an element of sexual desire on the part of the perpetrator, but that is built on a kind of 'knowledge' (to use Foucault's language) about sex and the way that humans relate to one another sexually. Of course, it is possible to argue that this is not knowledge as much as an assumption—however, according to Foucault, because that assumption is seen as true it is treated as true.

[2]For example, my alma mater, Cambridge University, did not bring in specific policies against sexual harassment until 2018.

- The same, equally, could be said about race, disability, religion, and so on. However, when we think about gender harassment, it's important to remember that men can also be the victims of harassment as well as the perpetrators.
- Harassment can often be understood as the actions of one individual against another, enabled by a power imbalance in the workplace, but in many cases, workplace harassment can be systemic and enabled by a culture of bullying and silencing.
- Legal frameworks do exist to protect the victims of harassment and (in theory at least) prevent it in the first place, but there are considerable gaps and disconnects, especially between laws and workplace policies.
- While theoretical work has gone some way towards explaining how and why people are harassed at work, such work has also highlighted as much that we don't know about workplace harassment, as much as what we do.

References

Adams A (2014) Bullying at work: how to confront and overcome it. Virago, London

Bartlett JE, Bartlett ME (2011) Workplace bullying: an integrative literature review. Adv Dev Hum Resour 13(1):69–84

Besag VE (1989) Bullies and victims in schools. A guide to understanding and management

Brewis J (2001) Foucault, politics and organizations:(re)-constructing sexual harassment. Gender Work Organization 8(1):37–60

Brodsky CM (1976) The harassed worker. DC Heath & Co

Bureau CA (2021) Taking action about harassment. https://www.citizensadvice.org.uk/law-and-courts/discrimination/taking-action-about-discrimination/taking-action-about-harassment/. Accessed 1 May

Caldwell LA (2018) House unveils landmark sexual harassment overhaul bill. https://www.nbcnews.com/politics/congress/house-unveils-landmark-sexual-harassment-overhaul-bill-n838436. Accessed 12 May

Carbo J (2009) The right to dignity at work: critical management studies and corporate social responsibility insights into workplace bullying

Charles K (2018) Sexual harassment: remember that men can be victims too. https://www.personneltoday.com/hr/sexual-harassment-remember-that-men-can-be-victims-too/. Accessed 12 May

Clarke L (2007) Sexual harassment law in the United States, the United Kingdom and the European Union: discriminatory wrongs and dignitary harms. Common Law World Rev 36(2):79–105

Cockburn C (2018) In the way of women. Cornell University Press

Dahl RA (1957) The concept of power. Behav Sci 2(3):201–215

Davenport N, Schwartz RD and Elliott GP (1999) Mobbing: emotional abuse in the American workplace. Civil Society Pub

Ehrenreich R (1999) Dignity and discrimination: toward a pluralistic understanding of workplace harassment. Geo LJ 88:1

Fahie D (2014) Blackboard bullies: workplace bullying in primary schools. Irish Educ Stud 33(4):435–450

Foucault M (1980) Power/knowledge: selected interviews and other writings, 1972–1977. Vintage, New York

Foucault M (1982) The subject and power. Crit Inquiry 8(4):777–795

Foucault M (2012) Discipline and punish: the birth of the prison. Vintage, New York

Francis R (2013) Report of the mid Staffordshire NHS foundation trust public inquiry: executive summary. The Stationery Office
Franke KM (1997) What's wrong with sexual harassment? Stanford Law Rev, pp 691–772
Gardner S, Johnson PR (2001) The leaner, meaner workplace: strategies for handling bullies at work. Employ Relat Today 28(2):23
Gitlin J (2018) Study: Me Too Movement and its influence on work culture. Reportno. Report Number|, Date. Place Published|: Institution|
Glambek M, Skogstad A, Einarsen S (2016) Do the bullies survive? A five-year, three-wave prospective study of indicators of expulsion in working life among perpetrators of workplace bullying. Ind Health 54(1):68–73
Government U (1997) Protection from harassment act. In: Parliament U (ed)
Government U (2021) Workplace bullying and harassment. https://www.gov.uk/workplace-bullying-and-harassment. Accessed 16 Mar
Government Equalities Office (2019). Consultation on sexual harassment in the workplace: government response. C. Office. Online HM Government
Green EB (2021) The global impact of #MeToo movement. Lexology
Greenberg Z (2018) 'What happens to# MeToo when a feminist is the accused?' New York Times, 13
Gutek BA (1985) Sex and the workplace. Jossey-Bass, San Francisco, CA
Hearn J, Parkin W (1987) Sex at work: the power and paradox of organisation sexuality. Macmillan St Martin's Press, New York
Hillstrom LC (2018) The# metoo movement. ABC-CLIO
Holland KJ, Rabelo VC, Gustafson AM et al (2016) Sexual harassment against men: examining the roles of feminist activism, sexuality, and organizational context. Psychol Men Masculinity 17(1):17
Johnson SL, Rea RE (2009) Workplace bullying: concerns for nurse leaders. J Nurs Adm 39(2):84–90
Juvonen J, Graham S (2014) Bullying in schools: the power of bullies and the plight of victims. Annu Rev Psychol 65:159–185
Kale S (2020) The spectacular rise and fall of Unilad. https://www.vice.com/en/article/jgejag/unilad-vs-ladbible-online-publishing. Accessed 20 Apr
Keashly L and Harvey S (2005) Emotional abuse in the workplace
Leaver N (2019) Power and resistance: a Foucauldian analysis of workplace bullying and harassment in the National Health Service. University of Manchester
Leymann H (1996) The content and development of mobbing at work. Eur J Work Organ Psy 5(2):165–184
Leiter B (2018) 'Blaming the victim is apparently ok when the accused in a title ix proceeding is a feminist literary theorist' Leiter Reports, 10
Liu C, Bailey D (2018) 'The apprentice in theory: Fan, student, star' Los Angeles Review of Books. Available at: https://lareviewofbooks.org/article/the-apprentice-in-theory-fan-student-star/ (Accessed: April 19th 2021)
Lorenz K (2002) On aggression. Psychology Press
MacKinnon CA (1979) Sexual harassment of working women: a case of sex discrimination. Yale University Press
Messner M (2009) It's all for the kids: gender, families, and youth sports. University of California Press
Milano A (2017) If you've been sexually harassed or assaulted write 'me too' as a reply to this tweet. In: @Alyssa_Milano (ed). Twitter
Nielsen MB, Magerøy N, Gjerstad J et al (2014) Workplace bullying and subsequent health problems. Tidsskr Nor Laegeforen 134(12–13):1233–1238
Ohlheiser A (2017) The woman behind 'me too' knew the power of the phrase when she created it — 10 years ago. *The Washington post*, October 19th 2017
Olweus D (1987) Bully/victim problems among schoolchildren in Scandinavia

Paglia C (1992) Sexual aggression and nature. *Reprinted in sexual harassment: confrontations and decisions, edited by Edmund Wall.* 112-113

Pierson B (2020) Weinstein found guilty of sexual assault, rape, in victory for #MeToo Movement. https://www.reuters.com/article/us-people-harvey-weinstein-idUSKCN20I159. Accessed 12 May

Pitchford B, Sternadori M, Starkey J, Koerber A (2020) 'From f-bombs to kissing students: Media framing of male and female professors accused of sexual harassment' Journal of Communication Inquiry

Richman JA et al. (1999) 'Sexual harassment and generalized workplace abuse among university employees: Prevalence and mental health correlates' American Journal of Public Health, 89 (3), pp. 358–363

Rubin AJ (2017) 'Revolt' in France against sexual harassment hits cultural resistance. The New York Times

Schultz V (2003) The sanitized workplace. The Yale Law Journal, 112(8), p.2061

Solictors CE (2018) Transphobia rife among UK employers as 1 in 3 won't hire a transgender person Reportno. Report numberl, Date. Place publishedl: Institutionl

Thrasher SW (2019) Sexual freedom is at risk from these damning new bills passed by Congress. The Guardian. Accessed 29 Mar 2018

Trust YWs (2018) It's (Still) a rich man's World: inequality 100 years after votes for women. Reportno. Report Numberl, Date. Place Publishedl: Institutionl

Unison (2019) Factsheet: transgender workers right. Reportno. Report Numberl, Date. Place publishedl: Institutionl

Wilhelm H (2017) Where #MeToo goes off the rails. Chicago Tribune

Williams R (2011) The silent epidemic: workplace bullying. Psychol Today 3(5)

Wise S, Stanley L (1987) Georgie Porgie: sexual harassment in everyday life. Pandora Press

Wood JT (1994) Saying it makes it so: the discursive construction of sexual harassment. In: Bingham SG (ed) Conceptualizing sexual harassment as discursive practice. Praeger, Westport, CT, pp 17–30

Yildiz S (2007) A 'new' problem in the workplace: psychological abuse (bullying). J Acad Stud 34(9):113–128

Zapf D, Einarsen S (2001) Bullying in the workplace: recent trends in research and practice– an introduction. Eur J Work Organ Psy 10(4):369–373

Chris Waugh is a doctoral researcher at the University of Manchester. His research areas include masculinities, affect, radical left wing social movements and the politics of authenticity.

Part VIII

Identity Abuse

Domestic Violence and Abuse in LGBTQ+ Communities

Kirsty McGregor

Learning Objectives
Having read this chapter, you should be able to understand:

- Who lesbian, gay, bisexual, trans, and queer (LGBTQ+) communities are.
- How domestic violence and abuse manifests within LGBTQ+ communities.
- Risk and protective factors associated with domestic violence and abuse within LGBTQ+ communities.

Introduction

This chapter introduces readers to the phenomenon of domestic violence and abuse within lesbian, gay, bisexual, trans, and queer (LGBTQ+) communities. Domestic violence and abuse (DVA) is widely recognised as a significant global public health and human rights concern (World Health Organization 2021). Due to the success of the feminist movement in raising awareness of DVA within heterosexual relationships, it is most commonly understood as a gendered issue of male violence towards women. However, the existence of DVA within same-sex relationships has led to debate around how best to define and explain it. This chapter will explore who the LGBTQ+ communities are before defining DVA; considering the existing explanatory theories; and exploring the prevalence and impact of DVA in LGBTQ+ communities. The chapter concludes by outlining the implications for practitioners, policy, and research.

K. McGregor (✉)
School of Humanities and Social Science, University of Brighton, Brighton, UK
e-mail: k.e.mcgregor@brighton.ac.uk

P. Ali, M. M. Rogers (eds.), *Gender-Based Violence: A Comprehensive Guide*,
https://doi.org/10.1007/978-3-031-05640-6_34

Who Are the LGBTQ+ Communities?

The term LGBTQ+ communities refers to 'the multitude of individuals who do not conform to heteronormative, [and/or] cisnormative models of gender and/or sexuality' (Donovan and Barnes 2019: 742), in other words, anyone who does not conform with the culturally normalised heterosexual roles, assumptions, and discourses which specify that heterosexuality and essentialist binaries of gender and sex are 'natural' or 'normal' (Habarth 2013). This includes a diverse range of people who identify with minority sexual orientations such as lesbian, gay, or bisexual; gender identities such as trans, non-binary, or queer; or any other sexual or gender minority.

The term 'sex' refers to the biological characteristics labelled as belonging to male, female, or intersex bodies (Johnson and Repta 2012). Gendered identities are socially constructed and are ascribed to bodies which are perceived to be sexed in certain ways (Rogers 2019; Enke 2012). Those whose biological sex assigned at birth matches their gender identity are referred to as 'cisgender' (Enke 2012), whilst those whose gender identity does not match their biological sex assigned at birth are referred to as transgender. There are also gender identities (for example, non-binary, queer, or genderqueer—see Box 1) which are fluid and changing and/or do not fit within the assumption that sex and gender are binary (i.e. male/female, masculine/feminine). Trans, non-binary, and genderqueer identities challenge not only the assumptions that sex and gender are binary, but also the centrality of heterosexism and cisgenderism which are inherent in the dominant theories of DVA (Rogers 2019).

Box 1 Key Terms

LGBTQ+—Is an acronym used to refer to lesbian, gay, bisexual, trans, queer, questioning, and other minority sexual orientations and gender identities.

Lesbian—Refers to a woman who has a romantic and/or sexual attraction towards women. Some non-binary people may also identify with this term.

Gay—Refers to a man who has a romantic and/or sexual attraction towards men. Often used as a generic term for lesbian and gay sexuality—some women define themselves as gay rather than lesbian. Some non-binary people may also identify with this term.

Bisexual—An umbrella term used to describe a romantic and/or sexual orientation towards more than one gender. Bi people may describe themselves using one or more of a wide variety of terms, including, but not limited to, bisexual, pansexual, queer, and some other non-monosexual and non-monoromantic identities.

Trans—An umbrella term to describe people whose gender is not the same as, or does not sit comfortably with, the sex they were assigned at birth. Trans people may describe themselves using one or more of a wide variety of terms, including (but not limited to) transgender, transsexual, genderqueer (GQ), gender-fluid, non-binary, gender-variant, crossdresser, genderless, agender, nongender, third gender, bi-gender, trans man, trans woman, trans masculine, trans feminine, and neutrois.

Queer—Queer is a term used by those wanting to reject specific labels of romantic orientation, sexual orientation, and/or gender identity. It can also be a way of rejecting the perceived norms of the LGBT community (racism, sizeism, ableism, etc). Although some LGBT people view the word as a slur, it was reclaimed in the late 80 s by the queer community who have embraced it.

Questioning—The process of exploring your own sexual orientation and/or gender identity.

+ *or plus*—refers to the wide range of sexual orientations and gender identities not captured by the LGBTQ acronym. For further information please see the list of LGBTQ+ terms available at www.stonewall.org.uk.

Heteronormativity—The assumption that heterosexuality is the norm and should be privileged over any other form of sexual orientation. This operates within and across interpersonal relationships, as well as at the macro level via social and cultural norms. For example, it is expected that a cisgender man and a cisgender woman marry and procreate.

Cisnormativity/cisgenderism—The assumption that binary cisgender understandings of gender are fixed. Any departure from this gender identity binary is considered abnormal. This paradigm promotes the belief that people must identify and express their gender identity within the confines of the gender binary. This operates at the micro and macro level via social and cultural norms and institutions and arguably is akin to sexism and racism (Rogers 2020).

LGBTQ+ communities are often conflated, which obscures the heterogeneity of each community (Donovan and Barnes 2020a; Rogers 2019). Moreover, there is heterogeneity both within and across each of the communities represented by this term, relating to gender, ethnicity, socio-economic background, age, disability, religion, and so forth. As a result, individual experiences, including of DVA, within groups characterised by the same sexual orientation or gender status will vary (Fassinger and Arseneau 2007), requiring an intersectional analysis of DVA. A wholly intersectional analysis of DVA within relationships where at least one partner is not heterosexual or cisgender is in its infancy (Donovan and Barnes 2019), with many experiences—particularly those of non-binary and trans individuals—significantly under-theorised (Rogers 2019).

Large-scale surveys in several countries (Australia, Canada, Norway, the UK, and the USA) in the Global North suggest that between 1.2 and 6.4% of the population are LGB (ONS 2021; Gates 2011), with US-based surveys suggesting around 1% of the population are trans (Gates 2011). Due to the variation of acceptance and legal status of non-heterosexual and trans identities in many parts of the world, it is difficult to gauge a more accurate global picture (Poushter and Kent 2020). Indeed, homosexuality is criminalised in 71 countries, with 11 jurisdictions imposing the death penalty, and trans people are vulnerable to criminalisation in at least 26 countries (Human Dignity Trust 2021). This means that sexual or gender minority people hide their identities for fear of criminal sanction and even punishment that has a fatal outcome alongside everyday experiences of stigma, marginalisation, and/or discrimination.

Definition

There are various definitions of DVA available (Hester 2004) and various terms of reference (See Box 2). The UK government (Home Office 2013) defines it as: 'any incident or pattern of incidents of controlling, coercive or threatening behaviour, violence or abuse between those aged 16 or over who are or have been intimate partners or family members, regardless of gender or sexuality. This can encompass, but is not limited to, the following types of abuse: psychological, physical, sexual, financial[1] and emotional'. The United Nations definition builds on this by including any threats or actions which 'frighten, intimidate, terrorize, manipulate, hurt, humiliate, blame, injure, or wound someone' (United Nations 2021). Together these definitions recognise the variety of DVA experienced and are inclusive of all genders and sexualities, thereby including relationships when one or more partner or family member is LGBTQ+. This inclusivity is also embedded in the UK Serious Crime Act 2015 (which created the offence of Coercive Control—s.76; Stark 2007) and the Domestic Abuse Act 2021. In contradiction, the UK policy framework underpinned by this legislation is gender-specific, as it focuses on violence against women and girls [VAWG] (for example, the Tackling Violence Against Women and Girls Strategy (Home Office 2021)).

Box 2 Alternative Terminology

Domestic violence and abuse: Same-sex intimate partner violence; LGBTQ intimate partner violence; domestic violence; intimate partner violence; domestic abuse; partner abuse; intimate partner abuse.

LGBTQ+: Lesbian, gay, bisexual, trans, and queer (LGBTQ); lesbian, gay, bisexual, trans (LGBT); queer, intersex, lesbian, trans, bisexual, asexual, and gay (QUILTBAG) communities; lesbian, gay, bisexual, trans, queer, intersex, and asexual (LGBTQIA).

[1] The Domestic Abuse Act 2021 updated the definition from financial to economic abuse to accommodate the range of ways abusers might restrict how survivors acquire, use, and maintain money and economic resources, including accommodation, food, and clothing, even after a relationship has ended (for example by negatively affecting the survivor's credit history) (Adams et al. 2008).

Explanations

Whilst these definitions are broad, and inclusive of those within LGBTQ+ communities, there is consensus amongst feminist qualitative researchers that DVA is an issue of gendered power and control, which manifests in a pattern of behaviours rather than singular incidents (Pence and Paymar 1993; Dixon and Graham-Kevan 2011). This is represented in Johnson's (2006) Intimate Terrorism typology of DVA and Stark's (2007) concept of coercive control (later embedded in UK legislation).

However, there is a body of research (see, for example, Langhinrichsen-Rohling et al. 2012) using quantitative methods (such as the Conflict Tactics Scale (CTS) (Stets and Straus 1989) and the revised CTS-2 (Straus et al. 1996)) and informed by family violence and/or conflict theory, which finds symmetry in the gender of DVA perpetrators in heterosexual relationships. They argue that gender has no explanatory power, suggesting instead that DVA occurs as the result of conflict rather than an attempt to gain control (Straus 2010). This is represented in Johnson's (2006) Situational Couple Violence typology of DVA and bidirectional violence (see, for example, Bates 2016). However, these theories are based on data from heterosexual cisgender [het-cis] people and assumes binaries of both gender (male/female) and experience of DVA (victim/perpetrator) and therefore cannot be applied to LGBTQ+ communities without critique.

By centring het-cis people to the exclusion of all other identities and practices, the dominant understanding and rhetoric surrounding DVA can be understood as being 'located within the heteronormative framework' (Rogers 2019: 804). As a result of this 'heterosexual assumption' (Weeks et al. 2001: 39), the dominant understanding of DVA is one in which the physically larger, het-cis man is the perpetrator of physical violence against the physically smaller, het-cis woman (Donovan and Hester 2015; Donovan and Barnes 2020a). This *public story* (Donovan and Hester 2011, 2015) firmly locates DVA within heterosexual relationships and interlocks perceived strength and physical size differences associated with male/masculine and female/feminine bodies with the binary of perpetrator/victim. This works alongside several myths which invisibilise LGBTQ+ DVA (Messinger 2017):

- LGBTQ+ DVA is rare because traditional gender dynamics are not present; therefore, when it does occur, it is bidirectional abuse.
- LGBTQ+ DVA is less severe because it is a fair fight between those of the same gender, and they are less likely to be married or have children.
- The more masculine-looking/behaving LGBTQ+ partner is the perpetrator, and the more feminine-looking/behaving partner is the victim.
- Discussing LGBTQ+ DVA diverts attention and funding away from the issue of het-cis DVA, consequently further stigmatising LGBTQ+ people.

Subsequently, this has implications for how DVA within LGBTQ+ communities is perceived. In addition, the public story, perhaps more subtly, codes victims and perpetrators as white and able-bodied (Donovan and Hester 2015), highlighting the importance of an intersectional approach to understanding DVA.

Arguably the success of the feminist movement in raising awareness of the het-cis public story has unintentionally prohibited an intersectional discussion inclusive of experiences which fall outside of the defining binaries (female/male, feminine/masculine, and victim/perpetrator) and associated characteristics. This impedes the ability for those outside of this narrative to recognise their own experiences as DVA (Ristock 2002; Donovan et al. 2006; Barnes 2008; Donovan and Hester 2010) and for appropriate support to be provided to those who need it (Donovan and Hester 2015; Ristock 2002). The power of this public story makes it difficult for members of LGBTQ+ communities to recognise their experiences as abuse, to seek help without fear of homo/bi/transphobia, and to receive appropriate support.

Whilst official statistical data supports the notion that women are more likely to be victims of DVA (see, for example, ONS 2022), the existence of DVA within LGBTQ+ communities should not be ignored. By not asking participants about their gender or sexual identity, research has continued to utilise cisgender heteronormative data collection tools which work to keep the sexual orientation and gender identity of those reporting their experience hidden (Donovan and Barnes 2020a; Rogers 2019). This silencing and erasure of sexual minorities can be understood as a result of heteronormativity, whilst the invisibilisation of trans and non-binary people from official statistics can be understood as a consequence of cisgenderism (Kennedy 2013; Serano 2007; Brotman et al. 2003).

There is a growing body of work which problematizes the dominant heteronormative cisgendered framework of understanding DVA, highlighting the reality that people of all sexualities and genders can be victim/survivors and/or perpetrators of DVA (for example, Donovan and Hester 2015; Frankland and Brown 2014; Rogers 2019). Whilst this work is in its relative infancy, several explanatory theories have been proffered.

Meyer (2003) suggests that LGBTQ+ citizens who do not meet the 'heterosexual assumption' (Weeks et al. 2001) may experience a sense of minority stress due to living in a context of heteronormativity and cisgenderism (Balsam, 2001). Stresses may be internal (e.g. internalised homophobia) or external (e.g. homophobia from friends, family, and/or colleagues) (see Box 3) and are associated with implications to mental wellbeing and physical health (e.g. Hunt and Fish 2008; Kelly et al. 2011), educational outcomes, and life chances (e.g. Warwick et al. 2004; Russell et al. 2011) and have been linked to the use and normalisation of DVA (Mendoza 2011). However, Donovan and Hester (2015) argue that the links between minority stress and DVA are correlational, not causal, since the majority of LGBTQ+ communities experience minority stress but do not perpetrate DVA. Additionally, if both partners are experiencing minority stress, it does not explain why one partner may become a victim or perpetrator.

Box 3 Associated Concepts

Familial abuse: many LGBTQ+ people experience familial rejection and/or abuse as a direct result of their gender or sexual identity. This form of domestic abuse is complex and has many implications for the LGBTQ+ person, including homelessness, poor mental health, and substance misuse.

Honour-based violence (HBV): HBV is a crime or incident(s) which has or may have been committed to protect or defend the honour of the family and/or community. It is not bound by ethnicity, race, or religion; however LGBTQ+ people may be particularly at risk within communities with strong conservative ideals.

In their 2014 study of the similarities and differences of DVA in heterosexual and same-sex relationships, Donovan and Hester found that patterns of love and violence, power, and control were organised in similar ways for both groups. This suggests that power and control are the defining features of DVA rather than gender or the enactment of heterosexual femininity or masculinity (Donovan and Hester 2015; Donovan and Barnes 2019; Barnes 2013b). They argue that the social and cultural context of heterosexual relationship rules and practices structured around gendered binaries influences all relationships, regardless of gender or sexuality, including those experiencing DVA. Furthermore, they argue that the broader intersectional social and cultural context of inequality will position each partner differently and therefore must be considered when exploring experiences of DVA. For example, someone's age, gender, sexuality, race and ethnicity, parental status, income status, and educational level will coalesce differently for each individual and will shape their experiences of DVA and help-seeking.

DVA and LGBTQ+ Communities

There is growing evidence that LGBTQ+ communities experience DVA in similar and different ways to het-cis people (Donovan and Barnes 2020a). Many of the types of abuse experienced by het-cis people will also be experienced by members of LGBTQ+ communities, e.g. physical, sexual, psychological, economic, and emotional abuse. However, the relationship context will affect the ways DVA is experienced (for example, if people are cohabiting, have children, or if they are in a consensual bondage, discipline, sadism, and masochism [BDSM] relationship) as will the wider social and cultural context the relationship is being lived in and the intersecting identities of each partner (Donovan and Barnes 2020a). However, there are some tactics and presentations of different types of abuse that are specific to LGBTQ+ communities which will now be explored.

Physical Abuse

Physical abuse is the most widely accepted form of DVA and includes a range of behaviours including slapping, kicking, punching, and strangulation, which can be both fatal and non-fatal (Donovan and Hester 2015). For trans survivors this may include experiencing violence against body parts with gendered meaning (e.g., breasts and genitals) (Goodmark 2013; Messinger 2017) and disrupting or interfering with medical procedures linked to transitioning (Rogers 2019).

Sexual Abuse

Whilst various legal definitions of sexual violence and abuse exist internationally, it can be understood as a broad spectrum of acts the victim is threatened with, forced, or coerced to engage in (Donovan and Hester 2015). For example, non-consensual penetration with an object, digit, or penis; unwanted touching; sending and/or sharing images without consent; forced impregnation; purposefully giving sexually transmitted infections; and stealthing (intentionally disrupting contraception use, for example, by piercing a condom). As many jurisdictions consider sexual abuse to require physical violence, there is a dearth of global literature on sexual coercion, particularly within LGBTQ+ communities (Messinger 2017). That which does exist suggests that stereotypes around bisexuality and trans identities particularly are employed to condone sexual abuse. For example, Girshick (2002) found the trope that bisexual people are hypersexual is used by abusers to justify rape.

Psychological Abuse

Psychological abuse can include combinations of verbal abuse, threats, monitoring and stalking behaviours, isolating the survivor, and other controlling behaviours (Messinger 2017). There are several psychological abuse tactics linked to the sexual or gender identity(s) of LGBTQ+ people and the structural violence associated with living in heteronormative, cisgender societies. Such identity abuse can be understood as using someone's marginalised status to control or shame them (Rogers 2020; Messinger 2017). There are some specific ways in which LGBTQ+ identities can be weaponized by an abuser (Rogers 2019, 2020; Donovan and Barnes 2020a; Messinger 2017), such as:

- Outing—threatening or forcing someone to share their gender identity, sexuality, or HIV status before they are ready or directly telling others without consent.
- Closeting—forcing someone to hide their gender identity or sexuality from others.
- Undermining someone's sense of their gender or sexuality, for example, suggesting they are not gay 'enough'.
- Restricting or controlling access to LGBTQ+ spaces, information, or networks.
- Utilising myths about the LGBTQ+ community to convince the victim/survivor that no one they will believe the abuse is real, e.g. condoning rape by claiming bisexual people are hypersexualised.
- Manipulating the victim/survivor into believing DVA is a normal part of being LGBTQ+.
- If the survivor is living in the UK on a spousal visa, the abuser may utilise their knowledge of immigration law to threaten deportation to their country of origin, which might be unsafe due to their LGBTQ+ identity.

In addition, for trans survivors, abuse can include being shamed for their gender status by intentionally using incorrect pronouns, deadnaming them (intentionally using their birth name), and/or commenting on body parts with gendered meaning which make the survivor uncomfortable (Rogers 2019; Goodmark 2013). Specific abuses linked to transitioning may include preventing the survivor from realising their preferred gender appearance/performance; and/or disrupting access to their medication or treatment; and/or fetishizing trans peoples' bodies at specific points of their transition (Rogers 2019). This suggests that perpetrators utilise transphobic constructions of gender identities, roles, and norms within relationships to abuse trans survivors (Rogers 2019, 2020). This may result in trans women experiencing a higher risk of DVA, particularly from men, as a result of 'transmisogyny' (Serano 2007) which positions femininity as inferior to masculinity and trans identities as inferior to cisgender identities (Rogers 2019).

International Comparison: Prevalence

There is evidence that DVA occurs in relationships where at least one partner or family member identifies as LGBTQ+ (Donovan and Barnes 2019; Donovan and Hester 2015). International attempts to garner the frequency of DVA in LGBTQ+ communities find a range of prevalence rates depending on the community(s) under investigation, the definition of DVA utilised, time scales measured (e.g. within the last 12 months or across a lifetime), and the methodological tools used, i.e. qualitative or quantitative (Messinger 2017). As a result of this inconsistency, it is very difficult to gauge an accurate picture of prevalence for all LGBTQ+ communities.

Box 4 Countries Where LGBTQ+ DVA Is Prevalent

Domestic violence and abuse is a universal phenomenon and is likely to occur wherever there are LGBTQ+ people. However, it may be more hidden in some countries where LGBTQ+ rights are restricted or under attack.

In his 2017 international review of evidence regarding LGBTQ+ DVA, Messinger found a huge variety of prevalence rates, as shown in Table 1. Much of the evidence comes from the USA where such data is collected routinely; however smaller scale studies were identified in Australia, Canada, Japan, China, Latin America, South

Table 1 Lifetime prevalence of psychological, physical, and sexual domestic violence for all sexual minorities by country (Messinger 2017)

Country	Psychological abuse	Physical abuse	Sexual abuse
Australia	34–78%	17–48%	8–25%
Belgium	58%	15%	–
Canada	94%	16%	4–10%
China	34–81%	24–40%	23–29%
United States	69%	25–57%	22%
United Kingdom	66–72%	12–20%	4–15%
South Africa	–	26%	23%
Germany	–	–	3%

Africa, Belgium, Germany, the UK, and the Netherlands. Table 1 outlines the variation in lifetime prevalence rates of psychological, physical, and sexual domestic abuse (where available) for all sexual minorities by country. Whilst there is significant variation between countries for each form of abuse, there is a trend towards psychological domestic abuse being most prevalent for sexual minorities, followed by physical and then sexual domestic abuse, echoing the het-cis literature (Stark 2007).

Messinger noted a variety of sampling measures and categories of participants employed, for example, by self-identified sexual orientation, gender of perpetrator, history of sexual orientation and activities, and so on. In an attempt to overcome this, he grouped the evidence relating to all sexual minority men and men who have sex with men (MSM); sexual minority women and women who have sex with women; all sexual minorities, MSM, and WSW; and trans people (Table 2). Paradoxically, this grouping may also work to invisibilise people who have a history of having sex or relationships with more than one gender and those whose gender does not neatly fit into the binary of man/woman. The range of prevalence rates highlight the impact of different data collection tools and the variety of approaches taken to the research.

Table 2 suggests that psychological abuse is highly prevalent for all LGBTQ+ groups, conflicting with the physical violence focus of the public story of DVA (Donovan and Hester 2015). The prevalence range for physical and sexual abuse victimisation suggests that LGBTQ+ people, and particularly for trans people (Valentine et al. 2017), are also at significant risk of physical and sexual violence. Unsurprisingly, studies which explore shorter time periods (e.g. last 12 months) find lower prevalence rates (Hunt and Fish 2008).

In the UK, Donovan and Barnes (2020) conducted mixed-methods research on LGBTQ+ victimisation and perpetration of DVA, involving a self-selecting, non-clinical sample of 872 survey respondents and 36 follow-up interviews. Their survey findings (Table 3) show that there are significant differences in prevalence across each gender in the last 12 months of their most recent relationship; however they become much more similar across their lifetime. In addition, Ristock (2002) cautions us to take care when interpreting gender differences in reporting, as women may have learnt to recognise and name abuse as a result of the public story. Contrastingly, some women may be reluctant to identify other women as abusive

Table 2 International lifetime prevalence of psychological, physical, and sexual domestic violence by sexuality and/or gender (Messinger 2017)

	Psychological abuse	Physical abuse	Sexual abuse
Sexual minority men and MSM	18–94%	16–48%	1–29%
Sexual minority women and WSW	46–84%	12–58%	4–33%
All sexual minorities, MSM, and WSW	58–81%	7–40%	8–17%
Trans people	57%	43–46%	8–47%

Table 3 Victimisation prevalence of combined DVA types by gender and timeframe (Donovan and Barnes 2020a)

	Men	Women	Trans+
Prevalence of combined types of DVA the last 12 months of most recent relationship	63.1%	62.3%	74.1%
Prevalence of combined types of DVA over lifetime	68.6%	71.9%	66.7%

and therefore underreport (Hassouneh and Glass 2008), whereas men might understand DVA as physical violence (Hester et al. 2007), and others might feel it is 'gender-typical behaviour' (Cruz 2003: 310). This suggests that gender may have a less consistent explanatory power when examining DVA in LGBTQ+ communities than for their het-cis counterparts.

When examining their survey findings by sexuality, Donovan and Barnes found that bisexuals were more likely than other sexual minorities to report at least one form of DVA in the last 12 months of their most recent relationship and had the highest rates of victimisation in all categories of DVA, supporting UK (ONS 2018) and US (Messinger 2011) research. However, it is not yet clear why this is the case or whether the perpetrator is the same or different gender and/or sexuality. In addition, they found a complex pattern of prevalence with age, suggesting that older (55 years+) and younger (16–25 years) LGBTQ+ people were most likely to report victimisation. Furthermore, queer respondents reported the highest rates of DVA perpetration, and younger respondents reported high rates of physically and sexually abusive behaviours. This strengthens the case for recognising the heterogeneity across and within LGBTQ+ communities, so that we can better understand and respond to these survivors and perpetrators.

Whilst there is great variation in the rates above, almost all research finds that LGBTQ+ people are at an increased risk of experiencing all forms of DVA than their het-cis counterparts (Walters et al. 2013; Harned 2002; Messinger 2011). Future research should also seek to explore how intersecting identities shape these experiences.

Impacts

The radiating impact of DVA (Riger et al. 2002) for het-cis survivors is well documented at both the individual and societal levels. For example, victimisation has been associated with increased fear and anxiety, injury, mental health issues (including PTSD, suicide ideation, and depression), substance misuse, economic-related outcomes (e.g. missing work), and sexual risk-taking (Messinger 2017). Many of these findings have been replicated in LGBTQ+ survivor research (see, for example, Koblin et al. 2006; Davis et al. 2015).

Specific impacts for LGBTQ+ survivors are less well documented, but several studies have identified an additional burden which negatively impacts LGBTQ+

survivors' social, psychological, and physical wellbeing as a result of heteronormativity and cisgenderism. For example, psychological abuse such as invalidating and/or belittling the relationship, the abuse, or a survivor's sexual and/or gender identity (identity abuse) works to marginalise the survivor in both the private and public spheres (Rogers 2020) and for trans survivors contributes to 'trans-erasure' (Serano 2007).

The impact of identity abuse can have a significant impact on trans people's safety and wellbeing, through the loss of relationships and employment, access to their children, social rejection, and discrimination and hate crime (Rogers 2019). Many techniques of abuse, including micro-aggressions, may undermine trans survivors' gender identity and disrupt their transition journey which can have significant and far-reaching impacts including a suppression of their gender identity, internalised transphobia, poor mental and physical health, and social isolation (Rogers 2020). This can have an isolating impact and acts as a barrier to seeking help (Messinger 2017). Isolation tactics such as this contribute to survivors' pre-existing sense of marginalisation and isolation due to their gender identity or sexual orientation (Walters and Lippy 2016) which may worsen their mental health.

Research suggests that 76% of trans people (Roch et al. 2010), 3–42% of sexual minority men (Pitts et al. 2006), and 20–46% of sexual minority women (Walters et al. 2013) have experienced mental health problems as a result of an abusive intimate relationship, including suicide ideation and attempts (Pantalone et al. 2010). Furthermore, Dickerson-Amaya and Coston's (2019) analysis of the 2011 National Intimate Partner and Sexual Violence Survey found that bisexual male survivors were more likely than gay men and significantly more likely than heterosexual men to rank their mental health as poor.

Cisgenderism and heteronormativity exacerbate the experience and outcomes of DVA for LGBTQ+ people (Rogers 2020) and may act as an additional barrier to LGBTQ+ victim/survivors asking for and receiving appropriate support (Donovan and Barnes 2020a). For example, they may anticipate experiencing discrimination from the agencies they seek help from and may fear being disbelieved as they fall outside of the het-cis public story of DVA. As a result, LGBTQ+ survivors are more likely to seek help from informal sources (e.g. friends or therapists) rather than DVA specialist organisations or the police (Donovan and Barnes 2020b). Additionally, silencing and erasure of DVA experiences within LGBTQ+ communities is likely to negatively impact survivors' capacity to recover due to a dearth of awareness within, and support available to, LGBTQ+ communities.

The UK government estimates that the annual cost of DVA is £66 billion per year, including preventative and consequential costs (Home Office 2019). Since this figure is based on official statistics, it represents the financial impact of reported DVA and does not fully represent the true prevalence of DVA, including within LGBTQ+ communities who are even less likely to report their experiences. Furthermore, as a result of the dominance of the public story of DVA and pervasive heteronormative and cisgendered societal structures, there are few services designed explicitly for LGBTQ+ survivors, or perpetrators, of DVA (Santoniccolo et al. 2021).

Risk and Protective Factors

Relatively little research has explored the risk and protective factors for LGBTQ+ DVA. From an ecological perspective of DVA (Heise 1998), there appears to be several personal, situational, and sociocultural level factors at play, such as gender and age. In contrast to the het-cis literature, Donovan and Hester (2014) found that many risk factors were more marked than gender in their survey of 746 LGBTQ+ people in the UK, including being under 35 years old, lower income levels, lower education levels, and having a disability (factors also identified in the het-cis data, although with less weighting than gender, e.g. Stripe 2020).

Donovan and Barnes (2020a) found that LGBTQ+ people are more vulnerable to DVA when coming out and/or being in their first intimate relationship, especially if they are young (16–25 years) or older (55+ years). Arguably this first relationship, particularly when with someone more experienced, creates a power dynamic whereby the more experienced partner has more experiential power and social capital with the LGBTQ+ community and can therefore set the tone of the relationship. The survivor may feel less confident with being out and the norms and expectations of LGBTQ+ relationships. In other words, they may have less community knowledge, including knowledge about where to go for help. This vulnerability may be particularly marked when the person is disconnected with their family of origin, especially due to familial abuse (as a result of poly-victimisation) (Donovan and Barnes 2020a). Similarly, for trans survivors, Rogers (2019) identifies the onset of transitioning as a vulnerable and risky time, where DVA may begin or escalate, akin to the risk associated with the onset of pregnancy for heterosexual couples (little research has considered the onset of pregnancy or parenting on LGBTQ+ DVA as yet).

LGBTQ+ people rarely seek support from formal agencies, e.g. police or DVA services (Donovan and Hester 2011, 2014; Donovan et al. 2014; Ristock 2002; Irwin 2006; Barnes 2013a), because of specific barriers at individual (e.g. identity-specific positioning), community (e.g. wider understandings about what constitutes DVA), and societal (e.g. local law) levels (see Box 4). Against the backdrop of these barriers, Donovan and Barnes (2020b) found that help-seeking is a non-linear process requiring an LGBTQ+ survivor to firstly recognise their experience as DVA, decide to seek help, and identify a suitable source of help (Liang et al. 2005). Consequently, LGBTQ+ survivors wait longer than het-cis survivors to seek support and/or report to police (Donovan 2010; SafeLives 2018; Donovan and Hester 2015) due to a fear of not being believed, their experiences being minimised, or for fear of homo/bi/transphobia from professionals.

Whilst an LGBTQ+ survivor is undergoing this process of help-seeking, the abusive relationship continues, and the survivor is likely to seek space for re/action to the abuse (Kelly 2003). This may increase the risk of escalation in frequency and severity of the abuse and consequently increases the risk to the survivor. Consequently, when LGBTQ+ survivors do seek help, they often present with high levels of risk and complex needs (SafeLives 2018). Care must be taken not to frame this help-seeking delay as the result of an individual failure; instead it is the result of heteronormative and cisgendered societal structures and the neoliberal tendency to responsibilise individuals, which pushes LGBTQ+ victim/survivors to view their experiences as private, therefore requiring a private source of support (Donovan and Barnes 2020a, b).

Whilst DVA within LGBTQ+ communities is the focus of this chapter, it is important to recognise the multiple oppressions experienced by the LGBTQ+ community which might pre- or co-exist with experiences of DVA. Donovan and Barnes argue they may experience 'structural factors which render LGB and/or T oppression invisible, insignificant, or which reinforce its perpetuation' (2019: 747). For example, LGBTQ+ people are more likely to have experienced multiple childhood adversities (Dempsey et al. 2020) including conflict, abuse, and deprivation in the home which may lead to homelessness and increase the risk of future poly-victimisation (Sterzing et al. 2017). As a result LGBTQ+ peoples' intersecting experiences of oppression are multifaceted and will have implications for their perpetrator's choice of abuse tactics, survivors' awareness and recognition of their experience as DVA, and their help-seeking and availability of appropriate support.

LGBTQ people frequently seek out connection with like-minded people, building informal LGBTQ+ communities of support locally and online, often referred to as their families of choice (Donovan et al. 2001). When faced with adversity, including DVA, having the support of trusted peers, a supportive family, access to counselling, and appropriate professional support (Valido et al. 2021) appears to act as a protective factor for LGBTQ+ DVA and is the first choice for many LGBTQ+ survivors of DVA (Donovan and Barnes 2020b). This highlights the importance of building awareness of DVA within LGBTQ+ communities, the professionals who work with them, and wider society to ensure victim/survivors receive appropriate support every time they ask for it. Further research is required to examine additional protective factors and opportunities for both prevention and intervention.

Implications for Policy, Practice, and Research

Whilst legislation and policy in certain jurisdictions acknowledges DVA, and LGBTQ+ rights, many have yet to fully consider DVA within LGBTQ+ communities (Messinger 2017). As a result, formal support is largely influenced by the public story of DVA and is based on evidence from heterosexual relationships. This may obscure the circumstances of LGBTQ relationships and how DVA might operate within them (Donovan and Hester 2015: 9), making practitioners less equipped to appropriately support LGBTQ+ survivors. Therefore policy-makers, practitioners, and researchers should be aware that a one-size-fits-all approach to DVA within LGBTQ+ communities is not coveted nor achievable. Rather, the heterogeneity within and across LGBTQ+ communities, the range of DVA experienced, and the variety of potential impacts on the individuals involved need to be understood so that the LGBTQ+ community can be supported to acknowledge and address the challenges DVA poses.

Internationally, LGBTQ+ communities are currently, and/or have historically been, pathologized by the state, forcing them to develop self-reliance and creating a gap of trust of mainstream services (Donovan and Hester 2010). Living within the isolating heteronormative cisgender framework (Rogers 2019) and/or within neo-liberal jurisdictions, which promotes narratives of the rational responsible citizen, creates a context in which risk of DVA management is individualised (Homes 2011). As a result of this forced self-reliance and the dominance of the public story of DVA, LGBTQ+ survivors and perpetrators struggle to recognise their experience, and when they do they tend to seek support from a friend, private counselling, or therapy rather than specialised DVA support, which may work to further individualise the problem (Donovan and Barnes 2019; Donovan and Hester 2015) (see Box 5). Therefore, awareness raising within LGBTQ+ communities, and wider society, is vital. Inclusive policies and services which encourage recognition of the full repertoire of DVA behaviours and where to go for support are important so that LGBTQ+ people can challenge the minimisation and/or denial of abuse, even in their first relationship. This is particularly vital given that growing evidence suggests that when LGBTQ+ people seek support for DVA it often is not helpful, with research (e.g. Goodkind et al. 2003) finding that friends and family may collude with the abuser by denying or minimising DVA or by blaming the survivor.

Alongside awareness raising within adult populations, young people must be provided with access to effective and inclusive sex and relationship education which represents the realities of their lives, including their gender identities and sexual orientations (Donovan and Barnes 2020a). Furthermore, Donovan and Hester (2014) argue that a complete cultural shift is required to ensure LGBTQ+ people normalise discussing relationship problems and can more easily access appropriate support. It is likely that, with increased awareness, demand for services will also increase, and therefore funding must be extended to support services to deliver these vital services.

Given the prevalence of DVA within LGBTQ+ communities, practitioners are expected to deal with cases regularly; therefore training is essential (Rogers 2016). Practitioners, including the police, must develop the knowledge and skills to address the barriers to help-seeking for LGBTQ+ people and support them in appropriate and inclusive ways which recognise the intersecting social locations and identities of each partner and how they might be implicated in the relationship dynamics (Donovan and Hester 2010). Practitioners should be aware of the causes, symptoms and impacts of DVA, and the barriers to help-seeking LGBTQ+ communities face so that they can provide appropriate support at the first encounter (Rogers 2016). This includes disengaging understandings of DVA from het-cis binary identities so that power dynamics within the problematic relationship can be analysed and addressed effectively (Donovan and Barnes 2020a). Additionally, services should have clearly inclusive language in their literature, websites, images, etc. so that members of LGBTQ+ communities are confident they can access the support on offer (Rogers 2016; Donovan and Barnes 2020a, b).

Further research is also required to investigate the gaps in existing knowledge. For example, intersectional research which tests the links between DVA victimisation and perpetration and the positionality of members of LGBTQ+ communities would ensure that policy and practice can better respond to the multifaceted experiences of the LGBTQ+ communities. Additionally, further work is required to test our theoretical understandings of DVA with LGBTQ+ communities and to explore suitable support mechanisms and risk assessments for LGBTQ+ communities.

Box 5 When LGBTQ+ Domestic Abuse Is Fatal

Özge Bilir was a 25-year-old Turkish trans woman living in supported housing for people with addiction and mental health problems in Utrecht in the Netherlands. She had a difficult childhood and began using drugs with boyfriend Ilias in their teens. At 19 years old, Özge transitioned. Özge was a keen vlogger, documenting her transition on the Internet. Although her family found her transition difficult, her friends were very supportive.

Ilias and Özge had known each other since they were 13 years old. Their relationship was described as tumultuous, involving drugs, crime, and domestic abuse. Whilst it is not clear exactly what role Özge's gender transition played in the abuse, since her transition the police were called on numerous occasions, including for Ilias' violence against her, leading to a restraining order being placed against him. It was reported that Ilias had threatened Özge with a knife during an argument on several occasions. They later ended their intimate relationship.

On 11 November 2020, Ilias turned up at Özge's property after he had been drinking and taking cocaine. Özge asked Ilias to sleep it off in the bedroom which he objected to. An argument ensued. Witnesses left as the argument escalated, and Özge was heard asking 'you're not going to stab me, are you?' to which he replied, 'maybe I will'. Ilias stabbed Özge multiple times. She died outside the entrance to her flat as she tried to escape.

Ilias was prosecuted for Özge's murder, although he claimed it was an accident and was not premeditated. Perhaps controversially, the judge stated that due to his childhood experiences of domestic abuse and his addiction issues, he should be convicted of manslaughter rather than murder. He was subsequently sentenced to 8 years in prison, mandatory addiction treatment, and ordered to pay Özge's mother 24,000 euros in compensation.

More information about Özge's case: https://www.rtvutrecht.nl/nieuws/2184972/om-eist-8-jaar-en-tbs-na-fataal-steekdrama-onder-invloed-van-drank-en-drugs-in-leidsche-rijn.html

Further cases:

Brian (Bri) Golec (United States), who was gender-fluid, was murdered by their father who claimed that a cult had broken into their home and killed them. This was found to be untrue, and Brian's father was charged with their murder. Link: https://tdor.translivesmatter.info/reports/2015/02/13/bri-an-golec_akron-ohio-usa_9c62aefc

Sabi (Beka) Beriani, a transgender woman from Georgia (Europe), was murdered by her boyfriend who then set her apartment on fire in an attempt to cover up his crime. Link: https://sova.news/2017/01/04/13355/

Raina Aliev moved from Chechnya to Russia where they transitioned and married their cis-husband. Raina's Muslim family discovered this and went on local TV calling for her murder. Authorities confirmed she had been murdered but have not released details. Link: https://www.gaystarnews.com/article/transgender-muslim-woman-hacked-death-russia-days-marrying-man/#gs.cO0Bo5s

Summary

- DVA within LGBTQ+ communities is highly prevalent and has significant implications for victims and wider society.
- Our understanding of DVA within and across the multiple communities represented by the LGBTQ+ umbrella is in its infancy, yet significant differences in prevalence and aetiology exist.
- The social and cultural context of the relationship is key to understanding DVA.
- Due to the multifaceted nature of DVA and the LGBTQ+ communities, there are many challenges in preventing and addressing it.
- Further research which explores the intersectional factors impacting on DVA is required.

References

Adams AE, Sullivan CM, Bybee D, Greeson MR (2008) Development of the scale of economic abuse. Violence Against Women 14(5):563–587

Balsam KF (2001) Nowhere to hide: lesbian battering, homophobia, and minority stress. Women Therapy 23(3):25–37

Barnes R (2008) 'I still sort of flounder in a sea of non-language': The constraints of language and labels in women's accounts of woman-to-woman partner abuse. In: Throsby K, Alexander F (eds) Gender and Interpersonal Violence: Language, Action and Representation, Basingstoke: Palgrave Macmillan, pp. 29–43.

Barnes R (2013a) 'I'm over it': Women's accounts of life after woman-to-woman partner abuse. Partn Abus 4(3):380–398

Barnes R (2013b) 'She expected her women to be pretty, subservient, dinner on the table at six': Problematising the narrative of egalitarianism in lesbian relationships through accounts of woman-to-woman partner abuse. In: Sanger T, Taylor Y (eds) Mapping intimacies: relations, exchanges, affects. Palgrave Macmillan, Basingstoke, pp 130–149

Bates E (2016) Current controversies within intimate partner violence: overlooking bidirectional violence. J Fam Violence 31:937–940

Brotman S, Ryan B, Cormier R (2003) The Health and Social Service Needs of Gay and Lesbian Elders and Their Families in Canada The Gerontologist 43(2):192–02 https://doi.org/10.1093/geront/43.2.192

Cruz M (2003) "Why Doesn't He Just Leave?": Gay Male Domestic Violence and the Reasons Victims Stay. The Journal of Men's Studies 11(3):309–23

Davis A, Best J, Wei C, Luo J, Van der Pol B et al (2015) Intimate partner violence and correlates with risk behaviours and HIV/STI diagnoses among men who have sex with men and men who have sex with men and women in China: a hidden epidemic. Sex Transm Dis 42(7):387–392

Dempsey D, Parkinson S, Andrews C, McNair R (2020) Family relationships and LGB first homelessness in Australia: What do we know and where should we go? Journal of Sociology 56(4): 516–34 https://doi.org/10.1177/1440783320927087

Dickerson-Amaya N, Coston BM (2019) Invisibility Is Not Invincibility: The Impact of Intimate Partner Violence on Gay Bisexual and Straight Men's Mental Health. American Journal of Men's Health 13(3) https://doi.org/10.1177/1557988319849734

Dixon L, Graham-Kevan N (2011) Understanding the nature and etiology of intimate partner violence and implications for practice and policy. Clinical Psychology Review 31(7);1145–155 https://doi.org/10.1016/j.cpr.2011.07.001

Donovan C, Hester M, Holmes J, McCarry M (2006) Comparing domestic abuse in same sex and heterosexual relationships: Initial report from a study funded by the ESRC. Available at: https://equation.org.uk/wp-content/uploads/2012/12/Comparing-Domestic-Abuse-in-Same-Sex-and-Heterosexual-relationships.pdf

Donovan C, (2010) Barriers to Making Referrals of Lesbian, Gay, Bisexual and Transgendered (LGBT) victim/survivors to the MARAC and Recommendations for Improvement: A Study of IDVAs, MARAC Coordinators and PPU Detective Inspectors Within the Northumbria Police Force Area. Project Report. University of Sunderland. Available at: http://sure.sunderland.ac.uk/id/eprint/2895/

Donovan C, Barnes R (2019) Domestic violence and abuse in lesbian, gay, bisexual and/or transgender (LGB and/or T) relationships. Sexualities 22(5–6):741–750. https://doi.org/10.1177/1363460716681491

Donovan C, Hester M (2010) 'I Hate the Word "Victim"': An Exploration of Recognition of Domestic Violence in Same Sex Relationships Social Policy and Society 9(2):279–89. https://doi.org/10.1017/S1474746409990406

Donovan C, Barnes R (2020a) Queering narratives of domestic violence and abuse. Palgrave Macmillan, Basingstoke

Donovan C, Barnes R (2020b) Help-seeking among lesbian, gay, bisexual and/or transgender victims/survivors of domestic violence and abuse: The impacts of cisgendered heteronormativity and invisibility. J Sociol 56(4):554–570

Donovan C, Hester M (2011) Seeking help from the enemy: help-seeking strategies of those in same sex relationships who have experienced domestic abuse. Child Fam Law Q 23(1):26–40

Donovan C, Hester M (2015) Domestic violence and sexuality: what's love got to do with it? Policy Press, Bristol

Donovan C, Heaphy B, Weeks J (2001) Same sex intimacies. Families of Choice and Other Life Experiments, Routledge, London

Donovan C, Barnes R, Nixon C (2014) The Coral Project: exploring abusive behaviours in lesbian, gay, bisexual and/or transgender relationships interim report ESRC ES/J012580/01. https://www2leacuk/departments/criminology/documents/coral-project-interim-report. Accessed 7 Jul 2021

Enke A (2012) Transfeminist perspectives in and beyond. Temple University Press, Philadelphia, PA

Fassinger RE, Arseneau JR (2007) "I'd Rather Get Wet Than Be Under That Umbrella": differentiating the Experiences and Identities of Lesbian, Gay, Bisexual, and Transgender People. In: Bieschke KJ, Perez RM, De Bord KA (eds) Handbook of counselling and psychotherapy with lesbian, gay, bisexual, and transgender clients. American Psychological Association, Worcester, MA, pp 19–49. https://doi.org/10.1037/11482-001

Frankland A, Brown J (2014) Coercive Control in Same-Sex Intimate Partner Violence Journal of Family Violence 29(1) 15-22 10.1007/s10896-013-9558-1

Gates GJ (2011) How many people are lesbian, gay, bisexual and transgender? Williams Institute, UCLA, Los Angeles

Girshick LB (2002) Woman-to-woman sexual violence: does she call it rape? University Press of New England, Lebanon, NH

Goodmark L (2013) Transgender people, intimate partner abuse, and the legal system. Harvard Civil Rights Civil Liberties Rev 48:51–104

Goodkind JR, Gillum TL, Bybee DI, Sullivan CM (2003) The Impact of Family and Friends' Reactions on the Well-Being of Women With Abusive Partners Violence Against Women 9(3) 347–73 https://doi.org/10.1177/1077801202250083

Habarth JM (2013) Development of the heteronormative attitudes and beliefs scale. Psychol Sex 6(2):166–188

Harned MS (2002) Abused women or abused men? An examination of the context and outcomes of dating violence. Violence Vict 16(3):269–285

Hassouneh D, Glass N (2008) The influence of gender role stereotyping on women's experiences of female same-sex intimate partner violence. Violence Against Women 14(3):310–325

Heise LL (1998) Violence against women: An integrated, ecological framework. Violence Against Women 4(3):262–290

Hester M (2004) Future Trends and Developments Violence Against Women 10(12):1431–448 https://doi.org/10.1177/1077801204270559

Hester M, Pearson C, Harwin N (2007) Making an Impact - Children and Domestic Violence: A Reader. London: Jessica Kingsley Publishers

Holmes C (2011) Troubling Normalcy: Examining 'healthy relationship' discourses in lesbian domestic violence prevention. In J Ristock (ed) Intimate Partner Violence in LGBTQ Lives. Abingdon: Routledge

Home Office (2013) Definition of domestic violence and abuse: Guide for local areas. Published 18 March 2013. www.gov.uk/government/publications/definition-of-domestic-violence-and-abuse-guidefor-local-areas

Home Office (2019) The economic and social costs of domestic abuse. Home Office Research Report 107. Published 21 January 2019. https://www.gov.uk/government/publications/the-economic-and-social-costs-of-domestic-abuse

Home Office (2021) Tackling violence against women and girls strategy. Published 21 July 2021. https://www.gov.uk/government/publications/tackling-violence-against-women-and-girls-strategy Accessed 22 Jul 2021

Human Dignity Trust (2021) LGBT and the law. https://www.humandignitytrust.org/lgbt-the-law/. Accessed 8 Jul 2021

Hunt R, Fish J (2008) Prescription for change: Lesbian and bisexual women's health check. London Sigma Research. https://wwwstonewallorguk/resources/prescription-change-2008 Accessed 31 May 2021

Irwin J (2006) Lesbians and domestic violence: Stories of seeking support. Women Welfare Educ 8:28–36

Johnson MP (2006) Conflict and control: gender symmetry and asymmetry in domestic violence. Violence Against Women 12:1003–1018

Johnson JL, Repta R (2012) Sex and gender: beyond the binaries. In: Oliffe JL, Greaves L (eds) Designing and conducting gender, sex, and health research. SAGE, London

Kelly L (2003) The wrong debate: reflections on why force is not the key issue with respect to trafficking in women for sexual exploitation. Fem Rev 73(1):139–144

Kelly BC, Izienicki H, Bimbi DS, Parsons JT (2011) The intersection of mutual partner violence and substance use among urban gays, lesbians and bisexuals. Deviant Behav 32(5):379–404

Kennedy N (2013) Cultural cisgenderism: consequences of the imperceptible. Psychol Women Sect Rev 15(2):1–7

Koblin BA, Torian L, Xu G, Guilin V, Makki H, Mackellar D, Valleroy L (2006) Violence and HIV-related risk among young men who have sex with men. AIDS Care 18(8):961–967

Langhinrichsen-Rohling J, Misra TA, Selwyn C, Rohling ML (2012) Rates of bidirectional versus unidirectional intimate partner violence across sample, sexual orientations, and race/ethnicities: a comprehensive review. Partn Abus 3(2):199–230

Liang B, Goodman L, Tummala-Narra P, Weintraub S (2005) A Theoretical Framework for Understanding Help-Seeking Processes Among Survivors of Intimate Partner Violence. American Journal of Community Psychology 36(1–2): 71-84 https://doi.org/10.1007/s10464-005-6233-6

Mendoza J (2011) The impact of minority stress on gay male partner abuse. In: Ristock JL (ed) Intimate Partner Violence in LGBTQ lives. Routledge, New York, pp 169–181

Messinger AM (2011) Invisible victims: same-sex IPV in the national violence against women survey. J Interpers Violence 26(11):2228–2243

Messinger AM (2017) LGBTQ Intimate Partner Violence. Lessons for policy, practice, and research. University of California Press, California

Meyer IH (2003) Prejudice, social stress, and mental health in lesbian, gay, and bisexual populations: conceptual issues and research evidence. Psychol Bull 129(5):674–697

Office for National Statistics [ONS] (2018) Women most at risk of experiencing partner abuse in England and Wales: years ending March 2015 to 2017. Published 31 May 2018. Available at: https://www.ons.gov.uk/peoplepopulationandcommunity/crimeandjustice/articles/womenmostatriskofexperiencingpartnerabuseinenglandandwales/yearsendingmarch2015to2017

Office of National Statistics [ONS] (2021) Sexual Orientation, UK: 2019. https://www.ons.gov.uk/peoplepopulationandcommunity/culturalidentity/sexuality/bulletins/sexualidentityuk/2019. Accessed 8 Jul 2021

Office for National Statistics [ONS] (2022) Domestic abuse in England and Wales overview: November 2022. Published 25 November 2022. Available at: https://www.ons.gov.uk/peoplepopulationandcommunity/crimeandjustice/bulletins/domesticabuseinenglandandwalesoverview/november2022

Pantalone DW, Hessler DM, Simoni JM (2010) Mental health pathways from interpersonal violence to help-related outcomes in HIV-positive sexual minority men. J Consult Clin Psychol 78(3):387

Pence E, Paymar M (1993) Education Groups for Men Who Batter. Springer Publishing Company, New York NY

Pitts M, Smith A, Mitchell A, Patel S (2006) Private lives: a report on the health and wellbeing of GLBTI Australians. Australian Research Centre in Sex, Health and Society, La Trobe University, Melbourne

Poushter J, Kent NO (2020) The global divide on homosexuality persists. Pew Research Centre. https://wwwpewresearchorg/global/2020/06/25/global-divide-on-homosexuality-persists/. Accessed 0 Jul 2021

Riger S, Raja S, Camacho J (2002) The radiating impact of intimate partner violence. J Interpers Violence 17(2):184–205

Ristock J (2002) No more secrets: violence in lesbian relationships. Routledge, London

Roch A, Ritchie G, Morton J (2010) Out of sight, out of mind? Transgender people's experiences of domestic abuse. LGBT Youth Scotland and the Scottish Transgender Alliance, Edinburgh. https://www.scottishtrans.org/wp-content/uploads/2013/03/trans_domestic_abuse.pdf Accessed 29 Oct 2021

Rogers M (2016) Breaking down barriers: the potential for social care practice with trans survivors of domestic abuse. Health Soc Care Community 24(1):68–76

Rogers M (2019) Challenging cisgenderism through trans people's narratives of domestic violence and abuse. Sexualities 22(5–6):803–820. https://doi.org/10.1177/1363460716681475

Rogers M (2020) Exploring the domestic abuse narratives of trans and non-binary people and the role of cisgenderism in identity abuse, misgendering and pathologizing. Violence Against Women 27(12–13):2187–2207. https://doi.org/10.1177/1077801220971368

Russell S, Ryan C, Toomey R, Diaz R, Sanchez J (2011) Lesbian, gay, bisexual, and transgender adolescent school victimisation: implications for young adult health and adjustment. J Sch Health 81:223–230

SafeLives (2018) Free to be safe: LGBT+ people experiencing domestic abuse. https://safelives.org.uk/sites/default/files/resources/Free%20to%20be%20safe%20web.pdf. Accessed 29 Oct 2021

Santoniccolo F, Trombetta T, Rollè L (2021) The help-seeking process in same-sex intimate partner violence: a systematic review. Sex Res Social Policy 20:391. https://doi.org/10.1007/s13178-021-00629-z

Serano J (2007) Whipping girl: a transsexual woman on sexism and the scapegoating of femininity. Seal Press, Berkeley, CA

Social Ecological Correlates of Polyvictimization among a National Sample of Transgender Genderqueer and Cisgender Sexual Minority Adolescents Child Abuse & Neglect (2017) 671–12 https://doi.org/10.1016/j.chiabu.2017.02.017

Stark E (2007) Coercive control: how men entrap women in personal life. Oxford University Press, Oxford

Stets JE, Straus MA (1989) Gender differences in reporting marital violence and its medical and psychological consequences. In: Straus MA, Gelles RJ (eds) Physical violence in American families: risk factors and adaptations to violence in 8,145 families. Transaction Publishing, New Brunswick, NJ, pp 227–244

Straus MA (2010) Thirty years of denying the evidence on gender symmetry in partner violence: implications for prevention and treatment. Partn Abus 1(3):332–362

Straus M, Hamby S, Boney-McCoy S, Sugarman DB (1996) The revised conflict tactics scales (CTS2): development and preliminary psychometric data. J Fam Issues 17(3):283–316

Stripe N (2020) Domestic abuse in England and Wales overview: November 2020. https://www.ons.gov.uk/peoplepopulationandcommunity/crimeandjustice/bulletins/domesticabuseinenglandandwalesoverview/november2020. Accessed 8 Jul 2021

United Nations (2021) What is domestic abuse? https://www.un.org/en/coronavirus/what-is-domestic-abuse. Accessed 23 Jul 2021

Valentine SE, Peitzmeier SM, King DS, O'Cleirigh C, Marquez SM, Presley C, Potter J (2017) Disparities in exposure to intimate partner violence among transgender/gender nonconforming and sexual minority primary care patients. LGBT Health 4:260–267

Valido A, Rivas-Koehl M, Espelage DL, Robinson LE, Kuehl T, Mintz S, Wyman P (2021) Protective factors of homophobic name-calling and sexual violence perpetration and victimisation among LGB, trans, and heterosexual high school students. Sch Ment Heal 13:602–615

Walters ML, Lippy C (2016) Intimate partner violence in LGBT communities. In: Cuevas CA, Rennison CM (eds) The Wiley handbook on the psychology of violence. Wiley, Chichester p, pp 695–714

Walters ML, Chen J, Breidling MH (2013) The National Intimate Partner and Sexual Violence Survey: 2010 findings on victimisation by sexual orientation. National Centre for Injury Prevention and Control, Atlanta Centres for Disease Control and Prevention https://wwwcdc-gov/violenceprevention/pdf/nisvs_sofindingspdf. Accessed 21 Oct 2021

Warwick I, Chase E, Aggleton P, Sanders S (2004) Homophobia, sexual orientation and schools: a review and implications for action. Research report RR594. Department of Education and Skills, London. http://webarchive.nationalarchives.gov.UK/20130401151715/https://www.education.gov.UK/publications/RSG/AllPublications/Page1/RR594. Accessed 21 Oct 2021

Weeks J, Heaphy B, Donovan C (2001) Same-sex intimacies: families of choice and other life experiments. Routledge, London

World Health Organisation (2021) Violence against women fact sheet. https://www.who.int/news-room/fact-sheets/detail/violence-against-women. Accessed 23 Jul 2021

Kirsty McGregor is a Senior Lecturer in Criminology at the University of Brighton. Her research examines domestic and sexual violence and abuse using an intersectional perspective, with a focus on victimisation and help-seeking experiences.

Older Adult Mistreatment

Silvia Fraga Dominguez, Jennifer E. Storey, and Michaela M. Rogers

Learning Objectives
Having read this chapter, you should be able to understand:

- The characteristics of older adult mistreatment.
- Risk factors for older adult mistreatment relating to victims and perpetrators and priorities for case management.
- That vulnerability to older adult mistreatment is multifaceted and may not always be visible.
- That many barriers may prevent older adults from reporting mistreatment.

Introduction

In this chapter, we introduce the reader to the phenomenon of older adult mistreatment (also known as elder abuse, and older adult abuse; see Box 1), which is estimated to affect one in six adults aged 60 and older and which has major consequences for victims and society (Dong 2015; Yon et al. 2017). In order to avoid any negative

S. Fraga Dominguez
Department of Psychology, Birmingham City University, Birmingham, UK
e-mail: Silvia.fragadominguez@bcu.ac.uk

J. E. Storey
School of Psychology at the University of Kent, Kent, UK
e-mail: j.storey@kent.ac.uk

M. M. Rogers (✉)
Department of Sociological Studies, University of Sheffield, Sheffield, UK
e-mail: m.rogers@sheffield.ac.uk

P. Ali, M. M. Rogers (eds.), *Gender-Based Violence: A Comprehensive Guide*,
https://doi.org/10.1007/978-3-031-05640-6_35

or culturally specific connotations associated with the term 'elder' (Lithwick et al. 2000) and with the aim of including both abuse and neglect (O'Keeffe et al. 2007), we adopt the term older adult mistreatment. In this chapter, we define and describe older adult mistreatment, as well as its types, and provide a historical context for this phenomenon. We also introduce the reader to explanatory theories and discuss evidence-based risk factors and case management. We outline worldwide prevalence estimates and the impact that older adult mistreatment has on victims and society. We finish with a discussion of available approaches to address older adult mistreatment and illustrate some challenges to intervention, including barriers to reporting for victims, by discussing a high-profile case.

Definition and Types

Older adult mistreatment (OAM) can be defined in multiple ways, and definitions remain a source of much disagreement in the field. A frequently used definition is the one coined by the UK charity Hourglass in 1995 (formerly known as Action on Elder Abuse) and which has been adopted by the World Health Organization (WHO) (Action on Elder Abuse 1995; O'Brien et al. 2016; WHO 2022). According to this definition, OAM is a 'single or repeated act, or lack of appropriate action, occurring within any relationship where there is an expectation of trust, which causes harm or distress to an older person' (WHO 2022, para. 2). However, we acknowledge that researchers and practitioners may have different conceptions which may not coincide with older adults' perceptions of mistreatment (Fraga Dominguez et al. 2021).

The five most commonly acknowledged types of OAM are financial abuse or exploitation, physical abuse, psychological or emotional abuse, neglect and sexual abuse (Lachs and Pillemer 2015; WHO 2022). They are defined by Lachs and Pillemer (2015: 1947) as follows:

- Financial abuse or exploitation: 'misappropriation of an older person's money or property'.
- Physical abuse: 'acts carried out with the intention to cause physical pain or injury'.
- Psychological or emotional abuse: 'acts carried out with the aim of causing emotional pain or injury'.
- Neglect: 'failure of a designated caregiver to meet the needs of a dependent older person'.
- Sexual abuse: 'nonconsensual sexual contact of any kind'.

Victims may suffer several types concurrently (Jackson and Hafemeister 2011; Rosen et al. 2019): a phenomenon known as poly-victimisation. Another type of mistreatment frequently considered in definitions is self-neglect or failure to care for oneself (Lachs and Pillemer 2015). However, self-neglect does not fit within the understanding of OAM as a type of interpersonal violence that takes place between two people (a victim and a perpetrator). It is the latter which is the position adopted in this chapter.

OAM is a diverse type of interpersonal violence (Butchart and Mikton 2014; Lithwick et al. 2000). It can happen at the older person's home, or be institutional, occurring at residential facilities, such as care or nursing homes (Yon et al. 2017, 2018). In addition, it can be perpetrated by a variety of individuals: family members—most commonly adult children and/or partners of the victim—friends, neighbours and professionals, with evidence suggesting that the prevalence of different perpetrator types may vary by type of abuse (Jackson 2016; Lithwick et al. 2000). For example, adult children have been identified as the most common perpetrators of neglect and partners as the most common perpetrators of physical abuse (Jackson 2016).

Although there is no agreement among researchers, practitioners or organisations as to when 'older age' begins and, thus, who is considered an older adult, this chapter will consider those persons aged 60 and above, which is consistent with the WHO (2022). However, we recognise that this age cut-off is not universal, that it is dynamic and may change as the population ages and vulnerabilities change and that population-specific age expectancy may also need to be considered (Fraga Dominguez et al. 2021).

Prevalence

Many prevalence studies have been conducted on OAM, usually at national level, and have obtained quite varied estimates (Yon et al. 2017). This disparity may be explained by geographic variation and sample size or could arise from the use of different measures or definitions of OAM and different time periods considered (e.g. in the past year, since becoming 'older') (Pillemer et al. 2016; Yon et al. 2017). Despite being understood as a worldwide issue, there is a lot of variation across countries in terms of awareness and perceptions of OAM (Butchart and Mikton 2014). It is important to acknowledge that the perceptions of older adults about mistreatment are understood to be dependent on cultural considerations (Dong 2015; Pillemer et al. 2016). Hence, the same behaviour (e.g. abandonment) may be perceived as abusive in one country but not in others, and this will likely affect prevalence estimates. A systematic review and meta-analysis of research on older adults living in the community indicated that 15% of older adults had been victimised in the past year (Yon et al. 2017). Extrapolating that figure to the worldwide population at the time, the authors estimated that 141 million adults aged 60 and older could be the victims of OAM every year (Yon et al. 2017). This estimate will only increase with the ageing of the population. Yon et al. (2017) also found that abuse varied by type with the most common type being psychological, followed by financial, while sexual abuse had the lowest prevalence.

In a subsequent study, researchers reviewed the available data for OAM occurring in institutions such as hospitals and care homes (Yon et al. 2018). They reviewed studies that were based on staff or older adults reporting abuse. Yon and colleagues found that 64% of staff self-reported engaging in mistreatment in the past year, most commonly psychological abuse. There were too few studies based on older adult reporting to estimate prevalence (Yon et al. 2018). Nevertheless, given the relatively large prevalence estimates from available studies on staff, it is suggested that professionals, both in social services and healthcare, may routinely encounter OAM cases (Pillemer et al. 2016).

Despite global research efforts, it is also worth noting that these prevalence estimates may underestimate the true population prevalence of OAM; both because of the under-reporting of abuse by older adults and because those potentially most at risk from mistreatment—people with a cognitive impairment—are generally excluded from prevalence studies (Fraga Dominguez et al. 2021; Pillemer et al. 2016; Rosen et al. 2019). To illustrate under-reporting to formal services, Lachs and Berman (2011) compared self-reported data by older adults with the number of cases referred to services (i.e. social services, law enforcement) and found that the number of self-reported cases was nearly 24 times greater than the number of referred cases, meaning only about 1 in 24 victims reports abuse.

Prevalence and Gender

In terms of variation by gender, there is disagreement as to whether women are more at risk of OAM than men. Yon et al. (2017) found no significant difference in prevalence estimates by gender in their systematic review, suggesting both men and women are equally likely to suffer OAM. However, there is some evidence indicating that women may be more at risk of mistreatment than men (Pillemer et al. 2016). It is arguable that this may be due to the fact that women live longer than men and thus spend more time at risk of OAM (O'Brien et al. 2016). Yon et al. (2017) indicated that, given the bias in the literature towards high-income countries, the gender symmetry found in their systematic review may no longer apply once there is more availability of studies in low- and middle-income countries. In particular, in patriarchal cultures or countries where women have an inferior social status, they may be more at risk than men of suffering specific types of abuse (Krug et al. 2002; Pillemer et al. 2016). See the next section for a further discussion of international differences.

In the most extreme cases, OAM can be fatal; however, most of the available research on the homicide of older adults have not reported data on whether the older adults were previously the victims of OAM (Rogers and Storey 2019). In a systematic review of homicide of older people, overall, Rogers and Storey (2019) found some variation by gender. Older women were more likely than older men to be killed at home and by someone known to them. Thus, it is possible that older women are more likely to fall victim to extreme violence resulting in homicide.

International Comparison

Different countries and cultures have divergent understandings and perceptions of OAM (Dong 2015; Zannettino et al. 2015) which are likely to affect reporting rates and the findings of prevalence studies. Thus, it is important to consider that definitions of OAM exist in a cultural context (Zannettino et al. 2015). This also applies when studying OAM among ethnic minorities within countries (Dong 2015). There are practices affecting older women in middle- and low-income countries that may not be perceived as abusive in those cultures or countries, but which result in harm (Krug et al. 2002; Pillemer et al. 2016). For example, mourning practices for widows in certain parts of the world (i.e. parts of Africa and India) involve behaviours, such as expulsion from their homes or forced marriages, that would be considered abusive elsewhere (Krug et al. 2002). Relatedly, there are different risks for older adults, particularly older women, depending on their social status in those countries or cultures. For instance, limited access to financial resources or universal pensions—only available to 30% of the older adult population—may place older adults at higher risk of harm in middle- and low-income countries by leading to higher dependency on their families for support (Krug et al. 2002). Older women may be especially affected by these structural factors due to lack of access to financial resources and having experienced oppression or marginalisation throughout their lives, likely leading to increased dependence in later life (Krug et al. 2002; Zannettino et al. 2015).

Box 1
Definition

Older adult mistreatment is a 'single or repeated act, or lack of appropriate action, occurring within any relationship where there is an expectation of trust, which causes harm or distress to an older person' (WHO 2022, para. 2).

Alternative terminology

Elder abuse, elder mistreatment, elder maltreatment, elder neglect, older adult abuse, domestic violence, abuse of older people.

Historical Context

OAM is not a new phenomenon; however, it has only recently received increased attention and been studied with more rigour, partly resulting from a wider concern due to the ageing of the population (Lachs and Pillemer 2015; Storey 2020; Yon et al. 2017). Nevertheless, research and awareness of OAM have not moved at the same pace worldwide. The issue started to garner more attention in the 1970s (O'Brien et al. 2016). Initially, it was understood as an issue occurring primarily in the context of caregiving relationships, particularly between a vulnerable older adult and their family members, with caregiver stress and burden regarded as the major causes for its occurrence (Anetzberger 2000). However, theories on caregiver stress have been sidelined as OAM has been recognised as a more complex and multifaceted type of interpersonal violence, with multiple contributing causes and consequences, as well as heterogeneity in perpetrator and victim characteristics (Jackson 2016; Lithwick et al. 2000). Despite growing attention, research on OAM has not been uniform, with a bias towards Western and high-income populations, resulting in a gap in our knowledge of the mistreatment of diverse older populations (Butchart and Mikton 2014; Dong 2015; Pillemer et al. 2016). Nonetheless, there are no reasons to understand OAM as an issue specific to certain countries, and it is currently recognised internationally as a major problem (Pillemer et al. 2016).

Explanatory Theories

A variety of explanatory theories have been forwarded to understand and explain OAM. Many are adaptations of theories from fields previously used to explain other phenomena such as child abuse or intimate partner violence (O'Brien et al. 2016). In early scholarship, one of the major explanatory theories of OAM was 'caregiver stress' (Anetzberger 2000). It was understood that perpetrators were frequently caregivers of the victim, particularly family members, and that the victim was dependent on them and others for meeting their care needs (e.g. personal care, feeding). Mistreatment occurred as a result of the stress of caregiving for a vulnerable older adult. This explanation has been critiqued due to a lack of empirical evidence (Jackson 2016). It is, however, currently regarded as a potential explanation for a subset of OAM cases, usually where a caregiver lacks adequate support (O'Brien et al. 2016).

The field has moved towards a more comprehensive range of theories that reflect the growing evidence demonstrating that OAM is a complex and multifaceted phenomenon. The ecological systems theory (Bronfenbrenner 1979) is a useful model for understanding OAM which identifies the influence of different environmental systems on the individual—for example, the family, workplace or community—as well as more structural influences such as dominant norms and beliefs (Bronfenbrenner 1979). Ecological approaches advance an understanding that, like with violence in general, no single factor can explain OAM as it is a complex problem resulting from the interaction of factors at individual, relationship, community and societal levels (Fraga et al. 2014; Krug et al. 2002).

At a macro or societal level, we should consider explanatory theories related to social and cultural norms, as well as institutions and policies that contribute to inequality (Fraga et al. 2014; Krug et al. 2002). At this level, ageism, as a prejudicial ideology which results in discrimination based on a person's age, has been increasingly discussed in the field of OAM as a contributing factor (Pillemer et al. 2021; WHO 2022). Recently, Pillemer et al. (2021) argued that the ways in which ageism could be linked to OAM are under-explored. Although they concluded that the evidence of the relationship between OAM and ageism was limited, they proposed a model with pathways that could explain this association and advocated for future research on the topic.

Risk Factors and Risk Management

Consistent with the ecological systems theory (Bronfenbrenner 1979), risk and protective factors for OAM are understood to occur at different levels including individual, relationship, community and society (WHO 2022). Highlighting individual risk, a recent study on OAM reviewed and synthesised 198 studies and identified several dynamic risk and vulnerability factors relating to the perpetrators and victims of OAM, respectively (Storey 2020). Dynamic risk factors are those that can be modified through intervention, and thus, their identification for assessment and change is an essential component in case management to reduce risk (Douglas et al. 2014). In this review, Storey (2020) identified eight common perpetrator risk factors that increase the risk of perpetrating mistreatment and victim vulnerability factors that place the victim at risk of mistreatment:

- Problems with physical health, including illness and functional impairment.
- Problems with mental health, including major mental disorder, personality disorder and cognitive impairment.
- Problems with substance abuse, including the use of illegal substances and misuse of legal substances, such as alcohol and prescribed medications.
- Problems with stress and coping, such as an inability to cope with life problems.
- Problems with attitudes: in the case of perpetrators, related to caregiving, older persons and the rights of others; in the case of victims, minimisation or inconsistent attitudes relating to the perpetrator and/or their behaviour.
- Victimisation: in the case of perpetrators, experienced or witnessed during childhood or adolescence; in the case of victims, during their lifetime and excluding the current case of mistreatment by the perpetrator.
- Problems with relationships, including conflictual relationships and social isolation.
- Dependency: victim's dependency on the perpetrator and perpetrator's dependency on the victim or other individuals.

In addition, Storey (2020) highlighted the importance of factors related to the mistreatment experienced and the community or institution in which the victim and perpetrator reside. Societal factors, such as inequality or ageism, are also understood to contribute to OAM occurrence, as explained in the previous section (Fraga et al. 2014; Pillemer et al. 2021).

In comparison, research on protective factors for OAM is limited. Nevertheless, social support and active social networks have been identified as lowering the risk of mistreatment (Pillemer et al. 2016). Informal and formal social support have also been identified as facilitators to help-seeking from the perspective of OAM victims (Fraga Dominguez et al. 2021).

Impact

The impact of OAM on victims has been well documented (Dong 2015). Studies have linked OAM to severe physical, psychological and economic consequences for victims (Dong 2015; Jackson and Hafemeister 2011). At a physical and psychological level, mistreatment has been associated with premature mortality and increased rates of healthcare use, long-term care placement, hospitalisation and depression (Dong 2015; Yunus et al. 2019). Significantly, a longitudinal study found that OAM victims were three times more likely to have died by the end of the 13-year follow-up period compared to non-victims (Lachs et al. 1998). Economic impacts identified include increased healthcare costs (Dong 2015), as well as direct financial loss in cases of financial abuse, averaging 100,000 dollars in one US study (Jackson and Hafemeister 2011).

OAM also has a societal level impact, with estimates of costs amounting to billions of dollars in the United States annually, encompassing the costs of services provided to victims, medical expenses and direct financial loss for victims (Dong 2015; Rosen et al. 2019). Apart from the impact on society more generally, recent research has identified that OAM can also have a negative psychological or financial effect on informal supporters of the victim, such as family members (Breckman et al. 2018; Fraga Dominguez et al. 2022).

Policy and Practice

The existence of legislation and interventions to prevent or address OAM varies geographically, with many countries lacking legislation, failing to enforce what legislation does exist or lacking dedicated services to facilitate interventions (Butchart and Mikton 2014; Pillemer et al. 2016; Rosen et al. 2019). From a legal and judicial perspective, and with the aim of identifying cases, many countries have developed mandatory reporting laws for OAM (Krug et al. 2002); however, the scope of these laws and the individuals who are designated as mandated reporters vary widely across and within countries (Donnelly 2019; Rosen et al. 2019). Countries like the United States have adopted a criminalisation approach to OAM, which has evidenced major challenges in prosecuting these cases, including a lack of support from victims and different degrees of success depending on the type of abuse prosecuted (Jackson 2016; Jackson and Hafemeister 2011).

In a worldwide survey, two-thirds of countries did not have adult protective services in place to assist vulnerable older adults (Butchart and Mikton 2014). Intervention for OAM has traditionally received less attention from the literature as compared to other areas of OAM (Lithwick et al. 2000). In a recent review of existing OAM programmes, it was found that most of the programmes reviewed focused on intervening in existing mistreatment cases, as opposed to prevention or identification (Rosen et al. 2019). In addition, many of the interventions available focus on the victim, with less focus on the perpetrator. When they do focus on the perpetrator, a common emphasis is on providing caregiver support (Jackson 2016; Rosen et al.

2019), which is problematic given the lack of support for the caregiver stress model. Overall, high-quality evaluation of existing intervention programmes is generally lacking (Rosen et al. 2019).

There is agreement that OAM cases should be managed by a multidisciplinary team—in countries where multiple services are available—with a focus on both victims and perpetrators (Lithwick et al. 2000; Pillemer et al. 2016; Storey 2020; Storey et al. 2022). Pillemer et al. (2016) reviewed available evidence and identified several promising interventions including caregiver interventions, money management programmes for older adults at risk of financial abuse, helplines for victims and emergency shelters. A more recent study by Storey et al. (2022) examined the efficacy of 12 intervention categories and 30 intervention strategies implemented by a Canadian multidisciplinary programme and identified several strategies with the most positive outcomes. These strategies focused both on the victim and the perpetrator and included supervision, removing access to methods of mistreatment, physical treatment for the perpetrator, mental health and substance abuse education for the victim and victim capacity assessment.

Implications for Policy, Practice and Research

Given the multifaceted nature and complexity of OAM, policy and practice are likely to benefit from a victim-centred approach (Spangler and Brandl 2007). A one-size-fits-all approach is unlikely to meet the needs of victims and effectively address perpetrator risk factors (Storey 2020). The use of a risk management approach focused on assessing and addressing dynamic risk factors is likely to be most successful in intervening in existing cases and preventing further mistreatment (Douglas et al. 2014; Storey 2020). Empirically based tools to support this practice are now becoming available (Storey et al. 2021).

Any type of intervention, including risk management, may meet with reluctance from victims and perpetrators, who may not be willing to accept support (Lithwick et al. 2000; Storey et al. 2022). A decision to intervene from the perspective of professionals may be dependent on mandatory reporting legislation, as well as on whether a victim has mental capacity, the latter of which may need to be determined through a formal capacity assessment (Fraga Dominguez et al. 2020; Storey et al. 2022). Where the victim lacks capacity to make their own decisions, the role of formal and informal supporters will be essential in ensuring victim safety (Fraga Dominguez et al. 2020). This is likely to be a common scenario, due to cognitive limitations being an important risk factor, and will be associated with particular challenges, such as victims' difficulty recalling the events of the abuse (Fraga Dominguez et al. 2020; Pillemer et al. 2016; see Box 2 for a case example involving cognitive limitations).

Given prevalence estimates, practitioners in health and social care are expected to encounter cases of OAM on a regular basis; thus, training is essential (Pillemer et al. 2016; Yon et al. 2017). Along with training on identifying signs of mistreatment, practitioners need to receive evidence-based information about barriers to help-seeking and work with victims to assess and address those barriers (Fraga Dominguez et al. 2020). A recent systematic review of the literature (Fraga Dominguez et al. 2021) identified that victims experience many barriers to help-seeking, relating to different areas (individual, community, societal). Some of the barriers that may need to be addressed are related to the victim's fear of consequences for themselves (e.g. institutionalisation) or the perpetrator (e.g. homelessness), individual feelings (e.g. shame), an ineffective social network, problems with access to formal services and the victim's lack of perception of mistreatment. A consideration of these barriers, which may or not be present depending on the specific relationship type between the victim and the perpetrator and OAM suffered, will be an important element of intervention design and implementation (Fraga Dominguez et al. 2020; Fraga Dominguez et al. 2021; Spangler and Brandl 2007).

In terms of research, there are many existing gaps in the field of OAM. Further studies on the effectiveness of current intervention approaches are a priority (Rosen et al. 2019). Similarly, further research on evidence-based risk management and its effectiveness is necessary (Storey 2020). Given the magnitude of under-reporting, continued research to understand its causes and to increase reporting is necessary. Because, traditionally, research on barriers to reporting has focused on professionals, continued research on the perspectives of victims is necessary (Fraga Dominguez et al. 2021). Given that research indicates that victims and perpetrators may reject intervention (Lithwick et al. 2000; Storey et al. 2022), a growing understanding of the views of victims and perpetrators towards third-party intervention will be essential in shaping professionals' approaches to combat OAM.

Box 2

Case Study

Brooke Astor (1902–2007) was an American philanthropist, socialite and writer and the subject of one of the first high-profile cases of OAM in the United States. In the last years of her life, she was financially abused by her son, who, after her death, was found guilty of stealing millions and tampering with his mother's state. Mrs. Astor's son allegedly neglected his mother's care in order to enrich himself. The case of Brooke Astor is one of many allegations involving well-known people such as comic book writer Stan Lee (1922–2018) and actor Mickey Rooney (1920–2014). Along with raising national awareness about OAM, these cases have also demonstrated that vulnerability to OAM is multifaceted and that even those in a privileged position (e.g. socially and financially) can be vulnerable to mistreatment and have difficulties reporting it. In the case of Brooke Astor, the abuse she experienced allegedly coincided with her diagnosis of Alzheimer's and increased dependency, making it harder for Mrs. Astor to notice and report the abuse. The abuse was also facilitated by the fact that Mrs. Astor's son was his mother's power of attorney. Other family members suspected mistreatment, and it was Mrs. Astor's grandson who eventually played a large role in the indictment of

Mrs. Astor's son (his own father), helped by other concerned family, friends and caregivers. This case highlights the critical role of other supportive family members and friends in cases where victims may not be able to disclose abuse and the difficulty of that role for family members who may need to challenge other relatives in order to protect their loved ones. As a result of his personal story with OAM, Mrs. Astor's grandson became an advocate for OAM and works to increase awareness and advance justice for older adults.

Summary

- OAM is a prevalent problem, affecting many older women and men worldwide, with major consequences for victims and society.
- The magnitude of OAM is likely underestimated and likely to increase as the worldwide population ages.
- There are many challenges to addressing OAM, due to its multifaceted nature, which does not suit a one-size-fits-all approach.
- Evidence on its aetiology, risk factors and barriers to help-seeking indicates that a victim-centred approach from services is likely to be the most successful in engaging victims and preventing further mistreatment for current and potential victims.
- Further research involving victims of OAM which amplifies their voices will be helpful in understanding barriers to reporting and guiding intervention.

References

Action on Elder Abuse (1995) New definition of abuse. Action on Elder Abuse Bulletin, vol 11. Action on Elder Abuse, London

Anetzberger GJ (2000) Caregiving: primary cause of elder abuse? Generations 24(2):46–52

Breckman R, Burnes D, Ross S, Marshall PC, Suitor JJ, Lachs MS, Pillemer K (2018) When helping hurts: nonabusing family, friends, and neighbors in the lives of elder mistreatment victims. Gerontologist 58(4):719–723

Bronfenbrenner U (1979) The ecology of human development. Harvard University Press, Harvard

Butchart A, Mikton C (2014) Global status report on violence prevention. World Health Organization, Geneva

Dong XQ (2015) Elder abuse: systematic review and implications for practice. J Am Geriatr Soc 63(6):1214–1238

Donnelly S (2019) Mandatory reporting and adult safeguarding: a rapid realist review. J Adult Protect 21(5):241–251

Douglas KS, Hart SD, Groscup JL, Litwack TR (2014) Assessing violence risk. Wiley, Hoboken, NJ

Fraga Dominguez S, Valiquette J, Storey JE, Glorney E (2020) Elder abuse detection and intervention: challenges for professionals and strategies for engagement from a Canadian specialist service. J Forensic Nurs 16(4):199–206

Fraga Dominguez S, Storey JE, Glorney E (2021) Help-seeking behavior in victims of elder abuse: a systematic review. Trauma Violence Abuse 22(3):466–480

Fraga Dominguez S, Storey JE, Glorney E (2022) Informal supporters of elder abuse victims: who are they and what is their experience seeking help? J Fam Violence 37:1013–1026. https://doi.org/10.1007/s10896-021-00347-5

Fraga S, Lindert J, Barros H, Torres-Gonzalez F, Ioannidi-Kapolou E, Melchiorre MG, Stankunas M, Soares JF (2014) Elder abuse and socioeconomic inequalities: a multilevel study in 7 European countries. Prev Med 61:42–47

Jackson SL (2016) All elder abuse perpetrators are not alike: the heterogeneity of elder abuse perpetrators and implications for intervention. Int J Offender Ther Comp Criminol 60(3):265–285

Jackson SL, Hafemeister TL (2011) Financial abuse of elderly people vs. other forms of elder abuse: assessing their dynamics, risk factors, and society's response. National Institute of Justice, Rockville

Krug EG, Dahlberg LL, Mercy JA, Zwi AB, Lozano R (2002) World report on violence and health. World Health Organization. https://apps.who.int/iris/bitstream/handle/10665/42495/9241545615_eng.pdf?sequence=1

Lachs MS, Berman J (2011) Under the radar: New York state elder abuse prevalence study, self-reported relevance and documented case studies. Lifespan of Greater Rochester, Inc., Weill Cornell medical Center of Cornell University, and New York City Department for the Aging, New York

Lachs MS, Pillemer KA (2015) Elder abuse. N Engl J Med 373(20):1947–1956

Lachs MS, Williams CS, O'Brien S, Pillemer K, Charleson ME (1998) The mortality of elder mistreatment. JAMA 280(5):428–432

Lithwick M, Beaulieu M, Gravel S, Straka SM (2000) The mistreatment of older adults: perpetrator-victim relationships and interventions. J Elder Abuse Negl 11(4):95–112

O'Brien M, O'Brien-Olinger S, Boccaletti L, Milianta S, Caciula I, Laurola H, Perttu S, Kadzik-Bartoszewska A, Canning K, Quinn S (2016) Elder abuse context and theory: Finland, Ireland, Italy and Romania, European Union Erasmus +

O'Keeffe M, Hills A, Doyle M, McCreadie C, Scholes S, Constantine R, Tinker A, Manthorpe J, Biggs S, Erens B (2007) UK study of abuse and neglect of older people: prevalence survey report. National Center for Social Research, London

Pillemer K, Burnes D, Riffin C, Lachs MS (2016) Elder abuse: global situation, risk factors, and prevention strategies. Gerontologist 56(Suppl_2):S194–S205

Pillemer K, Burnes D, MacNeil A (2021) Investigating the connection between ageism and elder mistreatment. Nat Aging 1(2):159–164

Rogers MM, Storey JE (2019) Elder homicide: a systematic literature review. Aggress Violent Behav 48:141–151

Rosen T, Elman A, Dion S, Delgado D, Demetres M, Breckman R, Lees K, Dash K, Lang D, Bonner A, Burnett J, Dyer CB, Snyder R, Berman A, Fulmer T, Lachs MS (2019) Review of programs to combat elder mistreatment: focus on hospitals and level of resources needed. J Am Geriatr Soc 67(6):1286–1294

Spangler D, Brandl B (2007) Abuse in later life: power and control dynamics and a victim-centered response. J Am Psychiatr Nurses Assoc 12(6):322–331

Storey JE (2020) Risk factors for elder abuse and neglect: a review of the literature. Aggress Violent Behav 50:101339

Storey JE, Hart SD, Kropp PR (2021) The harm to older persons evaluation (HOPE): user manual. Countering and Ending Abuse via Structured Evaluation (CEASE International Limited), Canterbury

Storey JE, Hart S, Perka MR (2022) Identifying interventions and their efficacy as used by a community agency managing and responding to elder abuse. J Appl Gerontol 41(1):103–112

World Health Organization (2022) Abuse of older people. https://www.who.int/news-room/fact-sheets/detail/abuse-of-olderpeople

Yon Y, Milton CR, Gassoumis ZD, Wilber KH (2017) Elder abuse prevalence in community settings: a systematic review and meta-analysis. Lancet Glob Health 5(2):e147–e156

Yon Y, Ramiro-Gonzalez M, Milton CR, Huber M, Sethi D (2018) The prevalence of elder abuse in institutional settings: a systematic review and meta-analysis. Eur J Public Health 29(1):58–67

Yunus RM, Hairi NN, Choo WY (2019) Consequences of elder abuse and neglect: a systematic review of observational studies. Trauma Violence Abuse 20(2):197–213

Zannettino L, Bagshaw D, Wendt S, Adams V (2015) The role of emotional vulnerability and abuse in the financial exploitation of older people from culturally and linguistically diverse communities in Australia. J Elder Abuse Negl 27(1):74–89

Silvia Fraga Dominguez, PhD is a Lecturer in Forensic Psychology in the Department of Psychology at Birmingham City University. Her research examines interpersonal violence with a focus on older adults, help-seeking, and service access for victims and offenders.

Jennifer E. Storey, PhD and HCPC Registered Forensic Psychologist is a Senior Lecturer in Forensic Psychology in the School of Psychology at the University of Kent. Her research examines interpersonal violence with a focus on older adult abuse (or elder abuse), stalking and intimate partner violence.

Michaela M. Rogers, PhD is a Senior Lecturer in Social Work in the Department of Sociological Studies at the University of Sheffield. Her research examines interpersonal violence with a focus on marginalised groups, impacts, help-seeking, service access and service responses.

Violence Against Disabled People

Debbie Hager

Learning Objectives
Having read this chapter, you should be able to understand:

- Violence against disabled people.
- Power as a major driver of violence against disabled people.
- The social and economic changes required to address violence against disabled people.
- A twin track response to violence against disabled people.
- Why 'vulnerability' is not a useful concept in relation to violence against disabled people.

Introduction

In 2021, the World Health Organization (WHO) stated that violence against women is a global epidemic. Estimates published by WHO indicate that globally about 1 in 3 (30%) of women worldwide have been subjected to either physical and/or sexual intimate partner violence or non-partner sexual violence in their lifetime.

Violence against disabled women and men is significantly more of an epidemic with, in some studies, over 90% of disabled participants disclosing physical, sexual, and emotional/coercive violence (Hughes et al. 2012).

The term 'disabled people' is the language used by disabled people in New Zealand to reflect a social model of disability (see Box 1). In this model, disability is understood as an interaction between impairments that people have (physical, mental, intellectual, or sensory), and the disabling environmental and attitudinal

D. Hager (✉)
School of Population Health, University of Auckland, Auckland, New Zealand
e-mail: d.hager@auckland.ac.nz

P. Ali, M. M. Rogers (eds.), *Gender-Based Violence: A Comprehensive Guide*,
https://doi.org/10.1007/978-3-031-05640-6_36

barriers within society that limit disabled people's full and effective participation (United Nations Convention on the Rights of Persons with Disability (UNCRPD) 2007).

Box 1 Understanding Disability

Disabled person—language used in New Zealand to express that people have impairments, and are disabled by an inaccessible environment/society.

Terminology

Person with disability/persons with disability—language used in the United Nations Covenant on the Rights of Persons with Disability and a number of countries around the world to express the same understanding of society as disabling, rather than disability as individual deficit.

Explanation

Impairments can be: cognitive (the way people think and how their brains work); physical (the way people's bodies function and/or physical illness that impedes people's functioning); sensory (such as blindness or deafness); experienced as mental distress/psychosocial disabilities; and/or age-related impairment. Put simply, impairments can affect a person's mobility, senses, moods, physical health, and the way their brain functions.

Impairment can be caused by accident, illness, emotional or physical trauma, a genetic condition, aging, and it may be congenital or happen at birth (Domestic Violence and Disability Working Group 2010).

Disabled people share experiences and understandings of the world that are related to their perspective as a disabled person. They also often share experiences of: marginalisation; a world that is not constructed to be accessible to them; stigma and discrimination related to misunderstanding of disability; poverty; abuse; lack of voice and agency; and political and institutional processes that do not invite or listen to the voices of disabled people.

In relation to the diversity of disabled women, the Committee on the Rights of Persons with Disabilities (2016) state:

> Women with disabilities are not a homogenous group. They include: indigenous women; refugee, migrant, asylum seeker and internally displaced women; women in detention (hospitals, residential institutions, juvenile or correctional facilities and prisons); women living in poverty; women from different ethnic, religious and racial backgrounds; women with multiple disabilities and high levels of support; women with albinism; and lesbian, bi-sexual, transgender women, and intersex persons.

Disability is often stereotyped as an individual deficit. The definitions above challenge this and remind us that disabled people are valued members of every family and community.

Disabled people inhabit a complex intersection of age, ability, ethnicity, gender/sexual identity, gender roles and expectations, culture, and socioeconomic position. Some people are privileged by these intersections; for others, intersectional disadvantage is potentially complicated by discrimination related to racism, sexism, classism, homo/bi–/transphobia, and ableism. For indigenous people, there are also the disabling effects of colonisation.[1] Coupled with this intersectional dis/advantage is the stigma related to societal, cultural, and religious misunderstandings, and fear, of disability.

This complexity increases the risk of violence. The prevalence figures are higher for disabled people who have intersecting marginalisation—indigenous people, women, people who belong to lesbian, gay, bisexual, transgender, intersex and queer (LGBTIQ+) communities,[2] people who live in residential services where their autonomy and choices are limited, and disabled people who have less access to education, employment, and sufficient income than non-disabled people.

This means that solutions and responses to violence against disabled people cannot simply be additional to mainstream responses, but must be designed by disabled people to ensure that the intricacies of disabled people's lives are incorporated into mainstream and specialist prevention and service delivery.

Historical Context

Historically, disabled people across the world have been stigmatised, denied basic human rights, isolated, institutionalised, and have suffered multiple forms of violence, abuse, neglect, exploitation, and discrimination. One source of stigma against disabled people is the equating, in some societies, of impairment, including mental distress, with punishment for personal or parental wrongdoing and sin, the influence of evil spirits, or actions committed in previous incarnations (Covey 2005; Livneh 2012; Makasiale and Williams 1997; Nikora et al. 2004). There is also socialised mistrust of disabled people, partly as a consequence of the way that they have been portrayed in literature and other arts—for example, 'hunchbacks', the 'mentally retarded', or people with a limb missing are associated with evil (Margolis and Shapiro 1987: 18), with total helplessness, as undesirable and pitiable, or with incomplete bodies and minds (Margolis and Shapiro 1987: 21; Peters 1996).

Myths about disabled people (such as they are innocent and dependent), combine with social stereotypes about gender and disability (Shakespeare 1999) to reinforce concepts of the inferior status of disabled people, leading to significantly increased risk of sexual and other violence. This risk is exacerbated by ideas that disabled people—and in particular people with learning disability—are not affected by sexual violence and other abuse, as they are used to it and/or do not understand it (Calderbank 2000; McCarthy and Thompson 1997), enabling perpetrators to justify the abuse.

[1] Indigenous people are the first people of an area or country and colonisation means coming from another land and stealing and taking control of Indigenous people's land and other resources. '...in the simplest sense colonisation is the violent denial of the right of Indigenous peoples to continue governing themselves in their own lands' (Jackson, 2021). https://e-tangata.co.nz/comment-and-analysis/moana-jackson-decolonisation-and-the-stories-in-the-land/.

[2] LGBTIQ+ is shorthand for lesbian, gay, bisexual, trans, intersex, queer, and other minorities identities.

These discriminatory perceptions of disabled people result in reduced access to the determinants of health (for example, education, income, employment, and housing) (Ministry of Health 2021) causing poverty (Pinilla-Roncancio 2015); lack of social connections and relationships; loneliness (Hunt 2021); reduced fulfilment of individual potential; increased rates of violence, neglect, and exploitation (Krug et al. 2002); and increased rates of disability (Pinilla-Roncancio 2015). This inequity, and disregard of disabled people's human rights, was recognised in 2006 with the adoption of the United Nations Covenant on the Rights of Persons with Disabilities (UNCRPD).

Violence and Disability

Violence and disability intersect in two ways. People can be impaired by violence and disabled people are more likely to experience abuse than non-disabled people. These two things are not exclusive, as disabled people are harmed by the violence they experience, just as non-disabled people are.

Violence Causes Impairment

Any person who is abused, neglected, and/or exploited can be physically or emotionally damaged by physical, sexual, and emotional/coercive violence (Committee on the Rights of Persons with Disabilities 2016). Disabling effects of violence include:

- Physical injuries resulting in impairment, including blindness, hearing impairment, and impaired mobility.
- Physical illnesses that result in physical impairment.
- Brain injury and neurological disorders causing short and long-term impairment.
- Self-harming behaviours such as alcohol and substance abuse, eating disorders, sexual promiscuity, and lack of self-care that can result in physical and emotional harm.
- A range of mental health problems, particularly, significant mental distress, depression, anxiety, and post-traumatic stress disorder. All of these can seriously impair people's functioning.
- Physical injuries and mental distress can result from sexual violence.
- Chronic illness, pain, and loss of mental and physical functioning can be caused by both deliberate and unintentional neglect and abuse. (Domestic Violence and Disability Working Group 2010).

All of these things can lead to emotional distress, low self-esteem, and impact on people's ability to function, and therefore their ability to remove themselves from harm, or be perceived as credible when they disclose violence (Hager 2001). For example, research from New Zealand (Fanslow and Robinson 2004, Gulliver and Fanslow 2013) found that across the population, women (18–64 years) who had experienced severe physical violence were three times more likely to have suicidal thoughts and eight times more likely to attempt suicide, compared to women who had not experienced violence; moreover, they were almost four times more likely to report current symptoms of emotional distress and suicidal thoughts. The harms that accrue from violence and abuse also affect the health and well-being of families, particularly children and those who are caring for/supporting disabled and/or elderly people (Greer and Hunt 2020).

Forms of Violence Against Disabled People

Disabled people experience the range of violent abusive behaviours common to all abusive relationships—physical, sexual, verbal, emotional, and financial (Powers and Oschwald 2004), including patterns of power, control, and coercion (Powers and Oschwald 2004; Walter-Brice et al. 2012). However, there are forms of abuse that are more specific to disabled people, or that have more debilitating effects if people are disabled. The Committee on the Rights of Persons with Disabilities (2016) describe these as:

> ...physical force; economic coercion; trafficking; deception; misinformation; abandonment; the absence of free and informed consent and legal compulsion; neglect, including...withholding or denying access to medication; removing or controlling communication aids or refusal of assistance to communicate; denying personal mobility and accessibility such as removing or destroying accessibility features such as ramps, or assistive devices such as a white cane or mobility devices such as a wheelchair, refusal of caregivers to assist with daily living such as bathing, menstrual and/or sanitation management, dressing and eating, thus denying the right to live independently and freedom from degrading treatment; denial of food or water, or threat of any of these acts; bullying, verbal abuse, and ridicule on the grounds of disability; causing fear by intimidation; harming or threatening to harm, removing or killing pets or assistance dogs, or destroying objects; psychological manipulation; and controlling behaviours involving restricting face-to-face or virtual access to family, friends, or others.

It can also be:

- Keeping people short of money, making financial decisions for people, misusing their money or abuse of power of attorney.
- Never letting a disabled person be alone with a health practitioner or other helping professional.
- Preventing disabled women having children by, for example, forcing a woman to have an abortion or be sterilised (without consent), or preventing disabled women accessing IVF treatment.
- Rape.
- Undesired touching and/or disrespect for intimacy and privacy.
- Overmedicating—so people are sedated and unable to function.
- Restraint.
- Unwarranted/unwanted control.
- Deprivation of independence and autonomy.

- Isolation—emotional and social deprivation, loneliness.
- Seeking consent under duress.
- Threats to withdraw care or institutionalise people (Barbuto and Napolitano 2014; Domestic Violence and Disability Working Group 2010; Harpur and Douglas 2014; Healey et al. 2008; Powers and Oschwald 2004; Radford et al. 2006; Schulze 2017; Walker 2021).

Abuse can be intentional—doing something to hurt, frighten/threaten/intimidate, or upset a disabled person-or it can be caused by either intentional or unintentional neglect, such as forgetting to collect or provide medication (which could risk killing the person or make a person endure pain for much longer than necessary); not providing adequate care; leaving an immobile person alone for long periods of time; not providing meals; not helping a person to the toilet; not enabling a person to be hygienic and clean; or failing to provide support that is required, resulting in further harm such as bed sores, malnutrition, and pain (Domestic Violence and Disability Working Group 2010).

Women with Disabilities Australia say that:

> …violations of women's sexual and reproductive health and rights (such as forced sterilisation, forced abortion, forced pregnancy, criminalisation of abortion, denial or delay of safe abortion and/or post-abortion care, forced continuation of pregnancy, forced contraception, and abuse and mistreatment of women and girls seeking sexual and reproductive health information, goods and services), are forms of gender-based violence (2021: 6).

The majority of this harm goes unnoticed, undisclosed, and unreported as disabled people are ignored, silenced, lack resources and networks to disclose, and are treated as unfit, non-credible witnesses when they attempt to report their circumstances (Roguski 2013).

Prevalence

Around the world, it is very difficult to establish prevalence rates for the abuse of disabled people because of the lack of systematic data collection (Hughes et al. 2012). Thiara et al. (2012: 25) say 'The first thing the research literature tells us is that there is not very much of it in any country'. The research that does occur provides indications of prevalence, but no definitive rates, as the studies are all methodologically different, with different study populations (McCarthy and Thompson 1997).

Global studies yield conservative estimates that:

- Disabled adults face 1.5 times the risk of violence than the non-disabled population (Hughes et al. 2012) .
- Adults experiencing mental distress, or who have psychosocial illnesses, are at nearly four times the risk of experiencing violence (Hughes et al. 2012).

- Disabled children are almost four times as likely to experience violence than non-disabled children; and this rises to being five times more likely for children with intellectual disabilities (UNFPA 2018).

Despite the significantly higher rates of violence against disabled men in relation to non-disabled men (Ballan et al. 2017), disabled women are more likely to experience violence than disabled men; that is, there is still a gender disparity (Special Rapporteur on the Rights of Persons with Disabilities 2017). For example, in many studies, more than 90% of intellectually disabled women disclose sexual abuse (see, for example, Curry et al. 2011).

Contexts for Abuse

Disabled people experience violence perpetrated by people in a wider variety of settings and from a wider range of perpetrators than non-disabled people. They are abused by close family, friends, intimate partners, and wider family, and also by professionals and people in institutional and civil society settings. People who provide often very intimate care and support for disabled people in their homes, either paid or unpaid, abuse disabled people (Appleton-Dyer and Soupen 2017).

Abuse in residential and organisational settings can be perpetrated by staff, including health and welfare professionals, or other clients; in educational settings, by teachers and others such as caretakers and drivers; in home-based environments, by landlords, caregivers (Otkay and Tompkins 2004), and health and welfare professionals; and in community settings, by strangers, employers, neighbours, people in faith communities, in cultural groups, in the street, in businesses, and people in other civic environments (Roguski 2013).

Historically, institutions have been sites of violence and abuse for disabled people. Sir Robert Martin, one of the disabled people who participated in the development of the UNCRPD, was one of the many disabled children who, as babies or children, were put into institutions and there suffered many forms of violence, abuse, and neglect. Martin (McRae 2014: 13, 15) states

> The Farm earned itself a reputation for brutality…I don't remember being touched and cuddled like other kids are. I was never loved as a child. Me and all those other kids…People say these things didn't happen, but they did. Or they say that if these things did happen then they were unusual. That it was just a few people who did bad things. I've spoken to people all over New Zealand who lived in Kimberley and places like it. In fact, all over the world people have told me their stories and they are all the same: institutions are places of abuse. (McRae 2014: 34).

For many people, institutional abuse is not historical—it is a current reality. People with psychosocial illness and others who are placed under 'compulsory treatment orders' and disabled people put into institutional and/or residential care, report violence, sexual abuse, institutional cruelty and neglect, forced treatment, the use of seclusion and restraint, indefinite detention, lack of autonomy, and inadequate access to justice to challenge these abuses (Barnett 2015; Mirfin-Veitch and Conder 2017; Roguski 2013; Royal Commission of Inquiry into Historical Abuse in State Care and in the Care of Faith-based Institutions 2020; Van Eden 2013).

Power: An Underlying Cause of Violence Against Disabled People

At its core, violence is an abuse of power.
(Paula Tesoriero, New Zealand Disability Human Rights Commissioner, 2020)

To understand why the rates of violence against disabled women, men, and children are so high, we need to look at who is primarily harmed by family and gender-based violence. Those who are harmed are women, children, older men and women, people in the LGBTIQ+ community, and disabled people of all ages. As you look at this list, what you see are decreasing levels of societal power, respect, prestige and influence, and increasing levels of powerlessness (Murphy 2009) and social stigma.

Underpinning this harm are hierarchies of power—patriarchy, ableism, sexism, ageism, homo/bi–/transphobia, racism, religious intolerance, classism and, particularly, hegemonic masculinity (Connell 2005). The dominant hegemonic attributes in many Western countries are white, English-speaking, able-bodied, heterosexual, nominally Christian, wealthy or middle-class, independent, strong, competitive, powerful men. Some of these attributes (white and/or Christian, for example), are changed in other cultural contexts, but being a powerful, dominant man is ubiquitous. Hegemonic men are accorded the highest power in society—they are the respected voices and hold the most respected positions, attitudes, and attainments to be aspired to (Murphy 2009). The rewards for achieving this position are honour, prestige, recognition, respect, acceptance, and heroic status. Men who achieve this status frequently misuse power to control others (all others) simply because they can—and because being seen as powerful and controlling cements their positions at the top of the hierarchy.

Other men—those unable to achieve this heroic status—may use power to control and harm others—other men, women, and children—to prove themselves worthy of acceptance and respect. Men who are marginalised in the hegemonic hierarchy can feel powerless and, consequently, may misuse power to control others and make themselves feel more powerful by harming those they perceive to have less power—including disabled partners or family members.

In the hierarchy of masculinity, subordinated men are those perceived to have traits associated with hegemonically normative female gender roles, for example, some elderly frail or disabled men, and men who are rendered powerless by illness. These men are perceived to be hegemonically aligned with unvalued traits associated with women (for example, as helpless, subservient, or dependant) and therefore are accorded no power and respect in this hierarchy. These are men who can be, and are, harmed.

Note that nowhere on the above list are there women; women are not part of the hegemonic project (Murphy 2009). They are not valued, and consequently, are available to be harmed. Yet women see this behaviour modelled as the way to gain power and some will use the same or similar behaviours against those they have power over/perceive as powerless. There are men who are harmed, and women who abuse, but primarily, globally, interpersonal violence is men's violence against women and other men. It is these usually invisible and unchallenged power hegemonies that create increased risk of violence for those who are positioned as undervalued, under-resourced, and powerless and that, combined with myths and stigma about disabled people, create circumstances of increased violence, neglect, and exploitation.

Protection

When applied to disabled people, the concept of protection is often interpreted as paternalistic, frequently denying people agency and choice, and replacing people's own needs and wants with those imposed by others (for example, the difference between substituted decision-making and supported decision-making (UNFPA 2018). Disabled people report being protected against making independent decisions, such as trying something new or doing things differently, if others feel that it may put them at risk. Schulze (2017: 11) explains:

> Inhibiting the possibilities for persons with disabilities to make a mistake, to take a risk, is part of a larger pattern that contributes to a sense of lacking possibilities, of being violated in one's opportunities… 'the right to make a mistake' is part of a human being's dignity; there is something akin to the 'dignity of risk'.

When talking about violence against disabled women, Frohmader (2015: 5) talks about the concept of protection as rights rather than paternalism:

> … protect their [women and girls] rights to live free from violence, abuse, exploitation and neglect.

If disabled people are unable to enact these rights in their everyday lives, they lose autonomy; and the risk of violence increases as they are increasingly unable to remove themselves from harm.

Responding to Violence and Abuse

Disability is not a straightforward concept. The disabled community includes people with a variety of physical, cognitive, sensory, and other impairments and intersecting identities. In response to this diversity, disabled people recommend a twin-track, intersectional approach to both the prevention of violence and the response to it (Schulze 2017). A twin-track approach to prevention means eliminating structural barriers to disabled people's full participation in society and the full realisation of their rights, aligned with specific strategies to prevent violence. The twin-track approach to response encompasses ensuring that mainstream services are fully accessible, with staff who understand working with disabled people, and specialist services for those who require them. This means that government strategies to prevent and respond to violence against disabled people must focus both on structural drivers of violence and abuse as well as responses to individuals and their families.

Violence Prevention

A structural governmental response requires the inclusion of disabled women and men at all levels—the development of legislation, government policy, organisational policy and practice, service, and prevention responses. In order for disabled people to have the autonomy to make their own choices and participate fully in society, government must ensure equitable access to:

- Adequate income (not minimal income).
- Warm, safe, accessible, affordable housing.
- Lifelong education.
- Legislation that prescribes reasonable accommodation to ensure that disabled people can be employed in positions matching their interests and skills.
- Adequate support services that enable all disabled people to achieve independence, and access to all societal domains.
- Resources and services co-designed with disabled people for disabled people, for prevention activities, ensuring that funding is sufficient to produce resources in accessible formats.

For this to be achieved, ableism must be challenged and addressed. Disability activists (Feminists with Disabilities for a Way Forward 2010) use the term ableism (see Box 2) to describe:

> …discrimination against people with disabilities, including the expression of hate for people with disabilities, denial of accessibility, rejection of disabled applicants for housing and jobs, (and) institutionalised discrimination in the form of benefit systems designed to keep people with disabilities in poverty.

and

> The effect of a system of classification based on ableist beliefs is to assist dominant, non-disabled groups to render the existence and concerns of disabled people either invisible, or subject to the exercise of patronage and benevolence. At the same time the benefits of being not disabled remain invisible and seldom acknowledged (McLean 2005: 65).

Addressing ableism necessitates the recognition of disabled people as legitimate, integral participants in society, and the resourcing of structural changes designed to enable their full participation.

Box 2 Ableism

Ableism

Ableism is '*discrimination or prejudice against people with lived experience of disability*' (King 2019: xii) and a value system that considers certain typical characteristics of body and mind as essential for living a life of value (United Nations Human Rights Council 2020: 3).

Ableism leads to social prejudice, discrimination against, and oppression of, persons with disabilities, as it informs legislation, policies and practices. Ableist assumptions lie at the root of discriminatory practices (United Nations Human Rights Council 2020: 3).

Service Delivery and Intervention

A twin-track approach to service provision and interventions responding to violence means ensuring mainstream services and supports are inclusive of, and fully accessible to, disabled people, and that specialised services and supports that are specific to disabled people, including for disabled children of victims, are also available. Being an accessible violence prevention or response service means providing not only physical access to buildings (toilets, bathrooms and all other spaces) but offering fully accessible information in a range of formats, including access to sign language speakers and interpreters. It means all organisations must develop policies and procedures in conjunction with disabled people that specify and teach the competencies required to understand who disabled people are; the dynamics and dimensions of violence against disabled women, men, and children; and how to constructively respond to this violence, including a knowledge of available services and processes. This will require:

- Support for victims to remain in a home that is adapted to their needs.
- Ensuring that relevant, up-to-date information about support and services, including information about legal processes, is available in accessible formats.
- Including disabled people in ongoing evaluation and development of services to better meet needs.
- Ensuring that mainstream refuges are fully accessible for disabled women who do not require 24 hour support and for women with disabled dependent children of any age.
- Training all service providers, the police, and justice services to understand disabled people, the dynamics of violence against disabled people, and ensuring that disabled people are perceived as autonomous and credible and are believed when they disclose abuse.

Improving the accessibility of mainstream services should proceed alongside the development of a range of specialist services. These must include, but not be limited to:

- Specialised refuges with 24-hour on-site support for women with significant mental distress/psychosocial illness.
- Specialised refuges with 24-hour on-site support for women with substance abuse problems.
- Accessible refuges with 24-hour on-site support for disabled women who require it [3] and/or women with dependent disabled children of any age.
- Services for disabled men and boys. It is not acceptable or safe for men and women to be housed in the same services.
- Specialist interagency safeguarding services for those who are unable to remove themselves from harm and/or require safe support for decision-making.

The Language of Vulnerability

The concept of vulnerability is frequently used to explain the high rates of violence against disabled people (Hager 2017). That is, a disabled person is abused because they are vulnerable. This chapter has deliberately not used this language. The concept of vulnerability as an uncontested descriptor of various non-hegemonic populations is increasingly being used in policy, legislation, and practice in Western nations (Fawcett 2009), and is strongly rooted in social work and related human service practices.

The perception of disabled people who require some level of support for daily living as vulnerable is, in many countries, enshrined in law. For example, the New Zealand Crimes Act (1961: section 2.1) defines a vulnerable adult as 'a person unable, by reason of detention, age, sickness, mental impairment, or any other cause, to withdraw himself or herself from the care or charge of another person'. However, when the adjective vulnerable is applied to a person or group of people, the meaning of the word is generally unexamined. Consequently, vulnerability is treated as objective and uncontroversial, applicable across a range of situations (Fawcett 2009). Most commonly, this word describes a person who is 'vulnerable' because of some reason or weakness inherent to themselves, for example, age, disability, or minority status.

The Oxford Dictionary defines the word vulnerable in two ways. One definition is that vulnerable means someone or something is open to attack or harm because of forces 'exposed to the possibility of being attacked or harmed, either physically or emotionally' (Oxford Dictionary undated). The other definition is that a person or group of people can be harmed because of some inherent weakness within

[3] This could be physical support, or support for women experiencing mental distress, for example.

themselves: '(of a person) in need of special care, support, or protection because of age, disability, or risk of abuse or neglect' (Oxford Dictionary undated). A further definition is that a vulnerable person is 'weak and without protection' (Collins English Dictionary undated).

Findings from New Zealand research (Hager 2017) suggest that labelling a disabled woman as vulnerable increases the chance that she will be physically, sexually, or emotionally abused—that the label enhances the risk of violence occurring. This can result in a vicious cycle of harm. This cycle describes disabled women labelled as vulnerable, which means they are seen as being available to be harmed. An outcome of this is that they become targets of predators who seek out perceived powerlessness and lack of protection. They are then more likely to be physically, emotionally, and sexually abused. Very few, if any, resources are provided by the state to protect disabled women from violence and abuse or to respond constructively when they are harmed. Therefore, disabled women can be harmed, which in turn means they will be seen as vulnerable.

Rather than using this language and alerting predators to an under-protected group of women and children, it is more constructive to describe the context that is creating the heightened risk. This would require a reframing of language (and thinking) from dis/abled women/people as the problem, to situating the problem within inadequate systems and social attitudes—such as hegemonic male/able-bodied privilege, ableism, and norms about gender roles—that enable violence. It would mean talking and writing about social and institutional structures and systems that enable violence against dis/abled women, and women who are endangered by inadequate systems, structures, and social attitudes, rather than vulnerable women. It takes a few more words to emphasise, but these distinctions clearly describe where responsibility for the violence lies.

Summary

- Disabled people of all ages experience higher rates of abuse than non-disabled people, but there is still gender inequity—disabled women experience higher rates of violence and abuse than disabled men.
- The violence experienced by disabled people is similar to that experienced in all abusive relationships—but more extensive, with impairment-related and institutional abuse common. Perpetrators of violence against disabled people include family, friends, professionals, people in the community, and paid and unpaid care and support people.
- It is more difficult for disabled people to disclose violence and receive help and support, because of their perceived lack of credibility.
- Violence against disabled people is about power—and the perception of the powerlessness of disabled people.
- If disabled people were resourced to fully participate in society—with access to adequate income, housing, education, employment, and autonomy—the opportunities for violence and abuse would be reduced.

- Responding constructively requires fully accessible mainstream services and access to a range of specialist services, ensuring that all those who interact with disabled people receive education about who disabled people are, the dynamics of violence against disabled people, and how to constructively respond.

References

Appleton-Dyer S, Soupen A (2017) Rapid review of the Waitematā safeguarding adults from abuse (SAFA) pilot report for the Waitematā police. Synergia, Auckland

Ballan M, Freyer MB, Powledge L (2017) Intimate partner violence among men with disabilities: the role of health care providers. Am J Mens Health 11(5):1436–1443

Barbuto R, Napolitano E (2014) Women with disabilities: from discrimination and violence towards an ethic of reciprocity. Mod Italy 19(2):161–168

Barnett H (2015) Report to the special rapporteur on the rights of persons with disabilities. United Nations Geneva. Disabled People's Assembly New Zealand, Wellington

Calderbank R (2000) Abuse and disabled people: vulnerability or social indifference? Disabil Soc 15(3):521–534

Committee on the Rights of Persons with Disabilities (2016) General Comment No. 3 Women and girls with disabilities. UN Doc CRPD/C/GC/3

Connell R (2005) Masculinities, 2nd edn. Allen & Unwin, Crows Nest, NSW

Covey HC (2005) Western Christianity's two historical treatments of people with disabilities or mental illness. Soc Sci J 42(1):107–114

Curry MA, Renke P, Robinson-Whelen S et al (2011) Facilitators and barriers to disclosing abuse among women with disabilities. Violence Vict 26(4):430–444

Domestic Violence and Disability Working Group (2010) Domestic violence and disabled people. It's Not OK Campaign, Ministry of Social Development, Wellington

Fanslow J, Robinson E (2004) Violence against women in New Zealand: prevalence and health consequences. N Z Med J 117(1206):1–12

Fawcett B (2009) Vulnerability: Questioning the certainties in social work and health. International Social Work. 52(4):473–484

Feminists with Disabilities for a Way Forward (2010) What is ableism? Five things about ableism you should know. http://disabledfeminists.com/2010/11/19/what-is-ableism-five-things-about-ableism-you-should-know/

Frohmader C, Dowse L, Didi A (2015) Preventing violence against women and girls with disabilities: integrating a human rights perspective. Women With Disabilities Australia (WWDA), Lenah Valley, TAS

Greer G, Hunt R (2020) Options paper: an options paper providing a range of options and recommendations on how the disability rights commissioner can best use her role, and the functions and resources of the human rights commission to address violence and abuse experienced by disabled people. New Zealand Human Rights Commission

Gulliver P, Fanslow J (2013) Exploring risk factors for suicidal ideation in a population-based sample of New Zealand women who have experienced intimate partner violence. Aust N Z J Public Health 37(6):527–533

Hager D (2001) He drove me mad: the relationship between domestic violence and mental illness. Master's thesis. University of Auckland. Auckland

Hager D (2017) Not inherently vulnerable: an examination of paradigms, attitudes and systems that enable the abuse of dis/abled women. PhD thesis. University of Auckland. Auckland. https://researchspace.auckland.ac.nz/handle/2292/36826

Harpur P, Douglas H (2014) Disability and domestic violence: protecting survivors' human rights. Griffith Law Rev 23(3):405–433

Healey L, Howe K, Humphreys C et al (2008) Building the evidence. Victorian Women with Disabilities Network Advocacy Information Service, Melbourne, Australia

Hughes K, Belli MA, Jones L et al (2012) Prevalence and risk of violence against adults with disabilities: a systematic review and meta-analysis of observational studies. Lancet 379(9826):1621–1629

Hunt R (2021) A community alone: why loneliness is a disability issue. The Spinoff. https://thespinoff.co.nz/society/14-04-2021/why-loneliness-is-a-disability-issue-and-how-our-societies-are-making-it-worse/ Accessed 6 Nov 2021

King PT (2019) Wai 2575, #B22. Māori with lived experience of disability part I. (p. xii). Waitangi Tribunal for Stage two of the Wai 2575 health services and outcomes Kaupapa inquiry

Krug EG, Dahlberg LL, Mercy JA, Zwi AB, Lozano R (eds) (2002) World report on violence and health. World Health Organisation, Geneva

Livneh H (2012) Psychological and social impact of physical disability. In: Marini I, Stebnicki MA (eds) The psychological and social impact of illness and disability, 6th edn. Springer, New York

Makasiale C, Williams P (1997) A Pacific Islands reflection. In: O'Brien P, Sullivan M (eds) Human services: towards partnership and support. Dunmore Press, Palmerston North, New Zealand

Margolis H, Shapiro A (1987) Countering negative images of disability in classical literature. English J 76(3):18–22

McCarthy M, Thompson D (1997) A prevalence study of sexual abuse of adults with intellectual disabilities referred for sex education. J Appl Res Intellect Disabil 10(2):105–124

McLean M (2005) Emancipatory understandings for allies: recognising ableism. In: O'Brien P, Sullivan M (eds) Allies in emancipation: shifting from providing service to being of support. Thomson Dunmore Press, South Melbourne

McRae J (2014) Becoming a person: the biography of Robert Martin. In: How an intellectually disabled man helped change the world. Craig Potton Publishing, Nelson, New Zealand

Ministry of Health (2021) Office of the Director of mental health and addiction services annual report 2018 and 2019. Ministry of Health, Wellington. https://www.health.govt.nz/publication/office-director-mental-health-and-addiction-services-annual-report-2018-and-2019 Accessed 6 Nov 2021

Mirfin-Veitch B, Conder J (2017) Institutions are places of abuse: the experiences of disabled children and adults in state care between 1950–1992. The Donald Beasley Institute, Dunedin. https://www.hrc.co.nz/files/3415/0103/3949/Institutions_are_places_of_abuse_The_experiences_of_disabled_children_and_adults_in_State_care_.pdf. Accessed 6 Nov 2021

Murphy C (2009) Men's intimate partner abuse and control: reconciling paradoxical masculinities and social contradictions. PhD thesis. Queensland University of Technology, Brisbane. https://library.nzfvc.org.nz/

Nikora LW, Karapu R, Hicky H et al (2004) Disabled Maori and disability support options: a report prepared for the Ministry of Health. University of Waikato and Ministry of Health, Hamilton

Otkay JS, Tompkins CJ (2004) Personal assistant providers' mistreatment of disabled adults. Health Soc Work 29(3):177–188

Peters S (1996) The politics of disability identity. In: Barton L (ed) Disability and society: emerging issues and insights. Longman, New York, NY

Pinilla-Roncancio M (2015) Disability and poverty: two related conditions. A review of the literature. Rev Fac Med 63:S113–S123

Powers LE, Oschwald M (2004) Violence and abuse against people with disabilities: experiences, barriers and prevention strategies. Oregon Health & Science University, Portland, OR

Radford J, Harne L, Trotter J (2006) Disabled women and domestic violence as violent crime. Pract Social Work Action 18(4):233–246

Roguski M (2013) The hidden abuse of disabled people residing in the community: an exploratory study. Tairawhiti Community Voice, Gisborne, New Zealand

Royal Commission of Inquiry into Historical Abuse in State Care and in the Care of Faith-Based Institutions (2020) Volume one: Tāwharautia: Pūrongo o te Wā—interim report New Zealand.

Abuse in Care, Royal Commission. https://wwwabuseincareorgnz/library/v/194/tawharautia-purongo-o-te-wa-interim-report. Accessed 6 Nov 2021
Schulze M (2017) Freedom from exploitation, violence and abuse of persons with disabilities: contribution to the Council of Europe Strategy on the rights of persons with disabilities. Council of Europe, London
Shakespeare T (1999) The sexual politics of disabled masculinity. Sex Disabil 17(1):53–64
Thiara RK, Hague G, Bashall R et al (2012) Disabled women and domestic violence: responding to the experiences of survivors. Jessica Kingsley, London
UN Special Rapporteur on the Rights of Persons with Disabilities (2017) Report on sexual and reproductive health and rights of girls and young women. A/72/133. https://wwwohchrorg/EN/Issues/Disability/SRDisabilities/Pages/ReproductiveHealthRightsaspx. Accessed 6 Nov 2021
UNCRPD Preamble (2007) Paragraph 5. https://www.un.org/development/desa/disabilities/convention-on-the-rights-of-persons-with-disabilities/preamble.html
UNFPA (2018) Young persons with disabilities: Global study on ending gender-based violence and realizing sexual and reproductive health and rights. https://www.unfpa.org/publications/young-persons-disabilities Accessed 6 Nov 2021
United Nations Human Rights Council (2020) Forty-third session. A/HRC/43/41 2020. Rights of persons with disabilities: Report of the Special Rapporteur on the rights of persons with disabilities. United Nations General Assembly. III/9/p. 3
Van Eden K (2013) Putting people first. A review of disability support services performance and quality management processes for purchased provider services. https://www.health.govt.nz/publication/review-disability-support-services. Accessed 6 Nov 2021
Walker H (2021) Still alone together. In: How loneliness changed in Aotearoa New Zealand in 2020 and what it means for public policy. Post pandemic futures series, vol 4. Helen Clarke Foundation and WSP, Auckland
Walter-Brice A, Cox R, Priest H et al (2012) What do women with learning disabilities say about their experiences of domestic abuse within the context of their intimate partner relationships? Disabil Soc 27(4):503–517
Women with Disabilities Australia (WWDA) (2021) Response to the 'violence and abuse of people with disability at home' issues paper of the Royal Commission into violence, abuse. Neglect and Exploitation of People with Disability, Hobart, WWDA
World Health Organization (2021) Violence against women: key facts. Newsroom fact sheets. https://www.who.int/news-room/fact-sheet. Accessed 6 Nov 2021

Debbie Hager, PhD is a Lecturer in Public Health/Health Promotion at the School of Population Health. Her research expertise is the gendered dynamics of domestic/family violence, the mental health effects of violence and violence against disabled people.

Part IX

Digital and Technology-Facilitated Abuse

Digital Sexual Assault: Understanding the Non-Consensual Sharing of Sexual Images

Signe Uldbjerg

Learning Objectives
Having read this chapter, you should be able to

- Understand digital sexual assault as the non-consensual distribution of sexual/sexualized images on digital media and identify types of digital sexual assault.
- Recognize the gendered aspects of digital sexual assault.
- Understand the impacts of digital sexual assault on victims in short- and long-term perspectives, and recognize ways of coping with these impacts.

Introduction

While many might have heard of digital sexual assault (DSA) in the context of 'revenge porn', the non-consensual sharing of intimate and sexual images covers a wide variety of abusive digital practices. Sexual images can be circulated on secret online fora, shared in private messages, uploaded to commercial porn sites and social media, or even used to create fake dating and escort profiles. The pictures and videos can be produced with consent or coercion; they can be taken without the victim's knowledge, they can be edited to show a sexual situation that never actually happened, or they can even document a physical sexual assault. Regardless of the

S. Uldbjerg (✉)
Department of Cultural Sciences, The Faculty of Humanities, Southern Danish University, Odense, Denmark

Aarhus University, Aarhus, Denmark
e-mail: siu@sdu.dk

P. Ali, M. M. Rogers (eds.), *Gender-Based Violence: A Comprehensive Guide*,
https://doi.org/10.1007/978-3-031-05640-6_37

origin and distribution history of an assaulting image, sharing of the image constitutes a type of gendered sexual violence that has specific mediated impacts on victims' lives and consequently requires specific coping methods and interventions.

This chapter aims to describe the variety of sexually assaulting digital practices that make up cases of DSA, and to consider their gendered character. First, it discusses different approaches to defining DSA in relation to the gendered, structural and mediated aspects of victimization as well as their attention and closeness to victims' lived experiences.

Second, the chapter draws on the discussions of DSA definitions to show how prevalence of DSA in relation to gender varies, depending on how many digitally assaulting practices are included in the defining framework of the studies. The argument is that while many assaulting digital practices are not necessarily gendered, current research strongly suggests that the broad, sometimes organized, sharing of non-consensual *sexual* images targets female and feminized victims disproportionately, and that the mental and social consequences of DSA are strongly gendered.

Finally, the chapter reports findings on the impacts of victimization, and the ways victims, in an in-depth qualitative study, described their experiences of coping with DSA; for example, by finding ways or reclaiming control of their social media presence and the narrative of the assaulting images, by seeking out other victims to share their experiences, and by negotiating misrepresentations of DSA and trying to shame perpetrators, thereby shifting shame away from themselves.

These considerations lead to the conclusion that DSA is a kind of gendered violence. Moreover, the considerations emphasize the need for prevention, legislation and victim-support that acknowledge DSA as sexual violence and allow victims, who frame their stories as sexual assault, to seek justice and support without having to reframe their experiences as cyberbullying, child pornography or reputational damage.

Definitions of DSA

The field of studies into digital sexual assault presents a large number of definitions and terminologies relating to the non-consensual sharing of intimate images (see Box 1). Henry et al. (2021: 4), for example, define 'image-based sexual abuse' as one or more out of three practices: the *non-consensual taking* of nudes or sexual images; the *non-consensual sharing* of nudes or sexual images; and *threats to share* nudes or sexual images. In addition to this definition, they understand these practices as part of the 'continuum of sexual violence' conceptualized by Kelly (1988), thereby pointing to how abusive digital practices are part of a broader cultural normalization of sexual violence.

A continuum is also used by McGlynn et al. (2017: 26) who argue that 'there is a continuum of practices which together form our concept of image-based sexual abuse'. Their continuum has five parameters: the sexual nature of the imagery; the gendered nature of perpetration and victimization; the sexualized nature of harassment and abuse; the harms to dignity, sexual autonomy and sexual expression and the minimization of these forms of abuse in public discourse, law and policy. In other words, image-based sexual abuse is defined as sexual violence in relation to these five criteria.

Understanding DSA as sexual violence on a continuum with other violent, gendered practices draws attention to its structural and underlying aspects and its existence in a culture, where many forms of gendered perpetration are normalized. However, it does little to offer insights into the various practices of producing, distributing and, most importantly, coping with DSA. In this way, these definitions can seem very far from the lived experiences of victims—especially as these experiences are intertwined with social and digital media.

The problem that definitions might sometimes be too distant from the lived, mediated experiences of victims is an underlying concern in many studies on DSA. In fact, several attempts to rename and define DSA start with a critique of the common term 'revenge porn' (Maddocks 2018; Ruvalcaba and Eaton 2020; Henry and Powell 2016). Maddocks (2018), for example, writes:

> The term 'revenge pornography' reduces these severe harms to a simple 'scorned exboyfriend' narrative. It suggests that perpetrators are motivated only by personal vengeance and implies that victims are to blame for causing perpetrators to seek revenge. (Maddocks 2018: 347)

In other words, 'revenge porn' indicates a narrative that distorts or simplifies victims' stories of DSA. Similarly, criticism has been directed towards understandings of DSA as cyberbullying; the argument is that viewing DSA as bullying ignores the gendered and sexual aspects of victimization (Dodge 2016).

When choosing between the various frameworks used to define DSA, we must consider which aspects (the cultural/structural, the mediated, the psychological/affective) are relevant and interesting in the specific context. The continuums offer a useful way to understand and discuss DSA as sexual violence within a broader cultural framework, the next section of this chapter presents an alternative framework, based on categories of DSA, which instead emphasizes the types of DSA and the mediated experiences of victims.

Box 1

Definition

Digital sexual assault is the digital distribution of sexually explicit or sexualized images when the person in the image(s) is identifiable (potentially through added data/doxing) and has not consented to the image distribution; and/or the harassment, stalking, shaming and bullying linked to this distribution of images.

Alternative terminology

Image-based sexual abuse, Technology-facilitated sexual violence, Revenge porn, Non-consensual sexting, Non-consensual pornography, Digital rape, Intimate image abuse.

Associated concepts

Voyeurism, up-skirting, down-blousing, creepshots, sextortion, drone porn, doxing, deep fakes, photoshop porn, grooming, sexploitation, hacking, identity theft, cyberbullying.

Types of DSA

There have been some suggestions of ways to categorize types of DSA. Powell et al. (2019) suggest a categorization framework that groups image-based sexual abuse into five subcategories: relationship retribution, sextortion, voyeurism, sexploitation and sexual assault. These five types of DSA focus on the acts of the aggressors. Relationship retribution is when images are non-consensually shared after a breakup or in an abusive relationship. Sextortion is extortion of victims for (more) images. Voyeurism is when a sexual voyeur shares images for social status or sexual satisfaction. Sexploitation is image sharing with economic interests, and sexual assault is when aggressors document physical sexual violence and share the images.

While these categories might be useful when focussing on the mediated practices and motivations of aggressors, they do little to understand victims' experiences of the assaults. In contrast, the framework presented below covers the mediated practices, which constitute DSA, from a victim perspective.

Figure 1 shows four categories of DSA based on three parameters. The parameters concern the issue of consent indicating which aspect(s)—distribution, production and sexualization—were non-consensual and thus assaulting in the respective types of DSA cases. Categorizing types of DSA in relation to the lack of consent creates categories that emphasize the events as sexual violence, and bring victim experiences of consent-violation to the front.

The first category, consensually produced sexual images, covers cases where the assaulting act was the image distribution, while the production of the image and the sexual situation were consensual. The second category, non-consensually produced images, covers cases where the distribution and production of the image were non-consensual, but there was, apart from the image production itself, no immediate non-consensual sexualization happening. The third category, repurposed images, covers cases where the image was produced with consent, but later edited or reused in sexualizing contexts, making the sexualization and distribution non-consensual. The fourth category, coerced images, covers cases where the distribution, production and sexualization were non-consensual, meaning that image production and distribution are part of, but do not solely constitute, a case of sexual violence.

Figure 1 shows examples of practices that fall under each category and additional DSA-related practices are named in Box 1. One person's experiences, however, might include more than one type of DSA.

In comparison to the definition of image-based sexual abuse by Henry et al. (2021), the definition presented above only includes cases where intimate images have been shared and not cases where they have been non-consensually produced

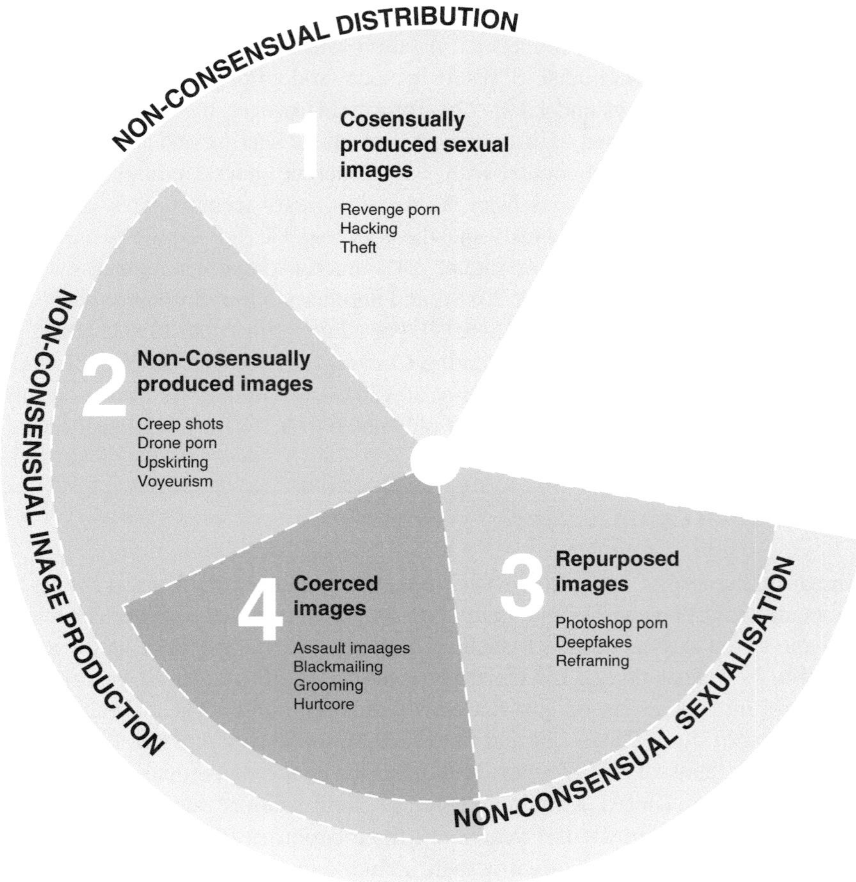

Fig. 1 Types of DSA. (Reproduced from Uldbjerg 2021a)

without being shared or where victims have been threatened without actual sharing taking place. Image-based sexual abuse, as Henry et al. define it, thus describes a broader range of related practices, while digital sexual assault, as defined here, refers specifically to non-consensual sharing of sexual images. This distinction is relevant when focussing on mediated aspects of assaults because the circulation and distribution of digital media shape victim experiences in very significant ways.

Prevalence

With the large number of types and definitions of DSA, research into its prevalence is complicated. Studies focus on everything from very general experiences of digital abuse to specific experiences such as having images uploaded to public Internet sites or shared among local peers. Further, a majority of studies focus on young people, excluding adult victimization.

Walker and Sleath (2017), in a systematic review of knowledge on non-consensual sharing of intimate images, found victimization rates among adults ranging from 1.8%–10.3% for men and 0.5%–3.3% for women, and among adolescents ranging from 2.1%–13% for boys and 1.3%–42% for girls. However, their review includes studies looking into a range of different kinds of image sharing and context.

In contrast, looking at a context with more coherent understandings of DSA as *sexual* violence, Danish surveys from the past few years seem to show consistent victimization rates for adolescents somewhere around 3%. For example, one large-scale study reports a victimization rate of 2.4% among students in their last year of primary school (Skolesundhed.dk 2018), and another study reports a rate of 3.3% among 15–20 year olds (Frisch et al. 2019). For adults (older than 18y) in a lifetime perspective, The Danish Crime Prevention Council (Heinskou et al. 2017) found a victimization rate of 0.5%, and Frisch et al. (2019) found that victimization rates drop with age from 3.3% for 15–19 year olds down to 0.5% for 35–39 year olds.

International Comparisons

Comparing the results above to surveys from other countries, the Danish results are low. In an Australian sample, one in ten (18–54 years) reported experiences related to image-based sexual abuse (Powell and Henry 2019), and in a study across Australia, New Zealand and the United Kingdom, one in five (16–64 years) report having had nude or sexual images shared without their consent (Henry et al. 2021). In an American study, Ruvalcaba and Eaton (2020) found a victimization rate of 8% among respondents of 18–97 years, and a European survey comparing Denmark, Hungary and the United Kingdom, reported victimization rates of 6% among 13–17 year olds within the last year in all three countries (Childnet et al. 2017). Depending on the types of digital assault included in the study and the extent to which informants have to *feel* offended to report as victims, numbers on prevalence vary even within the same population. Further, with emerging political focus on DSA in many countries, prevalence might change quickly from 1 year to another.

What is clear, however, is that the younger population is more vulnerable to DSA, and that experiences related to DSA are not uncommon in any of the countries mentioned above. Since DSA is, at this time, a relatively under-researched kind of sexual abuse, the global extent of the issue outside of Europe, Australia and the USA is mostly unknown. Furthermore, digital violence works across country borders, and while it is certainly relevant to look further into victimization in different national and cultural contexts, the offenders and the media infrastructures related to instances of DSA are rarely limited to one national context.

Prevalence and Gender

The types of DSA researched are vital for understanding its gendered nature. Studies focussing broadly on assaulting digital practices often find a larger victimization rate among men, as evident in the literature review by Walker and Sleath (2017).

However, studies looking at the large-scale public and organized sharing of intimate, and especially sexual, images find larger victimization rates among women. Uhl et al. (2018), for example, found that 92% of victims on revenge porn sites were female (or presenting as female), and a survey asking if the informants had images shared on social media (and not in private messages or other), found a larger victimization rate among women (2.6%) than men (1%) (Frisch et al. 2019).

Overall, the numbers indicate that while the non-consensual sharing of intimate images in general might not necessarily be gendered, the broad, sometimes organized (Jørgensen and Demant 2021), distribution of sexual images, and hence public humiliation and sexualization of victims, primarily targets women. This hypothesis is supported by Ruvalcaba and Eaton (2020); not only did they find a higher victimization rate among women than men when emphasizing the sexually assaulting nature of the image sharing, they also found that women victimized by DSA had a lower psychological well-being than non-victims, while for men, no significant connection was found. This indicates that non-consensual image sharing as sexual violence with psychological consequences is a gendered issue that targets women, while intimate image sharing with a range of (non-sexual) purposes and consequences is not gendered in and of itself.

Finally, it is relevant to mention that while there is very little research on victimization among gendered and sexual minorities, the studies that include categories outside the gender binary and consider sexuality strongly indicate a higher victimization rate among assigned-female non-binary people, bisexuals and homosexual men. One study, with a general victimization rate of 1.6% over a lifetime, reports victimization rates of 7.6% for non-binary female-assigned people, 5.6% for bisexual women, 2.4% for bisexual men, and 5.3% for homosexual men (Frisch et al. 2019). Another study, with a general victimization rate of 8%, reports rates of 17.19% for bisexual women, 12.82% for bisexual men, and 10.19% for homosexual men (Ruvalcaba and Eaton 2020).

Explanatory Theories

While quantitative studies into DSA indicate that at least some kinds of assault and their consequences are gendered, these gendered aspects of DSA are investigated and theorized in qualitative studies. Several studies researching intimate image sharing among youth point to an economic logic where girls are devalued when their images are shared, while the boys sharing them gain social status (Ringrose et al. 2013; Mandau 2020). Others show that intimate image sharing for girls and women is connected to experiences of sexual shame and the risk of 'failing' norms of feminine sexuality (Davidson 2014; Mann 2018; Rasmussen and Søndergaard 2020; Henry and Powell 2016). Meanwhile, when boys and men's images are shared, they are more likely to become objects of humour and homosocial pranking, or of ridicule focussed on bodily appearances or online behaviour (Paasonen and Sundén 2021; Corry 2021; Rasmussen and Søndergaard 2020).

The indication that sexual shame and shaming is essential to women's experience of non-consensual image sharing, but not necessarily to men's, resonates with theorizations around gendered shame. Mann (2018), for example, draws on Simone de Beauvoir in order to show how DSA can cause 'unbounded shame' because it displays an infinite failure in negotiating the boundary between ideal female attractiveness and virtue, thus making redemption, through the achievement of appropriate femininity, impossible. Others show that 'sexting prevention' campaigns for teens indicate the same sexual double standards trying to control girls' sexuality rather than seeking to stop non-consensual sharing (Salter et al. 2013; Döring 2014), and finally, studies into victims' experiences of DSA show that shame, and coping with shame, are central parts of female victims' experience (Uldbjerg 2020, 2021a).

Comparing these qualitative findings to those of prevalence from above, it becomes even clearer how the gendered nature of DSA lies not primarily in the image sharing itself but in its consequences; that is, in the long-term, widespread shaming and devaluation of female/feminized bodies, lives and sexual expressions.

Impact

Few studies investigate the impacts of DSA on victims, and those that do tend to focus on generalizable and measurable mental health effects. For example, Ruvalcaba and Eaton (2020) found a connection between victimization and higher rates of mental health issues, and Bates (2017: 22) reported that victims experience effects such as 'trust issues, posttraumatic stress disorder (PTSD), anxiety, depression, suicidal thoughts, and several other mental health effects' comparable to those experienced by victims of rape. Further, according to Henry et al. (2021), a majority (55.1%) of people who have experienced any kind of image-based sexual abuse reports that the assaults have impacted their health, affected their relationships, and/or resulted in harassment. These studies emphasize the seriousness of DSA as sexual violence, but more research is needed to learn about the specific, and mediated, impacts on victims.

In a qualitative study, including a small group of victims, the participants described and discussed the complex ways DSA had influenced their lives. They talked about the feeling of shame that followed their experiences of exposure, and they described how the anxiety attached to not knowing who had seen their images was always present when meeting new people on- or offline (Uldbjerg 2020). Further, they expressed frustration with the ways they sometimes felt urged to limit their online lives to stay safe and avoid harassment. For example, not being able to have recognizable profiles on social media can be a limitation both professionally, e.g. when applying for jobs and participating in online networking, and socially, e.g. when trying to engage in communities that use social media as part of their communication (Uldbjerg 2020, 2021a). In combination with the fear of shaming and exposure, being secluded from social media networking and peer-communities can cause victims to feel isolated and alone with their experiences. Finally, victims in the study pointed to a kind of endlessness to digital assaults, referring to how the images might potentially keep spreading online and new harassers or shameful confrontations continuing to appear.

Similar findings are reported by Henry et al. (2021), and include experiences of endlessness, social anxiety, isolation and constrained liberty. However, the participants in the qualitative study mentioned above also opposed the idea of 'the never-ending assault' by pointing to ways in which their experiences changed over time when the harassment gradually became less frequent or they found ways to intervene in and resist the assaults (Uldbjerg 2021a).

In addition to the impacts on victims, it is relevant to address their ways of coping with these negative impacts. In one study (see Uldbjerg 2020, 2021a, b), victims' coping strategies involved different ways of regaining control of their online identities, for example, some would implement strict data safety routines, while others would use social media to tell their stories openly and thereby be able to better control the narratives of the assaults and the ways people viewed them. Other strategies involved different ways of renegotiating (mis)understandings of DSA with families and friends and sometimes in public. For example, the participants would use their own experiences to argue against understandings of DSA as a 'youth problem' or something that only happens to 'ignorant girls' who 'carelessly share sexual images', and they would engage in 'counter-shaming' the aggressors and thereby turning shame away from themselves. Finally, some found a sense of empowerment in sharing their stories with other victims and in engaging in struggles related to sexual violence, e.g. through feminist activism or volunteering with victim-support organizations.

In general, DSA can have serious impacts on victims over a long time, because the assault risks being repeated every time an image is re-shared. The two case studies in Box 2 show examples of how the assaults might develop over long periods—sometimes despite organized efforts to end the image distribution. However, victims can find positive ways of coping, especially if they are in an environment where openness around assault experiences is encouraged and stories are met with care rather than suspicion and shaming. Since a central part of DSA victimization is the fear of recurring exposure, sharing one's story helps limit the concern that friends and family might find out, and it offers a chance to reclaim the narrative of the image.

Box 2

Two Case Studies

The Umbrella Case

The Umbrella case started in 2015 when a group of young boys filmed the (alleged) assault of a 15-year-old girl committed by a peer in Denmark. The video was circulated online, and 1 year later, two of the young boys were first convicted for sharing child pornography.

Despite the conviction, the video spread. Danish Police had it taken down from several platforms, but it continued to reappear with devastating consequences for the victims.

In 2017, Facebook detected the distribution of the video and notified authorities. In 2018, this resulted in prosecution of more than a thousand young people for distribution of child pornography. Consequently, public interest in the case spiralled, increasing awareness of DSA on one side, but also intensifying the circulation of the video on the other. The video was circulated widely in Europe, Russia, the USA and Australia mostly.

The Image Folder Case

The second case, made public in 2019, concerns a folder with intimate images of 720 women dating back several years. Unlike in the Umbrella case, the majority of the victims were older than 18 and only one perpetrator was prosecuted, while the instigator(s) were never identified. This case had few legal and political outcomes, but it showed the diversity of DSA victimization. While discussions of the Umbrella case had been on young people's digital sharing practices and morals, this case showed the variety of ways in which DSA can happen to women of all ages. Some had images shared by abusive (ex)partners, some had everyday-images edited to look sexual, some had images shared that they were not aware had been taken.

Despite the differences in media coverage and legal justice given in the two cases, they share the circumstance that in both cases, some of the assaulting images are still in circulation.

Policy and Practice

In many academic debates today, DSA risks being treated primarily as a problem concerning youth culture, and adult victims are forgotten (Henry and Powell 2015), while the experiences of underage victims are often viewed as cases of cyberbullying, ignoring the gendered and sexual aspects of victimization.

The issue of DSA being discussed primarily in relation to young people is evident in prosecution and press coverage as well. Legally, only few countries acknowledge DSA as a form of sexual violence, and if prosecuted, it is often under child pornography legislation (if the victim is underage) or as civil lawsuits. The two case studies described in Box 2 illustrate how a case concerning adolescent victims and perpetrators gained extensive press coverage and more than a thousand offenders were prosecuted, while another case concerning organized sharing of hundreds of adult women's images received limited press coverage and only one offender was prosecuted.

Implications for Research and Practice

As might have become clear from the above, digital sexual assault is a kind of gendered violence that has only recently been given political, academic and legal attention. There is still a need for further research into the basic characteristics of DSA such as prevalence, related practices and impacts. Particularly, adult victimization and global perspectives are under-researched, as are the long-term impacts on and coping methods of victims.

To prevent DSA and increase the chance of victims getting justice, measures must be taken to include digital sexual offences into legislation, prevention work and treatment related to sexual violence. Rather than reducing these harms to narratives of relationship drama, cyberbullying and stories of naïve, innocent youth, we must take victims' framing of their own experiences seriously and not adhere to processes that deprive them of sexual agency through the infantilizing stigma of child pornography, or ignore the harms done to their digital, sexual and emotional lives.

Summary

- DSA refers to the non-consensual sharing of sexual or sexualized images. Image production and distribution can happen in a number of ways, but essential for this kind of assault are the mediated forms of harassment, exposure and constraints that victims often experience.
- While the non-consensual taking and sharing of intimate images is not gendered in relation to prevalence, the widespread distribution of sexualized images and shaming of victims target women (and likely other feminized people) disproportionately. Further, the mental and practical impacts of DSA are gendered through sexual shaming and double standards.
- DSA victims experience consequences such as recurring or constant fear of shaming and exposure. They might also need to limit their social media presence resulting in social as well as practical constraints.
- However, victims can find ways of coping, including, but not limited to, implementing data safety measures in their everyday lives, coming forward with their experiences, renegotiating common misunderstandings of DSA, shaming aggressors, seeking out other victims and engaging in social and political initiatives about sexual violence.
- The above calls for approaches to DSA within law, politics, prevention work and victim aid that acknowledge victims' experiences as those of sexual violence (when victims themselves frame it this way). DSA should not be treated exclusively as a children's problem, nor should it be reduced to purely reputational harm. The consequences of DSA go beyond such concerns and reveal a particularly gendered kind of sexual harm.

References

Bates S (2017) Revenge porn and mental health: a qualitative analysis of the mental health effects of revenge porn on female survivors. Fem Criminol 12(1):22–42. https://doi.org/10.1177/1557085116654565

Childnet, KekVonal, SaveTheChildren, UCLan (2017) Young people's experiences of online sexual harassment. European Commission, Brussels

Corry F (2021) Screenshot, save, share, shame: making sense of new media through screenshots and public shame. First Monday 26(4). https://doi.org/10.5210/fm.v26i4.11649
Davidson J (2014) Sexting: gender and teens. Teaching gender. Sense Publishers, Rotterdam
Dodge A (2016) Digitizing rape culture: online sexual violence and the power of the digital photograph. Crime Media Cult 12(1):65–82. https://doi.org/10.1177/1741659015601173
Döring N (2014) Consensual sexting among adolescents: risk prevention through abstinence education or safer sexting. Cyberpsychology 8:9
Frisch M, Moseholm E, Andersson M, Andresen JB, Graugaard C (2019) Sex i Danmark - Nøgletal fra projekt SEXUS 2017–2018 (Sex in Denmark - Key findings from Project SEXUS 2017–2018). Statens Serum Institut og Aalborg Universitet, Aalborg
Heinskou MB, Schierff LM, Ejbye-Ernst P, Friis CB, Liebst LS (2017) Seksuelle Krænkelser: Omfang og karakter. Det Kriminalpræventive Råd
Henry N, Powell A (2015) Beyond the 'sext': technology-facilitated sexual violence and harassment against adult women. Aust N Z J Criminol 48(1):104–118. https://doi.org/10.1177/0004865814524218
Henry N, Powell A (2016) Sexual violence in the digital age: the scope and limits of criminal law. Soc Leg Stud 25(4):397–418. https://doi.org/10.1177/0964663915624273
Henry N, McGlynn C, Flynn A, Johnson K, Powell A, Scott AJ (2021) Image-based sexual abuse : a study on the causes and consequences of non-consensual nude or sexual imagery. Routledge critical studies in crime, diversity and criminal justice. Routledge, Taylor & Francis Group, London
Jørgensen KE, Demant J (2021) Shame, shaming and economy: a theory of image-based sexual abuse within different online sharing environments. First Monday 26(4). https://doi.org/10.5210/fm.v26i4.11670
Kelly L (1988) Surviving sexual violence. Feminist perspectives series, 1st edn. Polity Press, Oxford
Maddocks S (2018) From non-consensual pornography to image-based sexual abuse: charting the course of a problem with many names. Aust Fem Stud 33(97):345–361. https://doi.org/10.1080/08164649.2018.1542592
Mandau MBH (2020) Homosocial positionings and ambivalent participation. MedieKultur 36(67):55–75. https://doi.org/10.7146/mediekultur.v36i67.113976
Mann B (2018) Femininity, shame, and redemption. Hypatia 33(3):402–417. https://doi.org/10.1111/hypa.12432
McGlynn C, Rackley E, Houghton R (2017) Beyond 'revenge porn': the continuum of image-based sexual abuse. Fem Leg Stud 25(1):25–46. https://doi.org/10.1007/s10691-017-9343-2
Paasonen S, Sundén J (2021) Shameless dicks: on male privilege, dick pic scandals, and public exposure. First Monday 26(4). https://doi.org/10.5210/fm.v26i4.11654
Powell A, Henry N (2019) Technology-facilitated sexual violence victimization: results from an online survey of Australian adults. J Interpers Violence 34(17):3637–3665. https://doi.org/10.1177/0886260516672055
Powell A, Henry N, Flynn A, Scott AJ (2019) Image-based sexual abuse: the extent, nature, and predictors of perpetration in a community sample of Australian residents. Comput Hum Behav 92:393–402. https://doi.org/10.1016/j.chb.2018.11.009
Rasmussen P, Søndergaard DM (2020) Traveling imagery. MedieKultur 36(67):76–99. https://doi.org/10.7146/mediekultur.v36i67.113983
Ringrose J, Harvey L, Gill R, Livingstone S (2013) Teen girls, sexual double standards and 'sexting': gendered value in digital image exchange. Fem Theory 14(3):305–323. https://doi.org/10.1177/1464700113499853
Ruvalcaba Y, Eaton AA (2020) Nonconsensual pornography among U.S. adults: a sexual scripts framework on victimization, perpetration, and health correlates for women and men. Psychol Violence 10(1):68–78. https://doi.org/10.1037/vio0000233
Salter M, Crofts T, Lee M (2013) Beyond criminalisation and responsibilisation: sexting, gender and young people. Curr Issues Crim Just 24(3):301–316. https://doi.org/10.1080/10345329.2013.12035963

Skolesundhed.dk (2018) Ungeprofilundersøgelsen 2017/18, Landsplan [autogenereret]. Egedal Kommune

Uhl CA, Rhyner KJ, Terrance CA, Lugo NR (2018) An examination of nonconsensual pornography websites. Fem Psychol 28(1):50–68. https://doi.org/10.1177/0959353517720225

Uldbjerg S (2020) Defying shame: shame relations in digital sexual assaults. MedieKultur 36(67):100–120. https://doi.org/10.7146/mediekultur.v36i67.113960

Uldbjerg S (2021a) The rhythms of shame in Digitial sexual assault: rhythmic resistance and the repeated assault. First Monday 26(4). https://doi.org/10.5210/fm.v26i4.11660

Uldbjerg S (2021b) Writing victimhood: a methodological manifesto for researching digital sexual assault. Women Gender Res 29(1):27–39. https://doi.org/10.7146/kkf.v29i2.124893

Walker K, Sleath E (2017) A systematic review of the current knowledge regarding revenge pornography and non-consensual sharing of sexually explicit media. Aggress Violent Behav 36:9–24. https://doi.org/10.1016/j.avb.2017.06.010

Signe Uldbjerg , PhD is a research assistant at Aarhus University at the School of Communication and Culture. Her research focuses on victim experiences of digital sexual violence, and she works with participatory, activist methods within the fields of media and sexuality studies.

Online Text-Based (Sexual) Abuse

Olga Jurasz and Kim Barker

Learning Objectives
Having read this chapter, you should be able to understand:

- What online text-based (sexual) abuse is.
- The challenges to legal frameworks posed by the online text-based (sexual) abuse.
- The scale, impact and harms of online text-based (sexual) abuse.

Introduction

The large scale of vitriolic and gender-based online violence against women (OVAW) is no longer a niche issue. It is estimated that prevalence of OVAW globally reaches 85% of women, although it may be even higher due to underreporting (EIU 2021). Its scale and wide-ranging harmful effects have been acknowledged by international bodies as well as at domestic levels (UN 2018). Alarmingly, online spaces, which are in principle open to all, and enable equal participation, are also spaces where online gender-based abuse thrive. The UN Special Rapporteur on Violence Against Women, its Causes and Consequences, recognised in her 2018 thematic report that

O. Jurasz (✉) · K. Barker
Faculty of Business and Law, Law School, The Open University, Milton Keynes, UK
e-mail: olga.jurasz@open.ac.uk; kim.barker@open.ac.uk

P. Ali, M. M. Rogers (eds.), *Gender-Based Violence: A Comprehensive Guide*,
https://doi.org/10.1007/978-3-031-05640-6_38

> Despite the benefits and empowering potential of the internet and [information and communications technology (ICT)], women and girls across the world have increasingly voiced their concern at harmful, sexist, misogynistic and violent content and behaviour online. (UN 2018: 5)

Text-based (sexual) abuse (TBSA) is a prevalent form of OVAW. It frequently occurs on social media—such as Twitter, Facebook, Instagram—and takes forms of sexist and/or misogynistic comments, tweets, messages, but also threats of violence (both on- and offline). Although TBSA is only one of many forms of OVAW, its impact is sometimes overshadowed by the image-based forms of abuse. From a legal perspective, this has generally led to swifter legal regulation of image-based sexual abuse (Barker and Jurasz 2021b) across a number of jurisdictions worldwide,[1] leaving text-based forms of online abuse in the 'shadows' of bespoke, modern and adequate legal regulation.

This chapter explores the phenomenon of TBSA as a form of OVAW. It introduces the concept of TBSA as conceptualised by Barker and Jurasz (2019a, 2021b) and explores it in socio-legal and regulatory contexts.

Definition and Types

Online abuse, particularly that which takes the form of written, electronic abuse, is an emerging category of online violence against women (OVAW). Text-based abuse (TBA) is therefore definable as

> written, electronic communication containing threatening and/or disruptive and/or distressing content, such as, e.g., textual threats to kill, rape, or otherwise inflict harm on the recipient of such messages. (Barker and Jurasz 2019a: xiv)

Where TBA takes on other more extreme (and harmful) forms, especially sexualised threats and messages, this becomes text-based sexualised abuse (TBSA). Both TBA and TBSA are forms of OVAW, but unlike their image-based forms, are not often legally or judicially recognised. Given the overtly sexualised content of online communications amounting to TBSA, the predominant impact falls on women, and yet legal frameworks on OVAW omit TBSA from their purview (Barker and Jurasz 2021b: 248–249).

TBSA can be used as an umbrella term for numerous acts of online abuse and online violence directed at women through textual communications. For instance, TBSA may include acts such as the public tweeting of death and rape threats as seen

[1] France: Digital Republic Law 2016; Israel: Prevention of Sexual Harassment Law, 5758–1998, amended in 2014; Canada: section 162.1 Criminal Code (amended through Bill C-13 Protecting Canadians from Online Harm Act 2015); Japan: Shiji Seiteki Gazou Kiroku No Teikyotō Niyoru Higai No Boushi Nikansuru Hōritsu [Act on Prevention of Victimization Resulting from Provision of Private Sexual Image], Law No. 126 of 2014; England and Wales: section 33 Criminal Justice and Courts Act 2015; Scotland: Part 1, s2 Abusive Behaviour and Sexual Harm Act 2016; Northern Ireland: Part 3, section 51 Justice Act (Northern Ireland) 2016.

in *R* v *Nimmo and Sorley* (2014) or may be more nuanced posting of implied physical harms such as the advertising of a bounty posted on Facebook in *R* v *Viscount St Davids* (2017).

There are other terms and phrases used—often confusingly—to refer to acts and behaviours which can amount to TBSA. For instance, cyberbullying, online harassment, trolling and cyberstalking (amongst others) are all forms of online abuse. Crucially, however, they may—or may not—contain sexualised abuse (Jurasz and Barker 2021) and, as a result, are often descriptors that are more generic than TBSA. Such generic descriptors fail to capture the gendered harm and dimensions of TBSA and, by extension, continue to overlook the impact it has on recipients of such communications (Barker and Jurasz 2021b: 250; Jurasz and Barker 2021).

Box 1

Alternative Terminology and Associated Concepts

Online technologically facilitated violence against women, online violence against women, text-based abuse, online abuse, online misogyny, online gender-based abuse, cyberstalking, cyber harassment, trolling, flaming, doxing, dogpiling, image-based sexual abuse, sexist hate speech, sexism.

Continuing to use these generic descriptions also serves to ensure that TBSA is not treated with the same seriousness as image-based sexual abuse (IBSA), despite recognition that online sexualised abuse does not occur solely through images but can also take textual forms. The image-based variant of OVAW has been treated very differently to TBA and TBSA. This is, perhaps, due to the visual impact that arises where there is an instance of IBSA compared with the immediate impact of seeing TBSA. That said, TBSA is of equal seriousness, even where the legal system does not currently reflect such a situation.

IBSA, as the non-consensual sharing or creation of intimate images (McGlynn and Rackley 2017), especially private sexual images, has received a noticeably different response from law and policymakers, but also the judiciary. Legal reforms to tackle IBSA have seen their way rapidly on to the statute books in numerous jurisdictions—including England and Wales and Scotland. The speed of legislative action—despite the problems with the criminal offences capturing IBSA (Henry et al. 2020; McGlynn and Rackley 2015; Powell et al. 2020a)—stands in stark contrast to the lack of attention paid to textual forms of abuse online, and especially TBSA. There is therefore not only significant disparity in the measures available to tackle IBSA versus TBSA but also in the sentencing limits applicable in the event of successful prosecutions for the former. That said, it is only sexual imagery which is covered in the respective jurisdictions of the United Kingdom.

The impact and harm(s) of IBSA have been well documented and widely recognised (McGlynn and Rackley 2017). While the growth in severity and emerging recognition of TBSA continues to highlight its prevalence, the harms caused by TBSA continue to be overlooked. The 'shrug it off' or 'turn off the Internet' responses to claims of TBSA indicate that there is still some way to go in capturing and tackling it. This is despite the significant volumes of TBSA that is sent to women online.

The harms are also staggering, with courts recognising that victims of TBSA can face unprecedented economic harms from the so-called 'stranger danger' of anonymous yet invasive online threats of rape or other attacks. The steps taken by some victims to remove their online presences, seek alternative accommodation for their families or hire private security all come with costs—not just economic ones (*R* v *Nimmo and Sorley* (2014); Barker and Jurasz 2021b: 256–257) but psychological and physical harms too, amongst others. These have yet to be captured by the criminal justice system in a manner that is equivalent to the capturing of IBSA.

The Scale and Context of TBSA

OVAW is a serious problem in contemporary societies, but it is not a new phenomenon (Barker and Jurasz 2014). Online abuse against women has become an incredibly common experience (Amnesty International 2018), with research data highlighting that women who do not suffer some form of online abuse now fall into the minority. For example, the EU Fundamental Rights Agency reported that 'the risk of young women aged between 18 and 29 years becoming a target of threatening and offensive advances on the internet is twice as high as the risk for women between 40 and 49 years, and more than three times as high as the risk for women aged between 50 and 50 years' (European Union Agency for Fundamental Rights 2014: 96).

Box 2

TBSA: Victims and Perpetrators

It is generally acknowledged that gender plays a role in the type and form of online abuse experienced online, with women being more likely than men to experience sexualised forms of such abuse (Pew Research Centre 2021). Similarly, transgender individuals experience higher rates of online abuse and harassment overall and higher rates of sexualised and/or gender-based forms of such abuse than heterosexual cisgender individuals (Powell et al. 2020b; Amnesty International 2018).

Furthermore, experience from the United Kingdom shows that TB(S)A targets women irrespective of their views. For example, women from various parts of the political spectrum have been subjected to TBA online, with 58% of respondents in Europe and 42% of those surveyed globally reporting that they had online attacks directed at them because they are women, and women in politics (Barker and Jurasz 2021e). Similarly, the ongoing debate concerning sex- and gender-based rights between 'trans-inclusionary feminists' and 'trans-exclusionary radical feminists' (TERFs) has seen extreme forms of TBA directed at individuals on both sides of this debate by individuals from either side of the debate as well as other social media users.

The latter subverts one of the myths surrounding TB(S)A—namely, that it is directed solely by men against women. Studies carried out by DEMOS have shown not only that both men and women tend to use misogynistic language on Twitter (DEMOS 2014) but also that 50% of abusers analysed in the 2016 study were in fact women (DEMOS 2016).

As a gender-based form of violence, it is rooted in gender inequality, the structural discrimination of women and patriarchy and further reinforced by strongly embedded gender stereotypes. The offline abusive behaviours and gender-based violence directed at women has migrated to a new—online—environment, where it has taken on new forms specific to these environments, such as TBSA on social media platforms. For instance, the early forms of online TBSA can be traced back to online gaming and the abuse of women in these spaces—including gender-based, heavily stereotypical, image-based and text-based forms of abuse (Barker and Jurasz 2014; Jurasz and Barker 2021). As such, the underpinning, structural causes of OVAW and 'offline' VAW are shared and—just like its offline manifestations—undermine gender equality and non-discrimination of women (Barker and Jurasz 2020b), especially in the public sphere (Barker and Jurasz 2019b). For instance, 'women in countries with long-standing or institutionalised gender inequality tend to experience online violence at higher rates' (EIU 2021).

The intersectional aspects of VAW are also reflected in its online forms. For instance, a 2017 Amnesty International United Kingdom study of online violence against women in politics demonstrated not only the high volume of TBSA received by female MPs but also showed a significant increase in the volume of abuse directed at black and Asian women politicians (Dhordia 2017). In contrast, Kuperberg's small scale study of violence against women politicians in Israel suggest that whilst 'ethnicity, religion and age were small or non-existing factors, (...) abusive tweets included sexist, Islamophobic and racist language' (Kuperberg 2018: 687–688). This suggests that text-based forms of OVAW are reflective not only of the motivations of the perpetrators but also of various forms of oppression (Kuperberg 2018: 688). In turn, this is reflected in the wide-ranging, diverse types of harms flowing from TBSA (Fig. 1), which are only partially captured by the legal system (Barker and Jurasz 2021b).

Box 3 TBSA: A Global Perspective

TBSA—a global issue

TBSA takes place worldwide and manifests itself in a number of contexts, affecting different demographics and groups of women. As such, there is no uniform 'type', 'context' or 'victim' of TBSA. For instance, some of the specific groups of women that have been targeted by TBSA include (but are not limited to): feminists (Lewis et al. 2017), academics (Barlow and Awan 2016), politicians (Barker and Jurasz 2019d), journalists (UNESCO 2021) and human rights defenders (Kvinna till Kvinna 2018).

TBSA plays out in a number of contexts too, including elections (Bardall 2013), sport events (Observer Sport 2021) and even transitional political processes (LFJL 2021). It is also a tool in the perpetration of domestic and intimate partner violence. In particular, it is significant as a form of coercive and controlling behaviour, which can take the form of constant messaging by the abusive partner, using social media to post threatening or abusive content, including encouraging others to harass or abuse the victim.

TBSA directed at women is not only gendered but can also be highly contextual. Differences in languages, cultures and social norms that differ amongst countries are also reflected in the abusive content of messages, tweets or posts. For instance, a study on OVAW in Libya (LFJL 2021: 23) confirms that regional differences in Arabic dialect mean that certain words which are offensive to people in one region do not have the same meaning in another. However, the contextual and linguistic nuances are often disregarded in the context of moderation of abusive content by platforms, which poses a significant challenge in ensuring avenues of redress for such abuse (Barker and Jurasz 2021d).

The Impact of TBSA

The harmful impact of TBSA, fuelled by its hypervisibility, remains largely unaddressed by the legal system. Although some progress has been made in *R* v *Nimmo and Sorley* (see Box 4) and in *R* v *Viscount St Davids* to recognise the consequences of such abuse for the victims, the overarching categorisations of harms largely operate within the physical and psychological harms binary.

Box 4

R v Nimmo and Sorley (2014)

R v Nimmo and Sorley was a landmark case dealing with text-based (sexual) abuse directed against a Labour MP, Stella Creasy, and a feminist campaigner, Caroline Criado-Perez. It was the first judgement in England and

Wales where TBSA was successfully prosecuted, establishing accountability—however limited (Barker 2019)—for online, text-based and misogynistic abuse.

In 2013, Creasy and Criado-Perez campaigned for inclusion of more women on Bank of England banknotes, which attracted a significant amount of backlash in forms of abusive, threatening and violent tweets. At its peak, the abuse directed at Caroline Criado-Perez was reaching approximately 50 abusive tweets per hour for 12 h (Philipson 2013). John Nimmo and Isabela Sorley sent the most abusive tweets, including severe threats:

> *Fuck off and die, you should have jumped in front of horses, go die.*
> *Rape is the last of your worries.*
> *Rape?! I'd do a lot worse things than rape you.*
> *I will find you and you don't want to know what I will do when I do...kill yourself before I do* (R v Nimmo and Sorley 2014: 2).

The scale and impact of the abuse received by Creasy and Criado-Perez was judicially recognised by Judge Riddle who remarked that the effects of the harassment received by the women was 'life-changing', causing 'serious and entirely predictable harm' (R v Nimmo and Sorley 2014: 2). The long-lasting psychological effects of the abuse received were powerfully captured in Caroline Criado-Perez's statement: 'I don't think I will ever be free of them'.

As we argue elsewhere, harms arising from TBSA are much more nuanced and require a greater degree of conceptualisation, reflecting the diversity of contexts in which TBSA occurs and motivations behind the abuse. In doing so, it is crucial to note the possible—and in some contexts, very likely (see, e.g. LFJL 2021)—transference of harm between online and offline environments. Furthermore, the common occurrence and large scale of online TBSA, combined with its hypervisibility and limited avenues for redress, reinforce the notion that VAW—be it online or offline—is socially acceptable. This misperception causes a specific type of collective societal harm in that it contributes to the already existing normalisation of VAW. As a result, 'everyday' VAW, such as online TBSA becomes ironically 'unnoticeable' despite its scale and frequency (Barker and Jurasz 2019a), with only extreme cases of (O)VAW, such as deaths of Molly Russell or Caroline Flack, shocking the public conscience.

Figure 1 represents the diverse range of harms arising from TBSA, as proposed by the authors.

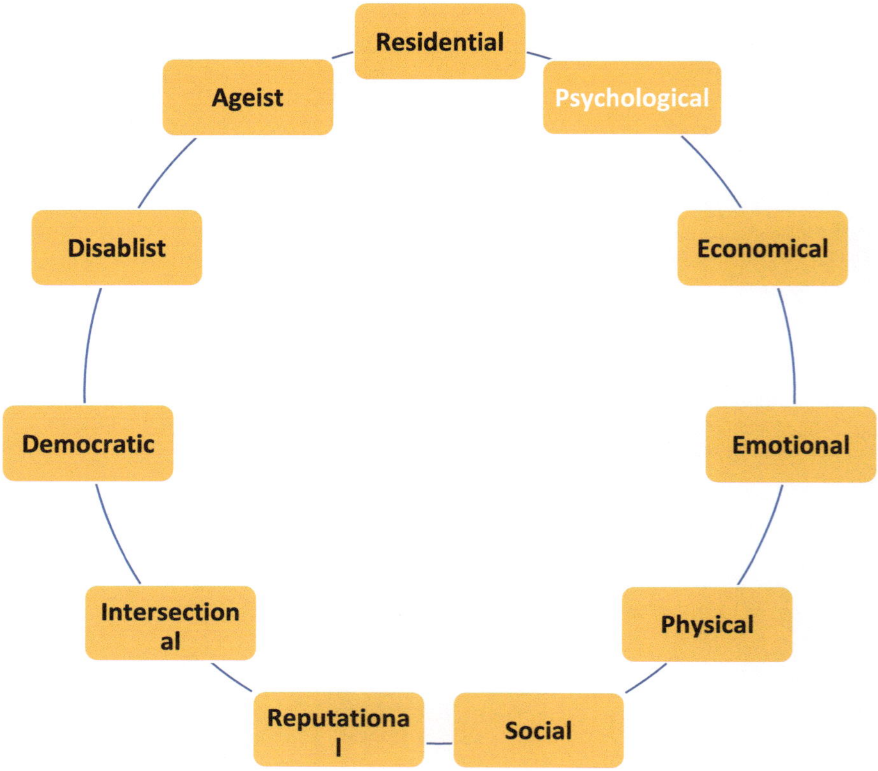

Fig. 1 The typology of harms arising from text-based (sexual) abuse, as proposed by Barker and Jurasz (2021b)

Law, Policy and Practice

The law has been very slow to respond to growth in instances of TBSA. The current capturing of TBSA (and TBA) aside, there have been some initiatives that have indicated some —albeit limited—willingness to address online textual abuse in its sexualised forms.

International and Regional Policy

Notably, the UN Special Rapporteur on violence against women has explicitly recognised the challenges posed by online gender-based abuse, including TBSA, and highlighted the need for action to address it: 'Online gender-based abuse and violence are undeniably a scourge, and governments and companies should be taking action against it' (OHCHR 2017). This recognition, while potentially an indicator of a change in law and policy responses, has not readily been matched at other regional or national levels.

In Europe for instance, there has been a lethargic reaction to addressing societal challenges such as IBSA. The focus, particularly at a European level, has fallen, instead, on taking steps to address connected albeit distinct challenges that fall within the broader VAW agenda. The policy agenda at a regional level focuses heavily on addressing forms of VAW, including sexist hate speech (Council of Europe 2016: 2), and misogyny (PACE 2017). Other initiatives suggest that issues such as IBSA fall within the anti-sexism agenda more broadly, especially when challenging perceptions of dominant masculinities, or misogynist hate speech (Council of Europe 2019).

National Law, Policy and Practice in England and Wales

At a more national level, there is a very different emphasis, particularly within England and Wales. The domestic response to TBSA and its harms is as woeful as the attention paid to it at a regional level. TBSA in England and Wales, Scotland and Northern Ireland's legal systems is treated as the poor relation of IBSA. Where attention has been given to TBSA, it has tended to arise in the context of either speech controls or hate crime discussions, especially those attached to either gender or to misogyny. The key legislative developments in England and Wales focus first on abusive and offensive communications, second on online harm/safety, and third, hate crimes (see Box 5).

Box 5 Summary of Relevant Legislation in England and Wales

Legislation/policy	Terms	Focus
Communications Act 2003	Electronic communication; grossly offensive	Misuse of a public communications network
Malicious Communications Act 1988	Communications; grossly offensive	Misuse of communications network
Criminal Justice and Courts Act 2015	Disclose; sexual photos; consent; intent to cause distress	Non-consensual sharing of intimate images
eCommerce Directive 2000	Liability shield	Limitation of liability for online platforms if not acting as editors of content
Online Safety Bill 2021	Safety; duty of care; illegal content; harms	Making the internet a safer place; imposing duties of care on websites and platforms for 'illegal' content
Digital Services Act 2020	Illegal content; harmful content; liability	Reform of the eCommerce Directive; liability shield
Communications Offences Review (Law Commission)	Communications; offensive; abusive	Updating the communications provisions
Hate Crime Review (Law Commission)	Hate crime; protected characteristics	Updating and reformulating the protected characteristics for hate crimes

Offensive Textual Communications

The leading current provision in England and Wales is that of the Communications Act 2003 (CA). Under s127, an offence may be committed where someone sends an electronic communication via a public communications network that is or could be 'grossly offensive'. This provision supplements the outdated (and soon to be repealed) Malicious Communications Act 1988 (MCA), which also includes a threshold of grossly offensive for an offence to be committed under s1.

There are several particular difficulties with the abusive communications provisions here. Firstly, neither provision expressly captures any element of sexualised abuse, nor text-based abuse. The CA and MCA provisions are also offences that only relate to the sending of a communication—there is no requirement that it be seen or received by the intended recipient (Barker and Jurasz 2019a: 69), which presents the second challenge. Thirdly, and perhaps most problematically, the standard which has to be satisfied for an offence to have been committed relates to the content of the communication which must be grossly offensive, not just offensive. This incredibly high standard has been widely criticised (PACE 2016; Barker and Jurasz 2019a: 40) because of how difficult it is to evidentially prove. Finally, even where that standard can be satisfied, there is no guarantee of a prosecution. Even where is a successful one, the resultant sentencing cannot be higher than 2 years, with most high profile (and repeat offenders) only receiving sentences of a handful of weeks—convicted abusers John Nimmo and Isabella Sorley received 8 weeks and 12 weeks, respectively after their 2014 trial (*Nimmo and Sorley* 2014), only for John Nimmo to reoffend 2 years later (Sommers 2016).

A successful prosecution and custodial sentence is little deterrent. Even where there is a successful prosecution, the Sentencing Council Guidelines make clear that the starting point for the most serious offence under s127 CA in the Magistrates Court, where there is higher culpability and greater harm, is a custodial sentence of 9 weeks, subject to (1) factors increasing seriousness, and (2) factors indicating a reduction (Sentencing Council 2017). The practice, therefore, when dealing with communication network offences triable summarily in a Magistrates Court that amount to or encompass TBSA is to not utilise the full range of custodial sentences despite the maximum potential penalties available in law. Reform proposals relating to the offensive communications provisions are currently ongoing by the Law Commission (Law Commission 2020a).

Online Harms/Safety

TBSA communications are currently the responsibility of the individual(s) sending the communication. There is no route of redress for the victim or target of the abuse against the platform which hosts or facilitates the communication. Platform operators such as Twitter, Facebook and TikTok are protected from such responsibility arising by virtue of the eCommerce Directive (2000) liability shield provisions. These provisions, which have been enacted into domestic law in the United Kingdom are currently the subject of reform by the European Commission through the Digital Services Act 2020—but it should be noted that this reform package retains and strengthens the liability shield protections (DSA Recital 18), rather than weakening them.

The provisions dealing with online content such as TBSA communications are subject to (at the time of writing) ongoing domestic law reform within the United Kingdom. The Online Safety Bill 2021 has been heralded as a potential solution to communications encompassing TBSA, and the harms that follow from such abuse. Within its provisions include the soon-to-be-introduced 'duty of care', which will be imposed on social media operators to ensure that certain harms do not arise from content which is shared, posted or sent via their platforms.

The proposed s5 duty of care includes 'illegal content duties' as well as 'adults' online safety protection duties'. While these duties may offer a fresh route for the tackling of offensive and/or abusive content, there has been no specific consideration made within the Bill for TBSA. This is despite the fact that the Online Harms White Paper (DCMS 2019) did acknowledge the problem posed by online abuse. Despite calls for TBSA to be explicitly recognised within this legislative reform package (Barker and Jurasz 2019c, 2021c, d), no such accommodation has been made. For the Online Safety Bill to capture TBSA, it would be necessary for harm to have arisen which falls foul of the duty of care obligations imposed on platform operators. Sexual imagery is the only sexualised abuse element captured by the Online Safety Bill—textual forms of sexual abuse remain notable by their omission (Barker and Jurasz 2021c).

Hate Crime

The current hate crime framework in England and Wales and Scotland focuses on protected characteristics. For TBSA to be captured within the hate crime framework, there needs to be a characteristic which is protected – such as, for example, race or religion. Gender/sex is not currently one of these characteristics, so there cannot be a gender-based hate crime capturing potential TBSA.

Similarly, for there to be an enhanced sentence applied to a criminal act—such as an underlying criminal offence, for example, a s127 grossly offensive communication—there also needs to be a protected characteristic which saw the offence be motivated by prejudice against that characteristic. For instance, a racially aggravated tweet can be prosecuted as a hate crime on the basis of racial hatred, (*Viscount St Davids* 2017), but a grossly offensive tweet which abuses a woman cannot be treated as a hate crime because there is no characteristic protecting sex/gender.

This leaves a somewhat problematic law and policy landscape whereby an offensive communication can comprise TBSA, but cannot be treated to an enhanced criminal sentence because there is no legal protection given to gender as a characteristic within the criminal law (Barker and Jurasz 2019a: 84). Reforms are ongoing in England and Wales as to whether sex/gender should feature as a characteristic in the hate crime framework (Law Commission 2020b). Discussions in Scotland focus on the development of a separate, stand-alone offence of misogynistic harassment, rather than the development of hate crimes motivated by sex/gender (Barker and Jurasz 2021a: 16).

Summary

- TB(S)A is a growing global phenomenon and a form of online violence against women.
- Law and policy responses in the United Kingdom have thus far prioritised image-based forms of online sexual abuse over those expressed in a textual form.
- TB(S)A gives rise to a number of different harms—both online and offline—which are not yet captured nor recognised by the legal system in the United Kingdom.

References

Abusive Behaviour and Sexual Harm (Scotland) Act (2016)

Amnesty International (2018) Toxic Twitter—a toxic place for women. https://www.amnesty.org/en/latest/research/2018/03/online-violence-against-women-chapter-3/#topanchor. Accessed 27 Oct 2021

Bardall G (2013) Gender-specific election violence: the role of information and communication technologies. Stability 60:1–11

Barker K (2019) R v Nimmo and Sorley (2014). In: Rackley E, Auchmuty R (eds) Women's legal landmarks: Celebrating 100 years of women and law in the UK and Ireland. Hart, Oxford, pp 608–610

Barker K, Jurasz O (2014) Gender, human rights and cybercrime: are virtual worlds really that different? In: Asimow M, Brown K, Papke D (eds) Law and popular culture: international perspectives. Cambridge Scholars Publishing, Newcastle upon Tyne

Barker K, Jurasz O (2019a) Online misogyny as a hate crime: a challenge for legal regulation? Routledge, London, New York

Barker K, Jurasz O (2019b) Online misogyny: a challenge for digital feminism? J Int Aff 72(2):95–113

Barker K, Jurasz O (2019c) Online Harms White Paper Consultation Response. http://oro.open.ac.uk/69840/. Accessed 27 Oct 2021

Barker K, Jurasz O (2019d) Violence against women in politics (#VAWP)—the antithesis of (online) equality. Scottish Policy and Research Exchange blog. https://spre.scot/violence-against-women-in-politics-online/. Accessed 27 Oct 2021

Barker K, Jurasz O (2020b) Online violence against women as an obstacle to gender equality: a critical view from Europe. Eur Equal Law Rev 1:47–60

Barker K, Jurasz O (2021a) Misogynistic harassment: a stumbling block for Scots hate crime reform? Juridical Rev 1(1):1–17

Barker K, Jurasz O (2021b) Text-based (sexual) abuse and online violence against women: toward law reform? In: Bailey J, Flynn A, Henry N (eds) The Emerald International handbook of technology facilitated violence and abuse. Emerald, Bingley, pp 247–264. https://doi.org/10.1108/978-1-83982-848-520211017

Barker K, Jurasz O (2021c) Gender-based abuse online: an assessment of law, policy and reform in England & Wales. In: Powell A, Flynn A, Sugiura L (eds) Handbook on gender, violence and technology

Barker K, Jurasz O (2021d) Online misogyny as a hate crime: an obstacle to equality? GenIUS

Barker K, Jurasz O (2021e) OVAW: recognising democratic harms and participatory exclusion. Conference paper presented at the suffrage now! International conference on Gender & Democracy, Stockholm University, 13–14 August 2021

Barlow C, Awan I (2016) 'You need to be sorted out with a knife': the attempted silencing of women and people of Muslim faith within academia. Social Media Soc 2(4):1–11

Communications Act (2003)

Council of Europe (2016) Combatting Sexist Hate Speech. https://rm.coe.int/CoERMPublicCommonSearchServices/DisplayDCTMContent?documentId=0900001680651592. Accessed 27 Oct 2021

Council of Europe (2017) PACE Resolution 2144 (2017). Ending cyberdiscrimination and online hate. http://assembly.coe.int/nw/xml/XRef/Xref-XML2HTML-en.asp?fileid=23456. Accessed 27 Oct 2021

Council of Europe (2019) Recommendation on Preventing & Combatting Sexism. https://rm.coe.int/prems-055519-gbr-2573-cmrec-2019-1-web-a5/168093e08c. Accessed 27 Oct 2021

Council of Europe Parliamentary Assembly Committee on Equality and Non-Discrimination (PACE). (2016). Ending Cyberdiscrimination and online hate, report by rapporteur Marit Maij. Doc 14217. https://assembly.coe.int/nw/xml/XRef/Xref-XML2HTML-EN.asp?fileid=23234. Accessed 27 Oct 2021

Criminal Justice Act (2015)

DCMS (2019) Online harms white paper (April 2019)

DEMOS (2014) Misogyny on Twitter. https://demosuk.wpengine.com/files/MISOGYNY_ON_TWITTER.pdf?1399567516. Accessed 27 Oct 2021

DEMOS (2016) The use of misogynistic terms on Twitter. https://demosuk.wpengine.com/wp-content/uploads/2016/05/Misogyny-online.pdf Accessed 27 Oct 2021

Dhordia A (2017) Unsocial media: tracking twitter abuse against women MPs. Medium. https://medium.com/@AmnestyInsights/unsocial-media-tracking-twitter-abuse-against-women-mps-fc28aeca498a. Accessed 27 Oct 2021

Digital Services Act (2020) Regulation of the European Parliament and of the Council on a Single Market For Digital Services (Digital Services Act) and amending Directive 2000/31/EC.COM(2020) 825

e-Commerce Directive (2000) Directive 2000/31/EC of the European Parliament and of the Council of 8 June 2000 on Certain Legal Aspects of Information Society Services, in Particular Electronic Commerce, in the Internal Market ('Directive on Electronic Commerce') [2000] OJ L178/1

EIU (2021) Measuring the prevalence of online violence against women. https://onlineviolencewomen.eiu.com/. Accessed 27 Oct 2021

European Union Agency for Fundamental Rights (2014) Violence against women: an EU-wide survey. Main results. Publications Office of the European Union

Henry N, McGlynn C, Flynn A, Johnson K, Powell A, Scott AJ (2020) Image-based sexual abuse: a study on the causes and consequences of non-consensual nude or sexual imagery. Routledge, London, New York

Jurasz O, Barker K (2021) Sexual violence in the digital age: a criminal law conundrum? German Law J 22(5):784–799

Justice Act (Northern Ireland) (2016)

Kuperberg R (2018) Intersectional violence against women in politics. Polit Gend 14(4):685–690

Kvinna till Kvinna (2018) #femdefenders. The hatred towards women human rights defenders—online and offline. https://kvinnatillkvinna.org/wp-content/uploads/2018/10/10-Femdefenders-the-hatred-against-women-ENG.pdf. Accessed 27 Oct 2021

Law Commission (2020a) Harmful communications: the criminal offences. A Consultation Paper. https://www.lawcom.gov.uk/project/reform-of-the-communications-offences/

Law Commission (2020b) Hate crime laws. A consultation paper. https://www.lawcom.gov.uk/project/hate-crime/

Lewis R, Rowe M, Wiper C (2017) Online abuse of feminists as an emerging form of violence against women and girls. Br J Criminol 57(6):1462–1481

LFJL (2021) 'We will not be silenced'. Online violence against women in Libya. https://wwwlibyanjusticeorg/news/urgent-action-needed-to-address-shocking-levels-of-online-violence-against-libyan-women. Accessed 27 Oct 2021
Malicious Communications Act (1988)
McGlynn C, Rackley E (2015) More than just 'revenge porn': tackling the misuse of private sexual images. The Holyrood. https://www.holyrood.com/comment/view,more-than-just-revenge-porn-tackling-the-misuse-of-private-sexual-images_6029.htm. Accessed 27 Oct 2021
McGlynn C, Rackley E (2017) Image-based sexual abuse. Oxf J Leg Stud 37(3):534–561
Observer Sport (2021) BBC's Sonja McLaughlan reveals online abuse over Owen Farrell interview. The Guardian. https://www.theguardian.com/sport/2021/feb/27/bbcs-sonja-mclaughlan-reveals-online-abuse-over-owen-farrell-interview. Accessed 27 Oct 2021
Office of the High Commissioner for Human Rights (OHCHR) (2017) UN experts urge States and companies to address online gender-based abuse but warn against censorship. https://www.ohchr.org/EN/NewsEvents/Pages/DisplayNews.aspx?NewsID=21317. Accessed 27 Oct 2021
Online Safety Bill (2021)
Pew Research Centre (2021) The State of Online Harassment. https://www.pewresearch.org/internet/2021/01/13/the-state-of-online-harassment/. Accessed 27 Oct 2021
Philipson A (2013) Woman who campaigned for Jane Austen bank note receives twitter death threats. The Telegraph. https://www.telegraph.co.uk/technology/10207231/Woman-who-campaigned-for-Jane-Austen-bank-note-receives-Twitter-death-threats.html. Accessed 27 Oct 2021
Powell A, Scott AJ, Henry N, Flynn A (2020a) Image-based sexual abuse: an international study of victims and perpetrators. Summary report. RMIT University, Melbourne
Powell A, Scott AJ, Henry N (2020b) Digital harassment and abuse: experiences of sexuality and gender minority adults. Eur J Criminol 17(2):199–223
R v Nimmo and Sorley (2014) (Westminster Magistrates' Court, 24 January 2014)
R v Viscount St Davids (2017) (Westminster Magistrates' Court, 11 July 2017)
Sentencing Council (2017) Communication network offences (Revised 2017), Communications Act 2003, ss.127(1) and 127(2). https://www.sentencingcouncil.org.uk/offences/magistrates-court/item/communication-network-offences-revised-2017/. Accessed 27 Oct 2021
Sommers J (2016) Troll John Nimmo faces second prison term for tweeting abuse to MP Luciana Berger. Huffington Post. https://www.huffingtonpost.co.uk/entry/twitter-troll-john-nimmo-faces-second-prison-term-for-tweeting-abuse-to-mp-luciana-berger_uk_5798d9cde4b0796a0b6139f5?guccounter=1. Accessed 27 Oct 2021
UNESCO (2021) The Chilling: Global trends in online violence against women journalists. https://en.unesco.org/sites/default/files/the-chilling.pdf. Accessed 27 Oct 2021
United Nations Human Rights Council (2018) Report of the Special Rapporteur on violence against women, its causes and consequences on online violence against women and girls from a human rights perspective, A/HRC/38/47. https://www.ohchr.org/EN/HRBodies/HRC/RegularSessions/Session38/Documents/A_HRC_38_47_EN.docx. Accessed 27 Oct 2021

Olga Jurasz is a Senior Lecturer in Law at the Open University. Her research focuses on legal responses to violence against women (including online violence), international law and human rights.

Kim Barker is a Senior Lecturer in Law at the Open University. Her research focuses on the legal regulation of online spaces, including online violence against women, internet law and online harms.

Technology-Facilitated Abuse

Colleen Fisher, Michaela M. Rogers, Lisa Fontes, and Parveen Ali

Learning Objectives
Having read this chapter, you should be able to understand

- The extent of technology-facilitated abuse in intimate partner relationships.
- The range of behaviours that constitute technology-facilitated abuse.
- The impact of technology-facilitated abuse on victim-survivors and their children.

Introduction

This chapter provides an overview of the ways in which technology-facilitated abuse has been defined and explored in the literature and framed in relation to intimate partner violence (IPV). It enables the reader to understand the range of

C. Fisher (✉)
School of Population and Global Health, University of Western Australia, Perth, WA, Australia
e-mail: colleen.fisher@uwa.edu.au

M. M. Rogers
Department of Sociological Studies, University of Sheffield, Sheffield, UK
e-mail: m.rogers@sheffield.ac.uk

L. Fontes
Department of Interdisciplinary, University of Massachusetts, Amherst, MA, USA
e-mail: lfontes@uww.umass.edu

P. Ali
Health Sciences School, University of Sheffield, Sheffield, UK
e-mail: parveen.ali@sheffield.ac.uk

P. Ali, M. M. Rogers (eds.), *Gender-Based Violence: A Comprehensive Guide*, https://doi.org/10.1007/978-3-031-05640-6_39

behaviours that constitute technology-facilitated abuse (TFA), drawing attention to the different technologies and varied strategies employed by perpetrators. The chapter provides a snapshot of the prevalence of TFA, although our knowledge about the extent of TFA perpetration is incomplete, and some countries lag behind in collecting data in this regard. However, available evidence clearly shows that digital technologies have opened up spaces for perpetrators to extend and expand their control over their partner beyond the physical world. We end by highlighting the range of impacts that studies on TFA have drawn attention to, including in relation to mental health, social impacts, economic consequences and in terms of the opportunities for perpetrators to create a sense of omnipresence.

Definitions and Explanations

In the United Kingdom, the USA and Australia, abuse facilitated through digital and communications technology has been increasingly raised as an important issue in the context of IPV (Woodlock et al. 2020b). Digital communication has heralded a revolution in the ways in which individuals seek out, commence, maintain and/or end intimate relationships. Perpetrators of IPV increasingly utilise these same technologies to exercise forms of power and control over victim-survivors and children not available before advances in digital and other new technologies were a reality and readily available. Thus, IPV is no longer exclusively perpetrated when the victim and perpetrator are face-to-face (Marganski and Melander 2018). Technology enables coercive control to transcend boundaries and fixed borders (Dragiewicz et al. 2018b), adding to victim-survivors feeling they are under constant surveillance by the perpetrator. Specifically, the research focus to date has centred on the increased use of technology (Henry and Powell 2015; Southworth et al. 2007) as a tactic of coercive control (Stark 2007) to abuse, intimidate, harass, monitor, humiliate, shame, stalk and punish women—both whilst in the relationship and post-separation (Woodlock et al. 2020a).

Technology-facilitated abuse is the original term used to capture the range of these behaviours (see Box 1). The term 'technology facilitated abuse', however, is subject to debate and not favoured by some researchers who argue it infers that technology, rather than the perpetrator, is implicated in the abuse (Vera-Gray 2017). Dragiewicz et al. (2018a, b), prefer to describe the behaviours as 'technology-facilitated coercive control'. They argue that this name more holistically captures the relational as well as the technological aspects of the diverse range of tactics (facilitated by technology) that perpetrators utilise to control their partner both within violent relationships and post-separation. This name is also grounded in understandings of IPV proffered by Stark (2007). That is, IPV is characterised by a pattern of coercive and controlling behaviours often reinforced by physical and/or sexual violence and threats.

Further, the term 'digital coercive control' was proposed by Harris and Woodlock (2018) as an alternative to both 'technology-facilitated abuse' and 'technology-facilitated coercive control'. Harris and Woodlock suggest that 'digital coercive control' is more appropriate for two main reasons—'digital' is preferred to 'technology-facilitated' as the term takes the focus away from the technology and firmly places the perpetrator's behaviour at the centre of the issue. 'Coercive control' is preferred over 'abuse' as it captures more aptly the 'spatially diffused' tactics that perpetrators engage in to exercise control over women in violent relationships (Stark 2007). Additionally, the term captures the 'borderless' nature of the behaviours and situates them within the broader context of gender-based violence and inequality (Harris and Woodlock 2018; Woodlock et al. 2020a).

Notwithstanding the importance of debates over the term used, in this chapter, we use the term 'technology-facilitated abuse' (TFA) (see Box 1). We do not consider that 'digital' adequately encompasses the myriad or hybrid forms of abuse experienced by victim-survivors and their children that are described in the literature and reported here. Using the term 'technology-facilitated abuse' is also a pragmatic decision. As the original term used to describe these behaviours, 'technology-facilitated abuse' is likely to be more widely recognised, rendering the information in this chapter accessible to a wider audience.

Box 1

Definition

Technology-facilitated abuse is a form of behaviour that involves the use of technology as a means to coerce, control, intimidate, stalk or harass another person.

Alternative terminology

Technology-Facilitated Violence and Abuse; Digital Coercive Control; Technology-facilitated coercive control; Cyber aggression; Cyber victimisation; Technology-Facilitated Domestic Abuse.

Behaviours Constituting TFA

The behaviours that constitute TFA are broad and may be either overt or covert, with strong evidence suggesting that it is experienced alongside physical, sexual and/or non-physical forms of violence in the physical world (see Box 2). In a national study conducted in Australia with professionals ($n = 515$) who work with victim-survivors, Woodlock et al. (2020a) found that almost all (99.3%) participants had supported clients who had experienced TFA in tandem with physical world abuse.

Repeated text messaging (Marganski and Melander 2018), including messages that contain threats (Dragiewicz et al. 2018a), is often the most commonly reported form of TFA (Woodlock et al. 2020a). Another commonly reported form is cyberstalking, or the use of digital communications to stalk another person (Hand et al. 2009; Logan et al. 2000; Marganski and Melander 2018; Woodlock 2017). The use of cyberstalking is concerning because we know that stalking in the physical world is a risk factor for both sexual violence and intimate partner homicide, but alarmingly, it is not often treated seriously (Scott et al. 2010). There is no reason to expect that because it occurs digitally that it will be treated any differently.

Cyberstalking is often reported as being more common after the relationship has ended (Hand et al. 2009), but this is by no means always the case. Cyberstalking includes: monitoring movements through GPS tracking devices (Dimond et al. 2011; Dragiewicz et al. 2018a), including perpetrators hiding a tracking device in the victim-survivor's vehicle (Woodlock 2017); tracking through location-based features on Facebook (Dimond et al. 2011) and telephones; and perpetrators engaging their friends and family members to expand the scope of abuse—referred to by Melton (2007) as 'proxy stalking'.

A straightforward solution for monitoring movements through GPS tracking would be to disable location tracking or remove the GPS device. To do so, however, may have implications for the safety of the victim-survivor as it could alert the perpetrator that she may be intending to leave the relationship (Woodlock 2017) or it could increase the risk of an escalation in the violence as the perpetrator attempts to wrest back control over her (Fraser et al. 2010).

The literature also reports victim-survivors' experiences of harassment and impersonation on social media (Dragiewicz et al. 2018a; Marganski and Melander 2018; Woodlock et al. 2020a). Social media provides a platform where the perpetrator can publicly harass, shame or humiliate the victim-survivor (Woodlock 2017). Where the abuse is not known outside the relationship, unwittingly family and friends can facilitate the abuse by disclosing information about the victim-survivor through these avenues (Freed et al. 2017). Blocking the perpetrator from social media accounts does not mean the abuse will cease as it can continue through the social media of shared friends or followers, or through those of their children (Freed et al. 2017). Where the perpetrator harasses family and friends of the victim-survivor, this can lead to her closing her social media accounts and potentially losing social media as a means of staying socially connected (Woodlock 2017). Being 'tagged' in photos on Facebook has the potential to diminish women's safety as it may compromise the privacy of her location (Dimond et al. 2011).

Box 2 Case Studies

A High-Profile Case Study: Matthew Herrick

In October 2016, Matthew Herrick was approached outside his home in New York City, USA, by a man unknown to him. The man claimed 'You were just texting me, dude'. The man held his phone up to Herrick showing a profile on his screen from the gay dating app Grindr. It featured a topless photo of Herrick on a fake profile. The man insisted that he and Herrick had been messaging and that Herrick had invited the man to his home for sex. Herrick knew the profile was not his and after a heated exchange, the man left. Herrick retreated into his home. Later that day, his doorbell rang. A different man was at the door insisting that he too had just made a sex date with Herrick via Grindr. A further two men showed up at Herrick's home that day expecting to have sex with him.

This happened numerous times over the course of the next few months. At the height of the abuse, 16 men showed up every day at Herrick's home or workplace; each man expected either degrading or violent sex. In total, over 1000 unknown men were involved in the abuse between October 2016 and March 2017. Fake profiles were set up on dating sites claiming that Herrick was HIV-positive and that he enjoyed aggressive, unprotected sex, with or without drugs. Adverts also claimed that potential sex partners should be persistent in their attempts to have sex with Herrick as this was part of his rape and role play fantasies.

Herrick's ex-boyfriend was found to be behind the fake profiles. Herrick described him as jealous and controlling. After filing more than a dozen complaints with the police, Herrick took out an 'order of protection' which stipulated that his ex-boyfriend should not have direct contact with Herrick nor attempt to do so through a third party. Herrick's experience is an example of *cyberharassment by proxy*; that is, harassment perpetrated through a third party. The ex-boyfriend was arrested in October 2017 and charged with stalking, criminal impersonation, identity theft and for breaching a court order (he was found hiding in a bush outside Herrick's home).

In an attempt to end the harassment, Herrick contacted Grindr and Scruff (another dating site which held fake profiles of Herrick) with a request to remove the fake profiles from their platforms. Scruff responded immediately and took down the accounts. Grindr did not respond and Herrick sought legal redress and took action under the Communications Decency Act 1996.Grindr claimed they had done nothing wrong, and a federal judge agreed. The case has drawn considerable public and media attention as Herrick went to the Court of Appeal then to the Supreme Court after the second circuit ruled in favour of Grindr.

An Everyday Case Study: Susan

Susan, 28, was a divorced mother of two girls, working as a paraprofessional in a school, when she met and fell in love with Tom, 38, a divorced auto mechanic with no children. They had a whirlwind romance, moved in together, married and had another child together within that first year.

During their decade together, Tom was physically violent on a dozen occasions. He terrorised Susan, humiliated her verbally, sexually assaulted her, and used technology to control and abuse her during and after their relationship. Tom constantly accused Susan of cheating on him, even with her family members, and used his jealousy as an excuse to steal Susan's phone, and monitor her messages and phone calls. He also tracked her whereabouts through a device in her car.

Tom would break into Susan's email, delete messages, and sometimes impersonate her in responses to her contacts. He hacked into her credit cards, ordered items for himself, then got into her computer to delete the evidence of his purchases. Tom also texted and harassed Susan's oldest daughter, Jenny. For instance, when Jenny was 16, Tom called her at her summer fast food job and told her that her mom was about to kill herself. She rushed home to discover that her mom was fine.

Eight years into their relationship, Susan began calling the police. Tom usually fled before they arrived. Almost 20 police reports of domestic violence, including TFA, were filed, yet Tom has not spent a night in jail. The cases are continued, and most are considered misdemeanours. Even when Tom threatened to kill Susan, and the police found ammunition in his car, he was not arrested. They told Susan that since Tom had not specifically said that he would shoot her, they did not have grounds to arrest him. This case is scheduled to be heard in court soon.

On social media, Tom harassed Susan by tagging her in posts with comments such as, 'snitches get stitches'. He also got other people to call her and text her threatening messages at all hours of the day and night.

Susan uses technology to protect herself. She installed 6 video cameras around her house to document Tom's stalking. She has video evidence of him beating her, throwing things at the house, attacking her car, and defecating on her front step. She has videos of Tom urinating on her car and breaking her daughter's toys and throwing them in different directions on the lawn. At one point, Tom hacked into Susan's computer and deleted most of the evidence. She now keeps evidence in a cloud-based application.

Ten years into their relationship, Tom was no longer living in the home, but would bang on the door demanding to take a shower. If Susan called the police, he would flee and then return angrier. She found it easier just to let him in to shower.

This ended when her 12-year-old tried to overdose on cold medicine and was hospitalised for 2 months. Child protective services got involved and initially charged Susan with failure to protect. When CPS became aware of the many times Susan had sought help, they dropped those charges and recommended that the courts award Susan full custody. Tom's lawyer pulls Susan into court frequently, demanding that he be allowed partial custody or visitation.

At one point, Susan moved. Tom found her in a week.

To this day, Tom regularly texts, instant messages, and emails Susan. Her efforts to block him on these various media have failed. When she blocks one avenue, he uses another. She has not responded to any of his communications in over a year and she reports them all to the DA's office.

Susan was forced to quit her job to stay home and care for her children, who are too afraid to be home alone or with other caretakers. She has gotten a large dog to add to their feeling of security.

Victim-survivors report having their emails monitored (Dragiewicz et al. 2018a) and their digital accounts, including online banking, accessed without authorisation (Dragiewicz et al. 2018a; Freed et al. 2017; Woodlock et al. 2020b). Keystroke logging hardware is used to learn the personal identification numbers (PINs) of victim-survivors (Douglas et al. 2019). Alternatively, because of the intimate nature of the relationship, perpetrators may be able to access online accounts through correctly answering security questions and re-setting account passwords. Once access is achieved, the perpetrator can exert control in a number of ways, including through activating or deactivating services. Unauthorised access to online banking could restrict the ability of a victim-survivor to leave the relationship or force her to return after leaving because of a potentially compromised financial position. Alternatively, the perpetrator may gain access to information that suggests she is saving money to leave the relationship. Apart from tracking, monitoring and restricting victim-survivors' access to banking and finances, banking apps are also used to monitor locations that they visit through details given in the actual apps (Woodlock et al. 2020a). Access to a mobile phone account enables a perpetrator to access incoming and outgoing calls and text messages.

Other digitally coercive and controlling behaviours engaged in by perpetrators include the publishing of private information ('doxxing') or intimate or sexual images (often referred to as image-based sexual abuse) without consent (Briggs 2018; Dragiewicz et al. 2018a; Henry et al. 2019). Often, the perpetrator publishes the information or image where the impact is most significant for victim-survivors: where the woman's family, friends, and potentially children, or employers have access to them (Woodlock 2017). Photo-shopped pornographic images have been reported to be used by perpetrators to shame women, particularly those from culturally and linguistically diverse backgrounds (Woodlock et al. 2020b). Perpetrators have also been reported as extorting money in exchange for taking the images offline; also known as 'sextortion' (Leitao 2021). Abusers may make covert and overt audio and video recordings to exert control over victim-survivors (Dragiewicz et al. 2018b).

Perpetrators abuse and control the victim-survivor indirectly through their children. Some of the tactics they use include altering children's possessions to monitor their mothers (George and Harris 2014), using their children's social media accounts to contact their mother or giving mobile phones to their children to monitor their mother's movements (Woodlock et al. 2020a). They also utilise child-minding apps for parents and 'find my phone' apps to covertly monitor the movements and activities of victim-survivors (Freed et al. 2017).

Prevalence of TFA

There are few studies that report the prevalence of TFA and none with representative or random samples. Where prevalence-related results are reported, however, the pervasiveness of TFA is apparent, including at the global level, where the United Nations suggests that 95% of abuse of women in the online environment is perpetrated by either their current or ex-partner (United Nations, cited in Baker et al. 2013) (see Box 3).

In the United Kingdom, Laxton (2014) surveyed 307 female IPV victim-survivors and found that 45% had experienced TFA from their current partner during their relationship and 45% from that same partner after the relationship had ended. In Australia, Woodlock et al. (2020a) undertook a national survey as a follow-up to research undertaken in 2015 (Woodlock 2015), examining the knowledge and experiences of frontline IPV professionals ($n = 442$) of TFA. The 2020 survey was used as a point of comparison to the earlier findings. The survey found that almost all respondents to the survey (99.3%) had provided support to clients for experiences of TFA (Woodlock et al. 2020a). The most commonly used forms used by perpetrators were reported as text messaging (60.7% of respondents seeing this 'all the time' representing a 28.5% increase from 2015) and through smartphones (36.1% seeing this 'all the time', again representing an increase since 2015). Text messages were reported as either being constantly sent, with a harassing intention, or worded specifically to instil fear in the victim-survivor.

The results also indicated an increase in the use of video cameras and GPS tracking devices (video camera use increased 183% over 2015 results to 35.4% in 2020). GPS tracking was seen in 16.2% 'all the time' and 45.6% 'often', representing an overall increase between the two time periods of 131% and 75%, respectively. The tracking, monitoring and restriction of women's access to banking and finances through technology, was also reported with 38.7% of respondents seeing it 'all the time' and 33.6% 'often'. The researchers also reported the Australian Government online accounts such as MyGov (the online federal government platform in Australia where Australians are able to complete their taxation returns, and access other government information and services) as also being misused to abuse women (27% seeing it 'all the time' and 37.8% 'often'). The 2020 findings showed a slight decline in the use of Facebook across the two surveys (36% in 2015 and 35.1% in 2020). The survey also identified new ways that victim-survivors are being stalked or monitored. Apps such as FaceTime (42% seen 'often'), and iCloud (42.2% seen 'often') were included in the survey for the first time in 2020 and results show they are commonly used by perpetrators. Apps such as TikTok should potentially be included in future surveys as they may account for some of the reduction in the misuse of Facebook.

The findings of this Australian study provide robust evidence for the co-existence of digital and physical world abuse. This has also been reported in other research. For example, Marganski and Melander (2018) found that nearly all respondents in their study who reported experiencing IPV (psychological, physical or sexual violence) also reported experiencing TFA (94.8%, 96.0% and 92.6%, respectively). Similarly, Woodlock (2017) found that victim-survivors who experienced cyberstalking simultaneously experienced emotional abuse (82%), sexual abuse (58%), physical violence (39%) and financial abuse (37%) from within the same relationship. There is also evidence that TFA increases the odds of in-person IPV, as threatening or harassing behaviours that have their genesis in the digital environment may continue when partners are together physically (Marganski and Melander 2018).

Perpetrators also use technology in hybrid forms. Woodlock (2017) reports instances where perpetrators use geolocation of Facebook posts to monitor their partner and use the information to turn up in person or to let her know that he knows where she is.

Specifically examining the involvement of children in IPV situations with TFA, research undertaken by the Australian eSafety Commissioner (eSafety Commission 2020) with 515 IPV professionals, found children's involvement was both through perpetrators directly abusing them, and through perpetrators involving them in the abuse, the aim being further abuse and control of their mothers. The overall findings of this study suggest that TFA involves children in 27% of IPV cases. Abuse is reported as largely occurring through devices that are readily available and have legitimate uses in contemporary society. Similar to the findings of the 2020 Australian survey undertaken by Woodlock et al. (2020a), the most commonly used technology was text messaging (75%). This was followed by Facebook (59%), Snapchat (43%), GPS tracking-enabled devices (36%) and spyware (28%) (eSafety Commission 2020).

Studies over smaller geographical areas also provide important information. Messing et al. (2020) undertook a study in an urban area in the Southwest of the USA with victim-survivors of IPV involving secondary analysis of two previous studies (one mixed methods and one quantitative) and found that 60–63% of the 1037 participants in the quantitative components reported experiencing TFA by an intimate partner. In a study undertaken in Queensland, Australia comprising 65 interviews with victim-survivors on up to three occasions over 3 years, TFA was part of the experiences of IPV for 85% of participants (interview 1), 34% at the second interview and 24% at the third (Douglas et al. 2019).

Although our knowledge about the prevalence of TFA is incomplete, the current evidence clearly shows that digital technologies have opened up spaces for perpetrators to extend and expand their control over their partners. The impact of this is significant.

Box 3
Countries Where the Issue is Prevalent

All countries where digital technology is readily available and affordable. Research largely emanates from Australia, the United Kingdom and the USA, but technology-facilitated abuse has been reported from around the world.

Impact of TFA

The body of research on TFA reveals significant impact on victim-survivors and their children (Anderson and Lee 2019; Dragiewicz et al. 2018b; eSafety Commission 2020; Woodlock et al. 2020a). Some research suggests that the impact is more severe than that of abuse that victim-survivors experience from their intimate partners in the physical world, (Woodlock et al. 2020a) or from TFA committed by peers or acquaintances (Bennett et al. 2011; Logan and Walker 2009; Scott et al. 2010). Additionally, the impact on the safety and mental well-being of victim-survivors is long lasting (Woodlock 2017). Victim-survivors report that they experience high levels of fear; they feel constantly unsafe (Dragiewicz et al. 2018a), exhausted, trapped and hopeless (Woodlock et al. 2020a).

The 'omnipresence' of the control is particularly debilitating (George and Harris 2014; Woodlock 2017). Victim-survivors believe they are unable to escape from the perpetrator. Perpetrators are able to track them internationally, control and isolate them, monitor their movements and contacts, and abuse their family and friends (Woodlock 2017). Technological advances facilitate perpetrator's monitoring and contact with victim-survivors anytime and anywhere (Katz and Aakhus 2002) and in ways that have not previously been possible, thus eroding the spatial boundaries of the relationship (Dimond et al. 2011; Hand et al. 2009).

The anonymity and immediacy of digital communications can further heighten the perceptions of victim-survivors that danger is all around them (Harris 2018). Each time a victim-survivor accesses a digital device or social media, they are potentially exposed to controlling behaviours. This is particularly the case for young women as they carry their devices with them wherever they go (Stonard et al. 2017). Victim-survivors are, however, reliant on these technologies for carrying out their daily lives: maintaining connections to family and friends, email for communication, paying bills, online shopping, relaxing or meeting others. These spaces are now infiltrated by a person whose aim is to control and instil fear in them. Shared children or parenting arrangements, social circles and extended family add further difficulties for victim-survivors to escape the perpetrator in the digital world (Freed et al. 2017). The difficulty of escape (Dragiewicz et al. 2018a) results in debilitating emotional and psychological impact (Anderson and Lee 2019).

Because of their dependence on their parents and their limited agency, children are particularly vulnerable to the impact of TFA. Research from Australia (eSafety Commission 2020) has demonstrated negative impact of the abuse on children's mental health, including depression and suicide ideation, on the relationship they have with the victim-survivor, on feelings of social isolation and on their ability to undertake regular daily activities. Like their mothers, children live with fear and the sense that they are constantly under surveillance. Children also experience a sense of guilt arising from the information they have disclosed to the perpetrator, often unwittingly. Their education is also negatively impacted through absenteeism.

Implications for Policy, Practice and Research

Research results compel all sectors, including governments, civil society organisations, technology and telecommunication companies and police and justice systems to take action against technology-facilitated abuse. While evidence suggests that experiences of TFA are increasing and IPV professionals are becoming more and more aware of it (Woodlock et al. 2020a), these same professionals find it difficult to stay abreast of the ever-changing ways that this abuse is perpetrated. Additionally, individuals, agencies and systems lack appropriate responses to perpetrators of TFA.

Across countries, some aspects of TFA are criminalised, but this is jurisdiction-specific. In some jurisdictions, forms of image-based sexual abuse and cyberstalking have criminal implications and convictions have been recorded. Other forms of TFA, however, are less amenable to intervention through the criminal justice system, despite their significant negative impact. Of concern, research findings suggest that there has been little change in the responses of the legal system over time [see, for example, Woodlock et al. (2020a) in an Australian context]. Breaches to protection orders perpetrated through technology are not taken as seriously as in-person breaches and are seldom enforced (Woodlock et al. 2020a). Disappointingly, an appropriate legal response often relies on the actions of individual police officers (Woodlock et al. 2020a) rather than a formal and systematic response protocol. The result is, at best, an inconsistent response between victim-survivors and, at worst, victim-survivors receive an inappropriate and potentially harmful response. Even in circumstances where victim-survivors receive an appropriate response, challenges remain for them as subsequent legal action remains problematic (Powell and Henry 2018; Woodlock et al. 2020a). Threats embedded in digital communication can have meaning solely to the victim-survivor. As such, victim-survivors may struggle to convince others, including the police and legal professionals, of their seriousness (Woodlock et al. 2020a).

Primary prevention of TFA may be achieved through the use of effective technology design, legislation, awareness and training for a range of professionals (human services, legal, justice, health), and resource development (such as the WESNET 'Stalking and Technology-Facilitated Abuse Log #knowtechabuse). Primary prevention campaigns also appear warranted. Collaboration with technology companies could be advantageous. The 'Framework for Inclusive Safety' developed by PenzyMoog provides a relevant example of positive outcome resulting from cross-sectoral collaboration in this space. The goal of PenzyMoog's framework is to support technologists to identify ways in which their product could potentially be misused, provide support to design against this misuse and look for opportunities for support or intervention with the user (www.inclusivesafety.com) (PenzeyMoog and Slakoff 2021).

IPV professionals who either support victim-survivors and their children or run programmes for perpetrators of IPV, would likely benefit from both information and practical support. There is limited information on effective responses to TFA to guide the practice of IPV professionals. Information on responses that do exist, and are evaluated as effective, needs to be disseminated broadly to professionals across human service, legal and justice, and health sectors who support and respond to victim-survivors and their children to enable their scaling up. Similarly, there is a dearth of literature reporting effective interventions for perpetrators of TFA. Once developed, implemented and evaluated, these interventions should be included as a component of perpetrator programmes, including men's behaviour change programmes. Practical support to guide evidence-based professional practice could include the development of screening tools that factor in technologies used in TFA and how best to mitigate the risks they pose. Practical information on cybersecurity for victim-survivors could be useful, as research suggests that it is common for the perpetrator to be more 'tech savvy' (Freed et al. 2017).

Whilst there is evidence to suggest that effective support and intervention for a mother has the potential to protect her children from TFA (eSafety Commission 2020), it is important that those developing and implementing interventions take the needs and experiences of children into account. The post-separation environment must also be fully considered in the development and implementation of interventions. It has been reported that TFA can escalate post-separation as the opportunities for control and physical violence have changed (eSafety Commission 2020). Situations such as co-parenting arrangements and visitation access to children provide ongoing opportunities for TFA, which can be directed at the children, the victim-survivor or both (Markwick et al. 2019).

It is important to note, however, that victim-survivors and their children are not passive recipients of control—rather they invoke a range of strategies in attempts to resist and prevent it—both through informal and formal channels. Informally, they block mobile phone numbers and replace compromised devices. They amend the settings and change their passwords. Where children are involved, victim-survivors monitor their children's online activities and engage in discussions with them about the abuse (eSafety Commission 2020). Children withhold information from the perpetrator. Research, however, suggests that children do not readily seek support for the abuse they are experiencing, but victim-survivors do seek police and justice system interventions (eSafety Commission 2020; Powell and Henry 2018). Given research that suggests that police responses are often unhelpful and inconsistent, developing appropriate support in this area appears important.

Disengaging from social media and discontinuing digital communications is not an appropriate response to TFA for both victim-survivors and their children (eSafety Commission 2020) – it is not the platforms per se that are the issue. Rather the issue is the perpetrator's behaviour and this is where the focus of intervention should remain. Because of the nature of digital media, texts and media objects can remain visible and connected to the identity of the victim-survivor long after her account has been closed (Anderson and Lee 2019; Dragiewicz et al. 2018a). Moreover, disengaging from technology will not ensure the perpetrator will stop; and indeed doing so could further isolate a victim-survivor and her children or prevent her from accessing appropriate support when needed (Anderson and Lee 2019; Woodlock et al. 2020b; Leitao 2021).

Finally, research into TFA remains in its infancy. Further research is clearly needed to better understand its prevalence and how it intertwines and compounds IPV in the physical world. There remains a dearth of research examining the issue and its differential impact for women with a disability, indigenous women, women from culturally and linguistically diverse backgrounds, older women and women who are geographically isolated. Research around the experiences of children and its impact is also needed as a priority. Evidence in these areas is imperative to guide appropriate and effective interventions. More broadly, undertaking research examining the impact and outcomes of TFA over the life course would provide vital evidence to inform policy and practice. The use of linked administrative data could enable this to commence in the short term. We also need research to improve the effectiveness of legal and justice responses and examine the potential for platforms such as Facebook, TikTok, Snapchat and Instagram to be part of primary prevention efforts.

Summary

- TFA is a pernicious form of abusive behaviour intended to coerce, control, intimidate, stalk or harass another person.
- Whilst prevalence data is limited, research shows that TFA is commonly perpetrated alongside abuse in the physical world.
- The consequences of TFA are wide-reaching and long-lasting, including impacts to mental health, to social networks and connectedness, to finances and employment, and in relation to a person's sanity and feelings of safety through the perpetrator establishing a sense of omnipresence.
- There are many implications for research to address the gaps in current knowledge, and for policy and practice in relation to current understandings, responses and professional confidence in tackling TFA.

References

Anderson J, Lee K (2019) The internet and intimate partner violence: technology changes, abuse doesn't. Crime Justice 31(2):28–33

Baker L, Campbell M, Barreto E (2013) Understanding technology-related violence against women: types of violence and Women's experiences. Learning network brief (6). Learning Network, Centre for Research and Education on Violence Against Women and Children, London, ON. www.learningtoendabuse.ca/learningnetwork/network-areas/technology. Accessed 28 Oct 2020

Bennett D, Guran E, Ramos M, Margolini G (2011) College students' electronic victimization in friendships and dating relationships: anticipated distress and associations with risky behaviors. Violence Vict 26(4):410–429

Briggs C (2018) An emerging trend in domestic violence: technology-facilitated abuse. Aust J Child Fam Health Nurs 15:1–2

Dimond J, Fiesler C, Bruckman A (2011) Domestic violence and lived experiences. Interact Comput 23(5):412–421

Douglas H, Harris BA, Dragiewicz M (2019) Technology-facilitated domestic and family violence: women's experiences. Br J Criminol 59(3):551–570

Dragiewicz M, Burgess J, Matamoros-Fernandez A, Salter M, Suzor NP, Woodlock D, Harris B (2018a) Technology facilitated coercive control: domestic violence and the competing roles of digital media platforms. Fem Media Stud 18(4):609–625

Dragiewicz M, Woodlock D, Harris B, Reid C (2018b) Technology-facilitated coercive control. In: De Keserley WS, Rennison CM, Hall-Sanche AK (eds) The Routledge International handbook of violence studies. Routledge, London

eSafety Commission (2020) Children and technology facilitated abuse in domestic and family violence situations. Full report. eSafety Commissioner, Government of Australia, Sydney

Fraser C, Olsen E, Lee K, Southworth C, Tucker S (2010) The new age of stalking: technological implications for stalking. Juv Fam Court J 61(4):39–55

Freed D, Palmer J, Minchala D, Levy K, Ristenpart T, Dell N (2017) Digital technologies and intimate partner violence: a qualitative analysis with multiple stakeholders. Hum Comput Interact 1(1):1–23

George A, Harris B (2014) Landscapes of violence: women surviving family violence in regional and rural Victoria. Deakin University, Geelong. https://www.deakin.edu.au/__data/assets/pdf_file/0003/287040/Landscapes-of-Violence-online-pdf-version.pdf. Accessed 22 Oct 2020

Hand T, Chung D, Peters M (2009) The use of information and communication technologies to coerce and control in domestic violence following separation (stakeholder paper 6). Australian Domestic and Family Violence Clearing House, UNSW, Sydney. https://advocacy4oromia.files.wordpress.com/2015/03/stakeholderpaper_6.pdf. Accessed 23 Oct 2020

Harris B (2018) Spacelessness, spatiality and IPV: technology-facilitated abuse, stalking and justice administration. In: Fitz-Gibbon K, Walklate S, McCulloch J, Maher JM (eds) Intimate partner violence, risk and security: securing women's lives in a global world. Routledge, New York

Harris B, Woodlock D (2018) Digital coercive control: insights from two landmark domestic violence studies. Br J Criminol 59(3):530–550

Henry N, Flynn A, Powell A (2019) Image-based sexual abuse: victims and perpetrators. Trends & issues in crime and criminal justice. No 572. Government of Australia, Australian Institute of Criminology, Canberra

Henry N, Powell A (2015) Beyond the 'sext': Technology-facilitated sexual violence and harassment against adult women. Australian & New Zealand Journal of Criminology 48(1):104–118. https://doi.org/10.1177/0004865814524218

Katz JE, Aakhus M (2002) Perpetual contact: mobile communication, private talk, public performance. Cambridge University Press, New York

Laxton C (2014) Virtual world, real fear: women's aid report into online abuse, harassment and stalking. Women's Aid, Bristol. https://www.womensaid.org.uk/wp-content/uploads/2015/11/Women_s_Aid_Virtual_World_Real_Fear_Feb_2014-3.pdf . Accessed 22 Oct 2020

Leitao R (2021) Technology-facilitated intimate partner abuse: a qualitative analysis of data from online domestic abuse forums. Hum Comput Interact 36(3):203–242

Logan T, Walker R (2009) Partner stalking: psychological dominance or "business as usual"? Trauma Violence Abuse 10(3):247–270

Logan T, Leukefeld C, Walker B (2000) Stalking as a variant of intimate violence: implications from a young adult sample. Violence Vict 15(1):91–111

Marganski A, Melander L (2018) Intimate partner violence victimization in the cyber and real world: examining the extent of cyber aggression experiences and its association with in-person dating violence. J Interpers Violence 33(7):1071–1095

Markwick K, Bickerdike A, Wilson-Evered E, Zeleznikow J (2019) Technology and family violence in the context of post-separated parenting. Aust N Z J Fam Ther 40:143–162

Melton H (2007) Stalking in the context of intimate partner abuse. Sociol Compass 1-2:530–535

Messing J, Bagwell-Gray M, Brown L, Kappas A, Durfee A (2020) Intersections of stalking and technology-based abuse: emerging definitions, conceptualization and measurement. J Fam Violence 35:693–704

PenzeyMoog E, Slakoff DC (2021) As technology evolves, so does domestic violence: modern-day tech abuse and possible solutions. In: Bailey J, Henry N, Flynn A (eds) The Emerald International handbook of technology facilitated violence and abuse. Emerald Group Publishing, Bradford. ISBN: 978-1-83982-849-2, eISBN: 978-1-83982-848-5

Powell A, Henry N (2018) Policing technology-facilitated sexual violence against adult victims: police and service sector perspectives. Policing Soc 28(2):291–307

Scott A, Lloyd R, Gavin J (2010) The influence of prior relationship on perceptions of stalking in the United Kingdom and Australia. Crim Justice Behav 37(11):1185–1194

Southworth C, Finn J, Dawson S, Fraser C, Tucker S (2007) Intimate partner violence, technology, and stalking. Violence Against Women 13(8):842–856

Stark E (2007) Coercive control: how men entrap women in personal life. Oxford University Press, London

Stonard K, Bowen E, Walker K, Price S (2017) 'They'll always find a way to get to you': technology use in adolescent romantic relationships and its role in dating violence and abuse. J Interpers Violence 32(14):2083–2117

Vera-Gray F (2017) Men's intrusion, women's embodiment: a critical analysis of street harassment. Routledge, London

Woodlock D (2015) ReCharge: women's technology safety, legal resources, research and training. Women's Legal Service NSW, Domestic Violence Resource Centre Victoria and WESNET, Collingwood. https://wesnet.org.au/research/recharge15/. Accessed 20 Oct 2020

Woodlock D (2017) The abuse of technology in domestic violence and stalking. Violence Against Women 23(5):584–602

Woodlock D, Bentley K, Schulze D, Mahoney N, Chung D, Pracilio A (2020a) Second National survey of technology abuse and domestic violence in Australia. WESNET, Perth

Woodlock D, McKenzie M, Western D, Harris B (2020b) Technology as a weapon in domestic violence: responding to digital coercive control. Aust Soc Work 73(3):368–380

Colleen Fisher, PhD is a professor of Public Health in the School of Population and Global Health. Her research expertise is domestic and family violence, particularly within communities of refugee background and across the lifespan.

Michaela M. Rogers, PhD is a Senior Lecturer in Social Work in the Department of Sociological Studies at the University of Sheffield. Her research examines interpersonal violence with a focus on marginalised groups, impacts, help-seeking, service access and service responses.

Lisa Fontes Aronson, PhD is a Senior Lecturer II in the Department of Interdisciplinary studies at the University of Massachusetts Amherst. Her research explores the intersections of culture and violence against women and children.

Parveen Ali, PhD Professor of Gender Based Violence and Professor of Nursing in the Health Sciences School, the University of Sheffield and Doncaster and Bassetlaw Teaching Hospitals. Her research examines gender-based violence, inequalities in health related to gender and ethnicity, and professionals preparedness to support victims of gender based violence.

Part X

Legal Responses

Domestic Violence: The Legislative Overview of South Asian Countries

Nasrin Rahman, Abu Naser Md. Wahid, and Nida Usman Chaudhary

Learning Objectives
Having read this chapter, you should be able to understand

- Approaches to address Domestic Violence (DV) by different countries in the South Asian region.
- Remedies to DV victims through DV legislation.
- The status of respondent/perpetrators in DV legislation.

Introduction

The United Nations defines Gender-Based Violence (GBV) as 'any act of gender-based violence that results in or is likely to result in, physical, sexual or psychological harm or suffering to women, including threats of such acts, coercion or arbitrary deprivation of liberty, whether occurring in public or in private life'

N. Rahman (✉)
Federation University Australia, Varendra University, Rajshahi, Bangladesh and Rajshahi Judges Court, Rajshahi, Bangladesh
e-mail: nasrin.r@vu.edu.bd

A. N. Md. Wahid
Department of Law, Rajshahi University, Rajshahi, Bangladesh
e-mail: anmwahid@ru.ac.bd

N. U. Chaudhary
Independent Researcher, Lahore, Pakistan
e-mail: nida@learnpak.com.pk

P. Ali, M. M. Rogers (eds.), *Gender-Based Violence: A Comprehensive Guide*, https://doi.org/10.1007/978-3-031-05640-6_40

(Assembly UG 1994). GBV manifests itself in various forms and in this way, it is a violation of fundamental human rights, including civil and political rights as well as economic, social, and cultural rights. Domestic Violence (DV) is a common form of GBV. Data show that one in three (30%) women are victims of DV worldwide (WHO 2021). To date, 189 countries have ratified the Convention on the Elimination of All Forms of Discrimination against Women (CEDAW) 1979, including the South Asian Countries that are the subject of this chapter, namely, Bangladesh, India, Pakistan, Nepal, Sri Lanka, Maldives, and Bhutan. These countries, being dualist nations, have incorporated the provisions of CEDAW by passing domestic laws, though the implementation and adoption has not been uniform. Several differences remain in the way different countries have chosen to incorporate CEDAW in their domestic law, depending upon their policies and approach. These countries are obliged to protect women against discrimination, diminish discrimination in the laws, improve women's situation through effective policies and programmes, and address gender inequality through individuals, legal, societal structures, and institutions (UN Women 2013). We will explore how DV is postulated in policy and the strategies adopted by the South Asian countries to respond to DV and support victims. We will also explore what constitutes DV under the laws of different South Asian Countries, the remedies available to the victims, and the implications of these among the South Asian Countries covered herein.

The South Asian region is highly populated, representing many ethnic and cultural groups, and consists of a highly patriarchal culture. South Asian women, across the region, are considered socially, culturally, and economically dependent on men and therefore subordinate to them (Fikree and Pasha 2004). 'Lived experiences of women in South Asia often navigate the volatility of individual and group rights, honour and shame, purity and pollution, customary practices and modern citizenship rights, extreme poverty, illiteracy, health vulnerabilities, armed conflict, gender-based violence, etc. These negotiations are deeply rooted in the social realities of religion, caste, race, ethnicity, class, age, and disability' (Mahanta et al. 2019, p. 150). Despite ratification of CEDAW by the countries of this region, instances of GBV, including DV, are still very high, as shown in Fig. 1 below.

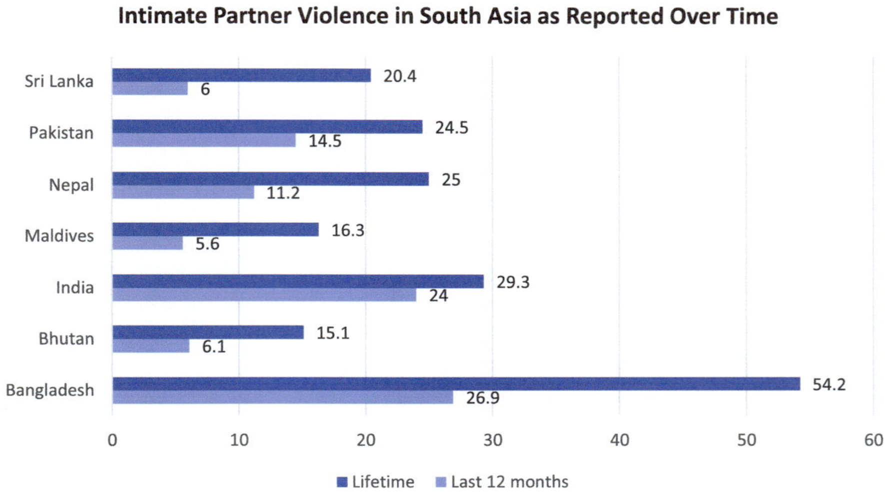

Fig. 1 Proportion of women disclosing experience of intimate partner violence of physical and/or sexual nature in South Asian Countries in the UNFPA Asia-Pacific region as of September 2022. Adapted from The United Nations Population Fund (UNFPA). Violence Against Women—Regional Snapshot (2022). (Proportion of women disclosing experience of Intimate partner violence of physical and/or sexual nature in South Asian Countries in the UNFPA Asia-Pacific region as of September 2022. Adapted from The United Nations Population Fund (UNFPA). Violence Against Women—Regional Snapshot (2022)—kNOwVAWdata [Internet]. [Place: Bangkok Thailand: Publisher: UNFPA]; [2022 September 6; cited 2022 September 26]. Available from: https://asiapacific.unfpa.org/sites/default/files/resource-pdf/knowvawdata_regional_vaw_map_september_6_2022.pdf)

Domestic Violence Legislation in South Asian Countries

We will explore how the legislation in different South Asian Countries defines, frames, and constructs the law and the redressal mechanisms available to the victims against the perpetrators. We use the term victim/aggrieved person to refer to the person who experienced violence and perpetrator/respondent/defendant to refer to the perpetrator of abuse. All South Asian countries have specific laws related to DV, as indicated in Box 1. It is pertinent to mention here that Pakistan, for example, currently has no law at the federal level that addresses domestic violence. The Bills were laid down in the National Assembly twice, once in 2012 and again in 2020; however, they lapsed before they could become an Act of Parliament. Post the 18th amendment of its constitution in 2010, the subject has devolved to its provinces. Sindh's provincial law, which was the first province to enact the law, will be the model law that we will refer to for the purposes of determining Pakistan's position in relation to the other South Asian countries.

Box 1

The DV legislation in the South Asian countries includes:

- Bangladesh: *The Domestic Violence (Prevention and Protection) Act, 2010.*
- Bhutan: *Domestic Violence Prevention Act of Bhutan 2013.*
- India: *The Protection of Women from Domestic Violence Act, 2005.*
- Maldives: *Domestic Violence Act, Act Number 3/2012.*
- Nepal: *Domestic Violence (Offence and Punishment) Act, 2066 (2009).*
- Pakistan (Sindh): *Provincial Laws on Protection of Women from Violence including Domestic Violence such as the Sindh Domestic Violence (Prevention and Protection) Act 2013 and the Punjab Protection of Women against Violence Act 2016.*
- Sri Lanka: *Prevention of Domestic Violence, Act, No. 34 OF 2005.*

How Is Domestic Violence Defined in the Countries in South Asia?

'Domestic violence' (DV) was traditionally understood as violence inflicted by a man on his wife/female partner or ex-partner (Laing 2000) in the private sphere, i.e. at home. In more recent discourse, domestic violence acknowledges that in addition to women, children could also be the primary victims of abuse (Murray and Powell 2011). The term 'family violence'(FV) is even broader and acknowledges that violence may happen between intimate partners and other family members, including aged parents, siblings, etc. (Murray and Powell 2011; Laing 2000). The terminology, therefore, matters because the appropriate labels and titles can be useful in determining the scope of such laws and the relationships that they would cover. Therefore, appropriate naming and framing of the issue is important as it can affect and obscure public response to the issue and can also have an impact on who is seen as a victim and who is not (Murray and Powell 2011). This would be one of the bases on which we would be comparing the legislations of the South Asian Countries under consideration. In that, we shall assess what labels they use to define instances of violence at home to determine the class of protected persons they cover. In other words, whether the law covers protection only for women or extends it to cover other family members as well, and whether or not it is gender neutral. Table 1 summarizes the scope of the class of persons under the various laws as follows:

All South Asian countries referred to in this chapter use the term 'domestic violence' in the title of their legislation which means violence by a husband/man against his wife/female partner or ex-wife/ex-partner. However, this meaning is more analogous to the term 'family violence' because the laws do not exclusively limit the violence between a husband and a wife. It means the operative parts of the definition are broad enough to encompass and cover all persons within the home. In this regard, the more appropriate phrasing or naming of the title could be 'family violence'.

Table 1 Naming, framing and defining DV in South Asian countries

Country	Name of the legislation	Framing of the legislation	Definition: what type of violence is included
Bangladesh	*Domestic violence (Prevention and Protection) Act, 2010*	Partly gendered: Women and children are the victims, and anyone in the family relationship can be the perpetrator	Physical, sexual, emotional/ psychological, and economic violence
Bhutan	*Domestic Violence Prevention Act of Bhutan 2013*	Gender-neutral: Anyone can be a victim and perpetrator	Physical, sexual, emotional/ psychological, and economic violence
India	*The Protection of Women from Domestic Violence Act (PWDVA), 2005*	Gendered: Women are the victims, and men are the perpetrators	Physical, sexual, emotional/ psychological, and economic violence
Maldives	*Domestic Violence Act Number 3/2012*	Gender-neutral: Anyone can be a victim and perpetrator	Physical, sexual, emotional/ psychological, and economic violence to others
Nepal	*Domestic Violence (Offence and Punishment) Act, 2066 (2009)*	Gender-neutral: Anyone can be a victim and perpetrator	Physical, sexual, emotional/ psychological, and economic violence
Pakistan	*Sindh Domestic Violence (Prevention and Protection) Act, 2013*	Gender-neutral: Women, children, and/or other vulnerable person (that means man and woman) are the victims, and anyone in the family relationship can be the perpetrator	Physical, sexual, emotional/ psychological, and economic violence to others
Sri Lanka	*The Prevention of Domestic Violence Act 2005*	Gender-neutral: Anyone can be a victim and/or perpetrator	Physical, sexual, emotional/ psychological with others

Bangladesh and Pakistan (Sindh) use the term 'prevention and protection' along with the term 'domestic violence' in the title. Sri Lanka and Bhutan only use 'prevention' in their title and India only uses the term 'protection' and the word 'women' specifically in its title. On the other hand, Maldives does not use any qualitative words like 'prevention' or 'protection'. Nepal's formulation of the title of the law is different from its counterparts as it expressly includes the terms 'offense and punishment' in the title itself. This formulation appears to focus on the 'crime' and 'punishment' aspect of DV, meaning they are criminalising the act of DV in the title as opposed to other countries who are using the term 'prevention' or 'protection' in their legislation. However, this is not to suggest that it is the only law with penal consequences for the perpetrator who is convicted under the law. In the laws of other South Asian countries also, in the substantive parts of their other penal legislation, DV falls under the definition of the offense of sexual or physical assault and prescribe the corresponding punishment; they have, however, adopted civil procedures and civil remedies against this act of violence in their specific DV law. It appears from the above discussion that the titles of the Acts denote a different emphasis on how to address the issue of domestic violence in the South Asian Region.

The 'Victim' and 'Perpetrator' Under South Asian DV Laws

In addition to the titles, another point of comparison between the laws of the different South Asian Countries as regards DV would be in how key terms such as 'victim' and 'perpetrator' have been defined under their respective laws. This may help us in understanding how these issues are seen and approached by the respective South Asian countries and in determining how progressive and inclusive their approach is in addressing the term of DV.

Through our review of the relevant legislation, we found that there are broadly two lenses with which these definitions have been approached:

1. Gendered.
2. Non-Gendered.

Countries that adopted the gendered lens, such as India and Bangladesh, see 'victims' as mainly women, and women and children in the home. As a result, they engaged with this issue within the underlying context of unequal power relations between members of a home. That inequality in power relations could be the result of gender, age, or other vulnerability; however, given that in patriarchal societies, the tilt of such power relations lies in favour of men, the approach of the lawmakers in such societies appears to be protective of those that are traditionally weaker in such a relationship. In other words, gendered framing centres on women as victims of violence (Murray and Powell 2011) and recognizes structural inequalities in power relations as the main cause of violence towards them. Such an approach aims to inform the society that women have the right to participate in society as equal citizens, and that they ought to be protected to ensure that they are able to enjoy their fundamental rights as equal citizens if those rights are threatened whether in the public or private sphere. On the other hand, the remaining South Asian countries, namely, Maldives, Bhutan, Sri Lanka, and Nepal chose to adopt a more gender-neutral and therefore inclusive lens to define these key terms. Under their law, a victim and a perpetrator could be any 'person' within the domestic relationship. These countries do not approach the law with the mindset of protecting a certain class of persons within the family context, but are open to the possibility of men being victims just as much. Pakistan (Sindh) adopted a partly gendered and child-sensitive lens, however, by adding 'vulnerable person' as victim themselves open to the possibility that a victim could be any person in the home.

Most countries provide a broader definition of 'family or domestic relationship or relevant person', which means a broader range of people can be classified as victims. In general, the definition includes couples, family members, adoption, domestic workers, carer, and shared residents/households[1] who live or have lived together in a shared household. In addition, the definition of a couple is further specified to include spousal relationship, cohabiting partner, intimate relationship, consanguinity, or marriage. The difference between Bhutan, Maldives, Sri Lanka, Nepal, and Pakistan (as discussed above) from Bangladesh, India is that the first group included all persons (family members) as victims. This includes couples and family members, including adopted children, parents of a child or carer, and domestic workers living together irrespective of their gender. In contrast, Bangladesh, India, and Pakistan define a 'Family Relationship' as a relationship between two persons related by consanguinity, marriage, adoption, or members of a joint family. That means women as victims refer to wives, partners, women who live together, mothers, sisters, girl child, or any other woman who is a joint family member. This suggests that regardless of framing, all countries define victims comprehensively.

As far as defining a 'perpetrator' is concerned, all South Asian countries adopt a non-gendered approach and define a 'perpetrator' as a person who is or has been in a domestic relationship with the aggrieved person and against whom which relief is sought under the law apart from India. The Indian law on DV remains true to its gendered approach even while defining 'perpetrators'. In that, a perpetrator can only be an 'adult man' who has been in a domestic relationship with the aggrieved person. This implies that women and children are not seen as 'perpetrators' to the extent of the DV law in India. This also appears to stem from the deeply patriarchal and unequal nature of the social relations in India because of which the state, by passing such a law, saw its role as that of protecting the party that is weak in the power relation within a domestic context. From a rights-based perspective, this approach may come across as discriminatory against men; however, this criticism is usually responded to by stating that the constitution allows for affirmative action and positive discrimination for the protection of women and children in the larger scheme of affairs of society with largely unequal power relations in the private sphere of which mostly women are at the receiving end.

What Is the Scope of Protected Relationships under the Respective Laws of South Asian Countries?

In our legislative review of the respective laws of the South Asian countries in relation to DV, we found that these countries do not confine DV to intimate partners and spouses only. All South Asian countries are aware that domestic violence has the

[1] 'Shared residence' means a residence is where, a victim and respondent may live either singly or jointly with the respondent in a family relationship, and either the victim or the respondent or both have the right to that residence.

potential to impact more than just the partner or spouse at home. Even in Pakistan (Sindh), where a gendered lens has been adopted, to define key terms like victims, are open to the possibility of children and/or other vulnerable persons at home (other than the wife) whether male or female could be aggrieved persons under the law. However, Bangladesh and India, where a gendered lens has similarly been adopted, define victims differently and limit that to the extent of 'women and children' and 'women' only, respectively. One of the factors for this could be that in South Asia, the concept of living together with families is still practised widely and, at any given time, the domestic setting would not just house the spouse/partner and children. In most cases, elderly parents, siblings, or even larger sets of families share the home. This socio-cultural context of South Asian societies is important to understand why across the board in all South Asian countries we found such similar range of protected persons in their respective laws and in how they all see domestic violence as impacting more than just the intimate partner. In the context of South Asia therefore, this approach is to be welcomed and encouraged as it promotes the concept of a healthy home and can accommodate and protect the rights of other persons living in the family home.

What Types of Violence Does DV Encompass?

In recent years, there has been a growing appreciation and realization of the fact that physical harm is not the only type of violence that vulnerable persons in a domestic setting can suffer. The same has been the position of the United Nations as well, that violence can take the form of economic violence, emotional and even psychological abuse amongst others (Assembly UG 1994).

Accordingly, we found that all South Asian countries, save for Sri Lanka, understand, and proclaim physical, sexual, emotional/psychological, and economic violence all as common forms of violence that can be meted out to the aggrieved person in a domestic context. Bangladesh, Nepal, Bhutan, and India provide details of the four types of violence. However, India emphasizes victims' health, safety, and physical and mental health and well-being. Nepal has emphasized psychological violence by adding the sentence about emotional harm. The Maldives listed 17 acts, including physical, sexual, verbal, psychological, and economic violence. In the definition, Pakistan included 15 acts, including sexual abuse, physical abuse, emotional abuse, economic abuse, harassment, stalking, trespass, mischief, abetment, assault, criminal force, and hurt. Entering someone's house without consent is also considered a form of abuse in Pakistan and Maldives. Interestingly, Sri Lanka's legislation list includes offenses such as culpable homicide, murder, assault, sexual harassment, kidnapping, abduction, rape, and others. Also, it named emotional abuse a form of violence, but does not include economic violence.

Comparative Analysis: DV Legislation Related to Victims and Perpetrators

It is possible to understand different approaches taken by South Asian countries relating to victims and perpetrators by comparing the legal response of those countries.

Response to DV Victims and Perpetrators

Legal response can be offered to DV victims by providing them with a remedy and/or a service. The legislation provides two kinds of remedies—civil or criminal, depending on how the legislation has articulated the problem. The legislation also states the support services and dictates how a victim will receive different services, such as support from shelter, police, legal system, counselling, and healthcare system. All the DV laws in South Asian Region offer both civil and criminal remedies for the victims in their DV legislation. However, the remedies offered by the countries—that use gender-neutral definition of DV—such as Pakistan, Bhutan, Maldives, Sri Lanka, and Nepal are complicated. With regards to civil remedies, primary legal remedy for victims of this region is the civil remedy in the form of an interim protection order and protection order. Other available remedies are custody of children, shared residence options, and compensation, as summarized in Table 2.

Protection Order

In general, protection orders are civil orders that can be used to prohibit contact between victims and abusers (Keilitz 1994). The specific provisions of protection orders may vary by jurisdiction and may offer differing levels of protection according to the needs of the victims. It also enables victims to access other resources to increase victims' independence and safety from their abuser (Durfee 2009). The protection order prohibits the perpetrator from committing or causing the commission of an act of domestic violence. There are two types of protection orders: interim protection order and permanent protection order. Interim Protection orders are provided on a temporary basis during the pendency of the proceedings before the courts if the aggrieved person is at risk. If the court finds that victims are at risk, the court may grant *an exparte* (by hearing the victim only) order to protect the victim if an emergent need to protect the victim is established.

A Permanent Protection Order, on the other hand, is provided after the conclusion of the proceedings. A protection order is provided to the DV victim/aggrieved person by obstructing the respondent from committing or aiding or abetting to commit any kinds of domestic violence either to the victims or to the dependents of the victim or any relatives or any person who assists the victims, prohibiting

Table 2 Civil remedies

Country	Interim protection order and protection order	Custody of children	Residence order	Compensation order
Bangladesh	A victim or any person or a police officer or an enforcement officer or a service provider can apply for a protection order on behalf of the victims	Because of gender framing, women get custody directly	Residence order which includes restraining the respondent from visiting the victim's residence or shared residence, disturbing the victim, directing the enforcement officer to arrange a safe shelter for the victim and her child/children, ordering the respondent to pay the rent for alternative accommodation, order accompanied by the enforcement officer to enter the offender's residence to collect the protected person's personal belongings, execute a bond for not conducting violence again, directing the officer in charge of the nearest police station to give protection to the aggrieved person exclude the perpetrator	The court may direct the respondent to pay expenses for personal injury, financial loss, trauma or psychological damage, and the maintenance of the aggrieved person and her children. In addition, in case of failure to pay, the court may direct the respondent's employer to pay the victim from the perpetrator's wages/ salaries
Bhutan	Before the court, a complainant can report DV to the police, a protection officer or service provider/ the social welfare officer or competent authority, or local government members. In addition, a victim or competent authority or protection officer or the complainant or the police or the service providers can apply for a protection order to the court on behalf of the victims	Temporary custody of any child or dependent is going to any person or institution as directed by the court Also, the court can deny the defendant to have access to the child in the best interest of the child. However, because of non-gender framing, if a woman becomes a defendant, there is the possibility of losing access to her child	Bhutan law prohibits the defendant from entering the victim's residence and directs the respondent to allow the victim to access the residence and the facilities. However, because of non-gender framing, if women become a defendant, the above-stated action will apply to her	The perpetrator has to pay monetary relief to the victim and any child or dependent of the victim. Also, the perpetrator has to pay compensation for personal and physical injury. However, because of the gender-neutral framing of the definition, there is a possibility that a man can be a victim of DV, so women may have to pay the compensation

India	A victim or any person or a protection officer can apply for protection on behalf of the victims	Because of gender framing, women get custody directly	Residence order prohibits the perpetrator or any of his relatives from entering any portion of the shared residence and disturbing the victim, alienating, or disposing of the shared household It requires the perpetrator to renounce his rights in the shared household It orders the perpetrator to pay the rent for alternative accommodation It can direct the perpetrator to remove himself from the shared household and execute a bond for not conducting violence again It can also direct the officer in charge of the nearest police station to give protection to the aggrieved person	The perpetrator is obliged to pay monetary reliefs, including the medical expenses, expenses for any property damage, and maintenance for the aggrieved person and their children The perpetrator has to pay the compensation to the victim. In case of failure to pay, the court may direct the perpetrator's employer to pay the victim from the perpetrator's wage/salary
Maldives	Any person or victim can give information about DV to the police A victim can make the application for protection order to the court	According to the law, a victim will get temporary custody of any child. However, because of non-gender framing, men or women can get the custody	The victim shall not be evicted or excluded from the shared household or any part of it by the perpetrator The court may order the respondent to pay the rent for the alternative accommodation of the victims or execute a bond for not conducting violence again or direct the nearest police officer to give protection to the victim and the children. However, because of non-gender framing, if women become a defendant, the above-stated action will apply to her	Maldives law notes that a victim will get compensation, but does not mention who will pay it. Because of the gender-neutral framing of the definition, there is a possibility that a man can be a victim of DV so that he will receive compensation

(continued)

Table 2 (continued)

Country	Interim protection order and protection order	Custody of children	Residence order	Compensation order
Nepal	A victim can lodge a written or oral complaint about DV to the police office, the National Women Commission, or local body. Next, a police officer or local body can forward the case to court with the victim's consent if they fail to settle the dispute through reconciliation for an interim protection order	Nothing is mentioned about the custody of a child	The defendant may allow the victim to continue to live in the shared house, not harass the victim by entering his/her separate residence, providing food, behaving decently, and bearing the expenses and maintenance of the victim. However, because of non-gender framing, if women become a defendant, the above-stated action will apply to her	The perpetrator has to pay treatment costs (physical and mental injury) and compensation. However, because of the gender-neutral framing of the definition, there is a possibility that a man can be a victim of DV, so women may have to pay the compensation
Pakistan	A victim or any person authorized by the victim can apply for a protection order on behalf of the victim	Because of gender framing, women get custody directly	A residence order includes a restraining order to prevent the perpetrator or any of his/her relatives from entering any household, disturbing the victim, ordering the respondent to pay the rent for alternative accommodation, executing a bond for not conducting violence again, directing the officer in charge of the nearest police station to give protection to the aggrieved person	The court may pass an interim order directing the respondent to pay monetary relief and compensation to meet the expenses incurred and losses suffered by the aggrieved person, such as medical expenses, compensation for economic abuse, expenses for damaged property, and the maintenance of the aggrieved person as well as her children In addition, in case of failure to pay, the court may direct the respondent's employer to pay the victim from the perpetrator's wages/salaries

Sri Lanka	A victim or a police officer can apply for a protection order on behalf of the victims. On behalf of a child, parent, guardian, or with whom the child resides, or a person authorized by the National Child Protection Authority	Because of non-gender framing, either men or women can get the custody	Prohibiting the defendant from entering a residence or any specified part of the shared residence, stopping the aggrieved person from entering the shared residnece or any part of the shared residence where the person ordinarily used to live, or any shelter in which the victim may be temporarily accommodated However, because of non-gender framing, if women become a defendant, the above-stated action will apply to her	The perpetrator has to provide monetary assistance to any person, where such respondent has a duty to support such a person The court may direct the employer of the respondent to directly pay the victim from the perpetrator's wages/salaries; however, because of the gender-neutral framing of the definition, there is a possibility that a man can be a victim of DV, so women may have to provide monetary assistance

interactions and communication, either physically or virtually with the victim or the children or prohibiting to entering the place of employment or child's school. Therefore, a protection order as a remedy does not hold the perpetrator accountable for their actions nor punish them.

Murray and Powell (2011) argue that 'in response to domestic violence a civil order effectively allows the perpetrator's past violence to go unacknowledged with a promise of future "good behaviour"' (p. 102). However, such orders can nevertheless offer civil remedies in a domestic context. The civil remedies offer greater flexibility and come with a lower threshold of the standard of proof as compared to criminal remedies that envisage imprisonment for the perpetrator. Given that the liberty of person is at stake, the case must be proved beyond reasonable doubt for a criminal sanction to be imposed. However, in civil matters, even if someone is able to prove a case on a balance of probabilities, s/he may get relief in shape of civil remedies that do not deprive the perpetrator of his/her own liberty, but still achieves the purpose of securing protection by such protective orders.

To get a protection order, the laws of the South Asian Countries vary slightly. According to the law of Bangladesh, Bhutan, India, Maldives, and Sri Lanka, a Protection Order can be requested before the court if an act of DV has been, is being, or is likely to be committed. It means that if anyone feels threat before violence, s/he can apply to the court for protection. Considering the patriarchal socio-cultural aspects of the South Asian region (Shankar et al. 2013), it may be a reasonable option for women victims to make an application when they feel threatened. However, Nepal has advanced a step forward by taking two approaches. Firstly, a victim (he/she) can directly file the complaint to the court. Or they can make a complaint to the Nepal Police Office, National Women's Commission, or a district court or local body.

The view of the DV laws of the Asian region, such as Bangladesh, is to keep the family intact (Rahman 2020). This is one of the main reasons to use the Civil Protection Order as a remedy. Nepal has institutionalized this reconciliation strategy by giving power to the Nepal Police Office, and National Women's Commission to act and conduct reconciliation between the parties. If they fail to settle their dispute through reconciliation, the case is forwarded to the court for an interim protection order. Considering women's situation in this region, this step is very victim-friendly as it saves time, money, and the harassment about going to court.

A victim or any person on behalf of the victim can make the application for a protection order in all countries. Besides, in Bangladesh, Bhutan, and Sri Lanka, a police officer, and for Bangladesh and India, an enforcement officer and a protection officer can apply for a protection order on behalf of the victims. A competent authority, protection officer, or the complainant can apply for a protection order in Bhutan. The service provider can also apply for a protective order. This is a victim-friendly option as sometimes they are not able to apply by themselves because of the trauma and or lack of knowledge.

However, one major legal concern in Bangladesh regarding a protection order is the possibility that a woman can be accused of making a false accusation against her husband or against any other person in the family for which the law provides a punishment (Rahman 2020). Therefore, unless she has evidence of violence in physical injury, she may hesitate to take the case to court, even for something like a protection order. The consequence of this, at least in Bangladesh, is women may be reluctant to report DV unless they have evidence of physical symptoms. This has severe implications for genuine victims of DV who are reluctant to come forward because of the fear of the punishment for a false complaint that they might get implicated in if they are unable to prove and/or establish physical injury or harm. This deterrence may be removed, and the law may be reformed to address this anomaly so that women are able to claim relief from violence other than of physical in nature.

Framing the DV legislation as 'domestic and family violence' may have implications for protection orders. Protection orders may be complicated to implement in practice if the legislation is framed as 'domestic and family violence' instead of 'domestic violence' because this includes a wide range of people in the definition of victim and perpetrator. For example, in Indian DV law, the definition of 'aggrieved person' is wide and gender-specific. It covers all the women who are related to the male of the family, including the wife, daughter, mother, sister, child (male or female), widowed relative, and even any woman who is the sexual partner of the male irrespective of whether she is his legal wife or not (Bhatia 2012). This gender-specific formulation also applies to Bangladesh and Pakistan.

Besides other countries, Nepal, Sri Lanka, Maldives, and Bhutan also added gender-neutral and a wide range of people in the definition as victims and perpetrators in DV law. Such definitions may make it difficult to impose protection orders considering the nature of relationships within the family; the remedy of the protection order is the same irrespective of the relationship between those concerned. For example, a scenario may arise where the victim is a mother, and the perpetrator is her adult son. It may be quite difficult to envisage a protective order asking the son to stay away from his mother in such relationships of blood within the socio-cultural context of South Asia. This situation may arise for other types of relationships within the family as well where the relationship is one of blood and not one by way of contract or marriage.

Custody of Children

Often, women tolerate violence due to the legal structures and systems of a country. Cases regarding the custody of children can be good examples. Women tolerate violence due to threats against children by partners, or concern for children's safety, or a fear of losing custody of their children (Ali 2003; Bhuiya et al. 2003; Ameen 2005; Meyer 2016; Overington 2017). The legislation of Bangladesh, India, Maldives, and Pakistan has made the custody of children straightforward for victims. The Law of Nepal does not mention about custody of children. Legislation in Sri Lanka is not clear in dealing with the custody of children. Although it talks about contact with the child of the aggrieved person, the court decides based on the child's best interest. According to the law of Bhutan, temporary custody of any child will go to any person or institution as directed by the court. The law does not clearly stipulate the person as such, but the court can deny the perpetrator access to the child in the child's best interest.

In Bangladesh and India under their respective legislation, only women are considered victims of DV. They are given immediate custody of the children, whereas a man can never be a DV victim. The implication of the differences of the legislation regarding custody of children is that in Bangladesh and India, women do not need to be concerned about the possibility of having to contest custody of their children until the court case of DV ends because the law has given her automatic custody. This can save her from additional psychological stress. However, complications may arise in Pakistan, Sri Lanka, Bhutan, and Maldives where a gender-neutral frame and definition is adopted. This allows a woman to be accused of being the perpetrator of DV, which may influence the decision on custody of children. This complication of definition is set out in Reeves (2017) who notes that when a woman is identified as a perpetrator, the resulting intervention order may cause the woman to temporarily lose custody of her child(ren).

Residence Order

Bangladeshi women face a lack of access to alternative economic and social options and a lack of alternative places to stay outside the family home (Bhuiya et al. 2003; Farouk 2005). The same condition prevails in the other six countries of this region (India, Pakistan, Nepal, Bhutan, Maldives, and Sri Lanka). The legislation in all countries confirms the right of the DV victims to share the family home with the respondent. India exclusively expresses the right of the victim to reside in a shared household. In Bangladesh, India, and Pakistan, the residence order may include, but is not limited to, a restraining order for the respondent or any of his relatives prohibiting them from entering or visiting a household or shared household without being accompanied by someone directed by the law, if necessary, disturbing the victims, ordering the respondent to pay the rent for alternative accommodation, executing a bond for preventing the commission of domestic violence, directing the officer in charge of the nearest police station to give protection to the aggrieved person, taking the possession of any immovable property such as dower,[2] any other property or assets of the victim.

Residence orders can meet different criteria to protect the victim of DV. These are:

1. Prohibit the respondent from entering the victim's residence or shared residence and allow the victim to access or share the residence (Bhutan, Nepal, Sri Lanka, Maldives, Bangladesh, India, and Pakistan).

[2] Dower (*Mehr*), a sum of money or any other valuables that a husband gives or undertakes to give to the bride upon marriage. In Islam, a dower is a dignified receipt by wives as a token of love and respect rather than their price (Chowdhury 2012). In addition, women's right to dower is prescribed under Muslim Family Law Ordinance, 1961.

2. With the court order, the respondent to pay the rent for the alternative accommodation of the victims or execute a bond[3] or direct the nearest police station to give protection to the victim (Bangladesh, India, Maldives, and Pakistan).
3. With a court order, the respondent to pay maintenance to the victim (Bangladesh, India, Maldives, and Pakistan).

With a court order, a respondent may be excluded from the home for the victim's safety (Bangladesh, Nepal, and India). However, the temporary exclusion is also problematic in this region. For example, in the case of Bangladesh, this woman-friendly initiative of law is difficult to implement in practice because a vast majority of people live below the poverty line. Thus, it may be impossible to provide the victim separate accommodation as the respondent may not pay for a separate residence despite court orders or provisions of the law. Their residence often consists of only one or two rooms (Huda 2016).

Residence right obviously is a positive step in this region where women are not economically independent. Bangladesh and India's DV Acts clearly confirm women's right to stay in residence as a usual victim, and they are not expected to leave the family home. However, for Pakistan (Sindh), Nepal, Bhutan, Sri Lanka, and the Maldives, because of the gender-neutral frame and definition, a woman may be identified as a perpetrator and may have to do the act according to the law.

Compensation Order

In all South Asian countries, DV legislation makes provision for the perpetrator to pay compensation to the victim, which is a strong marker for accountability for their behaviour. In case of failure to pay compensation, in Bangladesh, Pakistan, India, and Sri Lanka, the court may direct the respondent to the employer to directly pay the victim from the perpetrator's wages/salaries. This is an easier option for women of this region to get their rights, remedies, and even compensation because of patriarchal cultures, and it may save her money, time, and harassment. In addition, India, Bangladesh, and Nepal added mental torture, and Pakistan added economic abuse for compensation with other criteria, which establishes both as forms of DV. This is an advanced step. Bangladesh, Pakistan, and India also included the maintenance cost of the women with their children, which may help them live their lives as they are economically disadvantaged.

Alternatively, because of the gender-neutral framing of the definition of DV in Pakistan, Bhutan, Maldives, Sri Lanka, and Nepal, there is a possibility that a man can be a victim of DV. In that case, a woman may have to pay the compensation, which could be very difficult for them considering their economic condition as they tend to be economically less well off. In Bhutan, if the perpetrator is sentenced for the offence of DV, he/she may need to pay compensation. Similarly, in Nepal, if the perpetrator is unable to pay treatment costs (cost for physical or psychological injuries of the victim) due to economic reasons, the service centre provides the

[3] Executing a bond refers to a bond that needs to be signed by the respondent for not conducting violence again.

treatment expenses. It therefore appears that in Nepal, the state has taken the responsibility to ensure that costs don't hinder access to treatment of any physical or psychological injuries.

Summary

- All countries adopt the term 'domestic violence' in the name of the legislation.
- Except for India, all countries adopted mixed framing. India's framing is thoroughly gendered compared to the other countries. Bangladesh framed partly gender and partly non-gender as women are the victims and any person can be the perpetrator. In contrast, Maldives, Sri Lanka, Nepal, and Bhutan adopted non-gendered framing as they adopted gender-neutral definitions, therefore, it suggests that men, women, and children can be both victims and perpetrators. Pakistan broadly adopted a gender-neutral approach by inclusion of the term 'any vulnerable person' as an aggrieved person with the women and children as victims.
- All countries adopted a broader definition of family relationships, including intimate relationships, marriage, family relationships, shared householders, carers, and adopted children. Therefore, the framing refers to 'domestic and family violence' and is not limited to intimate partner or spousal violence.
- Except for Sri Lanka, all countries noted four kinds of violence. India, Maldives, and Pakistan added extra forms of violence with them.
- The civil remedy is available for all countries under the name of a protection order. In addition, there are different remedies that can be offered for the victims, such as custody of children, order to share residence, and compensation. However, because of the complication of gender-neutral frame and definition, women can be perpetrators in some countries and may lose their child custody and may also have to pay compensation.
- The law makes the perpetrator accountable for their behaviour by giving compensation to the victims amongst other things.

References

Ali S (2003) Violence against women in Bangladesh. Bangladesh National Women Lawyers Association (BNWLA), Dhaka

Ameen N (2005) Wife abuse in Bangladesh: an unrecognised offence, 1st edn. The University Press Limited, Dhaka

Assembly UG (1994) Declaration on the elimination of violence against Women (1993). In: In inter-American convention on the prevention, punishment, and eradication of violence against Women (convention of Belém do Pará). Organization of American States, Washington, DC

Bhatia M (2012) Domestic violence in India: cases under the protection of women from domestic violence act, 2005. South Asia Res 32(2):103–122

Bhuiya A, Sharmin T, Hanifi SMA (2003) Nature of domestic violence against women in a rural area of Bangladesh: implication for preventive interventions. J Health Popul Nutr 21(1):48–54

Chowdhury JA (2012) Pro-Women metamorphosis in legal discourses on matrimonial rights: is family mediation a speedway to reap its fruit? Dhaka Univ Law J 23(2):127–150
Durfee A (2009) Victim narratives, legal representation, and domestic violence civil protection orders. Fem Criminol 4(1):7–31
Farouk SA (2005) Violence against women: a statistical overview, challenges and gaps in data collection and methodology and approaches for overcoming them. UN Division for the Advancement of Women, Geneva
Fikree FF, Pasha O (2004) Role of gender in health disparity: the South Asian context. BMJ 328:823–826
Huda S (2016) Five years after Bangladesh's domestic violence (prevention and protection) act, 2010, is it helping survivors? A study by the Bangladesh National Women Lawyers' association (BNWLA), and plan International for the Protecting Human Rights (PHR) program. BNWLA and plan international Bangladesh. https://www.planusa.org/docs/phr-domestic-violence-2016.pdfb. Accessed 13 Apr 2018
Keilitz SL (1994) Civil protection orders: a viable justice system tool for deterring domestic violence. Violence Vict 9:79–84
Laing L (2000) Progress, trends and challenges in Australian responses to domestic violence. Australian Domestic and Family Violence Clearinghouse, University of New South Wales, Sydney
Mahanta U, Dalwai S, Shakil A (2019) Women and law in South Asia. Jindal Glob Law Rev 10(2):149–155. https://doi.org/10.1007/s41020-019-00105-1
Meyer S (2016) Still blaming the victim of intimate partner violence? Women's narratives of victim desistance and redemption when seeking support. Theor Criminol 20(1):75–90
Murray S, Powell A (2011) Domestic violence, Australian public policy, 1st edn. Australian Scholarly Publishing, Melbourne
Overington C (2017) Child custody: one mother's bitter lesson in sharing the kids with dad. The Australian. https://www.theaustralian.com.au/news/inquirer/child-custody-one-mothers-bitter-lesson-in-sharing-the-kids-with-dad/news-story/0807089cbc513954c6ebe68f1a726431. Accessed 10 Apr 2017
Rahman N (2020) A comparative analysis of domestic violence against women in Australia and Bangladesh: government policies, legislation and Organisational responses. A PhD thesis. Federation University Australia
Reeves E (2017) How Victoria's family violence system fails some victims—by assuming they're perpetrators. The conversation. https://theconversation.com/how-victorias-family-violence-system-fails-some-victims-by-assuming-theyre-perpetrators-87184. Accessed 12 May 2018
Shankar J, Das G, Atwal S (2013) Challenging cultural discourses and beliefs that perpetuate domestic violence in south Asian communities: a discourse analysis. J Int Women's Stud 14(1):248–262
UN Women (2013) Domestic violence legislation and its implementation, an analysis for ASEAN countries based on international standards and good practices. United Nations Entity for Gender Equality and the Empowerment of Women (UN Women), Regional Office for Asia and the Pacific, New York
World Health Organisation (WHO) (2021) Violence against women, key facts. https://www.who.int/news-room/fact-sheets/detail/violence-against-women. Accessed 28 Oct 2021

Nasrin Rahman received her PhD degree from the Federation University Australia where she examined the interrelationship between factors which contribute to DV along with government policies and legislation developed to deal with DV, and organisational responses by police and DV Crisis Support Services in Australia (Victoria) and Bangladesh. She is currently practicing law and is an Assistant Professor in the Department of Law and Human Rights at Varendra University, Bangladesh. Her research areas Include gender based violence, domestic and sexual violence, human rights and law and policy.

Abu Naser Md. Wahid is a Professor in Law and former Dean of the Faculty of Law at University of Rajshahi who received gold medals for his outstanding achievements in both LL.B (Honours) and LL.M examinations from the University of Rajshahi, Bangladesh. He did his LL.M (Research) from the University of Birmingham. His research areas include environmental law, gender-based violence and violent extremism.

Nida Usman Chaudhary is an award winning, diversity and inclusion advocate and founder of women in law initiative Pakistan. She holds LL.B (Hons) and LL.M in Law and Development from the University of London. She has over 12 years of experience in research, training and capacity building and has provided legislative and policy input on several key women and child rights laws including recent amendments to workplace harassment law in Pakistan. She is the author of Pakistan's first baseline report on 'State of Women's Representation in Law'. Her areas of focus include, amongst others, gender-based violence, fair representation and child rights.

The International Legal Framework on Gender-Based Violence

Julieta Marotta

Learning Objectives

- Having read this chapter, you should be able to understand:
- The law as a tool to change social conduct.
- How international and regional laws frame gender-based violence as a discriminatory act.
- The relationship established by international and regional laws between the right to a life free of violence, the right to access to justice, and the right to education as a way to overcome gender-based violence.
- The recognition given by international and regional laws to nations as being the main actors able to implement international standards.

Introduction

Gender-based violence is a global problem that societies have neglected historically and only in the last decades has it gained political attention. Gender-based violence (hereinafter, GBV) went from being left to be solved in the private sphere because it was a private problem between family members to being a societal problem

This chapter builds on portions of a larger work that was successfully defended as the PhD dissertation of the author (Marotta 2017).

J. Marotta (✉)
UNU-MERIT, United Nations University, Maastricht, The Netherlands
e-mail: julieta.marotta@maastrichtuniversity.nl

P. Ali, M. M. Rogers (eds.), *Gender-Based Violence: A Comprehensive Guide*,
https://doi.org/10.1007/978-3-031-05640-6_41

recognized by laws. Consequently, international and regional regulations were enacted, a number of countries amended their domestic laws to incorporate international standards, and various governmental and non-governmental organizations were mandated to enforce and advocate for the rights of victims of GBV to a life free of violence.

Despite numerous efforts, GBV remains a social problem that affects primarily women (World Health Organization 2021), and a number of international, regional, and national laws aim at protecting the rights of women (Flores 1998). These laws also consider that legal discriminatory actions can be carried out through the letter of the law and the actions of providers, and hence international laws require nations to challenge and reform the letter of the law and current customs. Moreover, laws highlight the social importance of creating a society free of discriminatory acts and enabling the full development of women in acknowledgement of their contribution to social capital and to the achievement of society's well-being and peace (UNTS 1981 Preamble). It is therefore in the best interests of nations to introduce policies that contribute to the full participation of women while also minimizing discriminatory practices.

In order to eradicate GBV, every level of government and every sphere in which society interacts needs to commit to promoting and respecting the laws that have been enacted. Moreover, the justice systems need to implement innovative methods to ensure access to justice and enforcement of rights. This chapter explores legal frameworks under the assumption that laws reflect social values that exist in societies. As a result, it begins by describing how GBV is defined in the international legal framework. Second, the chapter discusses how the international legal framework specifically addresses the right to access to justice. Third, the chapter looks at how the international legal framework addresses the right to education. Examples of how international law has been adopted by national laws are provided in all sections to help the reader understand the impact of international law on domestic law. The case of Argentina is used for that purpose.

Right to a Life Free of Violence

In 1981, the Convention on the Elimination of all Forms of Discrimination against Women (hereinafter, CEDAW) came into force. As shown in Box 1, by the year 2021, the majority of nations will have ratified this international treaty.

Box 1 Ratification of CEDAW

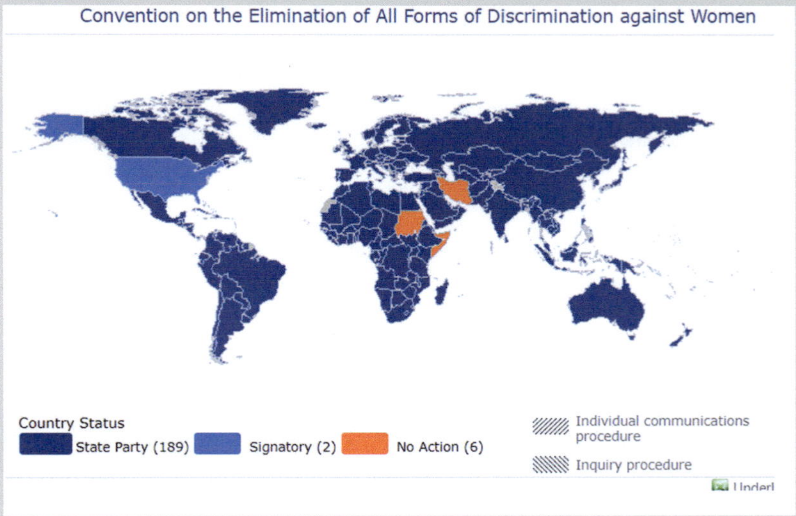

(United Nations Human Rights 2021)

CEDAW is a comprehensive recognition of the rights of women and an attempt to achieve global gender equality. It addresses the right to a life free of discrimination in all spheres of interaction[1] and defines violence against women as a discriminatory act (CEDAW General Recommendations Nos. 19 and 20 1992; General Secretariat Organization of American States 2007: paras. 49–50).

The importance of gender equality for the international community can be perceived by how gender was approached throughout the United Nations Millennium Goals, which had a target date of 2015 (UN 2021). The United Nations Millennium Goals represent a global compromise to work on a selected number of societal problems, and gender perspective was introduced to many of the millennium goals, such as in the educational, health, and employment spheres (Medina et al. 2013: 555–65). *The Road to Dignity by 2030: Ending Poverty, Transforming* report delivered by United Nations recognizes that 'gender parity in primary school enrolment, access to child and maternal health care and in women's political participation has improved steadily' (United Nations General Assembly 2014: para. 17). The demand for equality and non-discrimination is recognized by the post-Millennium Goals efforts as

[1] For example, it includes the rights of women within marriage and family relations and equates the rights of men and women when making decisions within the family environment.

one of the key aspects communities are called to work on,[2] and gender equality and empowerment of women and girls became the fifth Sustainable Development Goal. This demonstrates that gender equality remains an important global challenge (United Nations 2021).

In the Americas, the Inter-American Convention on the Prevention, Punishment and Eradication of Violence against Women (hereinafter Convention of Belém do Pará), which was adopted in 1994, incorporates the right of women to live in a world free of violence with the right to live in a world free of discrimination. According to Article 6 of the Convention of Belém do Pará:

> The right of women to be free from all forms of discrimination; and the right of women to be valued and educated free of stereotyped patterns of behaviour and social and cultural practices based on concepts of inferiority or subordination.

CEDAW and the Convention of Belém do Pará recognize the importance of nations in ending current discriminatory customs due to their ability to enact laws 'needed to prevent, punish and eradicate violence against women' (UNTS 1981 art 2, UNTS 1995 art 7(c)(e); UN Women 1996; General Secretariat Organization of American States 2007, para. 71). Moreover, these international documents directly address the role of nations in procuring proper mechanisms for victims of gender violence to benefit from a justice system that can deal with the characteristics of gender violence with due diligence (UNTS 1981 art 25, 1995 arts 7(d); 8(d); General Secretariat Organization of American States 2007, paras. 18; 24; 27). As a result, laws are positioned as social behaviour changers and nations as responsible actors, in order to achieve societal change.

The Convention of Belém do Pará requires states to implement specific measures and programmes to inform and train service providers who can enforce legal provisions (for example, judges, police officers) on issues of violence against women (art 8[c]). The states are also called upon to collect statistics in order to assess the effectiveness of the measures in place to punish those who commit violence against women (art 8[h]).

In the Americas, the Inter-American Commission on Human Rights[3] and the Inter-American Human Rights Court provide a comprehensive understanding of women's rights, highlighting the principles of equality and non-discrimination (Inter-American Court of Human Rights 2021; Organization of American States 2021). These regional bodies stress the importance of the nations in incorporating effective federal provisions and concrete policies to tackle gender violence and discrimination. It is worth noting the approach by the Inter-American Commission on

---

[2] Para. 54 reads: 'People have called for an end to all forms of gender inequality, gender-based discrimination and violence against women and against children and young boys and girls.' United Nations General Assembly, 'Integrated and Coordinated Implementation of and Follow-up to the Outcomes of the Major United Nations Conference and Summits in the Economic, Social and Related Fields. Follow-up to the Outcome of the Millennium Summit.'

[3] An organ of the Organization of American States, which performs together with the dependent Office of the Rapporteur on the Rights of Women.

Human Rights and the Inter-American Human Rights Court towards the role of legal provisions, not only as a set of standards and values but also as tools to change social conduct. Moreover, they recognize the importance of cooperation between every member state (Medina et al. 2013: 393–439).

At a national level, a number of nations in the Americas have incorporated the international standards into their domestic legislation. For example, Argentina enacted the Law on the Right of Women to Live Free of Violence in 2009 (hereinafter Law 26485). This law was meant to promote and ensure the abolition of discrimination and violence against women in all aspects of life. Argentina, with this law, fulfilled its international obligation to incorporate domestic laws to eliminate violence against women (UNTS 1981 art 7[c]). Law 26,485 also considers GBV to be a form of discrimination. It considers both discrimination and violence to be the result of socio-cultural patterns that feed upon expressions that stimulate and perpetrate violence against women.

Socio-cultural patterns are promoted and sustained through regulations, speeches, symbols, images, or any other means of expression that stimulate violence against women. Therefore, Law 26485 calls for a comprehensive analysis of all expressions that preserve gender inequality, practices, customs, and social and cultural conduct (for example, the promotion of assigned stereotypes of women and men and the use of images with a vexatious or discriminatory meaning) (Poder Ejecutivo de la Nación 2010).

Law 26485 understands that violence can be manifested in different ways, not limited to physical, physiological, and sexual violence, but also economic, patrimonial, and symbolic violence (Congreso de la Nación Argentina 2009 art 5; Medina et al. 2013: 98–108). The comprehensive approach to the concept offers a broad definition of violence against women with the goal of eliminating stereotypes about unequal power relations between men and women in the private and public spheres (Congreso de la Nación Argentina 2009 art 4). The active and proper state intervention also serves as a preventive measure (Comas de Argemir 2008: 279).

Right to Access to Justice

The right to access to justice, which is the right of people to seek and be granted justice by the justice system, is a fundamental driver in achieving the elimination of GBV. Moreover, discrimination against women can lead to social and organizational obstacles to access to justice and the claim of rights. Thus, the discriminatory factors in various communities can be assessed in the way in which the justice system and providers address domestic violence cases. This right was given legal certainty in 1994 as a result of international laws such as the American Convention on Human Rights (hereinafter Pact of San José). The Pact of San José introduced the right of victims to an expeditious and simple means of requesting protection from the justice system when a right is violated (UNTS 1978 art 25[1]). CEDAW and the Convention of Belém do Pará both address the right to access to justice for victims of GBV and highlight the importance of access to justice in eliminating GBV

(General Secretariat Organization of American States 2007, para. 6 [Executive Summary], 37–39 and 56; UNTS 1981 art 25, 1978 arts 7[d] and 8[d]).

The Brasilia Rules recognize that discrimination against women can lead to social and organizational obstacles for women victims of GVB to access to justice (XIV Ibero-American Judicial Summit 2008, para. 17). This discrimination is reduced when a nation introduces direct policies to facilitate access to justice and for victims of GBV (Comas de Argemir 2008: 283). Consequently, the Brasilia Rules require that the justice system develop appropriate tools for victims to understand and to ensure that those tools incorporate all formal procedural elements. Hence, an accessible system that is trained in dealing with GBV is essential in ensuring victims' right to access to justice (Medina et al. 2013: 468–69).

The global community recognized access to justice as a fundamental right when it was incorporated in the Sustainable Development Goals 16. The Sustainable Development Goals (SDGs) is the global policy agenda adopted in 2015 until 2030. With the inclusion of SDG 16, societies agreed to 'promote peaceful and inclusive societies for sustainable development, provide access to justice for all and build effective, accountable and inclusive institutions at all levels'. Moreover, ensuring the right to access to justice enables people to demand that their rights be enforced, and to hold the state accountable. For example, SDG 5 on gender equality can only be achieved when women are able to invoke their right to a life free of discrimination and violence within a responsive justice system.

Trained and informed employers working in the justice system can improve the participation of women victims of GBV in the justice process, whether during the formal process or when an alternative dispute resolution mechanism is chosen (XIV Ibero-American Judicial Summit 2008, para. 47). Alternative dispute resolution mechanisms are introduced as a means of broadening the spectrum of possibilities for parties to achieve conflict resolution through a tailor-made remedy (XIV Ibero-American Judicial Summit 2008). However, due to the power imbalance embedded in relationships with power disparities, most experts are cautious to introduce alternative dispute resolutions for GBV cases (Slaikeu 1996: 250). In addition to recommending a tailored justice system, the international documents require a holistic and multidisciplinary approach to the assistance provided to victims of GBV and family members. As a result legal remedies (such as child support, divorce, probation, or incarceration) have been expanded to include welfare, economic, and psychological health-related remedies (UNGA 2005 art 10).

Legal representation is recognized as a means of effectively guaranteeing the protection of rights and an important element for victims of GBV to obtain a remedy (Andreu-Guzmán and Courtis 2008: 54; Inter-American Court of Human Rights 1990). According to international instruments, legal assistance to victims of GBV should ideally be offered by specialized attorneys (XIV Ibero-American Judicial Summit 2008, para. 29). Furthermore, the Inter-American Court of Human Rights interprets and defines Articles 8 and 46.2 of the Pact of San José. According to the Court, when domestic provisions require legal representation and the person cannot afford it, the nation has a duty to overcome this economic limitation. If the nation fails to provide it, individuals can access regional courts without exhausting domestic procedures (Andreu-Guzmán and Courtis 2008: 54; Inter-American Court of Human Rights 1990, para. 28). Legal representation and assistance for victims of GBV should be provided by experts in the field and tailored to the needs of the various communities in a jurisdiction. Moreover, the Brasilia Rules recommend the commitment of the entire legal community, including participation by universities, organizations, and bar associations (XIV Ibero-American Judicial Summit 2008, para. 29).

The Brasilia Rules emphasize the importance of concrete actions to provide vulnerable populations with information on rights, as a necessary prerequisite to access to justice. On the one hand, the letter of the law needs to be understood by vulnerable groups; while, on the other, providers play a fundamental role in communicating legal provisions to people (XIV Ibero-American Judicial Summit 2008: paras. 26–27). Therefore, any means of communication, such as notices, summons, court resolutions, and oral hearings, need to be adapted to the understanding of the parties (XIV Ibero-American Judicial Summit 2008, paras. 58–61).

Box 2 Voice of Victims

A qualitative empirical study undertaken between 2012 and 2014 with 54 victims of domestic violence concluded the following regarding the understanding of victims of GBV of their rights:

- Few victims interviewed stated that they were aware of their legal rights following different interventions by the justice system. After being asked a second time, some victims mentioned specific rights. This group responded with the following specific rights they thought or assumed they were entitled to: *a right to a house and to dignity*, a right not to be yelled at on the streets and to work even without the permission of the accused, *a right to be respected as a woman, a right not to be insulted or shouted at,* a right not to be bothered; a right to be free, to do what they want without receiving threats and insults; a right to a tranquil and good life; and a right not to be hurt by the accused.
- Victims, at the time of submitting their complaints, perceived the justice system as a place to turn to for help. However, there was limited understanding of the implications of submitting complaints. It was also observed that, throughout the process, the majority of victims blindly followed instructions given by providers, still without understanding the consequences.
- Most victims perceived their problems in simple terms and not as falling within the realm of the law. However, in the majority of cases, victims expressed that their primary problems were the ones that compelled them to submit their complaints and the problems were expressed in a way that is assimilated to the law (for example, 'threats', 'harassment', 'child support', 'someone follows me', 'I want to separate'). Victims mostly submitted complaints with the simple desire to solve their problems.

- Victims mostly relied on the information provided and responded to suggestions made by organizations with limited understanding of what this information entailed. The risk in requiring victims to make decisions based on limited understanding of the legal information is that they could not exercise their own preferences or demand specific performance from service providers. Victims' limited understanding of rights hampered their ability to choose legal options merely because they were unaware of their existence or implications. The study found that there was no direct relation between why victims turned to the justice system and how they perceived themselves as holders of rights. These findings confirmed those of a previous study performed in Latin America by Antony García where victims ignored the legal provisions that protected them (Antony 2001; Marotta 2017)

Right to Education

Education is seen as a key element in overcoming discriminatory practices and ensuring awareness of rights. UNESCO stresses the importance of incorporating within educational plans an integrated approach to human rights and to all forms of discrimination. Education is viewed as a service that should be provided to every human being throughout their lives. However, the pre-school years are considered especially significant, because this is the time when people develop their fundamental attitudes (UNESCO 1974: para. 24). The education that nations need to promote, in order to prevent discriminatory behaviours, has to include the study of different cultures and the value enhanced in them to 'encourage mutual appreciation of the differences between [cultures]' (UNESCO 1974: para. 17).

As perceived by UNESCO, it is the awareness of diversity that fosters acceptance and non-discriminatory actions. Together with the performance of their social duties, education needs to prepare students 'to exercise their rights and freedoms while recognizing and respecting the rights of others' (UNESCO 1974: Para. 12). Similarly, CEDAW emphasizes the importance of revising school textbooks and programmes in order to eliminate discriminatory stereotypes and ensure access to them (UNTS 1981 art 10[c]). Special emphasis is placed on the opportunity for women living in rural areas to have access to those channels of information, as well as on providing that access beginning at an early age (UNTS 1981 art 14 and art 10[e]).

CEDAW recognizes the right of women to have access to information as a means to enable the exercise of rights. Access to information and awareness of rights are viewed as tools for exercising rights and achieving gender equality. As a result, it is suggested that both genders have equal access to those modes of communication (UNTS 1981 art 16e). For example, article 16(e) (h) emphasizes the importance of access to information and education of women as a prerequisite for free and responsible family planning.

According to the Convention of Belém do Pará, nations are required to create programmes to 'promote awareness and observance of the right of women to be free from violence, and the right of women to have their human rights respected and protected' (UNTS 1995, p. art 8[a]), as well as to 'promote and support governmental and private sector education designed to raise the awareness of the public with respect to the problems of and remedies for violence against women' (UNTS 1995 art 10[c]). Nations are required to provide victims with effective programmes that allow them to fully exercise their rights (UNTS 1995 art 8[f]). Furthermore, nations are urged to provide information and training to service providers in order to ensure the effective implementation of policies designed to tackle gender violence (UNTS 1995 art 8[c]).

The National Council of Women was established at the national level in Argentina by Law 26485. This Council is tasked with raising social awareness through the implementation of preventive measures. Scholars agree that it is through education and promotion of rights that long-term changes can be achieved when dealing with stereotypes that are embedded in society, stereotypes such as discrimination and gender violence (Medina 2011). Law 26485 also directs the Argentine Supreme Court to keep statistics on the socio-demographic characteristics of victims (for example, age, marital status, profession, and occupations of victims and of the accused). Statistics allow for a better understanding of the scope of the problem and, as a result, can aid in policy design.

Summary

- Gender equality and the empowerment of women and girls were added to the list of SDGs.
- International law addresses the right of women to a life free of violence to be a policy problem and considers it as a manifestation of a discriminatory act.
- Elimination of discriminatory stereotypes is considered a means of eliminating GBV.
- Discrimination is reduced when nations design and implement policies to facilitate access to justice for victims of GBV.
- International law perceives nations as the main actors in charge of providing opportunities for women to access information and, consequently, to become aware of their right to a life free of discrimination and violence.
- International documents stress the importance of educating children against non-discriminatory behaviours from an early stage in life.

References

Andreu-Guzmán F, Courtis C (2008) Comentarios sobre las 100 Reglas de Brasilia sobre Acceso a la Justicia de las Personas en Condición de Vulnerabilidad. In: Defensa Pública: Garantía de Acceso a la Justicia. La Ley, Buenos Aires, República Argentina, pp 51–60

Antony C (2001) Las mujeres confinadas: estudio criminológico sobre el rol genérico en la ejecución de la pena en América Latina y en Chile. Editorial Jurídica de Chile, San Diago

CEDAW General Recommendations Nos. 19 and 20 (1992) HRTB

Comas de Argemir M (2008) Violencia de género: Normativa internacional para combatirla y propuestas legales en España. In: Defensa pública: garantía de acceso a la justicia. La Ley, Buenos Aires, pp 279–295

Congreso de la Nación Argentina (2009) Ley de protección integral para prevenir, sancionar y erradicar la violencia contra las mujeres en los ámbitos en que desarrollen sus relaciones interpersonales

Flores MT (1998) Women's human rights in the framework of argentine domestic law: treatment since the return to democracy. J Gend Soc Policy Law 7:335–341

General Secretariat Organization of American States (2007) Access to justice for women victims of violence in the americas. Organización de los Estados Americanos. Comisión Interamericana de Derechos Humanos, Washington, DC. (No. OEA/Ser.L/V/II. Doc. 68)

Inter-American Court of Human Rights (1990) Opinión Consultiva OC-11/90 Excepciones al Agotamiento de los Recursos Internos

Inter-American Court of Human Rights (2021) Inter-American court of human rights [WWW document]. https://www.corteidh.or.cr/

Marotta J (2017) Access to justice and legal empowerment of victims of domestic violence through legal organisations in the City of Buenos Aires: a qualitative empirical legal study. Maastricht University/United Nations University, Maastricht

Medina G (2011) Ley de protección integral a las mujeres objetivo y derechos protegidos La Ley DFyP, p 3

Medina G, Yuba G, González Magaña I (2013) Violencia de género y violencia doméstica, 1st edn. Rubinzal—Culzoni Editores, Buenos Aires

Organization of American States (2021) Inter-American commission on human rights [WWW document]. https://www.oas.org/en/iachr/

Poder Ejecutivo de la Nación (2010) Decreto Reglamentario 1011/2010 a la ley 26485

Slaikeu KA (1996) When push comes to shove: a practical guide to mediating disputes. Jossey-Bass Publishers, San Francisco

UN (2021) United nations millennium development goals [WWW Document]. http: //www.un.org/millenniumgoals/. Accessed 27 Feb 2015

UN Women (1996) The United Nations fourth world conference on women. UN Women, Beijing

UNESCO (1974) Recommendation concerning education for international understanding, co-operation and peace and education relating to human rights and fundamental freedoms. UNESCO, Paris

UNGA (2005) Basic principles and guidelines on the right to a remedy and reparation for victims of gross violations of international human rights law and serious violations of international humanitarian law. UNGA, New York

United Nations (2021) Gender equality and empower all women [WWW document]. Httpssdgsunorgtopicsgender-Equal. Womens-Empower. United Nations, Tokyo

United Nations General Assembly (2014) Integrated and coordinated implementation of and follow-up to the outcomes of the major United Nations conference and summits in the economic, social and related fields. In: Follow-up to the outcome of the millennium Summit (No. A/69/700). United Nations General Assembly, New York

United Nations Human Rights (2021) Convention on the elimination of all forms of discrimination against women [WWW document]. www.ohchr.org. https://www.ohchr.org/EN/ProfessionalInterest/Pages/CEDAW.aspx

UNTS (1978) American convention on human rights. UNTS, Denton

UNTS (1981) Convention on the elimination of all forms of discrimination against women. UNTS, Denton

UNTS (1995) Inter-American convention on the prevention, punishment and eradication of violence against women. UNTS, Denton

World Health Organization (2021) Violence against women [WWW Document]. www.who.int. https://www.who.int/news-room/fact-sheets/detail/violence-against-women
XIV Ibero-American Judicial Summit (2008) Brasilia regulations regarding access to justice for vulnerable people

Julieta Marotta, PhD is Assistant Professor and Academic Programme Director of the Master Public Policy and Human Development Programme, at United Nations University-MERIT/. Her research interest is on inclusive forms of access to justice and legal empowerment with a focus on disadvantaged groups and through empirical legal research.

Part XI

Conclusion

Reflections and Way Forward

Parveen Ali and Michaela M. Rogers

Learning Objectives
Having read this chapter, you should be able to understand

- The diversity, complexity and pernicious nature of gender-based violence.
- That women and girls are the main victims/survivors of gender-based violence.
- The commonalities and differences across different types of gender-based violence.
- The implications for future policy and practice.

Introduction

This book aimed to provide a comprehensive understanding (as much as possible) of gender-based violence (GBV) and how it plays out in various parts of the world. The idea behind the book has been forming for many years in my head (Parveen). It all started from the time I was doing my PhD and realised that there is not a single source that postgraduate students, researchers or activists interested in the subject of GBV were able to pick up and learn about GBV as a complex, heterogeneous and entrenched global problem. Completing the PhD and working with like-minded colleagues further solidified this thought as well as a desire to fill this gap, hence myself

P. Ali (✉)
Health Sciences School, University of Sheffield, Sheffield, UK
e-mail: parveen.ali@sheffield.ac.uk

M. M. Rogers
Department of Sociological Studies, University of Sheffield, Sheffield, UK
e-mail: m.rogers@sheffield.ac.uk

P. Ali, M. M. Rogers (eds.), *Gender-Based Violence: A Comprehensive Guide*,
https://doi.org/10.1007/978-3-031-05640-6_42

and Michaela took up the challenge of inviting people to contribute to this edited book as the task is impossible to complete by one person. We were aware of the mammoth task we were signing up to but did not know if it would be possible. It took a lot of time, thinking, arguing, discussion, reflection, reading and revision to achieve the objective and we hope that readers find the book useful.

This has been a challenging, as well as rewarding, experience for us as authors and editors, mostly because of the realisation that GBV is embedded in every community and culture. We knew that forms of GBV are pervasive, but did not realise how varied and prevalent it is. GBV, in some communities, is hidden, and in others, it is more open and accepted by members. It is constantly evolving with new technology, meaning new opportunities to perpetrate abuse, and changes to our everyday living practices. It is both individual, group-based, systemic, institutional and widespread, affecting millions of individuals, families and communities across the world. This book attempts to explore and represent GBV, its explicit existence, as well as in its nuanced presentation. We also wished to illuminate its far-reaching impacts and to contemplate policy and practice responses. We are aware that still there are many GBV-related practices that we have not been able to capture in this book and this will be work for future editions of the book. We hope that by reaching this chapter, the reader will have grasped the breadth and depth of GBV, and here we aim to conclude the book, to reflect on the similarities and differences between various forms of abuse, identify issues that affect people's understanding of the problem and to discuss the implications for the future.

Definitions and Explanations

While the definition of GBV has been presented several times in this book, let's explore this one more time, especially reflecting on what has been presented in each chapter in the book. To recap, GBV refers to any acts or threats of acts intended to hurt or make women suffer physically, sexually or psychologically. These acts are directed towards women because they are women and impact women because they are women. It is also very clear that the term is used interchangeably to refer to violence against women (VAW). The chapters in this book show clearly that the main victims of GBV are women, although men and people with other gender identities can also experience forms of GBV. The violence and abuse experienced by women, however, is often systematic, repeated, and intense. Regardless of the form, violence and abuse is most often perpetrated by men and is often a product of gender inequality. The acts are often not unique episodes but are ongoing over time. Often, the violence is perpetrated by someone the woman knows, not by a stranger. It is no surprise that the 1993 Declaration on the Elimination of Violence Against Women also supports the notion that violence is rooted to the inequality between men and women which perisit across the world.

Nearly all definitions of GBV and VAW highlight the issue as one that is gendered, and our readers would have grasped while reading this book. Many opponents criticise these definitions, call them problematic and unsatisfactory, stating that these definitions highlight women as the weaker sex who lack autonomy, and that they depict society as patriarchal. They also argue that these definitions disregard violence

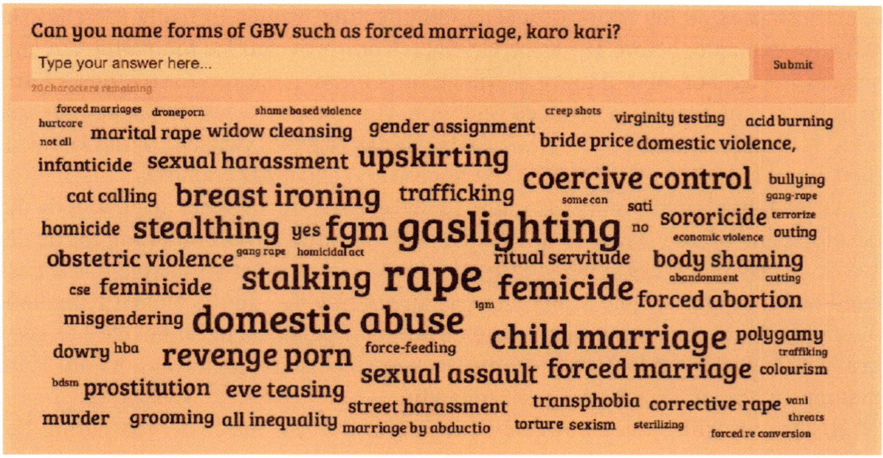
Can you name forms of GBV such as forced marriage, karo kari?
Type your answer here...
Submit
forced marriages
droneporn
shame based violence
creep shots
hurtcore
not all
marital rape
widow cleansing
gender assignment
virginity testing
acid burning
bride price
domestic violence,
infanticide
sexual harassment
upskirting
cat calling
breast ironing
trafficking
coercive control
bullying
gang-rape
some can
sati
homicide
stealthing
yes
fgm
gaslighting
no
sororicide
terrorize
economic violence
outing
obstetric violence
gang rape
homicidal act
ritual servitude
body shaming
cse
feminicide
stalking
rape
femicide
abandonment
cutting
forced abortion
igm
misgendering
domestic abuse
child marriage
polygamy
dowry
hba
revenge porn
force-feeding
traffiking
sexual assault
forced marriage
colourism
bdsm
prostitution
eve teasing
street harassment
transphobia
corrective rape
vani
threats
murder
grooming
all inequality
marriage by abductio
torture
sexism
sterilizing
forced re conversion

Fig. 1 Forms of GBV

against men and ask 'What about men? They experience abuse too'. However, as noted earlier, the majority of victims and survivors are women. Regardless of these criticisms, there is no definition that is free from these issues, or that captures all forms of violence and does not put men and women into two binary categories.

Here it may also be useful to share the findings of an activity that we undertook at the start of this book project. We distributed a call to colleagues, around the world, who were working on the issue of GBV asking them to provide us with the names of various examples of GBV as we wanted to ensure the book was comprehensive and represent all forms of GBV. People were generous, and we received about 490 entries naming varied practices and forms of GBV (see Fig. 1) - the vast majority of these were examples of GBV against girls and women- from around the world.

Historical Context of GBV

As mentioned earlier, GBV is deeply rooted in gender inequality as well as the ways in which women are positioned and viewed in society. It is clear that GBV, and especially VAW, is socially accepted and legally sanctioned in some instances as individuals or communities have used cultural and religious rationales to condone violence. Women, historically, have been seen as property and subservient to men. Culture, customs and societal expectations as well as religion (in its various interpretations) have often been and still are used as an excuse for GBV.

While GBV is prevalent in all cultures, countries and religions, countries may differ in their journey of acceptance/non-acceptance and some practices are more prevalent in some parts of the world than in others. However, the chapters in this book make it clear that similar harmful practices are prevalent across countries and regions, albeit there might be slight deviations and different terms applied. For example, honour-based violence, while seen as more of an issue happening in South Asian populations, has been practised since the time of the Roman Empire and, in some instances, is the result of legislation affecting women in many societies. In Italy, for example, before 1981, the Criminal Code provided for mitigating circumstances in cases of the killing of a woman or her sexual partner for reasons related to honour, providing for a reduced sentence. The practice seems to happen far and wide in Brazil, Canada, Iran, Israel, Italy, Jordan, Egypt, Sweden, Syria, Uganda, the United Kingdom (UK), the United States (US) and other countries.

An examination of history also shows how abusive practices are dealt with by the development of new laws or abolishment of harmful laws. For example, in the 1870s, courts in the US stopped recognising the common-law principle that a husband had the right to 'physically chastise an errant wife'. In the United Kingdom, the right of a husband to inflict moderate corporal punishment on his wife to keep her 'within the bounds of duty' was removed in 1891, although it was not until 1991 that rape within marriage was made unlawful.

History also illustrates how the women's movement that emerged during the 1970s is responsible for drawing attention to gender inequalities in its various forms, including VAW. At that time, researchers (mainly women), from various disciplines, including anthropology, law, philosophy, sociology and psychology, attempted to explore different dimensions of the phenomenon. Many of these scholars reflected a feminist perspective that regards patriarchy as responsible for VAW (Walker 1979). The movement built momentum with scholars working alongside activists and was successful in establishing shelters and safe houses for abused women and the organisation of advocacy groups.

Feminists, at the time, tended to view the issue from a criminal and judicial perspective. The movement called for reforms to the legal and judicial system and was successful in modifying 'criminal codes defining the crimes of sexual assault, criminal domestic violence, child abuse and neglect, and other crimes against women' (Kilpatrick 2004, p. 1210). During the 1990s, there was a shift as VAW was seen to be a public health concern with recognition that it was a major reason affecting women's mortality and morbidity (Tjaden 2005; Kilpatrick 2004). At the same time, the issue of VAW became an international concern that led the United Nations General Assembly to pass 'the Declaration on the Elimination of Violence against Women' in 1993 (United Nations 1994). Subsequently, the issue was highlighted through various agreements and declarations at important international events such as 'World Conference on Human Rights' held in Vienna in 1993, the 'International Conference on Population and Development' held in Cairo in 1994, and the 'Fourth World Conference on Women' held in Beijing, 1995. VAW was then declared to be a public health priority by the '49th World Health Assembly' and 'United Nations Population Fund' in 1996 and 1999, respectively.

At the same time, another paradigm shift took place and VAW was recognised as a human rights issue. This resulted in driving the world's attention towards other crimes against women such as women trafficking, prostitution, and traditional, but harmful, practices such as forced marriage, genital mutilation, honour killing and violence against incarcerated women. The human rights perspective also turned the lens towards structural violence, including state-tolerated and sponsored acts of violence against women, and any other discriminatory practice negating women's rights of inheritance, access to health, education and employment opportunities (Tjaden 2005; Human Rights Watch 1999). Human right activists argue that such discriminatory practices contribute to the vulnerability of women and increase the likelihood of psychological, emotional, social and gender-based discrimination and violence against women that, in turn, affects women's well-being (Human Rights Watch 1999). In combination, these perspectives (criminal justice, public health and human rights) led to the recognition of GBV as a major social, legal and public health problem that affects the lives of women. See Table 1, which details some of the most important milestones at an international level for the prevention of VAW.

Table 1 Milestones concerning the prevention of VAW

Year	Event
1979	The convention on the elimination of all forms of discrimination against women (CEDAW) recognised violence as a part of discrimination against women
1993	The world conference on human rights recognised VAW as a human rights violation. This contributed to the UN declaration
1993	UN declaration on the elimination of violence against women was the first international instrument explicitly defining and addressing VAW This declaration, as well as the world conference of the same year, is often viewed as a 'turning point' at which the consideration of VAW by the international community began to be taken seriously and countries started mobilising around the problem
1994	International conference on population and development linked VAW to reproductive health and rights, and provided recommendations to governments on how to prevent and respond to violence against women and girls
1996	The world health assembly (WHA) declared violence a major public health issue. It identified its types, including IPV and sexual violence. This was followed by a World Health Organization (WHO) report on VAW The UN created the trust fund to support actions to eliminate violence against women
1999	The UN adopted the optional protocol to the convention on the elimination of all forms of discrimination against women and designated 25 November as the international day for the elimination of violence against women
2002	The WHO published the first world report on violence and health addressing many types of violence and their effect on public health, including forms of VAW The report specifically noted the sharp rise in civil society organisations and activities directed at responding to VAW from the 1970s to the 1990s
2004	The WHO published its 'multi-country study on Women's health and domestic violence against women' involving over 24,000 women in ten countries from all regions of the world. The study assessed the prevalence and extent of VAW, particularly IPV, and linked this with health outcomes to women. The report also documented strategies and services that women use to cope with IPV
2006	The UN secretary general published the first comprehensive international document on all forms of GBV
2011	The Council of Europe Convention launched the second regional legally binding instrument on VAWG
2013	The United Nations Commission on the status of women (CSW) adopted agreed conclusions on the elimination and prevention of all forms of violence against women and girls The UN general assembly passed its first resolution calling for the protection of defenders of women's human rights. The resolution urges states to put in place gender-specific laws and policies for the protection of women's human rights defenders and to ensure that defenders themselves are involved in the design and implementation of these measures and calls on states to protect women's human rights defenders from reprisals for cooperating with the UN and to ensure their unhindered access to and communication with international human rights bodies and mechanisms

Structural and Individual Influences

Throughout this book, contributors have examined the causes of GBV, suggesting a variety of explanations and theories that are helpful. Various concepts such as patriarchy, culture, religion, media and individual characteristics intersect to explain GBV. The biological perspective sees the issue of GBV as being secondary to aggression, which results from structural and chemical changes in the brain due to, for example, trauma or head injury. Psychopathological theories consider that GBV results from psychopathology, mental illness, attachment problems, inability to manage anger and hostility, deficiency in various skills and abilities such as management of anger and hostility, lack of assertiveness, self-esteem, and communication skills. The feminist perspective blames the dominance of men, patriarchal structure of societies, as well as power and control issues. The sociological perspective assumes violence in the family of origin, differences in the possession of tangible and intangible resources of men and women in marital/intimate relationships, conflict in the family, and stress as the explanatory factors. Finally, the nested ecological framework looks at different factors at various levels in the family, community and society to explain the phenomenon of GBV.

It is clear, however, that no single theory or factor can fully explain the phenomenon of GBV. Every perspective contributes to the explanation of GBV and provides important insights into the issue. As the body of international research on GBV grows, understanding of the underlying causes and influencing factors is also increasing. For example, the role of family in preventing and perpetrating or perpetuating violence and abuse within a domestic context is significant and should be considered (Ali et al. 2019). A review of all previous chapters also highlights the important role of various factors at all levels of society. The impact of power imbalances, gender inequality is clearly evident. It is also important to acknowledge that there are intersecting issues or influences that should be included in the analysis and these include social problems such as poverty and substance misuse, as well as other social characteristics such as socioeconomic positioning, disability or age.

A Typology of Gender-Based Violence

Throughout the book, different forms of GBV which affect individuals at various stages of life are described. To capture all forms of GBV, whatever the context, we propose a typology of GBV. This typology organises these diverse forms into categories to capture the breadth of maltreatment, but also to show synergies, convergences and divergences across the three contexts of private, public and virtual environments. The categories are not discrete as some forms of abuse overlap and belong to more than one category: for example, in Table 2, we classify stalking as a harmful practice, but it is also found in intimate partner violence and may be used by someone perpetrating identity-related abuse. Another strain of stalking is used in virtual environments as cyberstalking.

Table 2 A typology of gender-based violence

Categories	Examples
Child abuse	Child marriage, child sexual abuse, child sexual exploitation, child trafficking, digital online (sexual) assault, familicide, FGM, forced marriage, rape
Intimate partner violence	Acid attacks, digital online (sexual) assault, familicide, economic abuse, honour'-based violence, older adult mistreatment, online text-based (sexual) abuse, intimate partner abuse, post-separation, abuse, rape, reproductive coercion and abuse, stalking, technology-facilitated domestic abuse, widowhood-related abuse
Non-partner sexual violence	Digital sexual assault, pornography, rape, sexual harassment, wartime violence, trafficking
Harmful practices	Acid attacks, abuse against female migrant domestic workers, bride abduction, colourism, dowry-related abuse, FGM, forced marriage, 'honour'-based violence, menstruation-related abuse, sexual harassment, spiritual abuse, stalking, street harassment, widowhood-related abuse
Human trafficking	Abuse against female migrant domestic workers, child trafficking, trafficking for sex work
Institutional violence	Child abuse, obstetric violence, older adult mistreatment, reproductive coercion and abuse, sexual harassment, wartime violence, workplace harassment
Identity abuse	Colourism, hate crime, LGBT communities and GBV, older adult mistreatment, spiritual abuse, violence against disabled people
Digital and technology-related abuse	Digital online (sexual) assault, online text based (sexual) abuse, pornography, online stalking, non-consensual sharing of sexual images, technology-facilitated domestic abuse

Prevalence and Various Forms of Practice

Another important aspect that clearly emerges from previous chapters is that knowing the exact prevalence of GBV is challenging. This is due to widespread underreporting, lack of recognition of experiences of abuse, and inaccurate or missed recording of incidents as GBV. Comparison across countries is problematised by issues such as the inconsistency of definitions, the absence of monitoring as well as by the adoption of different methodologies for data collection, analysis, and synthesis (Ali et al. 2015). Girls and women are the main victims of any form of GBV. This is not to say that boys and men do not experience abuse, but the number of girls and women experiencing abuse is much higher. While women can be perpetrators of various forms of GBV, men are the main perpetrators of abuse as highlighted in previous chapters. A review of all chapters also highlights that GBV can occur in any environment, including public, private and virtual (which can also be public or private) environments. In terms of the latter, digital and communication technologies now offer a new medium for perpetrating abuse, although the body of evidence with regard to prevalence is not fully accurate as we are still developing our understanding of the complexity and multiple forms virtual and online abuse takes. There are several chapters in this book that offer a foundation for understanding these newer types and practices that use online media and technology to cause harm and violate individuals.

Regardless of the particular environment in which it takes place, GBV appears to take the form of physical, psychological, emotional, sexual abuse and coercive control. It can manifest in various ways, as shown in Table 3. Coercive control and the deprivation of liberty is often a running thread. This has implications as to how various practices can be assessed and screened by professionals aiming to support

Table 3 Definition and examples of various forms of abuse, regardless of practice

Definition and examples
Physical violence or abuse: Use of physical force to inflict pain, injury or physical suffering to the victim • Slapping, punching or hitting with an instrument • Beating • Kicking • Pinching and scratching • Biting • Pushing and shoving • Dragging • Stabbing • Burning • Choking • Threatening or using a gun, knife or any other weapon
Sexual violence: Any sexual act, attempt to obtain a sexual act, unwanted sexual comments or advances, or acts to traffic, or otherwise directed, against a person's sexuality using coercion, by any person, regardless of their relationship to the victim, in any setting, including, but not limited to, home and work • Physically forcing someone to have sexual intercourse • Forcing someone to do something that they found degrading or humiliating • Harming someone during sex, forcing someone to have sex without protection
Psychological violence: Use of various behaviours intended to humiliate and control another individual in public or private • Verbal abuse • Name calling • Blackmailing • Constantly criticising • Repeatedly putting someone down such as telling them they are worthless • Embarrassing a person by saying something or doing something • Threats to beat women or children • Restricting economic independence and access to information • Restricting access to education or health services
Financial or economical abuse: Controlling a person's ability to acquire, use and maintain their own money and resources. • Not letting victims work • Sabotaging job interviews • Taking the welfare benefits the victim is entitled to • Using their money without consent • Building up debts in their name • Damaging their property and possessions • Withholding maintenance payment

Table 3 (continued)

Definition and examples
Coercive control: Often perpetrated in combination with other forms of violence, coercive control can include any act or a pattern of acts of assault, threats, humiliation and intimidation or other abuse that is used to harm, punish, or frighten their victim • Isolating a person from their family and friends • Monitoring their time and movements • Monitoring a person via social media or spyware • Taking control over aspects of their everyday life, such as where they can go, who they can see, what to wear and when they can sleep • Enforcing rules and activities which humiliate, degrade or dehumanise the victim/survivor • Forcing the victim/survivor to take part in criminal activities such as shoplifting, neglect or abuse of children • Making threats to hurt or kill, or to hurt or kill a child • Making threats to reveal or publish private information (e.g. threatening to 'out' someone) • Criminal damage (such as destruction of household goods or personal items) • Preventing a person from having access to transport or from working

victims of GBV. Understanding the complexities of GBV, how it impacts people, why it is difficult for victims to report is essential for everyone generally, but especially so for frontline professionals, including health and social care professionals, police, to name a few.

Power, Privilege and Positionality

Earlier, in chapter one, we introduced the concepts of power, privilege and positionality. We defined power as the ability, of anyone, to control and access resources, opportunities, privileges and decision-making processes of another individual or group. It refers to the ability of an individual or group to achieve their own goals or aims; however, it can be used negatively to prevent another (the victim/survivor in the context of GBV) from making their own decisions and exercising their personal right and powers on themselves. Privilege refers to a special right, advantage or immunity, granted or available, accessible only to a particular person or group, and this privilege is usually because of their position. This might refer to the elders of a community, or people in professional positions (such as police officers or politicians). Positionality, referred to as placement within a set of social relations as well as the practices or actions that enable identification (Anthias 2002, p. 501). This means that if someone performs or expresses themself in a particular way, others are enabled to identify them as one thing or another. For example, within the context of a hospital, through observation, it is possible to identify reception staff from nurses, and nurses from doctors, by the way people dress, behave and interact. This example highlights the concept of identity and of positionality, including an understanding of social positioning (as a process, practice or action) as well as social position (as an outcome).

'Positioning' is a useful conceptual tool in examining the synergy between social structures and individual agency (Rogers and Ahmed 2017). It is central to an analysis of GBV in which social structures and individual/community identities, practices and norms collide. For example, consider the power, privilege and positionality of a legal advocate plays a significant role in the experience of a rape survivor in court proceedings. Another example is of the difference of power, privilege and positionality between a woman and a girl in a community which accepts female genital mutilation (FGM) as part of its culture. Consider again the notions of power, privilege and positionality in this scenario, if it is known by the girl that the woman is a respected elder of the community who undertakes the practice of FGM herself. The woman is also the girl's aunt; again, reflect upon how this changes the levels and intersections of power, privilege and positionality in this scenario. These examples highlight the multiple positionalities that people have in terms of professional identity, personal identity, family identity and role, age and gender as well as the structures that affect people's experiences (the legal system, community culture and norms). Each chapter of this book focussed on a specific form of GBV and the role and interplay of power, privilege and positionality is evident.

GBV, Pandemics, Crises and Natural Disasters

At the time of compiling this book, the world was facing the COVID-19 pandemic and therefore, it is important to explore how pandemic and emergencies relate to GBV. We already know that any type of emergency (including the global pandemic, COVID-19, but also other phenomena such as tsunamis or earthquakes) can result in severe and adverse consequences for nations, communities and particular individuals, especially women and children. The incidence and prevalence of GBV increase in emergency situations, whether it is a natural disaster or a man-made one (Gearhart et al. 2018; Nguyen 2019; Sklavou 2019; Yoshihama et al. 2019).

During the COVID-19 pandemic, many countries reported increased rates of GBV. The surge was associated with restrictions on movement and social distancing as well as economic and social stressors resulting from the pandemic. For instance, the growth in unemployment, uncertainty around furloughing and job security as well as the effects of social isolation have been widely reported during the lockdown period. These resulted in higher levels of stress, economic difficulties, disruption of social networks and to everyday life (Talevi et al. 2020). Early data from the United Kingdom, the United States, France, Australia, Cyprus, Singapore, Argentina, Canada, Germany and Spain indicated an increase in GBV/DVA and increased demands for women's refuges and other support services (UN Women 2020). Women from marginalised backgrounds such as those from Black and Minority Ethnic (BME) backgrounds (Ali et al. 2021; Asunramu 2020; Fawcett Society 2020), people with disabilities (UN Human Rights 2020; World Health

Organization 2020), those from LGBTQ + communities (Galea et al. 2020; Green et al. 2020), older women, girls and women living in institutional settings, displaced women and women living in conflict-affected areas were affected badly and faced further barriers in accessing appropriate support services.

Lessons to be Learned in Adopting Best Practice: Using a Comprehensive Ecological Approach

As stated earlier, GBV is widespread and can happen in public and private. Tackling GBV and enabling recovery for victims/survivors is everyone's business. Supporting victims and survivors of GBV and holding perpetrators to account is everyone's responsibility, including family members, friends, neighbours, community, society, individual governments of each country as well as national and international organisations. A response at any of these levels should use a survivor-centred approach which encompasses an assessment of multiple needs, risk and vulnerabilities ensuring safety, security, confidentiality, privacy and non-maleficence (doing no harm) (United Nations 2015). Chapters in this book have highlighted various forms of GBV, explained their complexities and made recommendations to tackle the issue. Collating the main points from all chapters and using an ecological model, in the following, we suggest a best practice framework to suggest some strategies and actions for those working in frontline services. We have added an additional layer—that of family—into the model as it is a distinct and specific group that can play a critical role in condoning and condemning GBV (Fig. 2).

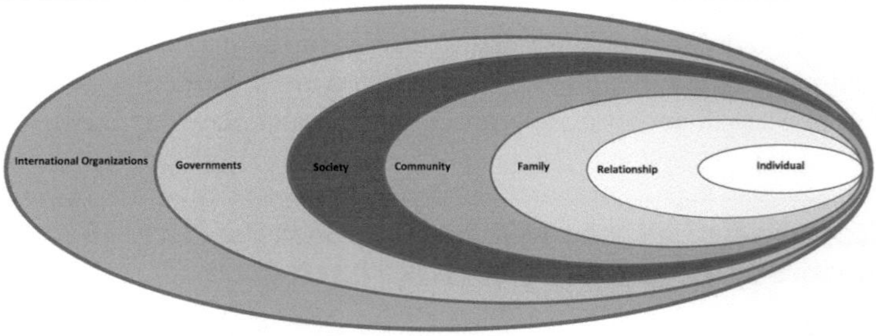

	International Organizations	Government	Society	Community	Family	Relationship	Individual
Monitor and analyse evidence from around the world to compare situations and develop uniform guidelines and policies to tackle GBV	✓						
Develop appropriate policies, laws to combat GBV and monitor implementation of these.	✓	✓					
Challenge gender stereotypes and gender role expectations that negatively affect women and contribute to GBV (e.g., greater childcare responsibilities, household responsibilities)	✓	✓	✓	✓			
Strengthen and develop innovative solutions using technology e.g., in the form of helplines, online counselling services, services through text messaging and social media outlets	✓	✓	✓	✓			
Increase women's representation and involvement in all aspects of policy development and implementation change, and monitoring in at all levels	✓	✓	✓	✓	✓		
Increase awareness about GBV, various forms, and its impact. Encourage dialogue about issues	✓	✓	✓	✓	✓		
Involve men in efforts related to the impact of gender stereotypes and the reduction of GBV and its various forms	✓	✓	✓	✓	✓	✓	✓
Provide appropriate and sufficient resources to address all forms of GBV in all circumstances generally and during pandemics and emergencies specifically		✓					
Strengthen the service provision for victims of GBV by capacity building of workers, rapid risk assessment, safety planning and case management, adapted to the crisis context, to ensure victim/survivors' access to support.		✓		✓			
Provide psychosocial and economic support for victims of GBV (face to face, virtual) at all levels		✓		✓	✓		
Expand the capacity of safe accommodation (e.g., refuges or shelters)	✓	✓	✓				
Develop and implement policies to support victims of GBV through their employers		✓	✓	✓			
Provide training to teachers, healthcare professionals on safety and referral information for children who may be exposed to GBV		✓	✓	✓			
Raise awareness of health and social care professionals, teachers, police and people in the criminal justice system		✓	✓	✓			
about GBV and provide training on how to respond, protect and refer victims/ survivors to appropriate services.							
Support women's rights organizations, especially those that provide essential services to hard-to-reach, remote and vulnerable populations		✓	✓	✓			
Implement bystander GBV prevention programme and measure their effectiveness				✓			
Develop skills to manage conflicts through discussion and dialogue				✓	✓	✓	✓
Sustain and value healthy relationships					✓	✓	✓
Respect choices and an individual's autonomy					✓	✓	✓
Believe and support of victims of GBV					✓	✓	✓
Show empathy, respect and a non-judgemental attitude					✓	✓	✓
If safe to do so, friends/ family members should intervene if they witness a conflict escalating between partners/spouses					✓	✓	

Fig. 2 Best practice framework using an ecological approach

Policy and Practice

Legal frameworks reflect social values. International legal frameworks help to frame social global problems and to summon nations to enforce actions to overcome those problems.

To tackle GBV, there is a need for nations to design and implement effective policies to define the problem, grant access to justice for victims through awareness campaigns, and design a justice system able to assist victims to solve their conflicts. Moreover, international law stresses the importance of educating children against non-discriminatory behaviours from an early stage in life. For this, they call for cooperation amongst different governmental sectors within nations (e.g. criminal justice systems, or education systems). It is through education and promotion of the rights that long-term changes can be achieved to inequalities, norms and stereotypes that are embedded in society; all which have a significant role in sustaining or addressing gender-based violence.

Summary

- GBV is pernicious, widespread and harmful at an individual, family, community and societal level.
- It is difficult to establish the extent of GV, however, due to methodological and reporting issues.
- There are various causes and correlations associated with GBV.
- GBV can occur in virtual, public and private settings and is ever-evolving in line with societal changes and developments, while there are still some traditional and well-established forms of GBV that remain prevalent.
- Theorising GBV can be helped by understanding the role of power, positionality and privilege.
- An ecological model for understanding also helps to examine the role of different social actions or influences and how these impact someone experiencing GBV.

References

Ali PA, Naylor PB, Croot E, O'Cathain A (2015) Intimate partner violence in Pakistan: a systematic review. Trauma Violence Abuse 16(3):299–315

Ali PA, O'Cathain A, Croot E (2019) Not managing expectations: a grounded theory of intimate partner violence from the perspective of Pakistani people. J Interpers Violence 34(19):4085–4113

Ali P, Rogers M, Heward-Belle S (2021) COVID-19 and domestic violence: impact on mental health. J Crim Psychol 11(3):188–202

Anthias F (2002) Where do I belong? Narrating collective identity and translocational positionality. Ethnicities 2(4):491–514

Asunramu Z (2020) The government's botched response to Covid-19 will set women back decades—and shows the need for more female leaders. Prospect, London. https://www.prospectmagazine.co.uk/politics/government-coronavirus-covid-impact-on-women-domestic-violence-jobs-childcare

Fawcett Society (2020) Coronavirus: Impact on BAME women. https://www.fawcettsociety.org.uk/coronavirus-impact-on-bame-women

Galea S, Merchant RM, Lurie N (2020) The mental health consequences of COVID-19 and physical distancing: the need for prevention and early intervention. JAMA Intern Med 180(6):817–818

Gearhart S, Perez-Patron M, Hammond TA, Goldberg DW, Klein A, Horney JA (2018) The impact of natural disasters on domestic violence: an analysis of reports of simple assault in Florida (1999–2007). Violence Gend 5(2):87–92

Green A, Price-Feeney M, Dorison S (2020) Implications of COVID-19 for LGBTQ youth mental health and suicide prevention. The Trevor Project, West Hollywood

Human Rights Watch (1999) The Enron Corporation: corporate complicity in human rights violations. Human Rights Watch, New York

Kilpatrick DG (2004) What is violence against women: defining and measuring the problem. J Interpers Violence 19(11):1209–1234

Nguyen HT (2019) Gendered vulnerabilities in times of natural disasters: male-to-female violence in the Philippines in the aftermath of super typhoon Haiyan. Violence Against Women 25(4):421–440

Rogers M, Ahmed A (2017) Interrogating trans and sexual identities through the conceptual lens of translocational positionality. Sociol Res Online 22(1):81–94

Sklavou K (2019) Violence against women in armed conflicts: pre, during and post. Dialogues Clin Neurosci Ment Health 2(4):254–258

Talevi D, Socci V, Carai M, Carnaghi G, Faleri S, Trebbi E, di Bernardo A, Capelli F, Pacitti F (2020) Mental health outcomes of the CoViD-19 pandemic. Riv Psichiatr 55(3):137–144

Tjaden P (2005) Defining and measuring violence against women: background, issues, and recommendations. Stat J U N Econ Comm Eur 22(3–4):217–224

UN Human Rights (2020) COVID-19 and the rights of persons with disabilities. https://www.ohchr.org/en/covid-19-and-persons-disabilities

UN Women (2020) COVID-19 and ending violence against women and girls. https://www.unwomen.org/en/digital-library/publications/2020/04/issue-brief-covid-19-and-ending-violence-against-women-and-girls. Accessed 3 June 2022

United Nations (1994) The declaration on the elimination of violence against women. United Nations, New York

United Nations, Women UN, UNFPA W, UNDP U (2015) Essential services package for women and girls subject to violence. UN Women, New York. https://www.unwomen.org/en/digital-library/publications/2015/12/essential-services-package-for-women-and-girls-subject-to-violence

Walker L (1979) The battered woman. Harper & Row, New York

World Health Organization (2020) Disability considerations during the COVID-19 outbreak. https://www.who.int/publications/i/item/WHO-2019-nCoV-Disability-2020-1. Accessed 3 Jun 2022

Yoshihama M, Yunomae T, Tsuge A, Ikeda K, Masai R (2019) Violence against women and children following the 2011 great East Japan disaster: making the invisible visible through research. Violence Against Women 25(7):862–881

Parveen Ali, PhD is a Professor of Gender Based Violence and Professor of Nursing in the Health Sciences School, the University of Sheffield and Doncaster and Bassetlaw Teaching Hospitals. Her research examines gender-based violence, inequalities in health related to gender and ethnicity, and professionals preparedness to support victims of gender based violence.

Michaela M. Rogers, PhD is a Senior Lecturer in Social Work in the Department of Sociological Studies at the University of Sheffield. Her research examines interpersonal violence with a focus on marginalized groups, impacts, help-seeking, service access and service responses.

Glossary

+ or plus Refers to the wide range of sexual orientations and gender identities not captured by the LGBTQ acronym.

Ableism Discrimination or prejudice against people with lived experience of disability. It also describes a value system that considers particular characteristics of the body and mind as essential for living a life of value.

Accessibility Refers to access to goods, services and information that can be used by people with disabilities on an equal basis with others.

Acculturation The process of assimilation into a different culture, usually the dominant one.

Acid attack An intentional act of violence in which perpetrators throw, spray or pour acid (a corrosive substance) onto victims' faces or bodies.

Adolescent stalking Stalking behaviours that occur during adolescence, typically between adolescent perpetrators and adolescent targets.

Aetiology A cause or the direction of causation of a disease, illness or behavioural pattern.

Ageism Prejudicial ideology which results in discrimination based on a person's age.

Ambivalent sexism A combination of hostile and benevolent sexism (see hostile sexism, benevolent sexism).

Anomie A social condition where the norms and values previously common to society disappear.

Anxiety A feeling of unease, worry or fear that can be mild, moderate or severe.

Arranged marriage The practice of parents selecting marriage partners for their offspring. While traditionally it has been found in many contexts, today it is mainly found in South Asia, the Middle East, North Africa and the Caucasus.

Assigned female A person who has been assigned the female gender at birth but does not necessarily identify with this gender throughout their whole life.

Asylum seeker A person who has left their country and is seeking protection from persecution but who has not yet been legally recognised as a refugee.

P. Ali, M. M. Rogers (eds.), *Gender-Based Violence: A Comprehensive Guide*, https://doi.org/10.1007/978-3-031-05640-6

Attachment-based therapy Interventions or approaches based on John Bowlby's Attachment Theory.

Autonomy The ability to make one's own decisions rather than being influenced by others.

Ayurvedic A healing and medicine system founded in India. The Sanskrit words Ayur means life and Veda, knowledge. The treatment relies on the use of natural products.

Benevolent sexism Sexist attitudes toward another gender (see also ambivalent sexism and hostile sexism).

Bible A holy book sacred to Christians.

Bilateral kinship A form of kinship in which relations between relatives are recognised on both mother's and father's 'sides' of families. Lineages are not usually formed in bilateral societies; rather, there is usually a 'web' of kinship relations.

Biopower A theoretical concept to explain the administration and regulation of human life at the level of the population and the individual body, e.g. the regulation of customs, health, reproductive practices or family.

Bisexual An umbrella term used to describe a romantic and/or sexual orientation towards more than one gender. Bi people may describe themselves using one or more of a wide variety of terms, including, but not limited to, bisexual, pansexual, queer, and some other non-monosexual and non-monoromantic identities.

Body dysmorphia A mental health condition related to body image, in which imagined or slight defects in physical appearance preoccupy the mind.

Borderline personality disorder A disorder of mood and the way in which a person interacts with others.

Bride abandonment The deliberate abandonment of a migrant bride abroad/or in their country of origin.

Bride price or bridewealth An amount of wealth in the form of money or valuable commodities (e.g. cattle) that is gifted to the bride's family by the groom's family (see also Lobolo).

Chestfeeding An alternative term to 'breastfeeding' to describe feeding an infant from a body. This term is usually used by people who are not female or identify as having breasts.Child marriage/early marriageThese terms are used interchangeably to refer to a forced marriage where one or more parties are under 18 years of age—unless the country they live in has a marriage age of younger than 18.

Child sex trafficking A form of child abuse that occurs when a child is advertised, solicited or exploited through a commercial sex act.

Child sexual abuse The involvement of a child in sexual activity that he or she does not fully comprehend, is unable to give informed consent to, or for which the child is not developmentally prepared, or else that violates the laws or social taboos of society.Child sexual exploitationA form of child sexual abuse which occurs when an individual or group takes advantage of an imbalance of power to coerce, manipulate or deceive a child or young person under the age of 18 into sexual activity.

Chronic mental health problems Persistent debilitating psychiatric symptoms that can impair function.

Cisgender Refers to people whose gender identity is the same as that which was ascribed at birth.

Cisnormativity/cisgenderism The assumption that binary cisgender understandings of gender are fixed. Any departure from this gender identity binary is considered abnormal. This paradigm promotes the belief that people must identify and express their gender identity within the confines of the gender binary. This operates at the micro and macro level via social and cultural norms and institutions and arguably is akin to sexism and racism (Rogers 2020).

Coercion The process of forcing someone to do something they are unwilling to do using threats or intimidation.

Cognitive behaviour therapy A common talking therapy aimed at changing thoughts and behaviour.

Colonialism A policy of control over people, land and/or country by a foreign state or nation.

Colourism A form of prejudice against dark skin tones, but can also be extended to facial features and hair texture (also known as shadeism).

Commodify To make into a commodity; i.e. something that can be bought and sold. A commodity can be tangible or intangible, e.g. labour.

Consent Simply defined, consent is voluntary or unforced agreement or permission.

Corporate land grabs (also known as land acquisitions) The buying or leasing of large parcels of land by transnational or national corporations (large, legally defined businesses) or by governments.

Counter-conventional The act of not adhering or conforming to, or rejecting conventional, accepted standards or norms.

Creepshots Images taken without the knowledge of the person photographed often depicting intimate or private situations.

Criminal justice The delivery of justice to those who have committed a crime.

Criminology The scientific study of crime and criminals, to identify the root causes of crime behaviour and to develop strategies to address it.

Cross-cultural studies Using data from multiple societies to examine the scope of human behaviour.

Customary marriage A marriage that is negotiated, recognised and conducted according to community norms, but not necessarily ratified by the state or state officials.

Customary tenure A form of land tenure in which land is held under 'custom and tradition'; i.e. (usually) uncodified norms, as opposed to statutory tenure. Customary tenure can vary, but in practice it is often communal, so that land is held by the whole group and is not privately owned. In much of Africa and in some other parts of the world among indigenous groups, land is thought to be held by group elders on behalf of ancestors.

Cyberbullying Bullying that takes place on and/or includes digital media and online platforms.

Cyberstalking The use of digital communications to stalk another person.

Decriminalisation The reclassification in law relating to certain actions to the effect that they are no longer considered a crime, including the removal of criminal penalties, e.g. the removal of all laws that criminalise consensual sex work for adults.

Deep fakes The use of photo editing to create fake, pornographic images of specific people used maliciously or to spread false information.

Depression A state of being persistently low in mood and feeling sad.

Digital sexual assault The non-consensual, digital distribution of sexual or sexualised images.

Disability Defined, in the United Nations Convention on the Rights of Persons with Disabilities, as the interaction between persons with impairments and attitudinal and environmental barriers that hinders their full and effective participation in society on an equal basis with others.

Disabled people A term in common usage to describe those people disabled by social arrangements that are not designed to include diverse ways of living.

Disciplinary power Power exercised over one or more individuals in order to provide them with particular skills and attributes, to develop their capacity for self-control, to promote their ability to act in concert, to render them amenable to instruction, or to mould their characters in other ways.

Dissociative disorder Disruption to memory, awareness, identity or perception. Often used as a defence mechanism.

Domestic violence and abuse Includes a range of incidents or pattern of incidents of controlling, coercive, threatening, degrading and violent behaviour, including sexual violence, between partners or ex-partners, family members or carers.

Domestic work Work which encompasses care services and managing the general housekeeping chores (such as cleaning, preparing and cooking meals or doing the household groceries shopping, amongst other tasks) in a private household or households.

Domestic worker Any person engaged in domestic work within the context of an employment relationship.

Down-blousing The practice of photographing someone's cleavage without their consent.

Dowry A form of payment via money, goods or estate paid at the time of marriage by the bride's family to the groom and his family.

Doxing/doxxing Sharing someone's private information online without their consent.

Drone porn The practise of using drones to film people in private settings without their consent and/or knowledge.

Dynamic risk factor A factor that can be modified through intervention and should be identified in case management to reduce risk.

Early marriage See child marriage.

Economic abuse Involves tactics or behaviours that can make an individual economically dependent on others and/or create economic insecurity.

End-demand criminalisation An approach to sex work regulation that criminalises the purchase but not the sale of sex. It is sometimes referred to as the Swedish Model or the Nordic Model.

Entrapment A state of being caught in a trap.

Epidemiology A branch of medicine dealing with incidence and prevalence of diseases and other factors relating to health.

Erotica Works of art that show or describe sexual activity, and which are intended to arouse sexual feelings.

External female genitalia Known as the vulva and includes mons pubis, labia majora and minora clitoris, urethra and vaginal opening.

False memory syndrome A situation where an individual wrongly 'remembers' things that happened to them in the past, including traumatic experiences such as physical and sexual abuse, with such memories often emerging during psychiatric therapies.

Familicide The case of a person killing a member or members of his own family and then commits suicide or attempts suicide.

Female genital surgery Surgery to address medical problems related to female genitalia, or carried out for aesthetic purposes.

Feminism An intellectual framework and a socio-political movement seeking justice for women and ending gender inequality.

Filicide The killing of a child by a parent, step-parent or de-facto parent.

Filicide-suicide The killing of a child by a parent, step-parent or de-facto parent followed by the perpetrator's suicide.

Financial abuse or exploitation Misappropriation of a person's money or property.

Flashbacks A symptom of post-traumatic stress, whereby a person can see and hear traumatic events they previously experienced.

Forced marriage A situation where duress is used to gain consent for marriage. Duress can include physical violence, emotional and psychological pressure, sexual and economic abuse.

Gay Refers to a man who has a romantic and/or sexual attraction towards men. Often used as a generic term for lesbian and gay sexuality—some women define themselves as gay rather than lesbian. Some non-binary people may also identify with this term.

Gay conversion therapy Therapies that aim to 'cure' someone of their homosexual, queer or trans identity.

Gender binary The system in which only two genders (male and female) are acknowledged.

Gender order A socially and historically constructed and accepted pattern of ideas, beliefs and behaviours through which gendered power relations between men and women are produced and reproduced. The gender order establishes a hierarchical difference between men and women, masculinity and femininity.

Gestational parent The parent that has carried and birthed a child. Often used for pregnant and birthing people who are not women.

Global North Refers to the regions of North America, Europe, Australia and New Zealand. Term developed by Wallerstein to refer to the global capitalist system that separates countries into core (Global North) and periphery (Global South) based on their economic participation.

Global political economy The field of study that deals with the interaction between political and economic forces and drives. It focuses on issues related to human welfare and how these might be related to state behaviour and corporate interests in different parts of the world.

Global South Refers broadly to identify regions of Latin America, Asia, Africa and Oceania.

Grooming The process of gradually manipulating people, often children, to perform sexual or sexualizing acts against their will.

Heteronormativity The assumption that heterosexuality is the norm and should be privileged over any other form of sexual orientation. This operates within and across interpersonal relationships, as well as at the macro level via social and cultural norms. For example, it is expected that a cisgender man and a cisgender woman marry and procreate.

Heterosexuality Romantic or sexual attraction, or sexual behaviour between persons of the opposite sex or gender.

Hidden crime Crimes which we are often oblivious to or underreported due to circumstances.

Homophobia, biphobia, transphobia Terms that refer to negative attitudes and/or behaviours toward homosexual, bisexual and/or transgender people.

Honour In the context of honour crime, honour is defined as a highly valued and fiercely protected currency in many social groups and communities across cultures that consider women and girls the objects of the currency.

Honour crime Violence, abuse and murder committed against anyone but predominantly against women and girls on the pretext of saving or restoring honour.

Honour-based violence Physical, psychological and economic harm and abuse committed against women and girls for the sake of family honour.

Hostile sexism A classic prejudice toward another gender (see also ambivalent sexism and benevolent sexism).

Hypersexual Something that has been made 'hyper' or extremely sexual in character or quality.

Identity abuse Identity abuse can be understood as using someone's marginalised status to control or shame them.

Image-based sexual abuse The publication of intimate or sexual images of another person on digital platforms without their consent (also known as revenge porn).

Immovable property Property tied to a fixed place such as land or housing.

Interpersonal violence Any violent act by a person, or persons, by another person, or persons.

Intersectionality The interconnected nature of race, class and gender creating overlapping and interdependent systems of discrimination.

Invalidating environment An environment in which communication of private experiences is met by erratic, inappropriate and extreme responses.

Joint ownership A form of property ownership (e.g. of housing or land) owned by more than one person, such as a wife and husband.

Juvenile delinquency The habit of committing criminal acts by a young person, especially one below the age at which ordinary criminal prosecution is possible.

Land reform This usually refers to the redistribution of land to agricultural smallholders or peasants, usually in state-backed schemes. Redistributive land reforms seek to improve the economic and social conditions of smallholders. More recently, however, the term 'land reform' has been used to refer to formalisation of land rights rather than to land redistribution.

Land tenure Refers to the relationship that individuals and groups hold with respect to land and land-based resources. Rules and expectations of land tenure define the ways in which rights to land are allocated, transferred, used or managed.

Land titling Codification and legalisation of land claims, usually with receipt of a document attesting to ownership or legal holding of the land/parcel of land.

Lesbian Refers to a woman who has a romantic and/or sexual attraction towards women. Some non-binary people may also identify with this term.

LGBTQ+ Is an acronym used to refer to lesbian, gay, bisexual, trans, queer, questioning and other minority sexual orientations and gender identities.

LMIC Low-income countries are nations that have a per capita gross national income of less than 1026 US dollars, and middle-income countries are those with a per capita gross national income of between 1026 and 4045 US dollars. LMIC therefore refer to countries with a per capita gross national income of 4045 US dollars or less.

Lobolo This refers to the property (in cash or in kind) which a prospective husband and/or the head of his family gives to the head of the prospective wife's family in consideration of a customary marriage (similar to bride price or bridewealth).

Longitudinal study A study involving the repeated observation or examination of a set of subjects over time with respect to one or more study variables.

Male proprietariness Male attitude of exclusive ownership and entitlement in relation to partners and children.

Male uxorial proprietariness Male attitude of exclusive ownership and entitlement in relation to his wife.

Mandatory reporting legislation Legislation that identifies specific individuals (e.g. healthcare professionals) as legally required to report abuse if they become aware of it or suspect it.

Marriage An important social institution in many places in the world, marriage is a socially and often legally recognised union and/or contract between two or more people, which often involves a long-term commitment and establishes certain rights and obligations including those to any children that may result from the union. Marriages can be concluded and recognised in terms of religious, customary, or civil and common law.

Matrilineal descent A form of kinship in which descent runs through the female line (e.g. grandmothers; mothers; daughters, sisters, brothers—and maternal uncles). The husband does not usually 'join' the matrilineal group; the brother-sister relation is important and brothers usually remain in sisters' matrilineage.

Medical abortion An induced abortion by means of abortifacient drugs.

Menarche Refers to the first experience of menstruation and to the age at which this occurs.

Menopause The cessation of the menstrual cycle.

Menses Refers to the time of menstruation (period) and the menstrual discharge.

Menstruation Refers to the physiological process of discharging blood and other material from the lining of the uterus through the vagina, which occurs in sexually mature women (except during pregnancy and for a time after pregnancy).

Mental health coercion Abuse tactics targeted towards a partner's mental health as part of a broader pattern of abuse and control.

Meta-analysis A combination of statistical results from multiple research studies.

Migrant A person who moves from one place to another, especially in order to find work or better living conditions.

Misogynoir A form of prejudice against black women, because of their gender and race.

Misogyny/misogynistic A deep-rooted prejudice against women.

Mobbing The bullying of an individual by a group, in any context, such as a family, peer group, school, neighbourhood, community etc.

Multi-systemic therapy An intensive family and/or community-based intervention, aimed specifically at children and young people.

Neglect The failure of a designated caregiver to meet the needs of a dependent person.

Non-binary An identity that does not relate to the binary gender system (see gender binary).

Non-consensual circumcision Refers to circumcision that is carried out on a person without the permission.

Nursing rooms A room, usually situated in a public area, such as a shopping centre or airport, which provides a private space for people to breastfeed or chestfeed.

Obstetric racism The intersection between obstetric violence and medical racism.

Obstetric violence A form of gender-based violence occurring within the obstetric institution that occurs during pregnancy, childbirth and/or the postpartum period.

Older adult mistreatment A single or repeated act, or lack of appropriate action, occurring within any relationship where there is an expectation of trust, which causes harm or distress to an older person.

Online violence against women (OVAW) Forms of abuse that are perpetrated against women in online environments or using social media.

Patriarchy A social system whereby men hold the power and are viewed as superior to women and other gender identities.

Patrilineage A lineage group formed through descent through the male line. In many societies, lineage groups were corporate entities with formal organisation and ability to act.

Patrilineal descent A form of kinship in which descent runs through the male line (e.g. grandfathers, fathers, sons); wives usually 'join' the husband's lineage or descent group.

Pelvic inflammatory disease An inflammation and infection of a woman's reproductive organs.

Perpetrator A person who carries out a harmful, illegal or immoral act.

Physical abuse Acts carried out with the intention to cause physical pain or injury.

Polyandry A system of marriage in which a wife can marry more than one husband.

Polygyny A system of marriage in which a man can marry more than one wife. Poly-victimisation: a situation in which a victim of abuse suffers more than one type of abuse concurrently.

Polyvictimisation Refers to the experience of multiple types of victimisation, for example sexual, psychological and physical abuse.

Pornography Presentations within media of sexually arousing material, including videos, film, writing, magazines and via social media.

Postnatal The time period after childbirth (also known as postpartum).

Post-traumatic stress The feelings, thoughts and behaviours that develop as the result of a traumatic experience.

Post-traumatic stress disorder A mental health condition that develops after an individual has experienced or witnessed a shocking, catastrophic or terrifying event.

Power Most definitions agree that power is the social production of an effect that determines the capacities, actions, beliefs or conducts of actors.

Power of attorney A legal instrument authorising one to act as the attorney or agent for another.

Procreation The sexual activity of conceiving and bearing offspring.

Psychological or emotional abuse Acts carried out with the aim of causing emotional pain or injury.

Psychopathology The study of mental disorders.

Psychosis An abnormal condition of the mind, resulting in difficulties determining what is real and not real.

Psychosocial evaluation An evaluation of psychological mental health and well-being.

Psychosocial history A thorough and comprehensive psychosocial evaluation of an individual's self-perception, past, present physical, mental and emotional health and ability to function within a family and community setting.

Psychosocial services Services that aim to respond to the psychological and social needs of individuals and communities in emergency contexts.

Public Health A discipline or profession concerned with ensuring people stay healthy and protected from threats to health.

Queer Queer is a term used by those wanting to reject specific labels of romantic orientation, sexual orientation and/or gender identity. It can also be a way of rejecting the perceived norms of the LGBT community (racism, sizeism, ableism etc.). Although some LGBT people view the word as a slur, it was reclaimed in the late 80s by the queer community who have embraced it.

Questioning The process of exploring your own sexual orientation and/or gender identity.

Quran The central religious text of Islam.

Rape Sexual penetration of the vagina or anus without lawful consent.

Rape culture A social environment where sexual violence is prevalent as a result of normalising male privilege and aggression and female subordination and objectification.

Rape myth acceptance The state of believing prejudicial, stereotyped or false ideas or claims about rape, rape victims and rapists.

Rape myths Myths about rape and other types of sexual violence that shift the blame from the perpetrator to the victim.

Refugee A person who has fled their country of origin due to war, violence, conflict or persecution, and has crossed an international border to find safety in another country.

Reproductive coercion and abuse Any deliberate attempt to dictate a woman's reproductive choices or interfere with her reproductive autonomy.

Revenge pornography/revenge porn The non-consensual distribution of private, intimate images with the purpose of revenge or control over an (ex)partner or close relation.

Risk factor Factor that increases the risk of an individual perpetrating mistreatment.

Scapegoating The practise of singling out a person or group for unmerited blame and consequent negative treatment.

Secondary trauma This results from a traumatic experience wherein one is not the direct victim oneself.

Sex trafficking The recruitment, transportation, transfer, harbouring or receipt of persons through force or other forms of coercion or deception, with the aim of sexually exploiting them for profit.

Sex work A term used to describe a wide range of direct and indirect activities, in which sexual services are negotiated and performed in exchange for monetary, or other, remuneration.

Sexting The sending and receiving of sexual or sexualised images.

Sextortion The practice of extorting money in exchange for taking intimate or sexual images offline that were uploaded without consent.

Sexual abuse The non-consensual sexual contact of any kind.

Sexual cleansing A traditional practice that requires a widow to have sex after widowhood as a cleansing.

Sexual harassment Refers to unwanted behaviour of a sexual nature which violates another person's dignity, and makes them feel intimidated or degraded, and/or creates a hostile and offensive environment.

Sexual violence Sexual violence is an umbrella term used to describe any sexual activity that happens without consent. There are different types of sexual violence, including child sexual abuse, rape and sexual assault.

Social ecology A field of study that explores how individuals interact with and respond to their environment and how these interactions in turn affect society.

Social model of disability This model refers to the belief that people are disabled, not by their impairment, but by systemic, environmental and attitudinal barriers within society that limit their full and effective participation.

Somatization The process whereby psychological issues are converted into physical health problems.

South Asia A geographical region comprising Pakistan, India, Nepal, Bhutan, Bangladesh, Sri Lanka, and Maldives. It can also include Afghanistan.

Stalking A persistent and repetitive pattern of intrusive behaviour which causes the target to feel alarm, distress or fear.

Stalking by proxy A stalking behaviour which involves the perpetrator engaging another individual, who may or may not be aware of the stalking, to contact or follow the target.

Street harassment Harassment or unwanted attention in the context of the street or public realm.

Structural violence The multiple ways in which social, economic and political systems expose particular groups of people to risks and vulnerabilities and prevent them from meeting their basic needs.

Substance use coercion The abusive tactics targeted towards a partner's substance use as part of a broader pattern of abuse and control.

Suicidality The risk of suicide, including ideation, plans, gesture and attempts.

Surgical abortion The induced abortion by means of a surgical procedure.

Surrogate relationship A scenario whereby a health professional acts as a substitute for another human being who is well known to the client, e.g. a parent.

Survivor A person who is going or who has been through a process of recovery following abuse.

Taboo A behaviour prohibited by social custom.

Technology-facilitated abuse A form of behaviour that involves the use of technology as a means to coerce, control, intimidate, stalk or harass another person.

Text-based abuse (TBA) Refers to written, electronic communication containing threatening and/or disruptive and/or distressing content, e.g. textual threats to kill, rape or otherwise inflict harm on the recipient of such messages.

Text-based sexual abuse (TBSA) A form of TBA, and online violence against women (OVAW), which frequently occurs on social media (e.g. Twitter or Facebook) and takes forms of sexist and/or misogynistic comments, tweets, messages, but also sexualised threats of violence.

Third sector organisations An umbrella term for a range of organisations that are neither public or private, and includes charities.

Tokophobia An extreme fear of childbirth.

Toxic masculinity A form of masculinity that adopts cultural norms around the idea of 'manliness' that are associated with harm to society and to men themselves.

Trans An umbrella term to describe people whose gender is not the same as, or does not sit comfortably with, the sex they were assigned at birth. Trans people may describe themselves using one or more of a wide variety of terms, including (but not limited to) transgender, transsexual, gender-queer (GQ), gender-fluid, non-binary, gender-variant, crossdresser, genderless, agender, nongender, third gender, bi-gender, trans man, trans woman, trans masculine, trans feminine and neutrois.

Transactional sex The act of having sex in exchange for money or drugs.

Transnational reproductive labour Refers to the remunerated, and also unpaid, activities across the global economy that reproduce the work force. This includes daily activities such as cooking, washing clothes but also bearing children.

Trauma-focused therapy A specific approach to therapy that recognises and emphasises understanding of a person's traumatic experience.

Typology The study and classification of artefacts according to their characteristics.

Up-skirting The practise of taking photographs up under someone's skirt without their consent and/or knowledge.

Vasectomy Refers to male sterilisation.

Victim This is a person harmed, injured or killed as the result of a crime, accident or other event/action.

Victimology The study of the impact of crime on victims, the interactions between victims and the criminal justice system and the relationships between victims and offenders.

Voyeurism The act of finding sexual or other kinds of satisfaction in watching and possibly photographing people without direct interaction.

Vulnerability/Vulnerabilities Refers to one or more factors that make an individual susceptible to a condition.

War This is armed conflict between two or more parties taking place within a nation or beyond national boundaries.

War-time violence Refers to violence from strangers and militant elements against the general population, witnessed or directly experienced, including physical violence, sexual violence, abduction, sexual exploitation, torture and killing.

Widow A woman who has survived or outlived the spouse.

Widow inheritance Is a practice whereby a widow is required to marry (to be 'inherited' by) a male lineage relative of her late husband, usually his brother or first cousin. The practice is also known as levirate marriage. This keeps the widow within the patrilineage.

Witch hunt An operation held against a person or group who are considered to be a threat to society.

MIX
Papier aus verantwortungsvollen Quellen
Paper from responsible sources
FSC® C105338

If you have any concerns about our products,
you can contact us on
ProductSafety@springernature.com

In case Publisher is established outside the EU,
the EU authorized representative is:
Springer Nature Customer Service Center GmbH
Europaplatz 3, 69115 Heidelberg, Germany

Printed by Libri Plureos GmbH
in Hamburg, Germany